Surgical Dressings and Wound Management

Surgical Dressings and Wound Management

A unique source of reference, providing detailed information on the development, key properties and clinical use of surgical dressings and modern wound management materials.

by

Stephen Thomas Ph.D.

Medetec Publications

Cardiff, South Wales

Copyright © 2010 Dr Stephen Thomas,

Medetec, Cardiff, South Wales.

Telephone +44 (0)79 74178077

Email: steve@medetec.co.uk

Visit our home page on www.medetec.co.uk

This publication is designed to provide accurate and authoritative information on the subject matter but it is sold on the understanding that the author is not rendering professional services. Persons who wish to use products described in this book should ensure that they only do so after first reading the instructions and specific guidance provided by the manufacturer concerned

Trademark Notice

Designations used by companies to distinguish their products are often claimed as trademarks. All brand names and product names used in this book are trade names, service marks, trademarks or registered trademarks of their respective owners and are used only for identification and explanation, without intent to infringe.

British Library Cataloguing in Publication Data

A catalogue record for this book is available from the British Library

ISBN-10   1-84426-834-9

ISBN-13   978-1-84426-834-4

Entirely produced by Medetec Publishing

Printed and bound in Great Britain by:

Copytech (UK) Ltd, trading as Printondemand-worldwide, Peterborough

Dedication

This book is dedicated with love to Cathy and Richard

'But most of all …to my best friend'

Acknowledgements

The author would like to acknowledge the help and cooperation given by a number of companies and individuals during the production of this book. These include the medical information departments of Convatec, Coloplast, Hartmann, Smith and Nephew, Synergy, Systagenix, 3M Healthcare amongst others for providing copies of references and publications for review.

Particular thanks to Peter Molan for reading and making detailed comments upon the Honey chapter, Dr Kosta Mumcuoglu for generously providing confocal microscopy images, and Martin Hall of the Natural History Museum for providing some images of flies.

Thanks also to the publishers of the Journal of Wound Care, HMP Communications, and World Wide Wounds for generously allowing me to reproduce substantial amounts of material I had previously submitted to those publications.

Also to Woodhead Publishing Ltd for permission to reproduce much of my chapter on dressings testing which was published in Advanced Textiles for Wound Care in 2009.

Finally to Peter Philips and other colleagues in SMTL for the considerable help and support they have provided to me over many years.

Dr Stephen Thomas

Contents

Preface

The production of this book represents the culmination of a working lifetime spent testing and evaluating surgical dressings and allied materials (with a few years off for maggot production).

When I first began working in the field in 1974 most of the materials then available consisted largely of cotton or viscose and were principally designed to absorb exudate or conceal the underlying wound in order to protect the delicate sensibilities of the patient and the public at large. Gradually, however, these simple materials were replaced by evermore sophisticated products which were claimed by the manufacturers concerned, not always entirely accurately, to represent a major advance on what had gone before. Some of these innovations have stood the test of time whilst others have fallen by the wayside to be replaced by the next generation of 'wonder dressings'.

During the last 35 years our understanding of the processes involved in wound healing at a biochemical and cellular level has advanced considerably, and some wound management materials are now available that have been designed specifically to influence these processes in some small way in order to facilitate healing.

This trend will undoubtedly continue, but what is less certain is that the products which result from this research will be produced at a price which will place them within the reach of most wound management practitioners or their patients. It is also by no means certain that these new developments, if and when they become available, will impact significantly on the management of hard-to-heal wounds such as those caused by circulatory disorders, diseases such as diabetes and cancer, or the pressure areas which will inevitably continue to plague some seriously ill patients.

It is likely, therefore, that the management of chronic wounds will continue to represent an increasing drain on financial and other resources for the foreseeable future and that the majority of problem wounds will continue to be dressed with variations of the types of dressings in current use.

If these materials are to be used in the most appropriate cost-effective manner it is essential that all those involved have a good understanding of the physical properties and key functions of the products concerned, combined with some knowledge of published evidence of their clinical effectiveness in normal use.

This book has been produced in an attempt to offer guidance in all these areas. It is important to note, however, that it does *not* attempt to provide the type of information commonly found in systematic reviews, most of which consume a considerable amount of time and money to produce, only to conclude that insufficient data is available upon which to make any useful recommendations that might influence clinical practice.

Rather it book sets out to describe the development, and where appropriate, the chemical and physical properties of the different dressing types. It then uses this information to provide the reader with some understanding of how these properties are likely to influence the clinical performance of the products concerned and attempts to support these predictions by reference to published clinical data describing the use of each type of dressing in a variety of clinical indications.

The text is divided into chapters most of which deal with particular types or classes of dressings. The classification system used is of necessity very simple and some products have perhaps not been classified in a way that their manufacturers would have wished. In some instances pseudoscientific 'generic' descriptions of certain types of dressings that have more to do with marketing or reimbursement issues than helping users understand the structure or function of the products concerned have been ignored in favour of alternative descriptions which more closely reflect their true nature.

Portions of the content have been published previously in various forms although I have tried to improve and update all previously published work were appropriate.

Some of the products described herein have been discontinued or are no longer available in specific markets. The inclusion of these products was deliberate, as in many cases they provide a useful indication of the way in which dressings have evolved. Their inclusion also provides the reader with a single convenient source of reference on wound management products past and present. When reviewing published literature, or reading an account of a trial conducted some years previously, it is helpful to have an understanding of the properties of the products involved in order to form a judgement on the relevance or otherwise of the clinical outcomes.

Many dressings have changed ownership over the years and some have also changed their names. Efforts have been made to ensure that the information provided is correct at the time of publication but it is possible that some information is out of date for which I apologise.

To save repetition, time and space, the commonly used practice of identifying the manufacturer of individual dressings as they are cited in the text has been set aside. This information has been collected together in a separate section of the book which also acts as a buyers guide.

I have attempted to make the book as international as possible by including products from markets outside the UK, in particular the United States. This unfortunately means that some dressings may not be familiar to all readers, or not available for purchase in some areas, but once again the inclusion of products from different countries should make it easier for the reader when considering studies undertaken in a different geographical location.

A significant and deliberate omission from this book is a chapter on cultured cell systems and tissue replacements. This has not been included as it is a specialist area which does not fall within the remit of this publication.

It is by no means certain that this publication will run to a second edition but if any dressing manufacturer from the UK or elsewhere identifies any serious omissions in terms of products or key publications which they believe should be included in a future edition, should this ever be produced, I would be pleased to hear from them. Similarly information on any errors, factual or otherwise, or comments on the content will be equally welcomed. Finally I sincerely hope you enjoy reading and using this book as much as I enjoyed producing it.

S. T.

1. Structure and function of skin

STRUCTURE OF SKIN

The skin, the largest organ of the human body, has an area of 1.5 - 2 m^2 and represents about one sixth of our total body weight. It performs numerous complex functions which are essential to our survival by acting as a barrier, protecting against harmful chemicals, UV radiation and pathogenic microorganisms, whilst regulating body temperature and moisture loss. It is also responsible for the production of Vitamin D. The structure of the skin changes with age and these changes can affect its moisture content and barrier function and also increase its susceptibility to irritant dermatitis. The ability of the skin to repair itself is also diminished with age which has important implications for wound healing.

Skin consists of three functional layers: the epidermis, dermis and subcutis or hypodermis. The principal structures contained within the skin are located in the dermis, but sweat glands and hair follicles communicate with the external environment through the epidermis. The structure of each of the skin is summarised below, but for more comprehensive information, the reader is advised to consult other more specialised texts[1-2] or internet resources.[1]

Epidermis

The epidermis, which forms the protective outer covering of the skin, has an average thickness of about 0.1 mm but varies from around 0.04 mm on the eyelids to 1.5 mm on the soles of the feet. It is differentiated into five layers.

Basal layer (stratum basale)

The *stratum basale*, the innermost layer, is principally composed of keratinocytes and is in intimate contact with the basal membrane that forms the junction or border between the dermis and epidermis. The basal cells act as 'mother-cells', responsible for the continuous regeneration of the skin and also contains the melanocytes, which are the pigment producing cells.

Prickle-cell layer (stratum spinosum)

The *stratum spinosum*, the prickle-cell layer, produces keratinosomes, membrane-bounded vacuoles, which contain the precursors of epidermal lipids.

---

[1] See http://www.nmsl.chem.ccu.edu.tw/tea/SKIN_910721.htm.

Figure 1: Basic structure of the skin

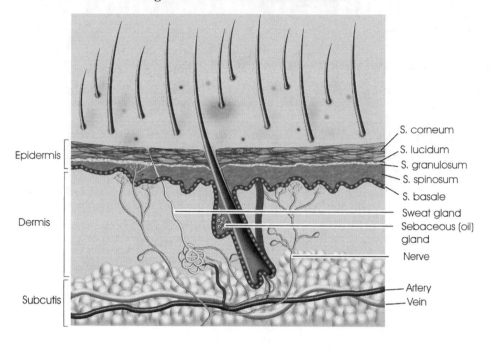

Epidermis

Dermis

Subcutis

S. corneum
S. lucidum
S. granulosum
S. spinosum
S. basale
Sweat gland
Sebaceous (oil) gland
Nerve
Artery
Vein

Granular layer (stratum granulosum)

Above the prickle-cell layer is the *stratum granulosum* where keratinization (cornification) of the keratinocytes begins. It contains keratohyaline granules, a precursor of keratin from which it derives its name, together with a mixture of several smaller protein units. In addition to keratohyaline it also contains filaggrins - the intercellular cement of the skin structure.

Clear layer (stratum lucidum)

The *stratum lucidum*, sometimes called the clear layer, as it is highly refractive, consists of flattened closely packed cells, the boundaries of which are no longer recognizable. It is only present in the palmoplantar skin, the thicker skin of the palms and soles, where it helps reduce friction and shear forces between the adjacent layers.

Horny layer (stratum corneum)

The *stratum corneum*, the outermost layer of the epidermis, composed of 15 - 20 layers of large, flat, polyhedral, dead keratin-filled cells, which have migrated up from the stratum granulosum. These cells are continuously shed, to be replaced by new cells which migrate upwards from the *stratum basale*. The thickness of the stratum corneum varies, but is typically between 10 - 40 microns and is thickest on the palms and soles of the feet which are sites particularly prone to injury.

Dermis (corium)

Like the epidermis, the dermis also varies in thickness from 0.3 mm on the eyelids to 3.0 mm on the back. The lower part of the dermis, which is adjacent to the subcutis, is the *stratum reticulare*. The upper layer is the *stratum papillare* which is clearly demarcated from the epidermis by an undulated border. This wave-like interface increases the contact area with the epidermis, thus ensuring optimal nourishment of the basal cells of the epidermis.

The bulk of the dermis consists principally of collagen together with other gel-like and elastic materials. Embedded in this layer are lymph channels, blood vessels, nerve fibres, and muscle cells, together with hair follicles, sebaceous glands and sweat glands which are unique to the dermis. The principal structural components consist of arc-shaped elastic fibres and undulated, relatively inelastic, collagen fibres.

The space within the dermal meshwork is filled with long chains of mucopolysaccharides (sugar molecules) known as glycosaminoglycans. With the help of fibronectins a type of 'glue', they bind to the connective tissue matrix to form proteoglycans, a gel-like mass that can absorb and release water like a sponge. Young collagen fibres in particular can bind large amounts of water, but as the skin ages, the interweaving of the collagen fibres increases and the water-binding capacity diminishes, causing the skin to wrinkle.

Other constituents of the dermis include fibroblasts and mast cells, as well as a multitude of blood and lymph vessels, nerve endings, hot and cold receptors and tactile sensory organs. Hair follicles which originate in the dermis are found everywhere on the body except for the palms and soles, but the majority of the hairs produced are very fine, scarcely visible to the naked eye. Sebaceous glands attached to hair follicles continuously secrete sebum, an oily substance which lubricates and protects the skin. On most of the skin surface this is produced in relatively small amounts, and is therefore usually not noticeable, but in areas with a higher concentration of sebaceous glands, such as on the face and back, sebum production may be significant, giving the skin an oily appearance and sometimes leads to the formation of blocked pores (comedones).

The skin also contains two types of sweat-producing glands. Apocrine glands are found under the arms, around the nipples and navel, and in the anal-genital area. Apocrine glands in the breast secrete fat droplets into breast milk and those in the ear help form earwax. Most apocrine glands in the skin are scent glands, and their secretions usually have a detectable odour which may play a role in sexual attraction, but otherwise have no known physiological function.

The eccrine glands, which are distributed over the entire body, have the highest concentration in the palms, soles, forehead, and underarms and form an advanced temperature regulating system. Several million of these glands produce a dilute salt solution which evaporates from the skin's surface to cool the body. Although they primarily produce sweat in response to physical activity and high temperatures, emotional stress and spicy foods can also lead to sweating. The process of heat regulation is facilitated by the presence of a network of fine capillaries within the dermis which dilate in warm conditions to give off heat, causing the skin to flush. In cold weather, they constrict, conserving heat but causing pallor. These vessels also provide nutrients to the skin and provide protection for the cellular and fluid systems. Like the eccrine glands, the blood vessels in the dermis respond to emotional stress by dilating. In these circumstances the resultant flush may be called a 'blush'.

The nerve endings in the dermis are the source of the body's sense of touch. They sense heat, cold, and pressure, providing both pain and pleasure.

Subcutis (hypodermis)

The subcutis serves principally as the energy reservoir of the skin where nutrients in the form of liquid fats are stored in the adipocytes. It is heavily interlaced with blood vessels, ensuring a quick delivery of the stored nutrients to the rest of skin as required. The subcutis also provides insulation and shock absorption.

FORMATION OF SKIN

Formation of new skin begins in the lowest or basal layer of the epidermis where new cells are constantly being reproduced as older cell migrate up toward the surface. During this process they become flattened and shrink. They eventually lose their nuclei and move out of the basal layer to the horny layer (the dead epidermis) at which point they consist almost entirely of keratin. These keratinocytes, being dead, are largely unaffected by external influences and so provide a protective function until they are eventually sloughed off. This entire process takes about 3-4 weeks.

Keratinocytes, the actual epidermal cells or dead skin cells, represent about 90% of the epidermis the remaining 10% are melanocytes which manufacture and distribute melanin, the protein that adds pigment to skin and protects the body from ultraviolet rays. The major proteins formed by the keratinocytes are keratins, intermediate filament proteins that form the cytoskeleton of keratinocytes. Two types if keratins exist, Type I (acidic keratins) and Type II (basic keratins). During keratin assembly, an acidic and basic keratin molecule combine to form polymers which are subsequently assembled into filaments.

During epithelial differentiation the expression of keratins changes; basal cells express keratins 5 and 14, but as keratinocytes leave the basal layer, they become larger and synthesise keratins 1 and 10. An imbalance in the various types of keratins can lead to numerous dermatological conditions. In hyperprolific epidermis, such as psoriasis and atopic dermatitis, keratins 6 & 16 predominate but defects in keratins 5 & 14 result in separation of the skin at the basal layer causing the congenital blistering disease, epidermolysis bullosa simplex.

SKIN AS A BARRIER TO MOISTURE

Moisture content of normal skin

The total volume of fluid held in the skin of a 70 kg man is about seven litres, but the moisture content varies throughout its structure. The dermis contains about 80% water, and the *stratum corneum* about 30%. This is non-uniformly distributed, varying from around 40% in the inner layers to around 10-15% in the outermost horny layer.[3] This figure can increase to around 60% when the skin is immersed in water or exposed to a very wet environment.[4]

Moisture loss through normal skin

Moisture is lost through the skin not only by means of specialist structures such as sweat glands and hair follicles, but also through the intact *stratum corneum* itself. This is termed the transepidermal water loss(TEWL) In one study the measured TEWL of intact skin varied from an average of 154 $g/m^2/24$ h in young adults, to 106 $g/m^2/24$ h in those over 80 years.[1] An average value for TEWL of 154 $g/m^2/24$h for normal skin was also reported by Parish.[5] Slightly higher values were recorded by Akita,[6] and Lake et al.,[7] 182 ± 42.5 $g/m^2/24$ h and 200 $g/m^2/24$ h respectively. These results relate to 'normal' skin but microcirculatory changes or skin changes associated with a disease process can greatly affect measured TEWL values. Aschoff et al.[8] monitored changes in skin hydration and TEWL in patients with mild-to-moderate atopic dermatitis and found that during treatment with an immunomodulating agent, pimecrolimus cream 1%, TEWL reduced from 847 $g/m^2/24$ h to 516 $g/m^2/24$ h indicating some restoration of the moisture barrier function.

Measured values of TEWL are influenced by numerous factors, including ambient and body-induced airflows near the probe, probe size, measurement site and angle, and measurement range. Nuutinen et al.[9] therefore developed a closed chamber technique which, they claim, overcomes these problems when monitoring changes in skin physiology.

Moisture control mechanisms of skin

Although the *stratum corneum* consists principally of layers of non-viable keratinized cells, the water content of this layer is crucial and is determined by at least three important mechanisms; transport of water from the dermis to the *stratum corneum*, moisture loss by evaporation, which is determined by intercellular lipids orderly arranged to form a barrier to transepidermal water loss, and the water binding ability of the *stratum corneum* itself. This in turn is governed by the presence of intracellular water soluble hygroscopic substances formed within the corneocytes by degradation of the histidine-rich protein known as filaggrin.[10] Together these comprise around 30% of the *stratum corneum* and are known as natural moisturizing factor (NMF). This consists of 40% free amino acids, 12% prolidine carboxylic acid, 12% lactate and 7% urea together with minerals, electrolytes and sugars. For a more comprehensive review of the fluid control mechanisms of the skin see Agache and Black.[11]

According to Verdier-Sevrain and Bonte,[12] glycerol, a well-known cosmetic ingredient, has been discovered in the *stratum corneum* as a natural endogenous humectant, and hyaluronan, which is regarded principally as a dermal component, is also present in the epidermis where it helps to maintain the structure and epidermal barrier function. A water-transporting protein, aquaporin-3, has additionally been discovered in viable epidermis. All these findings have brought new insights into the mechanisms of skin water distribution and barrier function.

The NMF can be readily released or extracted with water from the cells of the *stratum corneum* after first treating it with solvents or detergents to extract protective polar lipids such as sphingolipids that exist in the intercellular spaces.[13] It has also been demonstrated that repeated exposure to water can also adversely affect the fluid control mechanisms of skin by depletion of NMF even without prior solvent extraction.[14]

Effect of excess moisture loss

If the normal fluid regulating ability of the skin is adversely affected, it makes it susceptible to dryness and scaling, particularly if the moisture content of the *stratum corneum* falls below about 10%. This can result in dryness,[15] leading to chapping or cracking, particularly on the fingertips or knuckles.

Every year pharmaceutical and cosmetic companies spend millions of pounds developing and promoting products designed to improve the moisture content of the skin and 'reduce the appearance of fine lines and wrinkles' in order to 'combat the signs of aging'. In many circumstances, however, the application of a simple oily skin preparation or skin protectant will be sufficient to reduce transepidermal water loss and thus facilitate the repair of dry or cracked skin. Alternatively, oily emollients added to the bath form a film upon the surface of the water which is transferred to the skin as the individual rises out of the bathtub. This thin oily layer helps to conserve any additional moisture taken up in the *stratum corneum* during bathing.

In extreme cases, total dehydration caused by death of the underlying dermal structures will lead to the formation of a dry black leathery eschar commonly associated with pressure ulcers.

If the integrity of the epidermis is seriously compromised, by trauma or some metabolic or physiological disorder, the healing rate of the resulting wound will be influenced by the moisture content of the surrounding skin and the local environment. If it becomes too dry epithelialization will be delayed, too wet and there is a risk of maceration and infection.[16]

These outcomes are determined principally by the choice of dressing,[17] for in addition to facilitating healing, a product that maintains a moist environment can also help to prevent secondary damage to a vulnerable area of tissue caused by dehydration. The capacity of deep partial thickness wounds to undergo spontaneous healing depends upon the survival of epidermal cells in hair follicles and sweat glands in the base of the wound; if these are allowed to become dehydrated and devitalised the wound may actually increase in size and convert from a partial thickness to a full thickness injury.

Work on burns reviewed by Lawrence,[18] showed that the application of an occlusive dressing will salvage not only dermal tissue but also certain epithelial elements in the zone of stasis surrounding the original injury. The use of traditional dry dressings in these situations can result in progressive dehydration of the threatened zone followed by devitalization and necrosis, with the result that this zone becomes indistinguishable from the original lesion. The prevention of dehydration by the application of a suitable occlusive or semipermeable dressing may limit or prevent these secondary effects.

Effect of excess moisture retention

As well as becoming dehydrated, the skin can also become excessively moist. Most people are familiar with the skin changes that occur after spending too much time immersed in a hot bath which are characterized by pronounced softening, swelling and wrinkling of the epidermis. This process is known as maceration, a term derived from the Latin '*maceratus*', the past participle of '*macerare*', variously translated as 'to make wet, soak, steep or soften' or the process by which an object or material 'becomes soft or is divided into its constituents by soaking'. The Online Medical Dictionary (http://cancerweb.ncl.ac.uk/omd/) goes further, and defines maceration as a softening of tissue by soaking, especially in acids, until the connective tissue fibres are so dissolved that the tissue components can be teased apart.

In a clinical context, maceration is commonly used to describe changes in the appearance of the skin resulting from prolonged exposure to moisture or wound exudate, the causes and treatment of which have been described comprehensively in a series of articles by Cutting, Cutting and White, and other authors.[19-24]

It has previously been argued that the widespread use of the term maceration can be misleading, and that it is sometime applied incorrectly, potentially leading to inappropriate treatment in some instances.[25] An alternative umbrella term, 'moisture-related skin changes' was therefore proposed which encompassed maceration, but which also included other types of superficial skin damage such as intertrigo, and the irritation or excoriation caused by irritant body fluids such as urine, wound fluid or faecal material, and/or the presence of pathogenic microorganisms, their toxins and metabolites and inflammatory cytokines.[24]

The changes induced by extended immersion in a bath are generally assumed to be caused by absorption of the bath water by the outer layer of the skin which permeates the intercellular spaces, crosses cell membranes and swells the corneocytes.[11] However, similar changes can also result from simple occlusion, for example by the extended use of rubber or plastic disposable gloves. The relatively impermeable nature of these materials prevents normal transepidermal evaporative water loss (TEWL) which in turn leads to the accumulation of moisture within the skin, and ultimately the same softening and wrinkling described above.

In fact it is probable that the skin changes that occur from prolonged immersion in a bath result not just from absorption of water by the outer layers of the *stratum corneum*, but also by the accumulation of moisture in the deeper layers of the epidermis caused by the skin's inability to transpire excess water away in the form of sweat. In a hot bath, the situation is actually exacerbated by the fact that the capillaries within the skin are dilated as the body attempts to produced increased sweat as part of its normal temperature regulating process. These two simple examples clearly illustrate that major changes in the water content of the skin can be influenced by both endogenous and exogenous moisture. Irrespective of the cause, in the two situations cited above, the obvious changes in the thickness and appearance of the skin are reversible and therefore do not normally represent a serious threat to the individual concerned, although whilst in this condition the skin is more susceptible to physical damage, and its protective barrier properties to chemicals and microorganisms are also impaired as occluded (macerated) skin has been shown experimentally to be more sensitive to irritants.[26]

When exposed to a warm dry environment the skin returns to normal in minutes and no further treatment is indicated or required. This desorption or water efflux is called Skin Surface Water Loss (SSWL), and is distinct from TEWL.[11] The application of any form of oily skin preparation or skin protectant to skin in this condition would impair water vapour loss and thus delay a return to normal moisture values.

The presence of liquid, be it urine, sweat or wound exudate, is undoubtedly a major cause of skin damage, but the skin does not have to be completely macerated in order for the damage to occur, which is why the term 'moisture-related skin changes' may be preferred.

Where skin is at risk from these corrosive agents, it is possibly to apply topical agents such as zinc paste or modern proprietary skin protectants,[27] which are easier and quicker to apply and remove,[28] and which have the additional advantage of being transparent. For routine management, given the multiplicity of dressings available and the clinical and financial implications of significant skin damage, it might be supposed that that the medical literature would contain a wealth of information on the prevention and treatment of this condition. In fact, this is not the case. In 2007, a systematic review of the literature relating to the management of maceration of the periwound skin,[24] identified nine relevant articles and in only six of these was maceration cited as a primary or secondary outcome variable. The authors also considered the evidence for the use of honey, negative pressure wound therapy, compression therapy and the use of a skin protectant. Whilst there was reasonably strong evidence to support the use of skin protectants, the authors found no supporting evidence for the other treatment modalities.

In the absence of hard evidence from controlled studies, best practice standards based upon expert opinion, supported where relevant by laboratory or other experimental data, must be used to guide clinical practice. It must also be remembered that 'absence of evidence of effectiveness' is not the same as 'evidence of ineffectiveness'. Despite the lack of published data, most clinicians accept that the use of compression, which reduces oedema and exudate production, will inevitably impact upon maceration. Similarly the application of topical negative pressure which continuously removes exudate from the immediate vicinity of a wound will reduce the possibility of skin damage caused by the spread of irritant wound fluid over the periwound skin. However, when using this technique, it is important to consider the moisture vapour permeability of the film component of the dressing system, for if this is too low it could actually cause maceration of the periwound skin by preventing TEWL.

Historically, the selection of a dressing was determined by a number of factors, the majority of which were related to the position and nature of the wound, with particular attention paid to the presence of infection, odour and the amount of exudate present. Relatively little attention was given to the management of periwound skin or the effect that the choice of dressing system might have on this potentially vulnerable area. It was often tacitly accepted that wound fluid would inevitably escape from a heavily exuding leg ulcer onto the surrounding skin under the effects of gravity and that there was relatively little that could be done to prevent this, other than apply large quantities of bulky padding in an attempt to absorb the excess fluid. Products made from alginate or carboxymethylcellulose fibre are particularly prone to this problem, particularly if they are not used with appropriate secondary dressings.[29]

Modern dressings with enhanced fluid handling capabilities such as new types of highly permeable foam/film combinations,[30] foams containing superabsorbents, and highly absorbent hydrogel sheets, offer substantial advantages over products used in the past and have done much to alleviate this problem. The situation has been further improved by the advent of effective skin-friendly adhesive systems which form an effective seal between the dressing and the skin around the wound margin, which also permit replacement of dressings without the production of pain or trauma sometimes encountered with traditional adhesive materials.[31]

It is likely, therefore, that in most instances periwound skin damage, regardless of its primary cause, may be prevented by the adoption of simple measures which include the application and frequent replacement of appropriate dressings, and the use of skin protectants or barrier creams combined with good nursing practice. These simple measures should impact favourably upon the patient's quality of life by reducing the pain and some of the inconvenience associated with a heavily exuding wound. As in many areas of clinical practice, prevention of moisture related skin changes is better (and cheaper) than cure.

POTENTIATION OF SKIN DAMAGE BY BODY FLUIDS

Wound fluid

The skin changes described thus far are very different from those often observed around the margin of chronic wounds such as leg ulcers. Whilst these skin changes may be partly due to maceration, which predisposes the affected area to traumatic injury (which may also be caused by some types of adhesive dressings), a second and potentially more important factor is the presence, within chronic wound fluid, of proteolytic enzymes that can chemically degrade exposed skin, resulting in a red, weeping surface. In such situations an effective barrier cream may be indicated to provide a protective function. In one study it was reported that exudate-induced skin damage occurred in 55% of ulcers under investigation.[32] Maceration is a particular problem in diabetic ulcers,[33] which in common with heavily exuding ulcers of all types, require frequent dressing replacement to avoid damage to the surrounding skin.[34-35]

Urine or faeces

The presence, on the skin surface, of urine or faeces, can also lead to superficial damage. Diaper dermatitis is a common condition of which there are several types. When the occlusive effects of a nappy are not matched by its absorbency, hyperhydration of the stratum corneum occurs, which progresses to maceration increasing the coefficient of friction of the skin and predisposing to epidermal damage caused by rubbing. Faecal enzymes (urease, proteases and lipases) also can have a deleterious effect upon the skin.[36]

Figure 2: Damage caused to the skin of buttocks by urine, pressure and friction

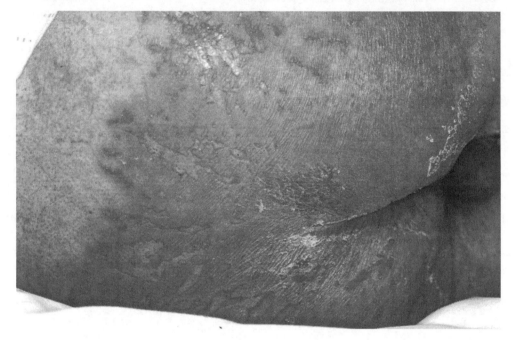

Fat or neglected children and adults are further subject to intertrigo - chafing or excoriation between moist skin folds or adjacent surfaces. All such areas are susceptible to infection with *Candida albicans*. In elderly or immobile patients, maceration secondary to incontinence of urine or faeces is sometimes regarded as a precursor to skin damage caused by pressure and shearing effects leading to ulcer formation or extension.[37]

References

1. Ghadially R, Brown BE, Sequeira-Martin SM, Feingold KR, Elias PM. The aged epidermal permeability barrier. Structural, functional, and lipid biochemical abnormalities in humans and a senescent murine model. *J Clin Invest* 1995;95(5):2281-90.
2. Fore J. A review of skin and the effects of aging on skin structure and function. *Ostomy Wound Manage* 2006;52(9):24-35; quiz 36-7.
3. Agache P. *Stratum corneum* Histopathology. In: Agache P, Humbert P, editors. *Measuring the skin*. Berlin: Springer-Verlag, 2004.
4. Bouwstra JA, Gooris GS, van der Spek JA, Bras W. Structural investigations of human stratum corneum by small-angle X-ray scattering. *J Invest Dermatol* 1991;97(6):1005-12.
5. Parish WE, Read J, Paterson SE. Changes in basal cell mitosis and transepidermal water loss in skin cultures treated with vitamins C and E. *Exp Dermatol* 2005;14(9):684-91.
6. Akita S, Akino K, Imaizumi T, Tanaka K, Anraku K, Yano H, et al. A polyurethane dressing is beneficial for split-thickness skin-graft donor wound healing. *Burns* 2006;32(4):447-51.
7. Lamke LO, Nilsson GE, Reithner HL. The evaporative water loss from burns and water vapour permeability of grafts and artificial membranes used in the treatment of burns. *Burns* 1977;3:159-165.
8. Aschoff R, Schwanebeck U, Brautigam M, Meurer M. Skin physiological parameters confirm the therapeutic efficacy of pimecrolimus cream 1% in patients with mild-to-moderate atopic dermatitis. *Exp Dermatol* 2008.
9. Nuutinen J, Alanen E, Autio P, Lahtinen MR, Harvima I, Lahtinen T. A closed unventilated chamber for the measurement of transepidermal water loss. *Skin Res Technol* 2003;9(2):85-9.
10. Rawlings AV, Harding CR. Moisturization and skin barrier function. *Dermatol Ther* 2004;17 Suppl 1:43-8.
11. Agache P, Black D. *Stratum corneum* Dynamic Hydration Tests. In: Agache P, Humbert P, editors. *Measuring the skin*. Berlin: Springer-Verlag, 2004.
12. Verdier-Sevrain S, Bonte F. Skin hydration: a review on its molecular mechanisms. *J Cosmet Dermatol* 2007;6(2):75-82.
13. Yamamura T, Tezuka T. The water-holding capacity of the stratum corneum measured by 1H-NMR. *J Invest Dermatol* 1989;93(1):160-4.
14. Visscher MO, Tolia GT, Wickett RR, Hoath SB. Effect of soaking and natural moisturizing factor on stratum corneum water-handling properties. *J Cosmet Sci* 2003;54(3):289-300.
15. Siddappa K. Dry skin conditions, eczema and emollients in their management. *Indian J Dermatol Venereol Leprol* 2003;69(2):69-75.
16. Winter GD. Formation of the scab and the rate of epithelization of superficial wounds in the skin of the young domestic pig. *Nature* 1962;193:293-294.
17. Winter GD. A note on wound healing under dressings with special reference to perforated-film dressings. *J Invest Dermatol* 1965;45(4):299-302.
18. Lawrence JC, editor. Laboratory studies of dressings. Symposium; 1982 1983; Birmingham. Oxford Medicine Publishing Foundation.
19. Cutting KF. The causes and prevention of maceration of the skin. *Journal of Wound Care* 1999;8(4):200-1.
20. Cutting KF. The causes and prevention of maceration of the skin. *Prof Nurse* 2001;17(3):177-8.
21. Cutting KF, White RJ. Avoidance and management of peri-wound maceration of the skin. *Prof Nurse* 2002;18(1):33, 35-36.

22. Cutting KF, White RJ. Maceration of the skin and wound bed. 1: Its nature and causes. *J Wound Care* 2002;11(7):275-8.
23. White RJ, Cutting KF. Interventions to avoid maceration of the skin and wound bed. *Br J Nurs* 2003;12(20):1186-201.
24. Gray M, Weir D. Prevention and Treatment of Moisture-Associated Skin Damage (Maceration) in the Periwound Skin. *J Wound Ostomy Continence Nurs* 2007;34(2):153-157.
25. Thomas S. The role of dressings in the treatment of moisture-related skin damage. *World Wide Wounds*: SMTL/MEP, 2008.
26. Basketter D, Gilpin G, Kuhn M, Lawrence D, Reynolds F, Whittle E. Patch tests versus use tests in skin irritation risk assessment. *Contact Dermatitis* 1998;39(5):252-6.
27. Campbell K, Woodbury MG, Whittle H, Labate T, Hoskin A. A clinical evaluation of 3M no sting barrier film. *Ostomy Wound Manage* 2000;46(1):24-30.
28. Cameron J, Hoffman D, Wilson J, Cherry G. Comparison of two peri-wound skin protectants in venous leg ulcers: a randomised controlled trial. *J Wound Care* 2005;14(5):233-6.
29. Thomas S. The importance of secondary dressings in wound care. *Journal of Wound Care* 1998;7(4):189-192.
30. Thomas S. Fluid handling properties of Allevyn foam dressing. *http://www.medetec.co.uk/Documents/Fluid%20handling%20properties%20of%20Allevyn%20foam%20dressing24-4-07.pdf* 2007.
31. Cunningham D. Treating venous insufficiency ulcers with soft silicone dressing. *Ostomy Wound Manage* 2005;51(11A Suppl):19-20.
32. Jorgensen B, Price P, Andersen KE, Gottrup F, Bech-Thomsen N, Scanlon E, et al. The silver-releasing foam dressing, Contreet Foam, promotes faster healing of critically colonised venous leg ulcers: a randomised, controlled trial. *Int Wound J* 2005;2(1):64-73.
33. Rodgers A, Watret L. Maceration and its effect on periwound margins. *Diabetic Foot (Suppl)* 2003;6(3):S2-S5.
34. Hilton JR, Williams DT, Beuker B, Miller DR, Harding KG. Wound dressings in diabetic foot disease. *Clin Infect Dis* 2004;39 Suppl 2:S100-3.
35. *European Wound Management Association (EWMA). Position Document: Wound Bed Preparation in Practice.* London: MEP Ltd, 2004.
36. Flagothier C, Pierard-Franchimont C, Pierard GE. [How I explore ... diaper dermatitis]. *Rev Med Liege* 2004;59(2):106-9.
37. Doughty D, Ramundo J, Bonham P, Beitz J, Erwin-Toth P, Anderson R, et al. Issues and challenges in staging of pressure ulcers. *J Wound Ostomy Continence Nurs* 2006;33(2):125-30; quiz 131-2.

2. Classification of wounds

DEFINITION OF A WOUND

For the purposes of this book a wound is defined as follows.

> *'A visible manifestation of an event that has caused disruption to the integrity of the skin, and/or a loss or impairment of its protective or physiological function'.*

Figure 3: The Wounded Man

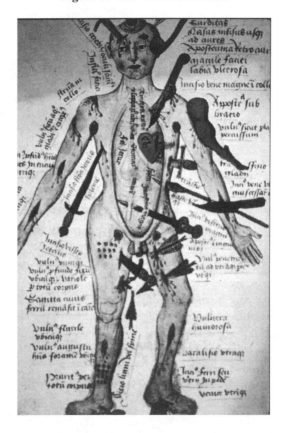

Hans von Gersdorff. Feldtbüch der Wundartzney (printed in Strassburg, by H. Schotten, in 1528).

Wounds can take many forms, and when assessing them to determine an appropriate form of treatment, it is useful to adopt a structured approach to facilitate the dressing selection process. Numerous classification systems have previously been described in the literature for this purpose, some of which are described briefly below.

WOUND CLASSIFICATION SYSTEMS

Classification by propensity to heal

In perhaps the most basic classification system, wounds are simply divided into acute and chronic wounds according to their observed (or assumed) ability to progress towards healing.

Acute wounds

Unless they become infected, most acute wounds heal in a timely and predictable fashion and are generally caused by some form of mechanical or thermal injury such as those summarized below.

Mechanical injuries

- Abrasions (grazes) are superficial wounds generally caused by friction from glancing or tangential contact between the skin and a second harder or rougher surface. By definition, abrasions are usually confined to the outer layers of the skin.
- Avulsions involve the loss of part or all of an entire structure or area of skin, usually caused by applied mechanical force which results in tearing or stripping.
- Bites, whether inflicted by animals or humans, which penetrate the outer layers of the skin, may look relatively trivial but can become infected by a range of pathogenic organisms, including spirochetes, staphylococci, streptococci and various Gram-positive bacilli. If untreated these infections can have serious sequelae, sometimes involving fascia, tendon and bone.
- Contusions (bruises) result from trauma that damages an internal structure without breaking the skin.
- Crush injuries result when an area of the body is subjected to significant compression, typically as a result of an accident with heavy or automated machinery. Usually such injuries result in splitting of the skin and in extreme cases, shattering of bone associated with damage to other internal structures.
- Cuts and incisions are wounds with cleanly cut even edges and range from minor injuries such as paper cuts to surgical incisions.
- Lacerations (tears) are more severe than abrasions and commonly involve both the skin and the underlying tissues. Such wounds generally have ragged uneven margins.
- Penetrating wounds may be caused by knives, bullets or other missiles, or an accidental injury caused by any sharp or pointed object.

Although the external appearance of wound may suggest that the injury is relatively minor, internal damage can be considerable, depending upon the site and depth of penetration, and/or the velocity of the bullet or missile.[1]

Burns and chemical injuries

There are several different types of burns: thermal, chemical, electrical, and those caused by radiation, thermal injuries being the most common. The severity of a thermal injury is governed by the temperature of the heat source, the thermal inertia (a function of the thermal conductivity, density and specific heat of the object), and the time of contact or exposure.[2] For example, a temperature of 70 °C will cause epidermal necrosis in one second but a temperature of 45 °C will require an exposure time in excess of six hours to induce tissue damage.

Burns and scalds (thermal injuries caused by moist heat) are generally classified into three types depending upon the degree of tissue damage.

- Superficial burns, which involve only the epidermis and superficial layers of the dermis, usually result from exposure to prolonged low intensity heat.
- Deep dermal (second degree) burns, result in destruction of the epidermis together with much of the dermal layer beneath. Only some isolated epidermal elements in the deeper layers remain viable, such as those within hair follicles and sweat glands.
- Full thickness (third degree) burns, result in destruction of all the elements of the skin.

A significant burn may have three identifiable zones: the innermost part of the injury, which has suffered irreversible damage, is called the zone of coagulation; the outermost zone, which has undergone minor reversible damage, is called the zone of uraemia and between these two is the area known as the zone of stasis. The eventual fate of the cells in the latter region is determined by the nature of the treatment provided.

Chronic wounds

Some wounds fail to progress through an orderly and timely sequence of repair and so are termed 'chronic' wounds. Examples of 'chronic' wounds include:

- Malignant wounds
- Leg ulcers, both venous and arterial in origin
- Pressure ulcers
- Ulcers associated with diabetes

Whilst it might reasonably be argued that malignant wounds, leg ulcers caused by ischemia, or ulcers associated with microvascular disease in individuals with diabetes are truly 'chronic' as they are caused or exacerbated by localized, irreversible histological or physiological changes, many pressure ulcers, including those caused by diabetic neuropathy without corresponding microvascular changes, heal uneventfully when properly managed. For this reason, it is probably incorrect to classify these as 'chronic' wounds. Similarly, a significant proportion of venous leg ulcers heal normally once the underlying problem has been addressed, by either surgical invention or the provision of adequate external graduated compression.

Some patients, however, have concomitant conditions such as poor nutritional status or incontinence, connective tissues disorders, osteomyelitis or systemic conditions such as sickle cell disease or end-stage renal or heart disease. All of these factors, individually or in combination, can lead to the formation of wounds that resolutely fail to respond to treatment. These may, therefore, be accurately described as 'chronic' wounds.

Whilst it is undoubtedly of paramount importance to obtain an accurate diagnosis for all wounds prior to initiating treatment, this in itself may do little to facilitate dressing selection. Knowing that a wound is caused by pressure damage or malignancy does not, necessarily, help with the selection of the most appropriate type of dressing.

Classification by intervention

In an alternative classification system, wounds are categorized according to the nature of the treatment provided:

- Sutured wounds, described as healing by primary intention
- Wounds left open for a few days then closed surgically - delayed primary closure
- Wounds closed with a skin graft
- Wounds closed with a flap
- Wounds allowed to heal by granulation and reepithelialization - healing by secondary intention

This classification is logical and easy to use, but is only of limited value if used as an aid to dressing selection.

Classification by depth

This approach has been widely adopted for the classification of pressure damage by organizations such as European Pressure Ulcer Advisory Panel (EUPAP) in 1998,[3] and the American National Pressure Ulcer Advisory Panel (NPUAP) in 2007.[4]

Table 1: The EUPAP pressure ulcer classification system

Grade	Description
Grade 1:	Non-blanchable erythema
Grade 2:	Blister or partial thickness skin loss involving epidermis, dermis, or both
Grade 3:	Superficial ulcer; full thickness skin loss involving damage or necrosis of subcutaneous tissue that may extend down to, but not through, underlying fascia
Grade 4:	Deep ulcer; extensive destruction, tissue necrosis, or damage to muscle, bone, or supporting structures with or without full thickness skin loss

Table 2: The NPUAP pressure ulcer classification system

Grade	Description
Grade 1:	Intact skin with non-blanchable redness of a localised area usually over a bony prominence. Darkly pigmented skin may not have visible blanching; its colour may differ from the surrounding area
Grade 2:	Partial thickness loss of dermis presenting as a shallow open ulcer with a red pink wound bed, without slough. May also present as an intact or open/ruptured serum-filled blister
Grade 3:	Full thickness tissue loss in which subcutaneous fat may be visible but bone, tendon and muscle are not exposed. Slough may be present but does not obscure the depth of tissue loss. May include undermining and tunnelling
Grade 4:	Full thickness tissue loss with exposed bone, tendon or muscle. Slough or eschar may be present on some parts of the wound bed. Often includes undermining and tunnelling
Suspected deep tissue injury:	Purple or maroon localised area of discoloured intact skin or blood-filled blister due to damage of underlying soft tissue from pressure and/or shear. The area may be preceded by tissue that is painful, firm, mushy, boggy, warmer or cooler as compared to adjacent tissue
Unstageable:	Full thickness tissue loss in which the base of the ulcer is covered by slough and/or eschar in the wound bed

In the European system, due to the need to effect debridement to determine the depth of a wound to complete the classification process, allocation of ulcer grading may be delayed or presumptive. Compared to the European classification, the American system recognizes two additional stages which are regarded as interim classifications before allocation to one of the other grades becomes possible once the wound has been fully debrided. Although these two classifications systems provide an effective way of recording the severity of pressure damage, once again they do little to facilitate dressing choice.

Classification by condition

In this system, based upon an approach described previously,[5] wounds are classified according to their condition and appearance rather than by their aetiology. Unlike the systems described previously, this classification system goes some way to identifying the properties of dressings that may be appropriate for a given wound at a specific stage of the healing process and will be used throughout the rest of this book.

Table 3: Classification of wounds by condition

Wound type	Required function(s) of dressing
Sutured wounds:	Physical protection, possibly provide waterproof barrier to enable bathing or showering
Black necrotic wounds:	Provide impermeable cover to facilitate rehydration and promote autolytic debridement
Dry sloughy wounds:	Facilitate rehydration and promote autolytic debridement by retaining moisture or donation of moisture.
Clean lightly exuding granulating wounds:	Absorb excess fluid whilst maintaining moist environment, to facilitate granulation, and be of low adherence.
Heavily exuding or slough covered granulating wounds:	Absorb excess fluid, promote autolytic debridement, facilitate granulation, be of low adherence and prevent exudate spreading onto periwound skin
Infected wounds:	Combat infection and prevent cross infection
Cavity wounds and sinuses:	Absorb excess fluid, prevent bridging of wound, promote drainage
Epithelializing wounds:	Maintain moist environment, be of low-adherence
Malodorous wounds:	Absorb odour or combat odour production
Dry superficial wounds, minor burns and donor sites:	Maintain moist environment, be of low-adherence
Overgranulating wounds:	Be permeable to oxygen, apply compression or combat inflammatory process (corticosteroid)

REFERENCES

1. Owen-Smith M. Wounds caused by the weapons of war. In: Westaby S, editor. *Wound Care.* London: Heinemann Medical, 1985:110-120.
2. Bull J, Lawrence JC. Thermal conditions to produce skin burns,. *Fire Mat* 1979;3:100-105.
3. EPUAP. European Pressure Ulcer Advisory Panel, Pressure Ulcer Treatment Guidelines. *http://www.epuap.org/gltreatment.html* 1998.
4. NUPUAP. Pressure ulcer stages. *http://www.npuap.org/pr2.htm* 2007.
5. Thomas S. The selection of dressings. *Primary Health Care* 1989;7:12-15.

3. Wounds: counting the cost

INTRODUCTION

It has been estimated that each year, in the UK, the NHS spends in the order of £2 - 3 billion on the management of an estimated 650,000 chronic wounds,[1-2] a figure takes no account of the suffering that such wounds cause to patients, or the negative impact they have on their quality of life and day-to-day activities.

COST OF TREATING 'CHRONIC' WOUNDS

Pressure ulcers

According to Bennett et al.,[3] approximately 412,000 individuals develop a new pressure ulcer every year in the United Kingdom. Of these, some 100,000 will be classed as Grade III or Grade IV according to the grading criteria adopted by the European Pressure Ulcer Advisory Panel, EPUAP (http://www.epuap.com).

The cost to the NHS of managing patients with such wounds they calculated to be in the range of £1.4 - 2.1bn, a figure derived using a 'bottom-up' costing method, based upon protocols of care, which reflect accepted good clinical practice and representative UK NHS costs at 2000 prices.

The costings assumed that patients were cared for in an institutional setting, but not admitted solely for the care of a pressure ulcer. Hotel costs were, therefore, not included in the calculation. The costings do include nursing time, dressings, antibiotics, diagnostic tests, support surfaces and hospital inpatient days where appropriate. The authors of this study chose not to include the costs of treating ulcers that develop on the heels of patients with peripheral vascular disease or pressure ulcers occurring in patients with diabetes.

Daily costs ranged from £38 to £196 per day with episodic costs ranging from £1,064 for a Grade I ulcer healing normally, to £24,214 for a Grade IV ulcer with bony involvement and osteomyelitis.

The presence of infection increased the projected daily treatment cost of all Grades of ulcers. For example, a period of infection raised the cost of treating a Grade III ulcer from £50 to £192 per day and increased the projected episodic treatment cost from £6,350 to £8,270.

In their paper, the authors quoted healing times from previously published studies and used these to derive mean values upon which they based their conclusions. This in fact introduced a significant source of error. Reference to the some of the original texts reveals that many of the ulcers in question had already existed for weeks or months before inclusion into the relevant studies. During this time they presumably had already been treated and therefore may have made some progress towards debridement and/or healing. This means that the figures quoted in the paper for the duration of the wounds probably represent a significant underestimate of the true values and therefore the actual treatment costs.

Diabetic ulcers

Diabetic ulcers also represent a major source of morbidity. According to Gordois et al.,[4] approximately 15% of the 1.4 million diagnosed diabetics in the UK develop at least one foot ulcer during their lifetime. They further state that the prevalence of foot ulcers in the diabetic population as a whole is estimated to be 5 - 7%, equivalent to around 84,000 ulcers, 76% (64,000) of which are primarily neuropathic or neuroischaemic in origin.

All ulcers, irrespective of Grade, can develop cellulitis or osteomyelitis, and 15% of all foot ulcers will result in an amputation of the toe, foot or leg. The authors calculated the total annual cost to the NHS of treating diabetic peripheral neuropathy (DPN) and its sequelae to be around £252m, or nearly £4,000 per patient, but if all types of diabetic ulcers had been included in this calculation, it is the opinion of the present author that the total figure would certainly have approached £300 m.

Some of the data used by Gordois et al.,[4] probably resulted in an underestimate of the true cost because they assumed that all ulcers were dressed primarily with relatively inexpensive dressings such as Melolin and Lyofoam, whereas in reality at the time the study was undertaken many wounds were dressed with more expensive interactive dressings such as alginates, hydrocolloids or hydrogels.

If this costing exercise were to be repeated in the current climate, the costs would be further inflated by the fashion for using dressings made from polysaccharide fibre, polyurethane foam, or dressings containing silver or other antimicrobials which are many times the price of the simple absorbents quoted by Gordois.

The costings assumed that patients were treated on an outpatient basis unless they developed osteomyelitis (when 50% would require a hospital stay) or they were specifically admitted to hospital for a surgical intervention (amputation).

The authors recognised that the total annual cost was very sensitive to changes in the prevalence of foot ulceration, and demonstrated that for every 10% change in prevalence, the total annual cost of DPN and its complications varied by approximately 9%. They concluded that the development of interventions by the healthcare industry to successfully treat DPN or to prevent or delay its long-term complications would lead to substantial cost savings in the UK.

Such innovations are clearly urgently needed for Nelson et al.,[5] in a systematic review on the treatment of infected diabetic foot ulcers reviewed twenty-three studies that investigated the effectiveness or cost-effectiveness of antimicrobial agents for DFU. Eight studied intravenous antibiotics, five oral antibiotics, four different topical agents such as dressings, four subcutaneous granulocyte colony stimulating factor (G-CSF), one evaluated oral and topical Ayurvedic preparations and one compared topical sugar versus antibiotics versus standard care. The authors concluded that 'the majority of trials were underpowered and were too dissimilar to be pooled. There was no strong evidence for recommending any particular antimicrobial agent for the prevention of amputation, resolution of infection or ulcer healing.'

Leg ulcers

It is also estimated that about 150,000 people in the UK suffer from active venous ulcers which costs the NHS between £300-£600 million a year[6]. No estimates are available for the cost of managing patients with critical ischaemia which leads to ulceration of the legs and feet, followed in many cases by amputation.

CONTAINING TREATMENT COSTS

In the pressure ulcer study referred to previously, expenditure on dressings and topical preparations represented between 2% and 10% of the daily costs depending upon nature and severity of the wound. Official figures reveal that in 2003, taken across the NHS as whole, salaries, and wages accounted for 58.6% of total health spending. Clinical supplies and services of all types accounted for 10.9%. According to one published estimate,[7] less than 5% of wound management costs are product related, the majority, circa 80%, are staffing costs.

In view of the contribution to overall treatment costs made by staff costs, it follows that any form of therapy that reduces treatment times or the total number of clinical interventions, should deliver a major cost benefit and enable nurses and other healthcare professionals to treat more patients with the same level of resources. The significance of this observation has been widely recognised, not only by clinicians, but also by manufacturers of dressings and wound management materials in the search for more cost-effective forms of therapy

As a result, numerous clinical studies have compared healing rates of specific wound types with different types of new dressings in an attempt to demonstrate increased cost-effectiveness.[8-11] The results of these investigations, which can sometimes involve hundreds of patients, often show no statistically significant difference in the healing rates achieved with the different regimens. In some instances differences are detected which, although statistically significant, are not clinically relevant.

This inability to demonstrate clinically meaningful differences in healing rates achieved with modern dressings in most non-infected wounds is simply explained. With a few exceptions, notably those products that contain growth factors or modify the biochemical processes taking place within a wound by some other means, most dressings can do nothing to stimulate or accelerate healing. At best it could be argued they simply provide a physical environment that permits healing to take place at the optimum rate and hopefully do not cause trauma upon removal. Simply put, the principal advantage of the best products is that they do the least harm.

Where differences in healing rates are encountered in clinical trials, these frequently involve comparators that cause dehydration or maceration of the wound bed or produce trauma to newly formed tissue upon removal. Paraffin gauze dressing is an excellent example of such a product, which has been widely used as a control in clinical studies involving new technologies, as will be described in the chapters which follow.

When this material is included in a study, the 'test' material, provided always that it does not have a major design flaw, will almost inevitably be shown to be superior in use. In contrast, comparative studies involving 'modern' wound management materials generally show minimal differences in healing rates, which is why alternative parameters or treatment outcomes are commonly selected to differentiate one product from another.

These parameters include exudate management, the status of the periwound skin, ease of application and removal of the dressing, wear time and an assessment of the pain produced during use or at dressing removal in addition to other quality of life issues.

The use of alternative outcomes is essential in studies involving wounds which are unlikely ever to heal and this issue has been comprehensively addressed by Enoch and Price.[12] They argue that either intermediate or surrogate endpoints, should be used as prognostic indicators of improvement in such wounds, and that 'controlling exudate, minimising or eliminating odour, preventing infection, and relieving pain should all be considered as legitimate non-healing endpoints'.

Regrettably few systematic reviews recognise or accept the importance of many of these parameters, and concentrate principally on healing rates thus greatly limiting their practical value.

The effective management of exudate, for example, has long been regarded as perhaps the most important function of a dressings but the importance of exudate itself and its value as a diagnostic indicator of changes in the healing status of a wound is often overlooked. For this reason the formation, composition and function of exudate forms the subject of a separate chapter.

REFERENCES

1. Thomas S. The cost of managing chronic wounds in the UK with particular emphasis on maggot debridement therapy. *Journal of Wound Care* 2006;15(10):465-469.
2. Posnett J, Franks PJ. The burden of chronic wounds in the UK. *Nurs Times* 2008;104(3):44-5.
3. Bennett G, Dealey C, Posnett J. The cost of pressure ulcers in the UK. *Age and Ageing* 2004;33:230-235.
4. Gordois A, Scuffham P, Shearer A. The healthcare costs of diabetic peripheral neuropathy in the UK - Cost-of-illness study. *The Diabetic Foot* 2003;6(2).
5. Nelson EA, O'Meara S, Craig D, Iglesias C, Golder S, Dalton J, et al. A series of systematic reviews to inform a decision analysis for sampling and treating infected diabetic foot ulcers. *Health Technology Assessment* 2006;10(12).
6. Simon DA, Dix FP, McCollum CN. Management of venous leg ulcers. *Bmj* 2004;328(7452):1358-62.
7. Smith and Nephew Sustainability Report 2003. *http://www.smith-nephew.com/sustainability2003/health_wm.html* 2003.
8. Thomas S, Banks V, Bale S, Fear-Price M, Hagelstein S, Harding KG, et al. A comparison of two dressings in the management of chronic wounds. *Journal of Wound Care* 1997;6(8):383-386.
9. Thomas S, Banks V, Fear M, Hagelstein S, Bale S, Harding K. A study to compare two film dressings used as secondary dressings. *Journal of Wound Care* 1997;6(7):333-336.

10. Banks V, Bale S, Harding K, Harding EF. Evaluation of a new polyurethane foam dressing. *Journal of Wound Care* 1997;6(6):266-9.
11. Cohn SM, Lopez PP, Brown M, Namias N, Jackowski J, Li P, et al. Open surgical wounds: how does Aquacel compare with wet-to-dry gauze? *Journal of Wound Care* 2004;13(1):10-2.
12. Enoch S, Price P. Should alternative endpoints be considered to evaluate outcomes in chronic recalcitrant wounds? *http://www.worldwidewounds.com/2004/october/Enoch-Part2/Alternative-Enpoints-To-Healing.html*, 2004.

4. Mechanisms of wound healing

INTRODUCTION

Irrespective of the nature or size of wound, the same basic biochemical and cellular processes are involved in the healing process. These are extremely complex, and are described here only in sufficient detail to explain how they may be influenced by the application of surgical dressings or the use of different wound management techniques. For additional information, readers are advised to consult more specialized texts.

As previously identified four types of wound healing are generally recognised: primary closure (healing by first intention), open granulation (healing by secondary intention), delayed or secondary closure, sometimes called healing by third intention and grafting or flap formation.

WOUND MANAGEMENT TECHNIQUES

Primary closure

Most clean surgical wounds and recent traumatic injuries are managed by primary closure. In this technique the surgeon approximates the edges of the wound and individually sutures the different layers of tissue together. The resulting wound contains minimal quantities of granulation tissue and once it has healed only a thin scar remains, which may be virtually undetectable when fully mature. Primary closure is generally not appropriate in the treatment of long-standing injuries, or wounds that are infected or contaminated with earth or other foreign material. The following brief outline of the healing process refers to sutured wounds and minor injuries involving minimal tissue loss which are allowed to heal naturally.

Healing begins with the acute inflammatory phase, which commences within a few minutes of the injury and lasts for about three days. As platelets liberated from damaged blood vessels flow into the wound, they come into contact with mature collagen, become activated, and aggregate together. During this process, granules within the cells liberate lysosomal enzymes, adenosine triphosphate (ATP), serotonin, growth factors, and other agents that potentiate further platelet aggregation. At the same time thromboplastin is liberated from injured cells in the vicinity of the wound, activating the clotting mechanism; this ultimately results in the cleavage of fibrinogen to form fibrin monomers, which polymerise to produce a fibrin network. Together these two mechanisms produce a plug or clot in the wound, which brings about haemostasis and gives strength and support to the injured tissue. In time this clot dries out to form the familiar scab.

Vasodilatory agents such as histamine and serotonin, liberated as a consequence of the original injury, increase the permeability of the local capillary bed, allowing serum and white cells to be released into the area surrounding the wound. The resulting accumulation of fluid in the tissue produces the characteristic swelling and sensations of throbbing and warmth that are experienced by the patient.

Within hours, polymorphonucleocytes (neutrophils) begin to appear in the wound, followed later by macrophages. Both neutrophils and macrophages play an important role in the removal of debris and the ingestion of bacteria. This is the beginning of the 'destructive' phase of healing, in which unwanted fibrin and dead cells are broken down by enzymatic activity. Neutrophils are primarily concerned with bacterial ingestion, and aid macrophages in wound debridement by the release of proteolytic, fibrinolytic and collagenolytic enzymes. In a series of studies in guinea pigs, Simpson and Ross[1] induced a selective neutropenia by administration of an antineutrophilic serum. They showed that, provided the animals were not exposed to significant numbers of pathogenic organisms, wound healing progressed normally, suggesting that neutrophils do not play an essential role in tissue repair. If, however, large numbers of organisms were introduced into their wounds, the animals died of septicaemia and bacteraemia.

The role of the macrophage is more complex. Like the neutrophil, it produces proteinases and other enzymes that break down clots and debris, forming fluid-filled cavities into which fibroblasts and endothelial buds can move. In addition, it produces factors that stimulate the formation of new vascular tissue,[2] and is also believed to play an important part in the initiation and control of fibroblasts - which are, in turn, responsible for the synthesis of collagen. Although the macrophage can function under both aerobic and anaerobic conditions over a range of pH and pO_2,[3] the cell is much less effective in destroying bacteria under hypoxic conditions.

After about 24 hours, the epithelial cells on the surface of the wound begin to turn down over the edge of the underlying dermis and grow across the defect under the dried scab. Depending upon the size and nature of the wound, this process may be complete within about two to three days. At about this time, some evidence of organisation may be detected within the body of the wound itself as fibroblasts begin to lay down strands of collagen, a major constituent of skin, and one which helps to give it strength and form. The production of collagen peaks around the 5th - 7th day, although this 'proliferative' phase of healing generally lasts about three weeks in total. It is followed by the final 'maturation' or 'remodelling' phase, which can take up to a year to complete.

During this phase, the nature of the final scar is determined and the cellular granulation tissue is changed to a relatively acellular mass. Many of the fibroblasts and capillaries formed during the early stages of healing disappear and the collagen fibres within the wound are reorganised and replaced. Collagen levels in a wound peak some two to three weeks after injury but the tensile strength of the scar tissue continues to increase for up to twelve months or more. This increase in strength corresponds to changes that occur in the structure of the collagen molecule as the material that is formed in the early stages of healing is replaced by a second more stable form as the scar matures. When first laid down, the collagen fibrils are distributed randomly within the wound area but as healing progresses they become orientated in the direction of maximum stress, resulting in an increase in overall wound strength. The closer alignment of the fibres also permits the formation of cross-links which lend further stability to the new tissue.

Secondary intention

In wounds that have sustained a significant degree of tissue loss as a result of surgery or trauma, it may sometimes be undesirable or impossible to bring the edges of the wound together. In these situations the surgeon may favour leaving the wound open to heal by secondary intention. A similar decision may be taken if there is considered to be a serious risk of infection, or if there is a likelihood of subsequent wound dehiscence. It has also been found that healing by secondary intention can sometimes give better results than primary closure or split-skin grafting, where the cosmetic results of the latter method can be marred by contraction, wrinkling and pigmentation.[4-6]

Although the basic mechanisms of healing of granulating wounds are similar to those that occur in wounds that heal by primary closure, there are significant differences, particularly in the relative duration of the various stages of the healing process. Like a sutured wound, a defect that is left to heal by secondary intention first undergoes an inflammatory response. During this time the exposed tissue or defect may become covered or filled with a layer of blood or serous fluid, which is released during or soon after the initial injury.

As a result of increased capillary and venous permeability, erythrocytes, leucocytes and platelets are liberated into the wound. Neutrophils predominate during the first two to three days but as these decrease in number they are followed by macrophages, which reach their maximum level on day five or six. As in a sutured wound, macrophages are responsible for the bulk of phagocytic activity but they also produce a host of complex proteins and extracellular products including a chemotactic factor, which is thought to attract fibroblasts to the wound area. Fibroblasts appear in the base of the developing wound as early as day four or five and are responsible for the production of intracellular precursors of collagen, which are eventually made into collagen fibrils extracellularly. This process of collagen production is thought to be at least partially under macrophage control.

Around the second or third day, endothelial cells appear in the developing inflammatory tissue as capillary buds. Knighton *et al.*[7] have suggested that the low oxygen tension in the centre of the wound in some way attracts macrophages, the only cells that are able to withstand the severe hypoxia in this situation. The macrophages clear away portions of the fibrous clot and liberate growth factors which stimulate the production of a capillary network. These capillaries retain their permeable nature and thus provide a constant source of cells and fluid for the developing tissue. When the process of repair is complete the demand for oxygen is substantially reduced and much of this new vasculature is lost.

During healing, the wound becomes progressively filled with granulation tissue, which is composed of collagen and proteoglycans, a complex mixture of proteins and polysaccharides together with salts and other colloidal materials which together produce a gel-like matrix contained within the fibrous collagen network. The production of granulation tissue continues until the base of the original cavity is almost level with the surrounding skin. At this stage, the epithelium around the wound margin becomes active and begins to grow over the surface of the wound, thus restoring the integrity of the epidermis. Occasionally the production of granulation tissue continues after the wound cavity has been filled, leading to the formation of 'hypergranulation tissue' or 'proud flesh'. This is sometimes associated with the use of occlusive dressings, and is often removed by the application of a caustic agent such as a silver nitrate pencil. A less traumatic method involves the short-term local application of a suitable corticosteroid cream or ointment, although this should only be done under medical supervision. Alternatively, a change to a more permeable dressing may be all that is required. The formation, causes and management of hypergranulation tissue have been reviewed previously.[8]

A further, and equally important, part of the healing process is contraction, a mechanism by which the margins of the wound are drawn towards the centre. This produces a small area of scar tissue, which may be only one-tenth of the size of the original wound. Contraction may take place in all healing wounds, but it is particularly important in large wounds that are left to heal by granulation and epithelialization. Although in many anatomical sites the process of contraction results in a wound with an acceptable cosmetic appearance, contraction of a wound on the face may result in distortion of the features due to the 'purse string' effect. Contraction takes place at a rate of approximately 0.6 - 0.7 mm/day and is not related to wound size, although it is known that rectangular wounds contract more rapidly than round ones. It has been shown that the contractile forces can be sufficiently powerful to cause severe loss of function,[9] and in wounds on the dorsum of the hand they have even been known to cause dislocation of the knuckles.[10]

Wound contraction generally begins about the end of the first week and may continue until the wound is completely closed. It is brought about by the action of a specialist cell called a myofibroblast which is formed from a normal fibroblast as a result of major structural and functional changes. Myofibroblasts show many of the properties of both fibroblasts and smooth muscle cells and will respond to agents that cause contraction or relaxation of smooth muscle tissue. The cells are joined together over the entire wound surface; when they contract they gradually pull in the edges of the wound. Some early evidence suggests that there may be a connection between the initiation of myofibroblast activity and the state of hydration (or dehydration) of the surface of the wound.[11] The process of contraction takes place most quickly if a wound is clean and free of infection and is slowed down or prevented altogether by the presence of eschar or adherent dressings.[12]

The healing of traumatic injuries, in which large areas of skin are lost, depends upon the extent of the damage. Superficial and shallow partial thickness burns, for example, heal as the surviving epidermal cells begin to grow and spread across the surface of the wound. In deep dermal burns, these epidermal cells can develop from small numbers of surviving cells present in the lower parts of hair follicles and sweat glands. These will grow up onto the surface of the wound and appear as isolated islands which gradually increase in size, eventually merging together. If a burn has been severe, the survival of these isolated areas of epidermis may be prejudiced by dehydration or an inappropriate method of treatment. In full thickness burns all epidermal elements are lost; without the application of a skin graft, resurfacing of the wound can only take place by migration of epithelial cells from the wound margins, and healing is therefore very slow.

Delayed primary closure

Less commonly used than the other methods of healing, delayed primary closure is generally carried out when, in the opinion of the surgeon, primary closure may be unsuccessful due to the presence of infection, a poor blood supply to the area, or the need for the application of excessive tension during closure. In these circumstances, the wound is left open for about three to four days before closure is effected. In these situations, sutures may be inserted at the time of the operation but left loose.

Grafting and flap formation

A skin graft is a portion of skin composed of dermis and epidermis that is removed from one anatomical site and placed onto a wound elsewhere on the body. If successful, grafting ensures that the wound will heal rapidly, thus reducing the chances of infection and the time spent in hospital. The major disadvantage of this technique is that the patient finishes up with two wounds instead of one, and it is often reported that the pain associated with the donor site is worse than that occasioned by the original injury. Most commonly used are partial thickness or split thickness grafts. These range in thickness from about 125 to 750 microns, although grafts 300 - 375 microns thick are typically employed. These are removed from a suitable donor site, such as the thigh or buttock, using a special knife which can be preset to ensure that the harvested material is of the required thickness. As elements of epidermal tissue remain in the base of sebaceous glands and hair follicles, the donor site heals rapidly, usually within 10-14 days.

For more specialist applications, such as facial reconstruction, full thickness grafts can be taken which may contain fat, hair and sebaceous glands. They have the advantages that they are cosmetically more acceptable and less likely to form severe contractures than split thickness grafts. Full thickness grafts are also used when a neurovascular bundle or cortical bone must be covered with tissue. They have the disadvantage that, in many cases, the donor site will itself require the application of a second, partial thickness graft, if the wound is too large to be closed by suture.

The success of a graft depends upon a number of factors, the most important of which is the presence of a good vascular bed to supply the metabolic needs of the transplanted tissue. Stress on the graft itself, infection, and the formation of seromas and haematomas are major causes of graft failure.

Skin flaps differ from grafts in that the relocated tissue is usually not completely separated from the body. In this technique a portion of skin and subcutaneous tissue is raised on three sides and rotated or transposed to cover an adjacent area of skin loss. In this way the entire flap continues to receive a supply of blood from its original vasculature until it becomes established elsewhere. The maximum size of the flap depends upon the anatomical site from which it is raised, and the nature and distribution of the major blood vessels. In a variation of this technique, a flap of tissue is relocated complete with its attached blood supply: this is known as a free flap transfer. A more detailed summary of the techniques of grafting and flap formation is given elsewhere.[13]

MONITORING PROGRESS TOWARDS HEALING

In both normal clinical practice, and more particularly in formal clinical trials designed to compare different forms of treatment, it is important to adopt some objective measures to monitor changes taking place within a wound to determine the effectiveness of a particular form of therapy.

These typically involve a record of changes in area or volume as the wound progresses towards healing, but equally important in some instances are the changes, both positive and negative, that occur in a wound's appearance. These may be due to the removal (or formation) of sloughy or necrotic tissue, the production of granulation tissue or new epithelium, or even the development of infection. Equally important are any changes that are visible in the periwound skin as these can sometimes provide an early warning of potential wound-related problems.

Monitoring wound area

Most practitioners record some basic information on wound dimensions. In its simplest form this simply consists of a simple sketch in the patients notes sometimes annotated with rough measurements of maximum length and breadth.

A more accurate procedure involves the production of a tracing of the wound on a piece of transparent plastic which may be marked with a grid to enable an estimate of the wound area to be made by counting the number of squares enclosed within the perimeter of the wound. A variation of this technique involves cutting out and weighing the wound tracing and calculating its area using a predetermined value for the weight per unit area of the tracing medium. More recently computer based systems have been described which facilitate calculation of wound area measurements from tracings or photographs. Numerous publications are available which describe these various techniques in some detail, and in some instance provide comparisons between them.[14-26]

Most planimetry techniques only provide two dimensional information, a measure of wound area. They do not facilitate measure of wound depth, which may be particularly important in cavity wounds. Historically this problem was addressed by measuring the volume of normal saline that could be introduced into a wound - a messy and inaccurate procedure, or by making a mould of the wound using something like alginate dental impression material[27] from which the wound volume could be determined indirectly by displacement or calculated by dividing the recorded weight by the density of the alginate. This procedure was said to be particularly useful for pressure sores and other irregular lesions which were difficult to measure by alternative means.

Once again, however, computer based systems have been described that facilitate such measurements. Plassmann[28-30] developed a system using colour coded light which projected a series of lines onto the wound and surrounding skin. Using a sophisticated computer algorithm the wound volume was calculated from the observed deformation in the pattern of these lines. A laser scanning method for measuring wound volumes has been described by Smith *et al.*[31]

Measurements of wound areas and volumes are not of any particular intrinsic value; it is the changes that take place in these values which are important to the patient and clinician. These changes may either be used to compare different products in a particular population, as in a clinical trial, or compare them with previously determined standard values for a similar patient population.

Marks *et al.*,[32-33] calculated the healing rates of hundreds of healthy surgical wounds from which they have derived simple equations which could be used to predict the likely time for such a wound of a given size to heal as follows:

$$Time\ to\ heal\ in\ days = (Wound\ depth\ in\ mm \times 1.23) + 3.6$$

They suggested that similar equations can be produced other wound types for example pilonidal wounds and wounds produced following surgery for hidradenitis suppurativa. Using these equations as a base line it is possible to monitor the progress of a wound and ensure that the rate of healing does not vary significantly from the norm; for example, due to the presence of a subclinical infection.

Similar exercises have been conducted with venous leg ulcers[34] and it has been suggested that the change in wound area during the first few weeks of treatment can in some instances can provide a useful prediction of eventual healing.[35-36] Similar opportunities also said to exist with pressure ulcers.[37]

Monitoring wound appearance

As previously indicated changes in the appearance of a wound can be as important as a change in area or volume, indicating, for example, the need for, or the success of, a period of debridement or a course of antimicrobial therapy.

Most people are familiar with the basic classification system in which wounds, or various portions of their surface, are described as Black, Yellow, Red or Pink, representing in turn necrotic tissue, slough, granulation tissue and new epithelial tissue. This simple classification although far from perfect, can provide a useful starting point to treatment or the dressing selection process.

The amounts of necrotic or sloughy tissue present in a wound are frequently determined in clinical trials involving debriding agents and so methods are required for determining these values with reasonable accuracy. Once again the simplest technique involves a visual estimate of the proportion of the total surface of the wound surface covered with necrotic material, but a more accurate value can be obtained using planimetry as previously described. Using this approach the amount of each tissue type present within the wound is individually recorded and calculated separately. Alternatively it is possible to photograph the wounds and determine the colour distribution by digital analysis[38-39]

Digital photographs themselves represent a useful method for recording changes in wound appearance, but it is important to produce these under standard conditions to maximise their value in this regard.[40]

PROBLEMS ASSOCIATED WITH WOUND HEALING

Delayed wound healing

Although the majority of wounds heal uneventfully, problems do sometimes occur. In most instances these are associated with delayed healing or scar formation. Some wounds, particularly those associated with malignant disease may never heal, and in such situations optimum control of exudate and odour may be all than can be offered to provide the best possible quality of life to the patient.

Infection

The isolation of microorganisms from a wound is not, of itself, an indication of the presence of an infection, as wounds of all types can rapidly acquire bacteria from any one of a number of sources. Such contamination may result from contact with infected or contaminated objects, the ingress of dirt or dust, either at the time of injury or later, or from the patient's own skin or gastro-intestinal tract. For example, it has been found that, unless effective measures are taken to prevent contamination, virtually all burns become colonized by bacteria within 12 to 24 hours.[41]

The consequences of bacterial contamination of a wound will depend upon a number of factors: these include the number of organisms, their pathogenicity (potential to cause disease), and the ability of the patient's own defence system to combat any possible infection. This in turn may depend upon the patient's age, general health and nutritional status, and other factors such as the administration of immunosuppressive drugs, which may inhibit the production of leucocytes.

Many wounds will yield a variety of organisms upon microbiological investigation but may never show the classical symptoms of infection - redness and swelling with heat and pain, which were described by Celsus nearly two thousand years ago. Indeed the presence of a whole host of different organisms is virtually inevitable in dirty or sloughy wounds such as leg ulcers or sacral pressure areas (particularly in patients who are doubly incontinent). However, a similar pattern of infection in a major burn could, if untreated, rapidly develop into a life-threatening septicaemia. Signs that a previously healthy wound may be developing an unacceptably high bioburden include a change in colour or odour, or an increase in exudate production. If adequate measures are not taken to control the infection, it may lead eventually to the formation of cellulitis and ultimately bacteraemia and septicaemia.

Lawrence, in a series of publications on the effects of bacteria on burns[42] and wound healing,[43-44] described the techniques available for detecting and quantifying the number of bacteria present in a wound, and outlined changes in the types of organism that have been isolated from infected wounds over a thirty-year period. The most common pathogen to be isolated from wounds of all types is *Staphylococcus aureus*.

This organism, which is found in the nose of 20-30% of normal persons, may be isolated from approximately one-third of all infected wounds. Other organisms that can cause serious wound infections include *Pseudomonas aeruginosa*, *Streptococcus pyogenes*, and some Proteus, Clostridium and coliform species. Gilliland *et al.* showed that the presence preoperatively of Pseudomonas sp. and *S. aureus* significantly reduced skin graft healing; they also demonstrated that in 16 ulcers which were slow to heal or which recurred after discharge, 15 (94%) contained *S. aureus*.[45]

The types of organism present in a given wound may not remain constant but vary as the condition of the wound itself changes.[41] Burns covered with a wet slough frequently contain an abundance of Gram-negative bacilli - including *P. aeruginosa*, *Proteus mirabilis*, Klebsiella spp., and *Escherichia coli* - together with *Streptococcus faecalis*, *S. aureus* and *S. pyogenes*. As the slough separates, however, the numbers of Gram-negative organisms decrease and the Gram-positive bacteria predominate. Of all these organisms, Lowbury and Cason[41] identified *S. pyogenes* and *P. aeruginosa* as being amongst the most serious pathogens in a burn. *S. pyogenes* will cause the total failure of a skin graft if present at the time of operation and *P. aeruginosa* has been found to be an important cause of systemic infections in patients with severe burns, although other organisms may also cause serious problems from time to time.

The number of organisms that might be considered to constitute an infection in a wound was discussed by Lawrence,[44] who considered that the level of 10^5 per gram suggested by Pruitt,[46] formed a useful guide - provided it was recognised that the bacteriological picture of a wound could change from day to day.

The management of an infected wound usually consists of a combined systemic and local approach, including the use of antibiotics where appropriate and the application of a suitable dressing, which may itself possess inherent antibacterial activity. The use of topical antibiotics is not generally encouraged, as it may cause sensitivity reactions or lead to the emergence of antibiotic-resistant strains of bacteria.

Metabolic factors

Metabolic changes, an imbalance between proteolytic enzymes and their inhibitors, and the presence of senescent cells can have a marked effect on the healing of chronic wounds.[47] Reduced or inadequate levels of growth factors may also be important, which is why much research activity has been focused on this subject in recent years

Another area that has attracted considerable interest is the excessive proteinase activity often encountered in non-healing or indolent wounds such as leg ulcers. This is believed to result from an over-expression of matrix metalloproteinases (MMPs) which are zinc-dependent endopeptidases.

Along with other similar enzymes, MMPs are capable of modifying the structure and therefore the activity of a number of bioactive molecules. They are known to be involved in the cleavage of cell surface receptors and cytokine activation and inactivation. They are also thought to play a major role in cell behaviour, determining proliferation, migration, differentiation, angiogenesis, apoptosis and host defence mechanisms. In the context of wound dressings, one of their most important actions may be that of degrading all kinds of extracellular matrix proteins and causing excoriation of periwound skin, effectively extending the size of an existing wound. For this reason, considerable attention has been focussed upon dressings which are described as 'protease modulators' that in some way 'mop-up', destroy or otherwise inactivate these important molecules.

Miscellaneous factors

A number of other local and systemic factors are well recognized causes of delayed or impaired wound healing. Foreign bodies introduced deep into a wound at the time of injury can, if not removed, cause a chronic inflammatory response and delay healing or lead to the formation of a granuloma or abscess. Long-standing wounds that heal by epithelialization, such as burns and leg ulcers, may develop Marjolin's ulcer, an uncommon slow-growing squamous cell carcinoma. Other major factors that have an important effect upon the rate of healing include the age and nutritional status of the patient, underlying metabolic disorders such as diabetes or anaemia, the administration of drugs that suppress the inflammatory process, radiotherapy, arterial disease which may be aggravated by smoking and the presence of slough and necrotic tissue.

Scar formation

Another long-term problem sometimes associated with wound healing is the formation of hypertrophic or keloid scars. These unsightly areas result from excess collagen production but the reason for their formation is not fully understood; they are most likely to occur in Negroes and in young people around puberty. Hypertrophic scars are limited to the site of the original injury but keloid scars may continue to grow and spread into the surrounding tissue for a number of years. The histological, epidemiological and aetiological characteristics of both types of conditions have been comprehensively described by Munro,[48] and a series of surgical techniques that may help to minimize scar formation were described by Pape.[49] Topical treatments that have been developed to treat or prevent hypertrophic scar formation are described in Chapter 18.

Wound pain

According to evidence reviewed by Price et al.,[50-51] six out of ten patients with chronic wounds suffer from persistent wound pain.

Many patients with acute wounds of all types can also experience significant pain, which is often associated with the removal or replacement of a dressing.[52-53] This problem can be particularly acute with burns and donor sites, where the application of an inappropriate dressing can cause serious discomfort or even significant rewounding upon removal as described in latter chapters.

Chronic wound pain can lead to depression and the feeling of constant tiredness. For this reason, prevention and treatment of wound-related pain should be a major priority when designing wound treatment plans for it has been suggested that unless wound pain is optimally managed, patient suffering and costs to health care systems will increase. To this end, a 'Wound Pain Management Model' has been described[51] that involves the proper assessment and recording of patients' experiences of pain based on six critical dimensions of the pain experience: location, duration, intensity, quality, onset and impact on activities of daily living.

This model recommends strategies for preventing and treating pain in a variety of wound types encompassing wound cleansing strategies, the use of compression or other measures to facilitate vascular flow, the use of appropriate dressings and various types of non-pharmacological and pharmacological and treatments including the use of the WHO Clinical Ladder for the control of pain originally derived for patients with cancer.

In 2007 a foam dressing containing a non-steroidal analgesic, ibuprofen, was introduced specifically to address the problems of localized wound pain and this is discussed in more detail in Chapter 10.

References

1. Simpson DM, Ross R. The neutrophilic leukocyte in wound repair a study with antineutrophil serum. *Journal of Clinical Investigation* 1972;51(8):2009-23.
2. Thakral KK, Goodson WH, 3rd, Hunt TK. Stimulation of wound blood vessel growth by wound macrophages. *J Surg Res* 1979;26(4):430-6.
3. Silver IA. The physiology of wound healing. *Journal of Wound Care* 1994;3(2):106-109.
4. Silverberg LI. Patient satisfaction. *J Fam Pract* 1987;25(3):220.
5. Barnett R, Stranc M. A method of producing improved scars following excision of small lesions of the back. *Ann Plast Surg* 1979;3(5):391-4.
6. Morgan WP, Harding KG, Hughes LE. A comparison of skin grafting and healing by granulation, following axillary excision for hidradenitis suppurativa. *Ann R Coll Surg Engl* 1983;65(4):235-6.
7. Knighton DR, Silver IA, Hunt TK. Regulation of wound-healing angiogenesis - effect of oxygen gradints and inspired oxygen concentration. *Surgery* 1981;90(2):262-171.
8. Dunford C. Hypergranulation tissue. *Journal of Wound Care* 1999;8(10):506-7.
9. Upton J, Mulliken JB, Murray JE. Major intravenous extravasation injuries. *Am J Surg* 1979;137(4):497-506.
10. Rudolph R. Contraction and the control of contraction. *World J Surg* 1980;4(3):279-87.
11. Thomas S. A new approach to the management of extravasation injury in neonates. *Pharm. J.* 1987;239:584-585.
12. Foresman PA, Tedeschi KR, Rodeheaver GT. Influence of membrane dressings on wound contraction *J Burn Care Rehabil* 1986;7(5):398-403.
13. Davies DM. Skin cover. *Br Med J (Clin Res Ed)* 1985;290(6470):765-8.
14. Bohannon RW, Pfaller BA. Documentation of wound surface area from tracings of wound perimeters. Clinical report on three techniques. *Phys Ther* 1983;63(10):1622-4.
15. Fuller FW, Mansour EH, Engler PE, Shuster B. The use of planimetry for calculating the surface area of a burn wound. *J Burn Care Rehabil* 1985;6(1):47-9.
16. Anon. Measuring devices for wounds. *Journal of Wound Care* 1994;3(1):16.
17. Taylor RJ. 'Mouseyes': an aid to wound measurement using a computer. *Journal of Wound Care* 1997;6(3):123-6.
18. Kantor J, Margolis DJ. Efficacy and prognostic value of simple wound measurements. *Arch Dermatol* 1998;134(12):1571-4.
19. Langemo DK, Melland H, Hanson D, Olson B, Hunter S, Henly SJ. Two-dimensional wound measurement: comparison of 4 techniques. *Adv Wound Care* 1998;11(7):337-43.

20. Taylor RJ, Taylor AD, Marcuson RW. A computerised leg ulcer database with facilities for reporting and auditing. *Journal of Wound Care* 1999;8(1):35-38.
21. Williams C. The Verge Videometer wound measurement package. *British Journal of Nursing* 2000;9(4):237-239.
22. Taylor RJ. Mouseyes revisited: upgrading a computer program that aids wound measurement. *J Wound Care* 2002;11(6):213-6.
23. Thawer HA, Houghton PE, Woodbury MG, Keast D, Campbell K. A comparison of computer-assisted and manual wound size measurement. *Ostomy Wound Manage* 2002;48(10):46-53.
24. Gethin G, Cowman S. Wound measurement comparing the use of acetate tracings and Visitrak digital planimetry. *J Clin Nurs* 2006;15(4):422-7.
25. Wang Y, Liu G, Yuan N, Ran X. [A comparison of digital planimetry and transparency tracing based methods for measuring diabetic cutaneous ulcer surface area]. *Zhongguo Xiu Fu Chong Jian Wai Ke Za Zhi* 2008;22(5):563-6.
26. Mayrovitz HN, Soontupe LB. Wound areas by computerized planimetry of digital images: accuracy and reliability. *Adv Skin Wound Care* 2009;22(5):222-9.
27. Resch CS, Kerner E, Robson MC, Heggers JP, Scherer M, Boertman JA, et al. Pressure sore volume measurement. A technique to document and record wound healing. *J Am Geriatr Soc* 1988;36(5):444-6.
28. Plassmann P. Measuring wounds. *Journal of Wound Care* 1995;4(6):269-72.
29. Plassmann P, Jones BF. Measuring leg ulcers by colour coded structured light. *Journal of Wound Care* 1992;1(3):35-38.
30. Plassmann P, Jones TD. MAVIS: a non-invasive instrument to measure area and volume of wounds. Measurement of Area and Volume Instrument System. *Med Eng Phys* 1998;20(5):332-8.
31. Smith RB, Rogers B, Tolstykh GP, Walsh NE, Davis MG, Jr., Bunegin L, et al. Three-dimensional laser imaging system for measuring wound geometry. *Lasers Surg Med* 1998;23(2):87-93.
32. Marks J, Hughes L, Harding K. Prediction of healing time as an aid to the management of open granulating wounds. *World Journal of Surgery* 1983;7:641-645.
33. Marks J, Harding KG, Hughes LE, Ribeiro CD. Pilonidal sinus excision--healing by open granulation. *British Journal of Surgery* 1985;72(8):637-40.
34. Cardinal M, Eisenbud DE, Armstrong DG. Wound shape geometry measurements correlate to eventual wound healing. *Wound Repair Regen* 2009;17(2):173-8.
35. Flanagan M. Wound measurement: can it help us to monitor progression to healing? *Journal of Wound Care* 2003;12(5):189-94.
36. Moore K, McCallion R, Searle RJ, Stacey MC, Harding KG. Prediction and monitoring the therapeutic response of chronic dermal wounds. *Int Wound J* 2006;3(2):89-96.
37. Wallenstein S, Brem H. Statistical analysis of wound-healing rates for pressure ulcers. *Am J Surg* 2004;188(1A Suppl):73-8.
38. Boardman M, Melhuish JM, Palmer K, Harding KG. Hue,saturation and intensity in the healing wound image. *Journal of Wound Care* 1994;3(7):314-319.
39. Greenwood JE, Crawley BA, Clark SL, Chadwick PR, Ellison DA, Oppenheim BA, et al. Monitoring wound healing by odour. *Journal of Wound Care* 1997;6(5):219-21.
40. Bellamy K. Photography in wound assessment. *Journal of Wound Care* 1995;4(7):313-6.
41. Lowbury EJL, Cason JS. Aspects of infection control and skin grafting in burned patients. In: Westaby S, editor. *Wound Care*. London: Heinemann Medical, 1985:171-189.
42. Lawrence JC. The bacteriology of burns. *J Hosp Infect* 1985;6 Suppl B:3-17.

43. Lawrence C. Bacteriology and wound healing. In: Fox JA, Fischer H, editors. *Cadexomer Iodine,*. Munich,: Stuttgart, Schattauer Verlag, 1983: 19-31.

44. Lawrence JC. The effect of bacteria and their products on the healing of skin wounds. In: Rue Y, editor. *A Biological Approach to the Wound Healing Process, Proceedings of a Symposium, Royal College of Physicians, 5 June 1987*. London: Andover, Medifax,, 1987:9-21.

45. Gilliland EL, Nathwani N, Dore CJ, Lewis JD. Bacterial colonisation of leg ulcers and its effect on the success rate of skin grafting. *Ann R Coll Surg Engl* 1988;70(2):105-8.

46. Pruitt BA, Jr. The diagnosis and treatment of infection in the burn patient. *Burns Incl Therm Inj* 1984;11(2):79-91.

47. Harding KG, Morris HL, Patel GK. Healing chronic wounds. *British Medical Journal* 2002;324:160-163.

48. Munro KJ. Treatment of hypertrophic and keloid scars. *Journal of Wound Care* 1995;4(5):243-5.

49. Pape SA. The management of scars. *Journal of Wound Care* 1993;2(6):354-360.

50. Price P, Fogh K, Glynn C, Krasner DL, Osterbrink J, Sibbald RG. Managing painful chronic wounds: the Wound Pain Management Model. *Int Wound J* 2007;4 Suppl 1:4-15.

51. Price P, Fogh K, Glynn C, Krasner DL, Osterbrink J, Sibbald RG. Why combine a foam dressing with ibuprofen for wound pain and moist wound healing? *Int Wound J* 2007;4 Suppl 1:1-3.

52. Thomas S. Pain and wound management. *Nurs. Times Community Outlook Suppl.* 1989;85:Nov-15.

53. Moffat CJ, editor. *Pain at wound dressing changes*. London: Medical Education Partnership Ltd, 2002.

5. Wound Exudate

INTRODUCTION

Wound exudate, also referred to as wound fluid, is a generic term used to describe the fluid produced by wounds of all types once haemostasis has been achieved.

PROPERTIES OF EXUDATE

Key functions

In acute wounds, exudate has numerous beneficial properties and is thought to assist healing by:
- Preventing the wound bed from drying out
- Aiding the migration of tissue-repairing cells
- Providing essential nutrients for cell metabolism
- Enabling the diffusion of immune and growth factors
- Assisting separation of dead or damaged tissue by autolysis

Fluid from acute wounds also has stimulatory properties and therefore makes an essential contribution to normal wound healing. It was perhaps with good reason that Paracelsus (1491-1541) described exudate as 'nature's balsam'.

Formation

Exudate is produced by diffusion of plasma, the aqueous component of blood, through the walls of small blood capillaries. In normal uninjured tissue the rate at which fluid passes through the vessel walls into the surrounding matrix is determined by the relative magnitude of the combined hydrostatic and osmotic pressures on both sides of the capillary wall, the net effect of the opposing pressures determining the direction and rate of flow (Starling's hypothesis).

The majority of fluid that leaves the capillaries in this way (about 90%), is normally reabsorbed directly back into the circulatory system, and the remainder is returned *via* the lymphatics. Following an injury, however, the permeability of the vessel walls increases under the influence of chemical mediators such as histamine and bradykinin released as part of the normal inflammatory process. This change in permeability also enables white blood cells to escape from the capillaries into the wound, but red blood cells and platelets are generally too large to pass through.

In an acute wound, as the inflammatory phase of healing comes to an end, exudate production normally diminishes, but in a chronic wound the inflammatory process is extended, perhaps indefinitely, so exudate production remains at a high level.

Other factors, notably clinical infection, or the presence of bacteria which produce metabolites such as histamine which act directly upon capillary permeability, can also increase exudate production.

Heparin, which is released from mast cells at the time of injury, has a potent anti-inflammatory effect in addition to its well known anticoagulant properties but neutrophils, attracted to the site of injury, trigger the release of heparin binding protein (HBP) which combines with heparin, preventing its anti-inflammatory action.[1] Lundqvist et al.,[2] reported that levels of HBP in exudate collected from chronic leg ulcers are increased compared with those found in acute wound fluid. They further showed that P. aeruginosa stimulates the release of HBP from neutrophils thus further aggravating chronic inflammation.

Appearance

Exudate is normally a pale straw-yellow colour but it can vary in colour and viscosity. The significance of these and other changes are summarized in Table 4.

Composition

Much work has been undertaken on the composition and biological activity of fluid collected from both acute and chronic wounds and many papers have been published in this important area. Whilst some of the major components of exudate are identified below, for more comprehensive information, interested parties are invited to consult more specialized texts or review articles.[3]

Exudate from acute wounds

May,[4] compared the chemical composition of normal blood with that of exudate collected from donor sites dressed with a semipermeable polyurethane film dressing and burn blister fluid (Table 5).

He reported that the number of white cells present in exudate was up to six times that of normal blood, but that the concentrations of electrolytes and most proteins in wound fluid were comparable with those of serum.

Glucose values in exudate were 30 - 50% of normal blood values, a difference which the author proposed was due to the metabolic activity of the elevated numbers of white cells present.

Acute wound fluid is also known to contain factors that induce cell proliferation such as platelet-derived growth factor like peptides, interleukin-6 and transforming growth factor-alpha and beta.[5] In an experimental pig model, Chen et al.[6] showed that fluid collected from wounds occluded with hydrocolloid dressings exhibited metalloproteinase activity; furthermore, when applied to cultured dermal fibroblasts, exudate also possessed mitogenic activity. They also showed the presence of platelet-derived growth factor-like and basic fibroblast growth factor-like factors causing them to speculate that the presence of growth factors, and the potential abilities of proteinases to activate latent growth factors and generate chemotactic peptides through connective tissue breakdown, could also contribute to the enhanced healing of occluded wounds.

Table 4: Significance of exudate appearance

Characteristic		Possible cause
Clear or amber coloured	.	Serous exudate, often considered 'normal', but may be associated with infection by fibrinolysin-producing bacteria such as *S. aureus*. Also may be due to fluid from a urinary or lymphatic fistula
Cloudy, milky or creamy	.	May indicate the presence of fibrin strands (fibrinous exudate - a response to inflammation) or infection (purulent exudate containing white blood cells and bacteria)
Pink or red	.	Due to the presence of red blood cells and indicating capillary damage (sanguineous or haemorrhagic exudate)
Green	.	May be indicative of bacterial infection, e.g. *P. aeruginosa*
Brown or yellow	.	May be due to the presence of wound slough, or material from an enteric or urinary fistula
Grey or blue	.	May be related to the use of silver-containing dressings
High viscosity, thick and/or sticky	.	High protein content due to infection or inflammatory process
	.	Necrotic material
	.	Enteric fistula
	.	Residue from some types of dressings or topical preparations
Low viscosity, thin or 'runny'	.	Low protein content due to venous or congestive cardiac disease or malnutrition
	.	Urinary, lymphatic or joint space fistula
Unpleasant	.	Bacterial growth or infection
	.	Necrotic tissue
	.	Sinus/enteric or urinary fistula

Exudate from chronic wounds

Compared with acute wound fluid, chronic wound fluid (CWF), has been shown to possess elevated levels of biologically active molecules including pro-inflammatory cytokines and matrix metalloproteinases (MMPs) that are released from neutrophils, macrophages and other cell types that orchestrate the normal wound healing process. The proteases have an adverse effect on wound healing, inhibiting proliferation of keratinocytes, fibroblasts and endothelial cells. Increased levels of proteolytic enzymes and reduced growth factor activity all contribute to a poorly developed extra cellular wound matrix.

Wysocki,[7] showed that chronic wound fluid can rapidly breakdown fibronectin, a structural protein has an important influence on cell adhesion and which also plays an important role in the healing process. This effect was not detected in blister fluid or fluid from mastectomy wounds. She also found elevated levels of MMPs in CWF compared with fluid from the acute wounds.

Phillips *et al.,*[5] demonstrated that fluid collected from chronic venous ulcers inhibits rapidly dividing newborn fibroblasts. Although the intensity of the inhibitory activity, which was reversible and heat sensitive, varied between the donors tested, all samples exhibited some evidence of activity. Interestingly, however, CWF exerted a mild stimulatory effect upon more slowly growing normal adult and wound fibroblasts.

Adverse effects of exudate

The production of large volumes of exudate can have undesirable consequences which are totally independent of any effects upon wound healing, impacting dramatically upon a patient's quality of life.

If exudate rich in proteolytic enzymes is allowed to spread onto healthy periwound skin, it can cause erosion or excoriation as previously described. Even in the absence of such enzymes, the presence of wound fluid on intact skin can lead to infection as a result of maceration which reduces the ability of the skin to form an effective barrier. Exudate soaked dressings are also an important potential vector for cross-infection.

Serious leakage can also result in soiling of clothing and bedding with considerable practical and economic consequences, as well as impacting upon other aspects of patients' lives and social interactions compounding other problems of pain, discomfort and malodour. The socio-economic problems resulting from a failure to manage exudate effectively have been summarised by Dowset.[8]

For all these reasons, exudate management consumes a significant proportion of healthcare resources and can also represent a significant practical problem for the healthcare professional or carer. As a consequence, each year manufacturers of dressings spend large amounts of money developing products with enhanced fluid handling capabilities.

Table 5: Composition of acute wound fluid

Parameter	Range of normal blood values (a)	Burn blister fluid (b)	Donor site exudate (b)	Significance p (c)
WBC ($\times 10^3$/μl)	4.8 - 10.8	1.4 ± 0.7	30.7 ± 33.6	0.02
RBC ($\times 10^5$/μl)	42 - 62	0.2 ± 0.1	3.1 ± 2.3	0.001
Platelets ($\times 10^3$/μl)	150 - 300	13.8 ± 10.8	14.0 ± 11.2	0.96
Na (mEq/l)	135 - 155	138.8 ± 2.1	139.4 ± 5.3	0.79
Cl (mEq/l)	99 - 111	103.7 ± 3.8	100.6 ± 5.8	0.20
K (mEq/l)	3.5 - 5.5	3.7 ± 0.4	4.6 ± 1.2	0.08
Ca (mEq/l)	8.6 - 10.6	7.8 ± 0.2	8.7 ± 1.6	0.21
HCO$_3$	22 - 32	27.5 ± 4.2	23.4 ± 6.8	0.14
Glucose (mg %)	65 - 110	99.0 ± 28.8	32.5 ± 27.7	< 0.001
Total protein (g %)	6.8 - 7.7	4.4 ± 0.7	5.5 ± 1.4	0.08
Albumin (g %)	3.5 - 4.7	3.1 ± 0.4	3.3 ± 1.0	0.74
Albumin: globulin ratio	1.4 - 1.6	2.5 ± 0.3	1.3 ± 0.4	0.001
Urea nitrogen (mg %)	8 - 25	15.9 ± 1.9	15.7 ± 6.2	0.93

Table reproduced from May 1982
(a) All non-cellular entries are normal serum values,
(b) Numerical entries are means and standard deviations
(c) Statistical significance of Student's t test (two tailed) comparing exudate and blister fluid

EXUDATE AS A DIAGNOSTIC AID

The need to monitor exudate

Despite the practical problems posed by excessive exudate production, its value as a diagnostic aid and the important role that it fulfils in normal wound healing is often overlooked.

Wounds do not exude at a common or consistent rate throughout their healing cycle and the condition of a wound is more important than its aetiology in determining exudate production. Wounds covered with black necrotic tissue, or a thick layer of adherent slough, are often very dry - to the point that they require additional fluid to promote rehydration and autolysis.

Wounds that are not covered with slough, particularly in the inflammatory phase of healing, may produce copious amounts of fluid, but once this has ended and epithelialization begins, exudate production decreases and once again it may be appropriate to use products that conserve or donate moisture. The importance of providing the appropriate environmental conditions for wounds at varying stages of the healing cycle was described previously.[9] This was facilitated by the design of a 'moisture balance' which illustrated graphically how different types of dressings influence the moisture content of a wound and the surrounding tissue.

Both the volume and appearance of exudate provide valuable information on the general health or condition of the wound as described previously, and a marked change in either may be indicative of a developing infection. The practice of 'taking down' dressings prior to a doctor's ward round therefore removes a potentially valuable diagnostic indicator of progress (or otherwise) towards healing.

Measurement of exudate

Despite all the problems caused by excess exudate, and the considerable resources devoted to its management, little information is available either on the quantity of exudate that is produced by different types of wounds, or the amount of moisture that is required in order to facilitate the optimal rate of healing. Even Winter's seminal work, conducted in the 1960s, that led to the concept of moist wound healing failed to address either of these issues.

The problem is compounded by the lack of any form of validated simple method for assessing or recording exudate production despite the fact that in many clinical studies, a semi-quantitative estimate of exudate production is required which usually results in the use of descriptors such as 'exudate +++' or 'wound heavily exuding'. As will be seen later, even highly experienced nurses cannot readily differentiate between lightly or heavily exuding wounds in absolute terms, so the value of simple descriptors must be seriously questioned. Some information on the amount of exudate produced by different types of wounds was generated by Lamke et al.,[10] who measured the evaporative loss from intact skin and a variety of wound types, (Table 6).

Table 6: Evaporative loss from different wound types

Wound type	No of measurements	Evaporative loss (g/m^2/24 h)
Normal skin	60	204 ± 12
First degree burn	12	268 ± 26
Second degree burn	30	4274 ± 132
Third degree burn	20	3437 ± 108
Granulating wound	21	5138 ± 202
Donor site	35	3590 ± 180

The importance of monitoring exudate both qualitatively and quantitatively was emphasized in a review published by White and Cutting,[11] which made reference to three tools or acronyms designed to record or modify exudate production as part of the general wound management process.

The Exudate Continuum Tool proposed by Gray seeks to remove some of the subjectivity attached to exudate assessment by generating a score relevant to volume and viscosity which is monitored on a regular basis.

The concept of Wound Bed Preparation,[12-14] also encompasses the need for effective exudate management, as does the T.I.M.E. acronym,[15] where 'M' represents moisture imbalance which must be corrected.

A consensus document on best practice principles on wound exudate has recently been developed by World Union of Wound Healing Societies (2007),[16] which describes the relationship between the exudate status of the wound and the dressing, which is a useful aid in clinical practice.

EXUDATE HANDLING MECHANISMS

Numerous mechanisms exist by which dressings remove or sequester excess fluid away from the wound surface. Whilst some simple products rely upon one of these mechanisms in isolation, other products with more complex structures may use two or more of these mechanisms in combination.

Evaporation

Arguably, the simplest way of dealing with an exuding wound is to do nothing. If a low to moderately exuding lesion is left exposed to the air, the aqueous component of the exudate will evaporate, resulting in a progressive increase in the concentration of dissolved solids such as proteins and electrolytes which eventually come out of solution, coalesce and dry out to form a scab – nature's own dressing. Scab formation is characteristic of minor traumatic injuries, heavily exuding wounds typically do not form scabs in this way.

Despite the valuable protective role of a scab, its presence delays healing as the newly-formed epithelial cells are forced to burrow down beneath the dry tissue to migrate over the surface of the wound.

Although a scab represents a reasonable barrier to infection, an exposed wound remains at risk of contamination until the process of scab formation is complete.

Most people who sustain a minor injury and virtually everyone with a more extensive wound seek to cover the lesion with some form of dressing. There may be several reasons for this, to keep it clean, hide it from view, or stop exudate or blood from soiling clothing etc. Historically, materials commonly used for this purpose included simple woven fabrics such as bandages or cloth. These dressings functioned principally by absorption, a mechanism that is described below.

Absorption

To 'absorb' literally means to 'take-in', 'suck-up' or 'incorporate as part of itself'. In a wound management context this may involve the passage of liquid into spaces formed within the structure of the product, such as gaps between fibres or pores within foams, and/or the uptake of liquid by individual fibres from which the dressings is constructed.

The simplest and most familiar surgical absorbents are absorbent cotton (cotton wool), lint, and cotton gauze, all of which have been used for over a century for this purpose, either alone or in combination, to absorb blood and tissue fluid during and after surgery.

The development of foam dressings represented a significant advance over simple cellulose-based materials, by eliminating the problems of fibre loss although adherence remained an issue with the earliest prototype foam dressings. This problem was subsequently largely overcome by the addition of a modified wound contact surface, and now hydrophilic foams made from polyurethane are amongst the most absorbent and widely-used dressings available.

In addition to its absorptive function, a simple dressing pad, being highly permeable to water, will also facilitate evaporation through the back which will further increase its fluid handling properties.

Providing it does not become saturated with liquid, a dense pad of gauze or cellulose fibres acts as a reasonable 'depth' filter, preventing the passage of bacteria through the dressing. If, however, exudate is transported from the inner to the outer surface of the pad, a continuous moist path will be established from the wound to the external environment.

This condition is termed 'strikethrough' and at this point the bacterial barrier properties of the dressing will be lost. For this reason, some early dressing pads included within their structure an impermeable outer layer to prevent strike-through although this also had the disadvantage that it also prevented evaporation.

Transmission

The apparent contradictory requirements for a product that could allow the evaporation of liquid whilst providing an effective bacterial barrier were addressed by the introduction of a family of dressings made from a thin plastic membrane. In their simplest form these consist of an adhesive polyurethane film that is placed directly over the wound and fixed firmly to the surrounding skin. The film permits the transmission of moisture vapour but prevents the passage of water or aqueous solutions and is therefore described as 'semipermeable'.

The moisture vapour permeability of the early versions of these dressings was limited to values that only just exceed the production of moisture from intact skin. As a result, wound fluid accumulated beneath the dressing and this had to be aspirated off using a needle and syringe.

More recently new hydrophilic polyurethane films and thin foam membranes have been introduced which, in the presence of liquid, allow much higher levels of evaporation. These are discussed in detail in the following chapters.

The addition of a semipermeable membrane to an absorbent pad immediately overcomes the problems of bacterial strike-through whilst maximising the fluid handling capacity (FHC) of the dressing. The FHC is defined as the sum of the absorbency and the moisture vapour transmission rate. The relative contribution made by these different mechanisms, as determined in laboratory studies, varies from product to product.

Gelation

Some absorbent dressings change their physical state as they interact with exudate, forming a semi-solid gel. Gel formation has the advantage that it increases the viscosity of wound fluid, thereby immobilizing it on the wound surface to form a moist environment that is claimed to facilitate healing without causing maceration. Examples of products that function in this way include dressings made from calcium/sodium alginate or carboxymethylcellulose fibre, and gel-forming sheets such as the hydrocolloids, both of which are described in detail later.

Some dressings, such as the hydrogels, may be applied to the wound in the hydrated form and some, but not all of these materials, have the ability to take up additional fluid whilst still retaining their semi-solid state.

Anhydrous gel-forming agents can be added to dressing pads to improve their performance, and CMC powder or superabsorbents made from acrylic polymers are sometimes used for this purpose. CMC is also an important constituent of most hydrocolloid dressings - products that rely upon gel formation and moisture vapour transmission for the management of exudate.

Some hydrocolloids are virtually impermeable to water vapour in their intact state and when applied to an exuding wound, do not become permeable until their absorbent limit is reached. This means that they can also safely be used on lightly exuding wounds without allowing them to become too dry. The impermeable nature of the hydrocolloids also means that they can be of considerable value in promoting rehydration and autolysis of necrotic tissue, a key stage in the process of wound debridement.

Important differences exist in the way in which different types of dressings interact with wound fluid. Most simple absorbent products act like a sponge, rapidly taking up exudate and removing it completely from the vicinity of the wound. Others act in a more selective fashion. In one laboratory study,[17] samples of Cutinova hydro, Granuflex (Duoderm) E, Comfeel Ulcer Dressing and Allevyn were incubated with artificial wound fluid. The total amount of fluid taken up by each was determined, but in addition the concentrations of total protein, albumin, immunoglobulin and growth factors were also measured after one day of incubation. As well as the expected differences in total fluid absorbency, it was also found that in the case of Cutinova hydro, there was an approximately two-fold increase over control values in the concentration of all proteins tested, indicating a selective absorption of water due, it is presumed, to the characteristics of the polyurethane matrix from which the dressing is manufactured. The authors suggested that this ability of the dressing to concentrate proteins within a wound could have a beneficial effect, citing the work of Jonkman *et al.*[18] to give support to this view.

Prevention

A further and as yet largely overlooked mechanism of coping with exuding wounds involves the use of pharmaceutical or other agents that prevent exudate formation. Examples of products that have been claimed to be of value for this application include hyocine,[19] eosin and potassium permanganate,[20] although none of these preparations has been formally evaluated in a clinical trial for this purpose.

In a study published previously[21] it was demonstrated that, under appropriate conditions, the application of a hydrocolloid dressing reduced the amount of fluid produced by leg ulcers by up to 50%.

The investigation was stimulated by the observation that the dressing, which appeared to possess limited fluid handling properties in laboratory tests, seemed capable of dealing with exuding leg ulcers, pressure ulcers and other such wounds in the clinical situation.

These apparently contradictory observations suggested that either the laboratory test method seriously underestimated the fluid handling capacity of the hydrocolloid (considered unlikely) or that the dressing somehow interacted with the wound to reduce the amount of exudate produced.

There are at least two possible mechanisms by which a dressing could function in this way. One is by the release of biologically active agents which reduce capillary permeability by means of a physiological/biochemical action; the second is by means of a simple hydrostatic effect.

It was postulated that a hydrocolloid sheet that adheres firmly to the periwound skin effectively forms a sealed chamber over the exposed tissue. With time this chamber gradually fills with exudate, increasing the pressure within the cavity to the point at which it approximates to that of capillary pressure, a process which is accelerated or enhanced by the presence of external compression such as that resulting from the application of a compression bandage. Once this point is reached, further exudate production will be inhibited as predicted by Starling's hypothesis.

For this pressure effect to occur, however, it is essential that the dressing is impermeable to wound exudate and that it forms a secure seal around the wound margin. It will not happen with simple absorbent dressing pads, non-adhesive dressings or very extensible products.

These two possible mechanisms were investigated in an open label, randomized, cross over study in which the amount of exudate produced beneath an intact Duoderm (Granuflex) wafer was compared with that produced by the same wound covered with an identical dressing that had been perforated to relieve the pressure and allow fluid to pass into an external absorbent layer. The use of the same dressing in each instance eliminated the possibility that a biochemical or physiological effect was responsible for the reduction in exudate formation.

Ten patients with venous leg ulcers were recruited to the study. Dressings were perforated over the area of the wound using a four mm biopsy punch immediately prior to application and a sterile nonwoven gauze swab was applied to the back of the dressing over the perforations and retained in position with a sheet of adhesive film of limited permeability to moisture vapour. Control wounds were dressed with an intact dressing, omitting the perforating of the hydrocolloid sheet.

All the components used for each dressing change, including the swabs, biopsy punch and adhesive film, were supplied sterile in a sealed outer plastic bag of known weight. Following application of the dressing, all unused components together with all packaging and release papers were returned to the outer plastic bag and reweighed. From these two values the weight of dressing applied to the wound could be accurately obtained by difference.

At the time of each dressing change, the hydrocolloid sheet was removed from the wound, together with the swab and film, and placed in a second bag of known weight. Any liquid remaining upon the surface of the wound was carefully removed with previously weighed sterile swabs which were also placed in the second bag that was subsequently reweighed. The combined weight of the dressing and exudate was then calculated by difference. From this value the weight of exudate was determined by subtracting the weight of the original dressing determined previously.

The dressing systems were applied alternately to each patient until a total of ten results were obtained. In this way each patient acted as his/her own control. The area of each wound was determined at intervals by a weighing method using tracings made on transparent plastic film. Appropriate compression therapy was provided for all patients and remained constant throughout the period of the study.

The interval between dressing changes for each patient was determined by the investigator based upon an initial assessment of the wound. Wounds that were judged to produce large volumes of exudate were changed daily; more lightly exuding wounds were dressed at 48 or 72 hour intervals. Once this time period was selected, however, it remained constant for each patient for the duration of the study. The results for a typical patient, patient number 2, are shown in Figure 1 [2]

---

[2] This information has been adapted from: Thomas S, Fear M, Humphreys J, Disley L, Waring MJ. The effect of dressings on the production of exudate from venous leg ulcers. *WOUNDS*. 1996;8(5):145–150, and is reproduced with kind permission of the copyright holder

Figure 4: Exudate produced by Patient 2

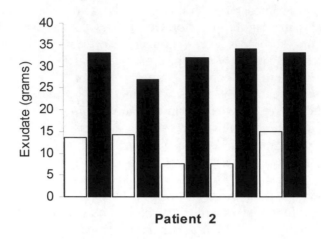

The weight of exudate produced by each wound was recorded both in absolute terms, and expressed as $g/cm^2/24$ h to facilitate comparisons between patients. These data are given in Table 7 and summarized in Figure 5 and Figure 6. The difference between the mean values for perforated and intact dressings was examined using a t-test, the results of which are also included in Table 7.

Table 7: Effect of hydrocolloid dressing upon exudate production

Patient Details		Wound area (cm^2)		Change interval	Mean exudate weight in grams (t)		Mean exudate weight in g/cm^2/24 h (t)	
No	Sex	Initial	Final	(hours)	Intact dressing	Perforated dressing	Intact dressing	Perforated dressing
1	M	17.7	13.7	48	13.5	27.5	0.43	0.9***
2	F	24.5	25.4	72	14.3	33.6	0.19	0.45***
3	F	11.8	0.5	72	7.7	6.7	0.36	0.5 (ns)
4	F	12.0	7.9	48	7.5	10.5	0.39	0.52*
5	F	39.8	31.3	48	15.0	29.5	0.21	0.41***
6	F	10.5	7.7	24	5.1	4.3	0.58	0.48*
7	M	7.4	5.2	72	15.8	21.9	0.83	1.20**
8	F	13.0	10.3	48	6.8	10.4	0.29	0.44*
9	M	33.9	43.6	24	8.0	18.4	0.20	0.47***
10	M	9.4	4.4	48	12.6	12.7	0.82	0.87 (ns)

each result represents the mean of five determinations.
*** = $p < 0.001$
** = $p < 0.01$
* = $p < 0.05$
ns = not significant,

The exudate rates for all patients appeared to fall into two groups. Seven were in the range 0.41 - 0.52 $g/cm^2/24$ h, the remaining three (where infection was suspected) were in the range 0.87 - 1.2 $g/cm^2/24$ h.

In seven of the ten patients the amount of exudate produced beneath the perforated dressing was statistically greater than that beneath the intact dressing. In two patients whose wounds were healing rapidly and thus reducing in size, the difference in exudate production, although still marked, failed to achieve statistical significance and in one patient, (Number 6), whose wound was very small and produced very little fluid, exudate production was not inhibited by the use of the hydrocolloid.

An analysis of variance (ANOVA) was performed which showed that the mean weight of exudate from all wounds dressed with intact dressings (0.43 ± 0.24) was lower than that from the wounds with perforated dressings (0.63 ± 0.29). These results are highly significant ($p < 0.01$).

The study results therefore strongly support the proposition that hydrocolloid dressings can, in specific circumstances, inhibit exudate production by a previously unreported mechanism which is entirely consistent with Starling's hypothesis.

From these results it is possible to calculate that a circumferential ulcer on a large leg could, in theory, produce in excess of 500 mL of exudate every day, representing a significant loss of plasma protein and electrolytes for the patient, and a significant management problem for them or their carer.

A further important finding of this study was that the subjective impressions of the clinical investigators and their classification of the wounds as light, moderate or heavily exuding are not supported by the experimental data when calculated on a $g/cm^2/24$ h basis. There is, however, some evidence that their predictions are based upon the total amount of exudate produced which is a function of wound area rather than capillary permeability. Simply put, large wounds appear to be more heavily exuding than small ones although this might not actually be the case when exudate rates are compared on a fixed area basis.

Figure 5: Total weight of exudate produced by each wound

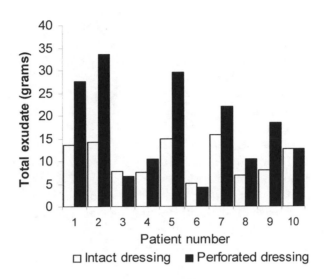

Figure 6: Exudate production expressed as function of wound area

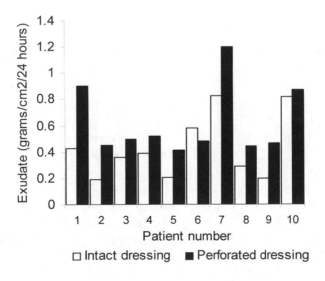

MANAGEMENT OF EXUDATE IN CLINICAL PRACTICE

Despite the fact that nursing staff are regularly required to make judgments concerning the amount of exudate produced by specific wounds in clinical records or documentation used during clinical trials of wound management materials, even experienced healthcare professionals experience considerable difficulty classifying wounds in this way as previously identified.

Their decisions generally reflect, or are influenced by, the **total** amount of exudate produced in a given period, irrespective of wound size. It is self evident that a small wound will produce (in total volume terms) much less fluid than a large wound exuding at the same rate but because the latter will represent greater problems in terms of day to day management, it will probably described as more heavily exuding.

This can have important implications for treatment, for whilst a significant increase in exudate production in a large ulcer caused by an episode of infection will be easily detected, a similar increase in a small wound may be overlooked, and therefore an important diagnostic indicator may be missed and appropriate treatment delayed as a result. Furthermore, some dressings are indicated or marketed for low, moderate, or heavily wounds but in the absence of an objective or scientific method for assessing exudate production such guidelines must be considered to be of limited value.

Healing wounds normally do not exude at a constant or standard rate, as fluid production gradually decreases to zero over time. In chronic wounds, or in the presence of infection, the inflammatory process will be extended and therefore exudate production can continue almost indefinitely.

The management of exudate remains a primary requirement of a modern dressing and is achieved by the use of products or combinations of products that meet the changing needs of the wound at it passes through the various stages in the healing process. Some, products, such the hydrocolloids, are complete dressings with a complex structure that are intended to be used alone, or in combination with a compression bandage. Others, such as the alginates, must be regarded primarily as wound contact materials and as such provide the opportunity to construct a dressing system that is appropriate to the nature and condition of a specific wound. In such situations the importance of the secondary dressing cannot be over emphasised if desiccation or maceration is to be avoided.[22-24]

Patient comfort and acceptability are also major factors when determining the success or otherwise of a dressing treatment. Simply applying layer after layer of absorbent pads may not be the best way of dealing with the problem. In such situations the use of highly permeable films may be preferred, providing that these do not lead to pooling of exudate under gravity.[25]

In the context of exudate management, the interactions that take place between dressings and the cellular and metabolic processes within a wound remain poorly understood for some of the research findings appear at first sight to be somewhat confusing and contradictory. Semipermeable film dressings, for example, produce an increase in the concentration of proteins and other solutes present in the wound, as the aqueous component evaporates. Similarly products such as Cutinova have been shown to increase the concentration of proteins and other solutes by selectively absorbing water. The consequences of this increase are not well understood. Alper et al.,[26] reported that chronic wound fluid collected from beneath a film dressing when added to human serum, caused stimulation of fibroblast cell division. Jonkman et al., suggested that the accelerated epithelialization associated with the use of film dressings that was observed in experimental wounds in guinea-pigs was due to increased precipitation of fibrin and fibronectin in the gelatinous coagulum beneath these films.[18,27] Products such as Promogran are claimed to facilitate wound healing by selectively removing proteolytic enzymes from the wound environment.[28]

Whilst it might reasonably be argued that, depending upon the nature and condition of the wound, there may be situations when one or other of these functions is to be preferred, it is probably true to say that given our current state of knowledge and the absence of a simple diagnostic test to measure the proteolytic activity of wound secretions 'in vivo', the decision on which treatment approach to take is likely to be arbitrary and therefore potentially incorrect.

Exudate management remains an art which is largely based upon some poorly understood science. Like most skills it requires practice and experience to achieve an acceptable level of competence but it should never be forgotten that the patient is the individual who is paying for the practitioner's education.

REFERENCES

1. Gautam N, Olofsson AM, Herwald H, Iversen LF, Lundgren-Akerlund E, Hedqvist P, et al. Heparin-binding protein (HBP/CAP37): a missing link in neutrophil-evoked alteration of vascular permeability. Nat Med 2001;7(10):1123-7.
2. Lundqvist K, Herwald H, Sonesson A, Schmidtchen A. Heparin binding protein is increased in chronic leg ulcer fluid and released from granulocytes by secreted products of Pseudomonas aeruginosa. Thromb Haemost 2004;92(2):281-7.
3. Field FK, Kerstein MD. Overview of wound healing in a moist environment. Am J Surg 1994;167(1A):2S-6S.
4. May SR. Physiological activity from an occlusive wound dressing. In: Lawrence JC, editor. Wound Healing Symposium. Birmingham: The Medicine Publishing Foundation, 1982:35-51.
5. Phillips TJ, Al-amoudi HO, Leverkus M, Park H-Y. Effect of chronic wound fluid on fibroblasts. Journal of Wound Care 1998;7(10):527-532.
6. Chen WYJ, Rogers AA. Characterization of biological properties of wound fluid collected during early stages of wound healing. Journal of Investigative Dermatology 1992;99(5):559-564.
7. Wysocki AB. Wound fluids and the pathogenesis of chronic wounds. Journal of Wound Ostomy and Continence Nursing 1996;23(6):283-90.
8. Dowsett C. Exudate management: a patient-centred approach. J Wound Care 2008;17(6):249-52.
9. Thomas S. Assessment and management of wound exudate. Journal of Wound Care 1997;6(7):327-330.

10. Lamke LO, Nilsson GE, Reithner HL. The evaporative water loss from burns and water vapour permeability of grafts and artificial membranes used in the treatment of burns. *Burns* 1977;3:159-165.

11. White RJ, Cutting KF. Modern exudate management: a review of wound treatments. *World Wide Wounds*, 2003.

12. Falanga V. Classifications for wound bed preparation and stimulation of chronic wounds. *Wound Repair Regeneration* 2000;8(5):347-352.

13. Sibbald RG, Orsted H, Schultz GS, Coutts P, Keast D. Preparing the wound bed 2003: focus on infection and inflammation. *Ostomy Wound Manage* 2003;49(11):23-51.

14. Schultz GS, Sibbald RG, Falanga V, Ayello EA, Dowsett C, Harding K, et al. Wound bed preparation: a systematic approach to wound management. *Wound Repair Regen* 2003;11 Suppl 1:S1-S28.

15. Dowsett C, Ayello E. TIME principles of chronic wound bed preparation and treatment. *Br J Nurs* 2004;13(15):S16-23.

16. Wound Union of Healing Societies (WUWS). Principles of best practice: Wound exudate and the role of dressings. A consensus document. In: MacGregor L, editor. London: MEP, 2007.

17. Achterberg V, Meyer-Ingold W. Hydroactive dressings and serum proteins: an in vitro study. *Journal of Wound Care* 1996;5(2):79-82.

18. Jonkman MF, Hoeksma EA, Nieuwenhuis P. Accelerated epithelization under a highly vapor-permeable wound dressing is associated with increased precipitation of fibrin(ogen) and fibronectin. *J Invest Dermatol* 1990;94(4):477-84.

19. Haisfield-Wolfe ME, Rund C. Malignant cutaneous wounds: a management protocol. *Ostomy Wound Manage* 1997;43(1):56-60, 62, 64-6.

20. Cutting KF. The causes and prevention of maceration of the skin. *Journal of Wound Care* 1999;8(4):200-1.

21. Thomas S, Fear M, Humphreys J, Disley L, Waring MJ. The effect of dressings on the production of exudate from venous leg ulcers. *Wounds* 1996;8(5):145-149.

22. Scurr J, H. , Wilson LA, Coleridge -Smith PD. A Comparison of the Effects of Semipermeable Foam and Film Secondary Dressings
over Alginate Dressings on the Healing and Management of Venous Ulcers. *Wounds* 1993;5(6):259-265.

23. Thomas S. Alginate dressings in surgery and wound management - part 3. *Journal of Wound Care* 2000;9(4):163-166.

24. Nielsen A. Management of wound exudate. *Journal of Community Nursing* 1999;13(6):27-34.

25. Grocott P. Exudate management in fungating wounds. *Journal of Wound Care* 1998;7(9):445-8.

26. Alper JC, Welch EA, Ginsberg M, Bogaars H, Maguire P. Moist wound healing under a vapor permeable membrane. *Journal of the American Academy of Dermatolgy* 1983;8(3):347353.

27. Jonkman MF, Molenaar I, Nieuwenhuis P, Klasen HJ. Evaporative water loss and epidermis regeneration in partial-thickness wounds dressed with a fluid-retaining versus a clot-inducing wound covering in guinea pigs. *Scand J Plast Reconstr Surg Hand Surg* 1989;23(1):29-34.

28. Vin F, Teot L, Meaume S. The healing properties of Promogran in venous leg ulcers. *Journal of Wound Care* 2002;11(9):335-41.

6. The development of dressings

INTRODUCTION

From the earliest times, mankind has had to cope with a variety of different types of wounds sustained during the battle for survival. According to Majno,[1] in a fascinating and comprehensive review of the early history of wound management, many different materials were used to treat these lesions in an attempt to staunch bleeding, absorb exudate or promote healing.

Originally these would have consisted of readily-available natural substances such as honey, animal oils or fat, cobwebs, mud, leaves, sphagnum moss or animal dung,[2] applied in the crude form in which they were found, but later some of these 'raw materials' began to be combined together, either to make them easier to handle, or to improve their clinical effectiveness. Whilst most of these early preparations probably conferred little real benefit, others, such as honey, used alone or mixed with oils or waxes, undoubtedly were of some practical value.

Even the use of cobwebs may impart some clinical benefits according to the results of a recent study[3] which investigated the feasibility of using recombinant spider silk protein as a dressing for deep second-degree burns using an animal model. Sixty rats were randomly divided into four groups and their wounds dressed with either one of two types of recombinant spider silk proteins or collagen as a positive control. Healing in the treatment groups was much better than that in the control group ($p < 0.01$), accompanied by an increase in the expression and secretion of the growth factor bFGF and hydroxyproline.

The practice of using whatever materials were conveniently to hand to cover wounds or remove exudate or absorb blood during a surgical procedure, continued well into the 19th Century and whenever dressings were required, practitioners of the time used old pieces of cloth or linen fabric which they often recycled for this purpose.

This fabric was sometimes first unravelled to form short ends of thread called 'charpie', or the surface of fabric was scraped with knives to produce 'soft lint' a soft fluffy material not dissimilar to absorbent cotton (cotton wool) which could be used to pack cavities and soak up exudate or blood.

Oakum, also widely used as a wound dressing, consisted of a fibrous mass produced by shredding tarred or untarred rope; the former, sometimes called 'marine lint', was regarded as a cheap alternative to soft lint. Oakum was often originally obtained from penal institutions where 'oakum picking' was considered an appropriate occupation for prison inmates, but by the early 1870s it was being produced commercially.

Oakum was used extensively in the American Civil War and its use was also favoured in Britain, for in 1870 the Lancet[4] reported that this material 'absorbs discharges, destroys bad odours and supersedes the use of lint, ointments and linseed meal or bread poultices'.

EARLY WOUND DRESSINGS

Lint

The first product to be manufactured specifically for use as a dressing is thought to be absorbent (sheet) lint, which was originally introduced to stop haemorrhage but gradually gained wider application as a general purpose dressing. Lint was formed by scraping sheets of old linen with sharp knives to raise a fibrous 'nap' on one surface, increasing the absorbency of the cloth but decreasing its tensile properties.

Initially a manual process, a lint making machine was developed in the first half of the 19th Century which used new, specially woven, fabric for the purpose. This resulted in a more consistent product with, it is assumed, a considerably lower bioburden. Originally lint was made from linen, but this was eventually replaced by cotton by the middle of the 20th Century.

Surgical Gauze

Lightweight open fabrics such as muslin or gauze also have a long history in wound management, although these were not originally produced specifically for this application. In 1871 Robert Lister described the use of such a fabric, sometimes medicated with carbolic resin and other medicaments, which he often folded into six or eight layers. The cloth which was of open texture could be 'washed and used over and over again'. Modern-day cotton gauze defined as a loosely woven fabric of plain weave, which is universally used in surgery, is said to have evolved from 'tiffany' a fine fabric used by nurserymen to stretch under the roofs of greenhouses.

Figure 7: Robinson's advert in a Chemist and Druggist diary 1895

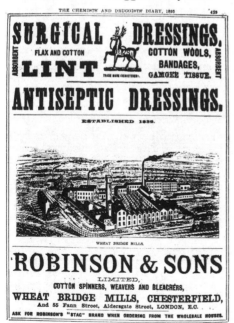

In 1870 a French surgeon, Alphonse Guerin, began to use cotton fibres which had been washed and carded to dress wounds, thereby protecting them from contamination from the air. Ten years later a British surgeon, Joseph Gamgee, became aware of this practice but found that although the cotton dressing was soft and comfortable, it was not absorbent. He discovered that by subjecting the cotton to a scouring process it was possible to remove the natural oils from the fibres and, by so doing, render them highly absorbent.[5] He later used this material, enclosed in a layer of bleached tiffany, to form 'Gamgee Tissue' the first proprietary composite dressing pad which was marketed by Messrs Robinson & Son of Chesterfield.

Gauze also became very popular in the United States, where it was manufactured by Johnson and Johnson Inc. of New Brunswick who, recognizing the importance of asepsis, began to produce fabric that had been sterilised by exposure to steam under pressure. Folded pieces of gauze called swabs or sponges sometimes stitched around the perimeter to retain their shape and structure remain the principal absorbents used during surgical procedures to this day. These swabs incorporate an X ray-detectable yarn or tab,

Figure 8: 'J&J advert in Chemist and Druggist diary of 1893'

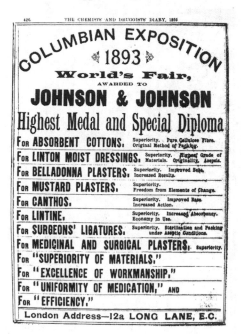

rich in barium sulphate, so that if a swab is inadvertently left inside a patient during a surgical procedure it may be readily located.

For general wound cleansing purposes outside theatre, swabs manufactured from nonwoven fabric composed of viscose or polyester are widely used to cleanse wounds and/or the surrounding skin at the time of dressing changes. They are also often employed as secondary dressings, providing a degree of absorbency when applied behind a low-adherent wound contact layer. Sometimes they contain a thin fleece of absorbent cotton to improve their fluid handling properties when they are known as filmated swabs. The absorbency and loss of fibres and particulate material from seven nonwoven swabs was compared with that of traditional woven gauze in a laboratory study.[6] .The nonwoven swabs were superior to the woven and filmated gauze swabs in terms of absorbency, and because they are manufactured from continuous extruded or filament yarns, not from yarns spun from individual cotton fibres each of limited length, they also have less propensity to shed small particles which can promote the distribution of microorganisms into the air when dried-out dressings are removed from infected wounds, thereby greatly increasing the risk of cross infection.[7] At the time this study was undertaken, the nonwovens were substantially cheaper than gauze, resulting in an estimated saving of between 35 and 40%. Swabs made from woven and nonwoven fabric and impregnated with sodium chloride, Mesalt, Mölnlycke, were compared in a small study published by Brown et al.,[8] who concluded that although the absorptive properties of the two products were similar, the nonwoven fabric appeared to promote, or delay less, the formation of new epithelial tissue.

Fibre loss from gauze

In 1913, in address to the Royal College of Surgeons,[9] Adams discussed how foreign bodies such as gauze swabs introduced into the peritoneal cavity could lead to the formation of a localized reaction and the resultant formation of granulomas and adhesions. Isolated native cellulose fibres, such as those released from swabs and disposable drapes (see Figure 9), have also been known to cause such a response which, in extreme cases, has lead to serious or even fatal reactions.[10]

Figure 9: Cotton gauze showing loose fibres and particulate material

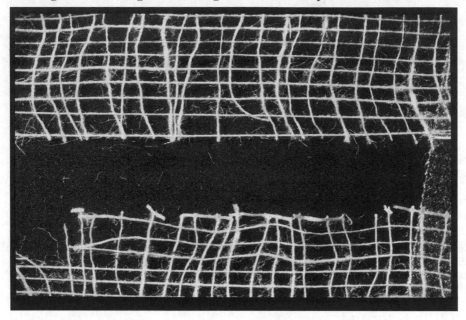

In an experimental study,[11] Sturdy *et al.* introduced a number of agents into experimental wounds in rats which were then monitored for the formation of granulomata or adhesions. 'Fuzz' formed by rubbing pieces of dry gauze together which were allowed to fall into the abdominal cavity was shown to be a potent stimulant of the formation of both gross and microscopic granulomas.

In the same paper, pathological samples consisting of foreign body granulomas collected over a seven year period were examined microscopically. Gauze residues were considered to be the cause of 23/32 peritoneal samples, and 22/23 samples collected from the skin and subcutaneous tissue. In a third group of six cases involving the cervix, five were found to contain gauze particles. Saxén and Myllärniemi[12] reviewed the findings of a series of 309 repeat laparotomies that showed evidence of intra-abdominal adhesions. They found foreign body type granulomas in 61% of cases, and in 26% of these, gauze lint was found and considered to be the causative agent. Talc, then used as a glove lubricant, was considered the principal causative agent in over 50% of cases.

Broadly similar results were reported by Weibel and Majno[13] who reviewed data collected during the course of 752 autopsies. Peritoneal adhesions were found in about one quarter of patients who had not undergone previous surgery but this figure rose to about 67% in those who had underdone a previous operation. Thirty eight adhesions were studied histologically of which seven (18%) contained filaments of dressings or related materials.

Tinker *et al.* identified cellulose fibres from disposable surgical fabrics as the cause of granulomatous peritonitis in two patients and showed that similar lesions could be induced in rats by the introductions of small amounts of cellulose fibre.[14] She later described a further 45 cases of cellulose granuloma, 27 of which were extraperitoneal and the remaining 18 intraperitoneal.[15]

Brittan *et al.*,[16] in 1984, published a case report in which they described a patient who developed granulomatous peritonitis caused by cellulose fibres, and in the same year, Janoff *et al.*[17] recorded that 24 cases of foreign body reactions associated with lint fibres had been identified in three hospitals over a five year period. Ten of these involved extraperitoneal granulomas and 14 an intraperitoneal granuloma. Six patients with intraperitoneal granuloma developed acute granulomatous peritonitis one of whom subsequently died. In one case, which they described in detail, cellulose fibres caused the failure of a surgical wound on the breast to heal in a satisfactory manner, resulting in prolonged drainage of serous fluid and scar formation. The authors reviewed the literature on the subject and suggested that the incidence of foreign body reactions is much more common than is generally realised.

One report,[18] described how, in seven female patients, the use of finely shredded gauze to reinforce berry aneurysms led to a series of events including headache, pyrexia, seizures, and cranial nerve deficits. One patient, with blindness and hydrocephalus, died and was examined at autopsy. It was found that the gauze had induced a foreign-body granuloma, accompanied by progressive occlusion of neighbouring small arteries.

Even in superficial wounds cellulose fibres may cause keloids and wound dehiscence. In 1976, residual cellulose fibres, embedded in granulation tissue in wounds previously dressed with cotton gauze, were found in about ten percent of patients examined in a specialist clinic.[19] The presence of foreign bodies will also predispose a wound to infection. In an experimental study using human volunteers, Elek[20] showed that more than 10^6 staphylococci had to be injected into the dermis to cause an infection. In the presence of a piece of silk stitch, however, only about 100 viable organisms were required to cause a comparable lesion.

Because nonwoven swabs release less particles, radio opaque nonwoven swabs (Sorbtex™, Vernon Carus) were developed for use in theatre, to replace the traditional woven products. Although in experimental studies these appeared to offer advantages over standard gauze in many respects,[21] they were not well liked by surgeons generally, and so failed to gain widespread acceptance.

Towards the end of the 19th Century a particular type of woven gauze was developed specifically for packing cavities, sinuses and small excised wounds to keep the wound open and allow it to granulate upwards from the base. Called 'ribbon gauze', it was produced both in a plain and an X-ray detectable form which incorporated a radio-opaque yarn for use in theatre.

In contrast to normal gauze, which was woven in wide form and subsequently slit to width, the official form of this new material, (as described in the British Pharmacopoeia), was woven in a range of narrow widths with a selvage so that it would not fray or ravel in use. A much less acceptable alternative was also produced called 'four-fold ribbon gauze' which consisted of standard gauze fabric which was cut into narrow strips and folded over four times (Figure 10). This material was a potent source of cellulose particles because of the extensive cut edges. Although still available, ribbon gauze is no longer widely used in routine wound care in the UK as it has been largely replaced by other more modern dressings.

Figure 10: Structure of official and non-official four-fold ribbon gauze

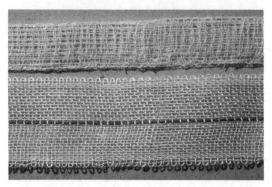 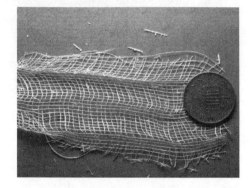

The loss of fine fibrous particles from gauze is easily demonstrated by gently agitating a sample in a suitable quantity of filtered water or saline, and passing it through a dark coloured membrane filter. Under a low power lens, the fibrous material lost from the fabric is easily detectable visible against the dark background. If examined under a microscope, the structure of the fibres and debris can be seen more clearly.

Figure 11: Fibre and particulate loss from cotton gauze on Millipore filter

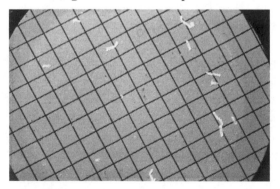 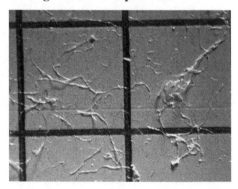

Historically, both plain and ribbon gauze have been employed impregnated with a variety of medicaments. Often aqueous solutions were used which, in the main, consisted of agents designed to kill or prevent the growth of bacteria, and included various types of dyes such as acriflavine, proflavine, scarlet red and brilliant green, salts of mercury, or solutions of sodium hypochlorite which were sometimes formed into a crude emulsions with liquid paraffin.

Gauze as a wound dressing

In contrast to gauze swabs that are used during the course of a surgical procedure, which are only in contact with a wound for a very limited period (minutes or a few hours at most) gauze or other fabrics applied to wounds healing by secondary intention (i.e. not sutured closed) may be left in place for several days. During this time there exists a very real possibility that the fabric will adhere to the new tissue and cause serious pain or trauma upon removal. There also exists the possibility that wounds dressed in this way will become excessively dry which in turn will delay healing.

For this reason, in many countries gauze is no longer recommended as a primary dressing. In the USA, however, the use of gauze for this application has remained popular, including the use of a technique called 'wet to dry dressings' in which a piece of saline soaked fabric is applied to a wound containing necrotic tissue, allowed to dry out, then ripped away to facilitate debridement, a practice that results in considerable pain or discomfort to the patient.

In a review of the use of gauze as a dressing Jones in 2006,[22] cited Stotts et al.[23] who surveyed 240 nurses in the US in 1993 and found that nearly 20% were using this technique and 26% were using moist gauze as the primary wound contact material.

Even in the USA, however, the use of gauze has generated some debate amongst nurses. One relatively recent article, published in 2000,[24] supported the use of gauze as a primary wound dressing for a variety of wound types but a second article by Ovington,[25] whilst acknowledging that gauze is still the most widely used wound care dressing, argued that it is inappropriate to regard it as the standard of care, citing extended healing times, disruption of angiogenesis during dressing removal, increased infection risk from frequent dressing changes and strike-through as good reason to abandon this particular practice.

The widely held UK view that gauze has no role in the routine management of wounds was eloquently expressed in a paper by a Tissue Viability nurse specialist,[26] produced in 2003 as part of an MSc/Postgraduate Diploma in Wound Healing. She concluded that;

> "The days of sitting a patient in a bath to soak off a gauze dressing should be history. We cannot allow a patient to drown in a bath before gauze packing is banned from wound care practice."

In a fascinating review article, Armstrong and Price[27] attempted to unravel the background to the use of gauze, identify what actually constitutes a wet-to-dry dressing, explain why it is used, and describe how specialist nurses interpret this technique. They also conducted a survey in which they sent a questionnaire to a sample of general surgeons in New Hampshire and Vermont and interviewed nine wound, ostomy, and continence nurses. A total of 127 questionnaires were sent out and 65 were returned.

An important finding of their research was that there was no clear understanding of, or differentiation between, the terms 'wet to dry gauze' and 'moist gauze'. Many respondents used them interchangeably although others understood them to mean different things.

The authors also found that despite the fact that three quarter of respondents had access to 'modern' dressings, wet-to-dry dressings and moist gauze were commonly prescribed even in situations where there was little evidence to support their use. The survey revealed that 30 of the 67 responders supported the use of wet to dry gauze for the treatment of open surgical wounds healing by secondary intention, and the majority of the remainder recommended moist gauze. Considerable variability was also revealed in the way in which the technique was performed, and a lack of agreement was uncovered on whether the gauze should be dry or moist upon removal.

Interestingly the Agency for Healthcare Research and Quality (AHRQ) guidelines supported the use of wet-to-dry dressings, stating that its use is supported by expert opinion, although this type of evidence is poorly rated on their hierarchy of evidence.

Armstrong and Price concluded that although the American journals contain many articles on modern dressings, surgeons have not been influenced by these, continuing to prescribe both wet-to-dry and moist gauze in preference to modern products, often inappropriately.

Although evidence is available to combat the use of gauze for many indications, it is disparate, and most nurses are not in a position to influence the practice of their surgical colleagues, many of whom cite cost as a reason to continue to use gauze. This issue had previously been addressed by Ovington,[25] who put forward an argument based upon cost-effectiveness as a reason for change. She described how, when the costs saline and gauze were compared with those of an advanced dressing (Tielle Johnson & Johnson) over a four-week period, the advanced dressing was found to be cheaper because of the reduced healing time and a requirement for fewer dressing changes.

DRESSINGS AND MOIST WOUND HEALING

The early days

The simple observation that dressings which are kept moist are less likely to adhere to the wound bed and cause trauma on removal contributed to the theory of 'moist wound healing'.

Although in the literature George Winter is almost universally given credit for introducing this concept, in reality this was not the case as 'wet' dressings had been used long before he published the results of his research in the 1960s.

According to Bishop,[4] in 1846 the surgeon Robert Liston provided a vivid picture of the dressing of wounds using dry dressings which he said was 'the routine practice long pursued'.

According to this technique, the cut edges of the wound were brought together and retained by sutures plaster or bandages after which the whole area was covered up for a number of days. At the end of this period Liston says;

> *"The envelope of cotton and flannel, the compress cloths, the pledgets of 'healing ointment' as it is called, and plasters are taken away loaded with putrid exhalations and a profusion of bloody, ill-digested, foetid matter."*

Liston's preferred technique was much simpler. After arresting bleeding and suturing, a simple fabric dressing (lint) dipped in cold water was applied to wounds which were subsequently kept moist by the application of oiled silk, a forerunner of modern film dressings.

Despite his enthusiasm for moist dressings, Liston also recorded a special use for dry lint which he employed for preventing or repressing granulation which had become 'too high and exuberant'. It is presumed that the fabric adhered to the rapidly forming new tissue and destroyed it when the dressing was removed.

Moist dressings were used in this way for decades until Lister introduced 'antiseptic surgery' in 1867, after which fashions changed and clean absorbent dressings began to be used to keep wounds dry to 'inhibit the growth of microorganisms'.

In the first part of the 20th Century several clinicians discovered once again the advantages of occlusion, following their early experiences with film dressings in the form of cellophane which attained particular prominence during the Second World War (see chapter on film dressings) but this practice failed to gain widespread acceptance for a variety of practical, clinical and commercial reasons.

The work of George Winter

In 1962 George Winter published his seminal paper,[28] which provided a scientific basis for the clinical benefits previously reported to result from the use of cellophane and other primitive film dressings.

Using an animal model, he demonstrated that the formation of a scab over a drying wound inhibited the migration of epidermal cells from the wound margin over the exposed dermis, forcing them to pass through the living fibrous tissue to which the scab was attached. As result, the upper surface of the original wound lay above the new epidermis, effectively deepening or extending the original injury

Winter,[29] described his observations thus: Figure 12 'shows a 1.4 mm length of the surface of a standard shallow wound magnified about 100 times. The wound is three days old and was not covered. This represents the base time for comparative purposes; healing under a dry scab. A layer of leucocytes lies within the dermis under the injury and a new epidermis is being formed beneath this. Measurements show that that more than 60% of the surface area of the wound is still bare of epidermis at this time.'

In a wound kept moist by the application of a piece of polyethylene film, epidermal cells were able to migrate easily through the serous exudate above the fibrous tissue of the dermis thus accelerating healing. Winter stated 'In contrast to the wound exposed to the air, more than 90% of this wound is covered by newly regenerated epidermis. In the absence of a scab the new epidermis is moving over the surface of the dermis in fluid exudate which has collected between the dressing and the wound' (Figure 13).

Figure 12: Shallow excised wound in the skin of a young pig, exposed to the air

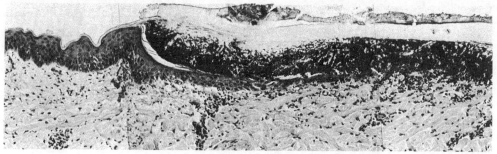

Note epidermal migration below scab on wound exposed to the air.[3]

Figure 13: Shallow excised wound in the skin of a young pig covered with plastic film

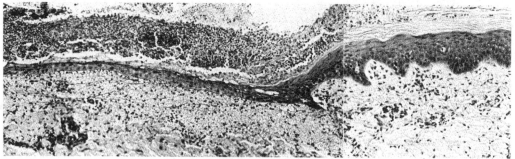

Note epidermal migration through moist exudate on wound surface.[4]

Winter further showed that the benefits of occlusion extended past the epithelial phase, as connective tissue under the regenerated epidermis appears earlier than normal. Despite the convincing nature of his results, Winter stressed that 'it would be unwise to draw conclusions about he specific effects of various substances on the rate of wound healing, where results may be complicated by occlusion of the wound, for example by dressings or greasy bases'. The clinical significance of Winter's finders was investigated by Hinman and Maibach,[30] in study conducted in San Quentin Prison. They produced small matched partial thickness wounds on the forearms of six volunteers which were either left exposed to the air or dressed with a polythene film. Biopsies were subsequently taken from the same lesions with an eight mm punch at three, five seven and nine day intervals for histological examination. Very marked differences were found between the treatments in term of reepithelialization rates but the authors also described how, in air exposed wounds, the epithelium had to move downwards at

---

[3] Reproduced from Winter 1975 with permission
[4] Reproduced from Winter 1975 with permission

right angles to the surface to find a plane of cleavage to proliferate under the eschar. Winter also described how dressings, including gauze, applied to an open granulating wound can become partially incorporated into a scab.[31-33] When such materials becomes soaked with exudate and dry out in contact with a wound, the proteinaceous components precipitate out, forming a scab or crust that adheres firmly to the wound bed. New blood vessels and tissue can also grow into the interstices within the structure of the dressing and thus incorporate some of the components of the dressing into the scab which act like reinforcing bars in concrete.

Figure 14: A shallow wound treated with gauze for 48 hours

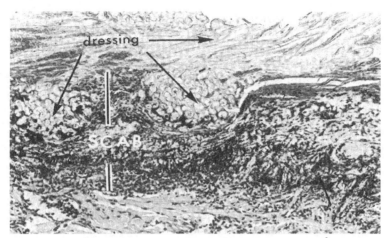

Note bundles of cotton fibres incorporated into scab.[5]

The mechanism by which gauze might adhere to a wound at a cellular level was investigated by Rogers *et al.*,[34] who showed in a laboratory study that the serum-derived proteins, fibronectins and vitronectin were readily adsorbed onto traditional fabrics. These in turn facilitated the adhesion of fibroblast cells in cell attachment/adhesion studies. This adhesion did not occur on co-spun fibres of viscose and gelling fibre

If significant adhesion occurs clinically, premature removal of the dressing inevitably leads to further damage to the wound, rupturing blood vessels and destroying some, or all, of the regenerating epidermis. The application of a continuous plastic film prevented this occurring, but the limited permeability of the early films to moisture vapour meant that there was a very real chance of excess fluid accumulating beneath the dressing. Small holes in the film could resolve the drainage problem but although the tissue adjacent to the film was kept moist and non-adherent, that opposite the holes became dehydrated and adherent.

---

[5] Reproduced from Winter 1975 with permission

Supporting evidence for moist wound healing

De Coninck et al.[35] repeated some of Winter's early work some thirty years later, when, using a pig model as before, they compared healing rates of 32 full-thickness wounds each 3 cm x 3 cm that were dressed with either a semipermeable polyurethane film dressing (Tegaderm) or a non-occlusive dressing (Melolin) in the presence and absence of an isotonic hydroxyethylcellulose gel, both of which were renewed twice a week.

The time required for wound closure was 19.2 ± 1.6 days and 26.6 ± 3.0 days (mean $\pm$ SD) for Tegaderm and Melolin respectively ($p < 0.001$). Histological evaluation was performed on full-thickness skin biopsies of the whole wound, harvested from the time of closure for a three month period. No significant histological variations were observed between the differently treated wounds. The authors concluded that in a porcine model for full-thickness wounds, occlusive dressings enhance healing rates and shorten the time for wound repair and they suggested that his reduction is primarily a function of the effect of occlusive dressing on epithelialization.

The effect of a moist healing environment provided by a foam dressing was investigated by Kunugiza et al.[36] who compared it with the much drier conditions associated with the use of gauze on the healing of excisional wounds in rats. The defects were examined histologically and gene expression of vascular endothelial growth factor (VEGF), fibroblast growth factor (FGF), hepatocyte growth factor (HGF) and hypoxia inducible factor-1 alpha (HIF-1a) in granulation tissue was examined by real-time reverse transcription polymerase chain reaction (real-time RT-PCR). VEGF protein was measured by ELISA. All of these investigations indicated that the foam dressing facilitated formation of granulation tissue and wound closure but that the scab formed in the gauze-treated wounds disturbed epithelialization and delayed healing.

The maintenance of a moist wound environment can have important implications for extensive partial thickness wounds such as burns which undergo spontaneous healing from epidermal cells in hair follicles and sweat glands which multiply and coalesce to form islets of epithelium upon the wound surface. If these structures are destroyed by desiccation, this process is seriously impaired with important consequences for the speed of wound healing.

As previously identified, a significant burn has three identifiable zones: the innermost part of the injury, which has suffered irreversible damage, is called the zone of coagulation; the outermost zone, which has undergone minor reversible damage, is called the zone of uraemia; and between these two is the area known as the zone of stasis. The eventual fate of the cells in the latter region is determined by the nature of the treatment given.

It was once believed that damage in the zone of stasis was irreversible, inevitably leading to necrosis, but Zawacki[37] demonstrated in the pig model that this was not the case, The provision of a relatively occlusive cover which prevented evaporation and desiccation of the damaged tissue facilitated complete reepithelialization from surviving hair follicles within the wounds. He suggested that prevention of desiccation probably explained the common observation that partial-thickness burns heal more rapidly with a better cosmetic effect when the blister is left intact or replaced by a homograft, heterograft or transparent adhesive tape.

The concept of moist wound healing also has relevance to the healing of deeper wounds. Dyson et al.,[38] compared the effects of an adhesive polyurethane film dressing and dry gauze in full thickness excised wounds on porcine skin. Quantitative studies were made of changes in the populations of neutrophils, macrophages, fibroblasts, and endothelial cells for a period of 21 days after surgery. During this time the number of inflammatory phase cells (neutrophils and macrophages) in wounds dressed with the film decreased more rapidly than in wounds dressed with gauze. Proliferative-phase cells, fibroblasts and endothelial cells, appeared sooner in the moist wounds and by day five after surgery 66% of the cells of the granulation tissue of the moist wounds were of this type, compared with only 48% of the cells of equivalent areas of the dry wounds. By day 21 the number of fibroblasts in the granulation tissue of the moist wounds had fallen below that in the dry wounds, suggesting that progress from the proliferative into the remodelling phase of repair was more rapid in the moist wounds. The authors concluded that, compared with a dry dressing, the moist environment provided by an adhesive polyurethane dressing resulted in more rapid and orderly healing of excised dermal wounds with both epidermal and dermal repair being accelerated.

In a second paper,[39] Dyson and her colleagues used the same dressings and experimental model to compare the effects of occlusion upon angiogenesis for up to 60 days following surgery. Quantitative studies, using computerised image analysis, were carried out on microfocal x-ray images of skin sections following perfusion in vivo with a radio-opaque medium. They found that in moist wounds there was an early increase in vessel development which peaked around days 3 - 5 followed by a gradual decrease around day one. In dry wounds, the vessel numbers in the upper part of the wound did not peak until day seven. The total percentage area of the wound bed occupied by blood vessels was also greater in the moist wounds.

This work of Winter and others work represented a watershed in the understanding and practice of wound management which, in the late 1970s and early 1980s, led to the introduction of important new groups of dressings, all of which maintain a moist healing environment. Many of these new developments are described in the following chapters. Early accounts of the benefits of occlusion using some of these new dressings were provided by Alper,[40] Alvarez,[41] Eaglstein,[42-43] and Hermans,[44] amongst others.

Not all publications have proved to be so positive for the value of modern dressings, however. Ubbink et al.[45] in a randomized clinical trial involving 285 hospitalised surgical patients with open wounds compared the effectiveness and treatment costs of gauze-based dressings with modern materials designed to provide a moist wound-healing environment. Primary end points were complete wound healing, pain during dressing changes, and costs. Secondary end point was length of hospital stay.

Overall, time to complete wound healing did not differ significantly between modern dressings and gauze-based products. Postoperative wounds, 62% of those included, healed significantly (p = 0.02) quicker with gauze dressings. Median pain scores were low and similar in the both groups. The cost of modern dressings was significantly higher than gauze but nursing costs per day were significantly higher when gauze was used due to reduced treatment times. The authors concluded that the use of modern dressings does not lead to enhanced wound healing, reduced pain or financial savings, as the lower costs resulting from the less frequent dressing changes do not balance the higher costs of occlusive materials.

Much of the early work on moist wound healing appears to suggest that the clinical benefits it imparts simply results from the ability of a dressing to prevent desiccation. There is a sense, therefore, in which these materials appear to accelerate healing by not actively delaying it! More recent research has demonstrated that in reality, the situation is much more complex, as retained wound fluid, as previously described, possesses a host of complex biochemical properties which may stimulate healing or delay it, depending upon the nature of the wound from which it is derived.

It follows, therefore, that although there is reasonable evidence to suggest that in the management of acute wounds significant benefits may result from maintaining the wound in a moist state, bathed in its own exudate, this approach may be less appropriate for the treatment of chronic wounds which produce fluid rich in proteolytic enzymes. The secret of successful wound management may simply be determining which is which. This issue has recently formed the subject of a consensus document,[46] prepared by an international group of experts, designed to stimulate interest in the production of new diagnostics for use in wound management to help inform the decision making process.

THE 'IDEAL' DRESSING

Numerous modern authors have made passing reference to the requirements of an 'ideal dressing' and almost all have incorrectly attributed this concept to George Winter. In fact the term was originated by John Scales of the Department of Biomechanics and Surgical Materials in the National Orthopaedic Hospital, Stanmore, Middlesex.

In a remarkable paper published in 1956, Scales and his co-workers,[47] possibly for the first time, proposed that surgical dressings should be developed that met specific performance criteria. They also described clinically relevant test methods which could be used to measure or monitor dressing performance in the laboratory.

Their recommendations were based upon the findings of earlier work published by Burch and Winsor in 1944,[48] who had measured the amount of water lost through intact skin, and from minor injuries such as blisters.

They showed that at a temperature of 24°C and a relative humidity of 50%, 1.63 g/m^2 of moisture is lost every ten minutes (equivalent to 235 $g/m^2/24$ h). From the floor of a blister raised by cantharides the measured loss was approximately ten times this value. Taking account of these findings, Scales and his co-workers proposed a series of properties that the ideal should possess, based upon the understanding of the wound healing process and the range of materials available at that time.

They suggested that the ideal dressing should have the following properties:

- It should ideally have a porosity to water vapour of at least 1,400 $g/m^2/24$ h, measured at 37°C with a relative humidity of 75%
- It should not adhere either to a blood clot or to granulating surfaces, nor should it allow the penetration of capillary loops. It must, however, absorb free blood or exudate and give protection to the wound
- It should be a barrier to the passage of microorganisms
- It should be capable of following contours around a joint during movement - for example flexing of a finger
- It should be unaffected by domestic or industrial fluids-for example detergents or oils
- It should not produce a tissue reaction when applied to normal skin or granulating surface nor a state of allergy or hypersensitivity
- It should be non-inflammable
- It should be capable of being sealed to the skin
- It should be capable of being sterilised
- It should be available at a low cost

Furthermore, they recognized the importance of matching the dressing to the condition of the wound, stating that;

> *'The properties which the dressing should possess depend upon the extent of the loss of the epidermal cell layer and of any damage to the dermis, and the events that occur following injury and during healing of the wound'.*

They also described the limitations of the materials available to them at that time, accepting that;

> *'With present materials it is impossible to produce the ideal dressing and it seems likely that future dressings will be a compromise ... Plastic film dressings have certain advantages over traditional fabric dressings but they also possess certain undesirable features – for example, the occlusive waterproof dressing causes maceration of the skin surrounding the wound and an increase in bacterial flora of normal skin. Both nylon and cellophane are insufficiently permeable and flexible'.*

The rest of their publication was devoted to the description of a first aid dressing consisting of a new microporous plasticized polyvinylchloride film backing layer, bearing an absorbent pad located centrally forming an island. This dressing was subsequently produced commercially by Smith and Nephew under the now familiar brand name Elastoplast Airstrip.

This was tested both clinically and in the laboratory using a bacterial barrier test which is very similar in concept to that which has recently been proposed as the basis of a new national or European standard. Perhaps somewhat surprisingly, however, Scales *et al.* apparently failed to recognise the potential value of this new film in the treatment of other types of wounds.

It is interesting to note that amongst the acknowledgements which appear in this publication is one for Mr G.D. Winter of the same department for 'invaluable technical help'. Winter must have maintained an interest in this field for some ten years later he published the work previously described, which established him as the founder of moist wound healing.

In a later publication, Winter,[29] revisited Scales requirement for the ideal suggesting that it should be:

1. Capable of providing good absorption of blood and exudate
2. Sterilizable
3. Non-toxic
4. Non-allergenic or sensitising
5. Constant in performance terms over a range of temperatures and humidities
6. Non-flammable
7. Of small bulk (hospital storage problem)
8. Stable with a long shelf life
9. Conformable to anatomical contours
10. Tear resistant
11. Able to create ideal microclimate for most rapid and effective healing (prevents dehydration and is permeable to oxygen)
12. Capable of protecting against secondary infection
13. Non-adherent
14. Fibre-fast (does not shed loose material into wound)
15. Capable of providing mechanical protection to wound
16. Soil resistant
17. Able to accept and release medicaments
18. Cost effective

Whilst gauze and other fabric dressings in common use at that time generally satisfied the first ten criteria, they performed badly or very badly against the remaining eight, including the key requirements for a surgical dressing numbered 11-14. (The items in Winter's original list have been reordered for convenience).

Recognising the deficiencies of the products available at that time, manufacturers of dressings expended considerable efforts in an attempt to develop new products which approximated more closely to Winter's requirements.

These developments, coupled with an increased understanding of the wound healing process, have been such that a new definition of the ideal dressing or dressing system is now required which reflects the fact that a combination of different components may be required to produce the optimum healing conditions for any given wound. It also recognises that the optimal conditions may change as a wound progresses towards healing. A modified definition of the ideal dressing is therefore proposed as follows:

> *'The ideal dressing or dressing system provides an environment within the wound in which the objectives of the current phase of treatment may be achieved in a timely and cost effective manner without compromising either the patient's safety or quality of life, or adversely affecting the integrity of the periwound skin or the final cosmetic appearance of the healed wound where this is relevant.'*

It will be seen that this definition applies equally to products designed to achieve debridement, combat odour or infection, or promote granulation or epithelialization. It also follows that for some wounds, but by no means all, optimal wound management may involve the sequential application of a number of different 'ideal dressings' which are selected according to the condition of the wound as it presents at that point in time.

A revised list of the requirements of a dressing is given in Table 8 which is divided into two parts. Primary requirements are those which are common to most wound management materials, secondary requirements relate to specific types of wounds or wounds in a particular condition or stage in the healing process.

In both groups the performance requirements have been further divided into those which are determined principally by the design and construction of the dressing, over which the clinician has little or no control, and those in which the ability of the product to perform in the required fashion is also influenced to a significant degree by the nature and condition of the wound.

Even a cursory review of this table will indicate that it is unlikely that a single dressing or dressing system will ever possess all of the required attributes, a view put forward by Scales half a century earlier. For example, a dressing that is ideally suited for the early stages of the treatment of an infected, malodorous or necrotic wound, may not be optimal for the later stages of healing. Similarly a film dressing, which may provide ideal conditions for the final stages of the healing process of an epithelializing wound, may not be suitable for a slough-filled heavily exuding infected leg ulcer.

Table 8: Performance requirements of the 'Ideal Dressing'

Primary requirements	How determined	How examined
Maintains the wound and the surrounding skin in an optimum state of hydration (this implies the ability to absorb exudate effectively under compression)	Design feature + wound related	Lab + Clinical
Provides protection to the periwound skin from potentially irritant wound exudate and excess moisture	Design feature + wound related	Clinical
If self-adhesive, forms an effective water resistant seal to the periwound skin, but is easily removable without causing trauma or skin stripping	Design feature	Clinical
Forms an effective bacterial barrier (effectively contain exudate or cellular debris to prevent the transmission of microorganisms into or out of the wound)	Design feature	Lab
Conforms well to wound and limb	Design feature	Lab + Clinical
Produces minimal pain during application or removal as a result of adherence to the wound surface	Design feature + wound related	Clinical
Free of toxic or irritant extractables	Design feature	Lab
Does not release particles or non-biodegradable fibres into the wound	Design feature	Lab
Requires minimal disturbance or replacement	Design feature + wound related	Clinical
Maintains the wound at optimum temperature and pH	Design feature + wound related	Clinical
Secondary requirements		
Possesses antimicrobial activity - capable of combating localised infection	Design feature	Lab + Clinical
Has odour absorbing/combating properties	Design feature	Lab + Clinical
Has ability to remove or inactivate proteolytic enzymes in chronic wound fluid	Design feature	Lab + Clinical
Possesses haemostatic activity.	Design feature	Lab + Clinical
Exhibits effective wound cleansing (debriding) activity	Design feature + wound related	Lab + Clinical

REFERENCES

1. Majno G. *The Healing Hand*. First Havard Paperback Edition ed. Cambridge, Massachusetts: Havard University Press, 1991.
2. Forrest RD. Early history of wound treatment. *J R Soc Med* 1982;75(3):198-205.
3. Baoyong L, Jian Z, Denglong C, Min L. Evaluation of a new type of wound dressing made from recombinant spider silk protein using rat models. *Burns* 2010.
4. Bishop WJ. *A history of surgical dressings*. Chesterfield: Robinsons & Sons, 1959.
5. Gamgee S. Absorbent and medicated surgical dressings. *Lancet* 1880;Jan 24:127-128.
6. Thomas S, Loveless P, Hay NP. Comparing non-woven, filmated and woven gauze swabs. *Journal of Wound Care* 1993;2(1):35-41.
7. Lawrence JC. Reducing the spread of bacteria. *Journal of Wound Care* 1993;2(1):48-52.
8. Brown M, Myers RB, Pasceri P. A new generation of gauze dressings. *Ostomy/wound management* 1991;34(My/June):57-59.
9. Adams JE. Peritoneal Adhesions (An experimental study) *Lancet 1990* 1913(March 8th):664-668.
10. Dixon MF, Beck JM. Multiple peritoneal adhesions related to starch and gauze fragments. *J Pediatr Surg* 1974;9(4):531-3.
11. Sturdy JH, Baird RM, Gerein AN. Surgical sponges: a cause of granuloma and adhesion formation. *Ann Surg* 1967;165(1):128-34.
12. Saxen L, Myllarniemi H. Foreign material and postoperative adhesions. *N Engl J Med* 1968;279(4):200-2.
13. Weibel MA, Majno G. Peritoneal adhesions and their relation to abdominal surgery. A postmortem study. *Am J Surg* 1973;126(3):345-53.
14. Tinker MA, Burdman D, Deysine M, Teicher I, Platt N, Aufses AH, Jr. Granulomatous peritonitis due to cellulose fibers from disposable surgical fabrics: laboratory investigation and clinical implications. *Ann Surg* 1974;180(6):831-5.
15. Tinker MA, Teicher I, Burdman D. Cellulose granulomas and their relationship to intestinal obstruction. *Am J Surg* 1977;133(1):134-9.
16. Brittan RF, Studley JG, Parkin JV, Rowles PM, Le Quesne LP. Cellulose granulomatous peritonitis. *Br J Surg* 1984;71(6):452-3.
17. Janoff K, Wayne R, Huntwork B, Kelley H, Alberty R. Foreign body reactions secondary to cellulose lint fibers. *Am J Surg* 1984;147(5):598-600.
18. Chambi I, Tasker RR, Gentili F, Lougheed WM, Smyth HS, Marshall J, et al. Gauze-induced granuloma ("gauzoma"): an uncommon complication of gauze reinforcement of berry aneurysms. *J Neurosurg* 1990;72(2):163-70.
19. Wood RA. Disintegration of cellulose dressings in open granulating wounds. *Br Med J* 1976;1(6023):1444-5.
20. Elek SD. Experimental staphylococcal infections in the skin of man. *Ann N Y Acad Sci* 1956;65(3):85-90.
21. Burgess NA, Moore HE, Thomas S. Evaluation of a new non-woven theatre swab. *Journal of the Royal College of Surgeons of Edinburgh.* 1992;37:191-193.
22. Jones VJ. The use of gauze: will it ever change? *Int Wound J* 2006;3(2):79-86.
23. Stotts NA, Barbour S, Slaughter R, Wipke-Tevis D. Wound care practices in the United States. *Ostomy Wound Manage* 1993;39(3):53-5, 59-62, 64 passim.
24. Hess CT. When to use gauze dressings. *Adv Skin Wound Care* 2000;13(6):266-8.
25. Ovington LG. Hanging wet-to-dry dressings out to dry. *Home Healthc Nurse* 2001;19(8):477-83; quiz 484.

26. Bethell E. Why gauze dressings should not be the first choice to manage most acute surgical cavity wounds. *Journal of Wound Care* 2003;12(6):237-9.

27. Armstrong MH, Price P. Wet-to-Dry Gauze Dressings: Fact and Fiction. *Wounds* 2004;16(2):56-62.

28. Winter GD. Formation of the scab and the rate of epithelization of superficial wounds in the skin of the young domestic pig. *Nature* 1962;193:293-294.

29. Winter GD. Methods for the biological evaluation of dressings. In: Turner TD, Brain KR, editors. *Surgical dressings in the hospital environment.* Cardiff: Surgical Dressings Research Unit, UWIST, Cardiff, 1975:47-81.

30. Hinman CD, Maibach H. Effect of air exposure and occlusion on experimental human skin wounds. *Nature* 1963;200:377-379.

31. Winter G. Healing of skin wounds and the influence of dressings on the repair process. In: Harkiss KJ, editor. *Surgical Dressings and Wound Healing.* Bradford: Bradford University Press, 1971:46--60.

32. Winter GD. A note on wound healing under dressings with special reference to perforated-film dressings. *J Invest Dermatol* 1965;45(4):299-302.

33. Winter GD. Epidermal wound healing under a new polyurethane foam dressing (Lyofoam). *Plast Reconstr Surg* 1975;56(5):531-7.

34. Rogers M. Treatment of 'angiomas': a modern commentary. *The Australasian Journal Of Dermatology* 2000;41 Suppl:S89-91.

35. De Coninck A, Draye JP, Van Strubarq A, Vanpee E, Kaufman L, Delaey B, et al. Healing of full-thickness wounds in pigs: effects of occlusive and non- occlusive dressings associated with a gel vehicle. *J Dermatol Sci* 1996;13(3):202-11.

36. Kunugiza Y, Tomita T, Moritomo H, Yoshikawa H. A hydrocellular foam dressing versus gauze: effects on the healing of rat excisional wounds. *J Wound Care* 2010;19(1):10-4.

37. Zawacki BE. Reversal of capillary stasis and prevention of necrosis in burns. *Ann Surg* 1974;180(1):98-102.

38. Dyson M, Young S, Pendle CL, Webster DF, Lang SM. Comparison of the effects of moist and dry conditions on dermal repair. *J Invest Dermatol* 1988;91(5):434-9.

39. Dyson M, Young SR, Hart J, Lynch JA, Lang S. Comparison of the effects of moist and dry conditions on the process of angiogenesis during dermal repair. *J Invest Dermatol* 1992;99(6):729-33.

40. Alper JC, Welch EA, Ginsberg M, Bogaars H, Maguire P. Moist wound healing under a vapor permeable membrane. *Journal of the American Academy of Dermatolgy* 1983;8(3):347353.

41. Alvarez OM, Mertz PM, Eaglstein WH. The effect of occlusive dressings on collagen synthesis and re-epithelialization in superficial wounds. *J Surg Res* 1983;35(2):142-148.

42. Eaglstein WH. Effect of occlusive dressings on wound healing. *Clin Dermatol* 1984;2(3):107-11.

43. Eaglstein WH. Experiences with biosynthetic dressings. *J Am Acad Dermatol* 1985;12(2 Pt 2):434-40.

44. Hermans MHE. Air exposure versus occlusion: merits and disadvantages of different dressings. *Journal of Wound Care* 1993;2(6):362-365.

45. Ubbink DT, Vermeulen H, Goossens A, Kelner RB, Schreuder SM, Lubbers MJ. Occlusive vs gauze dressings for local wound care in surgical patients: a randomized clinical trial. *Arch Surg* 2008;143(10):950-5.

46. Wound Union of Healing Societies (WUWS). Principles of best practice: Diagnostics and wounds. A consensus document. In: MacGregor L, editor. London: MEP, 2008.

47. Scales JT, Towers AG, Goodman N. Development and evaluation of a porous surgical dressing. *Br Med J* 1956;2(4999):962-8.
48. Burch GE, Winsor T. Rate of insensible perspiration (difffusion of water) locally through living and through dead human skin. *Arch Intern Med* 1944;74(6):437-444. .

7. Laboratory testing of surgical dressings

INTRODUCTION

As previously described, the use of materials to cover or treat wounds stretches back into antiquity. Lawrence[1] in an interesting early review of the structure and use of dressings and their effects upon wound healing, alluded to the importance of dressing design to prevent adherence and fibre loss, whilst providing the required degree of environmental control. Early test systems for measuring the absorbency of dressings were described by Piskozub[2] and Thomas et al.,[3] however, meaningful standards and specifications designed to characterize the performance of wound management materials have only been developed and widely adopted during in the last 10-20 years.

The first standards for dressings were very simple, concentrating primarily upon product composition and structure and intended to regulate the manufacture of materials that had previously been found to perform in a generally satisfactory manner in clinical practice. This typically involved counting the number of threads present in the warp and weft in gauze products for example.

Figure 15: A mechanical thread counter

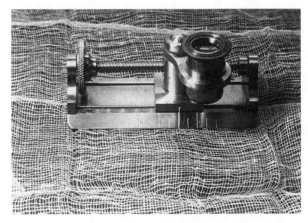

As more sophisticated dressings were developed, however, it became obvious that new standards and test systems were required to demonstrate that these innovative materials also performed a specific function in the required manner in a consistent and reproducible way.

Although the commercial success of a dressing is ultimately determined by its clinical performance, well designed laboratory tests can provide a useful rapid and cost-effective technique for obtaining objective information on how well a new product development functions in certain areas without having to embark upon expensive and time-consuming clinical trials.

This chapter discusses the need for dressing standards, describes how these have evolved, and briefly outlines test methods which can be used to assess key aspects of the performance of many different types of products.

IMPORTANCE OF LABORATORY TESTING

Laboratory tests for dressings are required for a number of reasons:

- To demonstrate compliance with national or international standards or specifications
- To ensure product meets 'in-house' manufacturing standards
- To facilitate objective comparisons between similar products
- To generate data to support allocation of shelf life (stability/storage)

STANDARDS FOR DRESSINGS

Types of standards

There are essentially three types of standards or specifications:

- Structural standards - which define the structure and/or composition of a product
- Performance standards - which characterise one or more functions of a dressing
- Safety standards – designed to ensure that a product, when used appropriately, is unlikely to adversely affect the health or wellbeing either of the individual to whom it is applied or the population at large

Early dressing standards

As new families of dressings were developed and the production of surgical materials became more sophisticated, it became necessary to develop formal standards to ensure that these products were consistently produced to an agreed of level of quality.

In the United Kingdom, the first of these appeared in two supplements to the British Pharmaceutical Codex (BPC) of 1911 and these were later incorporated into the 1923 edition of this publication. Over 80 products were described, the majority of which consisted of cotton fibre, both medicated and unmedicated, and a variety of cotton fabrics together with a few more complex products such as emplastrums (plasters) and oiled silk.

The BPC remained the principal source of standards for surgical dressings within the United Kingdom for over fifty years, but in 1980 these were transferred to the British Pharmacopoeia (BP). When, as a result of European legislation, dressings became classified as Medical Devices, monographs for these materials were subsequently omitted from the B.P.

The early monographs for dressings consist almost entirely of structural specifications, supplemented by limit tests for potential contaminants. The specification for gauze, for example, contains a requirement for tests for water or ether soluble extractives, determination of sulphated ash, and the presence of surfactants and optical brightening agents

Performance-based standards

Whilst the early standards undoubtedly had value as quality control checks to ensure that products were produced in a consistent way from a range of well-characterized materials, they did not facilitate comparisons between structurally different dressings designed to perform a common function. Furthermore, the proscriptive and inflexible nature of structural standards for many years prevented or delayed official acceptance of new and more innovative products which although different from the traditional materials were superior in performance terms.

Recognising these limitations, in the early 1990s the Surgical Dressings Manufacturing Association, (SDMA), set up a series of working groups comprising technical staff from the industry and the NHS, to devise a new family of performance-based test methods and specifications. These were based in a number of instances upon work that had been pioneered within the Surgical Materials Testing Laboratory (SMTL), an NHS facility that specialised in testing wound dressings and other medical disposables for the NHS in Wales.

These working groups published test methods for bandages, alginates, films, hydrocolloids and hydrogels, many of which subsequently became incorporated into the BP and/or adopted as European Standards. The types of investigations required to characterise the performance of a dressing are principally determined by the nature and condition of the wound to which the product is to be applied, but may include tests for:

- Absorbency
- Permeability,
- Control or prevention of infection (antimicrobial activity)
- Bacterial barrier properties
- Odour control
- Low-adherence
- Freedom from toxicity

FLUID HANDLING TESTS

Absorbency

In clinical practice, although some products such as hydrogels are applied to donate moisture in order to promote autolytic debridement, the majority of dressings are applied to remove excess wound fluid (exudate) from the immediate vicinity of the wound. With the exception of the vacuum assisted closure technique, in which fluid is actively withdrawn from the wound, with most conventional dressings exudate management depends upon the uptake of liquid by absorbent fibres or foam which is then retained within their structure. Depending upon the design of the dressing, this is then distributed throughout the body of the absorbent layer spreading both laterally and vertically towards to outer surface.

Some dressings also contain gel forming agents which may be derivatives of starch, or carboxymethylcellulose (CMC) or made from totally synthetic polymers which possess a remarkable affinity for liquid. Sometimes, as in the case of dressings made from alginate or CMC fibres, the absorbent and gel-forming layers are one and the same. The presence of these gel-forming agents greatly improves the ability of a dressing to retain liquid under pressure as the fluid is 'locked away' within its structure. This can be particularly important in the case of products made from foam which, although capable of taking up significant volumes of fluid, do not necessarily retain this well under compression.

Over the years numerous methods for measuring the absorbency of dressings have been described. The simplest consist of simple 'dunk and drip' tests, in which dressings or pieces of dressings and weighed, dipped into water and, after draining, reweighed to measure the weight of fluid retained.[4] More sophisticated techniques involve the application of an appropriate test fluid to a sample of dressing under controlled conditions.

Choice of test fluid

The choice of test solution is important when testing modern wound management materials, for some dressings chemically interact with ions or proteins present in blood or wound fluid. Foetal calf serum or blood are useful in a research environment, but are too expensive and impracticable for routine use. A standard test solution was therefore devised and adopted for all relevant European Standards for dressings. Called simply 'Solution A', it consists of sodium and calcium chloride solution containing 142 mmol of sodium ions and 2.5 mmol of calcium ions as the chloride salts. This solution has an ionic composition comparable to human serum or exudate. The presence of both sodium and calcium ions is required as these both have a marked effect upon the gelling characteristics of alginate fibres. In some situations the selection of an appropriate test solution can be critical, (see chapter on silver dressings).

Free swell absorptive capacity

This, the first standard test described in BS EN 13726-1, and a form of 'dunk and dip test', measures the uptake of fluid by fibrous dressings such as those made from alginate fibre presented either in sheet or rope form.

The dressing is placed in a Petri dish together with a quantity of 'Solution A' equivalent to 40 times the weight of the test sample, and held for 30 minutes at 37° C after which it is gently removed from the dish, allowed to drain for 30 seconds and reweighed. The absorbency is then expressed as the mass of solution retained per 100 cm^2, for sheet dressings, or per gram of sample for cavity dressings.

It will immediately be seen that this method may be criticised for two reasons. First the alginate is tested in the absence of any pressure, which means that the results obtained bear little relation to the volume of exudate that the dressing will take up under normal conditions of use. This point is returned to later. Secondly it ignores the possibility that the dressing will dissolve or disintegrate in the Petri dish.

In the presence of sodium ions, alginate fibres absorb fluid and swell, sometimes taking on a gel-like appearance. The degree of swelling and dispersion is determined by the chemical structure, ionic content and method of preparation of the dressing. Some alginate products with a high mannuronic acid content, appear to form an amorphous mass whilst others, with a high guluronic acid content, tend to retain their structure and swell to a much lesser degree.[5] These properties are quite important as they determine how the dressing will perform when introduced into a wound and BS EN 13726-1 describes two simple tests that help to characterise the alginate and determine its dispersion/solubility.

Permeability

It is self evident that the absorbent capacity of any dressing is finite, limited by size (area) and volume, and although in theory it is possible to increase the absorbent capacity by simply increasing dressing thickness, this impacts negatively upon conformability and patient comfort.

A second fluid handling mechanism is therefore often employed, which involves the use of a semipermeable film or foam layer. Such materials permit the loss of water vapour by evaporation whilst preventing the ingress or egress of liquid or microorganisms.

Unlike absorbent dressings where the absorption capacity is finite, the ability of a permeable dressing to cope with exudate by evaporation is relatively unlimited, determined only by the permeability of the membrane relative to the rate of exudate production by the wound.

Permeability is also an important factor in adhesive dressings which are to be applied to intact skin. In these situations the product must be sufficiently permeable to cope with normal transepidermal water loss. If the product is occlusive or the adhesive layer does not have the capability to absorb the required amounts of moisture, fluid will accumulate beneath the dressing, potentially leading to maceration of the skin and/or a failure of the adhesive bond.

Moisture vapour transmission rate (MVTR)

The permeability of a dressing may be determined using a simple piece of apparatus known as a Paddington Cup (so called because the working party that finalized the test met in a hotel in Paddington). The cup is described in detail in BS EN 13726-2,[6] but essentially consists of a cylinder with an internal cross-sectional area of 10 cm^2 having a flange at each end. To one end of the cylinder is fitted an annular ring the internal diameter of which is identical to that of the cylinder, and to the other a solid plate which can be clamped into position forming a water tight seal (.

A piece of dressing under examination is cut to shape and clamped between the annular ring and one of the flanges. Approximately 20 mL of test fluid is then added into the cup and the plate clamped in position. The cup is then weighed before being placed in an incubator capable of maintaining the internal temperature and humidity within specified limits, 37 ± 1°C and $< 20\%$ RH throughout the test.

After a predetermined period, usually 24 hours, the cylinder is reweighed and the amount of fluid lost through the back of the dressing by evaporation during the period of test is calculated by difference.

Although the official method specifies that the apparatus shall be incubated with the solution in contact with the test sample, it is also possible to undertake the test with the cylinder inverted so that the dressing is not in direct contact with the liquid but exposed only to moisture vapour.

Figure 16: A Paddington Cup

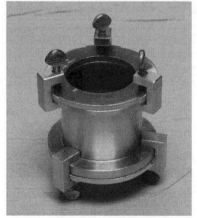

Photographs courtesy of P.Fram

This is important because the permeability of some types of polyurethane film will increase dramatically whilst in contact with liquid but revert back to previous values when this is removed – a characteristic that has obvious and important implications for its use as a wound dressing when in contact with intact periwound skin.[7]

When very permeable products are tested, the water loss from within the cup is sufficient to cause a partial vacuum which has the effect of drawing the film into the interior, an effect sometimes referred to as 'doming'. This has the dual effects of increasing the surface area of the plastic whilst causing it to reduce in thickness, both of which will tend to alter its permeability to moisture vapour and thus potentially provide an erroneous test result. Preliminary studies suggest that the formation of a small hole through the wall or the base of the cup *circa* 0.25 mm in diameter will relieve the vacuum and prevent this effect whilst producing a negligible effect on moisture vapour loss.

Dynamic MVTR

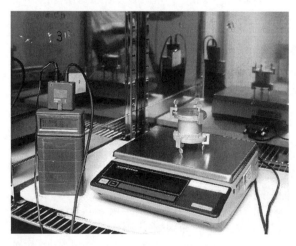

Figure 17: A dynamic MVTR test in operation

The fluid handling and moisture vapour transmission methods described previously, provide a single value for the amount of fluid which is lost from the dressing during the test period.

Whilst this may be suitable for film dressings, the permeability of which remains relatively consistent throughout the test period, the test has serious limitations for products such as hydrocolloids in which the permeability of the dressing changes with time as the adhesive mass on the wound contact surface gradually becomes hydrated.

This problem can be overcome by a modification to the standard test which is described in an earlier paper.[8] A Paddington Cup is set up as described previously and placed upon the pan of a top loading balance located in a controlled humidity cabinet which is connected to a data logger. In this way, the weight of the Paddington Cup can be continuous monitored over the test period, and from the recorded data the change in moisture vapour transmission rate may be determined. Depending upon the product this may be virtually zero for a number of hours, gradually increasing to reach a steady state sometime during the following 24-48 hours.[8-9]

Fluid handling capacity

Some dressings combine absorbency, gel formation and permeability to provide optimal exudate management. Together these determine the fluid handling capacity of the product (FHC). The relative importance of these individual mechanisms is governed by the structure, composition and physical characteristics of the various components from which the dressing or dressing system is constructed but the way in which fluid is distributed throughout the absorbent layer is also important and contributes to the dressing's performance.

A method for determining the FHC of dressings is described in BS EN 13726-1. This is based on the method published previously,[8] and provides information on the amount of test fluid both retained and transpired by hydrocolloid sheets or dressings made from foam or hydrogel provided that they incorporate an integral waterproof backing layer. The method is not suitable for testing fibrous products or permeable absorbents.

The test involves the use of a Paddington Cup as before. A piece of dressing under examination is cut to shape and clamped between the annular ring and one of the flanges. The cylinder together with all the associated parts is then weighed. Approximately 20 mL of test fluid is then added into the cup and the plate clamped in position. The cup is then weighed again before being placed in an incubator capable of maintaining the internal temperature and humidity within specified limits, $37 \pm 1°C$ and < 20% RH throughout the test.

After a predetermined period (usually 24 hours) the cylinder is reweighed, the plate removed and the excess fluid is allowed to escape after which the cylinder is reweighed once again. From these weighings it is possible to calculate the amount of fluid lost through the back of the dressing by evaporation during the period of test, and the weight of fluid retained within its structure. The sum of these two values represents the Fluid Handling Capacity of the dressing.

Limitations of existing fluid handling tests

Although the standard methods facilitate comparisons of the fluid handling properties of similar products within specific groups and provide useful quality control tests to confirm consistency of production, they do not permit comparisons between different groups of dressings such as alginates and hydrocolloids for example.

Importance of compression

The test methods described thus far also cannot be used to investigate the performance of the different dressings whilst under compression– a major factor in the treatment of venous leg ulcers where dressings are often subjected to pressures as high as 40 mmHg.

Some dressings, such as foam sheets, are like bath sponges, capable of taking up large volumes of fluid, but unable to retain this under even light pressure. Much research has therefore been devoted to maximising the performance of foam dressings by the inclusion of hydrophilic polymers or super-absorbents within the porous structure of the foam itself.

These developments have resulted in the formation of a family of dressings that are among the most absorbent and widely used products available. Test systems are therefore required which may be used to compare the fluid handling properties of these different families under varying levels of pressure.

Over the years, various laboratory 'wound models' have been described most of which consist of variations on a common theme. The dressing under examination is placed on a sinter or a metal or acrylic plate with a small hole or depression in the centre. A weight is applied to the back to simulate pressure applied by a bandage, and test fluid is delivered the dressing through a hole in the plate by some means of a peristaltic pump or syringe driver.

Passive versus active fluid delivery

In some test systems the fluid is not actively pumped into the dressing but is absorbed passively by the dressing itself from some form of constant head apparatus.[10] A particular example of such a test system is the 'demand wetability' apparatus that was developed to investigate how fibre pre-treatments and alignment can influence the uptake of water.[11]

A similar, more sophisticated version of this type of equipment was described in a series of publications by Ferrari et al.[12-15] in which they also measured the rheological properties of different dressings during the gelling process.

A far more complex system for monitoring the gelling properties of hydrocolloid dressings was described by Lanel et al.[16] This technique, which is considered to be far too complex for routine use, involved the use of a video camera to record changes in the physical appearance of a dressing held inside a transport chamber, followed by the application of advanced mathematics to predict the kinetics of uniaxial swelling of a cylindrical gel sample.

A simple demand test does not truly reflect the clinical situation because the production of exudate is an 'active' process which occurs whether a dressing absorbs fluid or not. Also some products have a slightly hydrophobic wound contact surface which may not readily initiate the 'take up' of an aqueous solution. The use of a peristaltic pump or syringe driver to apply the test solution addresses this problem,[3] but this approach also can be criticised. With a hydrocolloid dressing, for example, such a test may simply become a measure of the strength of the adhesive bond formed between the dressing and the surface of the wound model as fluid pumped into the system accumulates as a large bubble beneath the dressing surface.

Endpoints of absorbency testing

The absorbent capacity of a surgical dressing is generally taken to be that volume of fluid taken up by the test sample by the time at which strike-through occurs. This is defined as the point at which absorbed fluid reaches the outer surface or edge of a dressing and this may be determined in a number of different ways. In one early system devised by SMTL,[3] the distribution of liquid absorbed by the dressing was monitored electronically by means of sharp steel spikes which penetrated into the body of the dressing. The disruption to the structure of the test sample caused by the spikes cast doubt on the validity of this method and so it was abandoned.

Figure 18: Early form of absorbency testing apparatus

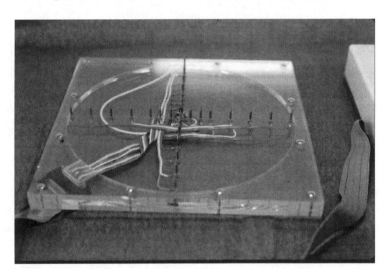

Many other early test systems used within the industry, and elsewhere, also suffered from a series of disadvantages.

- They were difficult to automate and therefore not suitable for running unattended over extended periods.
- The application of a weight and/or strike-through detector on the back of the dressing prevented the loss of moisture vapour, an important mechanism by which some dressings cope with exudate production.
- If moisture vapour transmission is to be measured, it was usually not possible to apply a weight or strike-through detector on the back of the dressing to simulate the effect of pressure.
- Most test systems provided a single value for the total absorbency of a dressing with little indication of how the product performed over a specified period of time (dynamic performance testing).
- Most wound models were not suitable for testing hydrogels or packing materials.
- They did not readily enable predictions to be made of clinical wear times of different types of dressings.

Dynamic fluid handling testing

Research undertaken in the SMTL, led to the development of a new test system (subsequently called the WRAP rig), designed to address these issues and facilitate comparisons of the fluid handling properties of most types of dressings irrespective of their structure and composition, even whilst subjected to compression.

Design requirements

In order to address some of the shortcomings of existing test systems and produce a system that more closely approximated to the clinical situation, a series of key design criteria for the new model were identified.[17]

- Fluid should be provided to the test sample by some form of pump or other suitable positive flow device. A passive uptake technique is not acceptable.
- The fluid should not be presented to the test sample under excessive pressure. Previous test systems have, in effect, injected fluid into the dressing under pressure, although there is no evidence that this occurs in wounds.
- There must be some suitable method for controlling the temperature of the system for the duration of the test, to reproduce the environmental conditions in the wound.
- The test should provide some indication of the dynamic performance of the dressing by measuring its fluid handling capacity profile over time, and not just resulting in a single total absorbency figure.
- The equipment should be capable of delivering test solution at a range of different flow rates, so that the effect of different rates of exudate can be examined.
- The apparatus should indicate when either vertical or lateral strike-through has occurred.
- The apparatus should be suitable for testing a wide range of different types of dressings to permit direct comparison of the results. Previous methods were frequently dedicated to one type of technology, such as alginates.
- The equipment should be compatible with a range of different test solutions
- Where appropriate, the apparatus should permit the application of varying loads to the test sample in order to determine the effect of external pressure.
- The apparatus should permit the measurement of moisture vapour transmission by the dressing as an integral part of the test.
- The test should be easy to perform and provide results that can be reproduced within and between laboratories.
- The equipment should not be excessively expensive to produce.
- The test should, ideally, provide an indication of the wear time of a dressing in normal clinical use.

In addition to the primary design criteria, a number of additional features were identified which although not essential, are considered desirable feature in a wound model.

- The apparatus should withstand sterilization or disinfection.
- The apparatus should permit analysis of wound fluid that has been in contact with the dressing to measure changes in ionic composition or changes in concentration of solutes such as proteins caused by selective absorption by the dressing.
- The apparatus should permit microbiological examination of the local environment during the course of the test.
- The test equipment should allow the pressure beneath the dressing to be varied if this is considered desirable.

A prototype test system was developed based upon these criteria, and following some early validation work, some minor modifications were made and a new version of the rig produced, the use of which was described in a publication which also clearly illustrates the effects of compression upon dressing performance.[7]

Whilst the WRAP rig is an excellent research tool, it has the disadvantages that it is expensive to construct, time consuming to set up and use, and can only test one dressing at a time. Nevertheless, the equipment is very flexible and probably provides results which are as relevant to the clinical situation as it is possible to achieve in the laboratory. The rig comprises a number of separate components described below.

The wound model

This consists of a two-part stainless steel plate, the 'wound bed', which is mounted on a Perspex table. An electronically controlled heating mat beneath the steel plate keeps the plate and test sample within a narrow temperature band. The central section of the plate is milled from solid stainless steel and includes a shallow circular recess bearing two ports on opposite ends of a 15 mm-long shallow channel. An inlet hole, three mm in diameter, and an outlet hole, seven mm in diameter, permits the introduction and unimpaired exit of test solution. The diameter and depth of the circular recess is sufficient to accommodate two thin absorbent pads that ensure the effective transfer of liquid from the channel to the dressing above.

Test fluid, introduced by means of a syringe pump, travels along the narrow channel and passes out through the second port, falling vertically down through a short, wide-bore tube. This tube discharges into a receiver placed on the pan of an electronic balance. The liquid in the receiver is covered with a layer of oil to prevent loss by evaporation. The balance is connected to an electronic data capture device that records changes in the balance reading at predetermined intervals throughout the period of the test.

A dressing sample typically measuring 10×10 cm is secured on to the test plate which is set to a predetermined temperature. Test fluid applied to the test rig passes along the open channel some or all of which will be taken up by the dressing. Any unabsorbed fluid continues to pass along the channel until it falls through the outflow pipe into the receiver, causing a change in the balance reading. The amount of fluid that accumulates in this way is inversely proportional to the absorbency of the dressing. A highly absorbent dressing may take up all the liquid that is applied to it, while less absorbent products will absorb only for a short time, or take a little while to reach maximum absorbency. During the course of the test, therefore, the maximum weight of fluid that can be taken up by a dressing is determined by the flow rate of the syringe pump.

As this test system is designed to simulate the normal use of a dressing it is important to ensure that the test conditions employed are as clinically relevant as

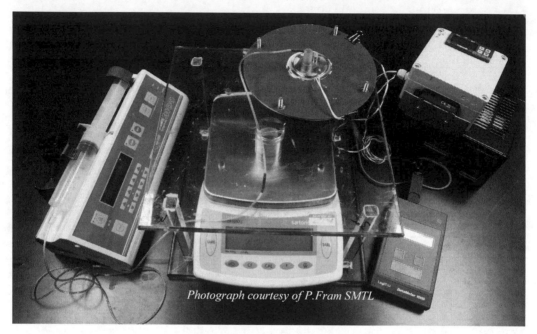

Photograph courtesy of P.Fram SMTL

Figure 19: The WRAP Rig

possible, particularly in relation to the production of exudate. According to the literature, a heavily exuding wound typically produces around 5 mL/10cm^2 per 24 hours,[18] but in the presence of infection this value can easily double.[19]

Although it is possible to run the test with these flow rates, for most tests the syringe pump is normally set to deliver a nominal one mL per hour as this value provides a reasonable compromise between clinical relevance and a need to keep testing times to a minimum for practical reasons.

When testing cavity wound dressings, alginate fibre or hydrogel dressings, a simple modification is made to the apparatus. A piece of stainless tube is fixed inside the recess in the centre of the plate to form a chamber into which the dressing is placed. Although strike-through measurements are not appropriate with such dressings, it is possible to apply pressure to cavity dressings such as alginate packing by means of a weighted stainless steel piston, which forms a sliding fit in the tube. In all other respects the test procedures remain the same. When testing hydrogel dressings, the open end of the chamber is sealed with a piece of aluminium foil held in place with impermeable plastic tape to prevent evaporation.

The pressure/ vertical strike-through plate

As previously described, a solid weight may be applied to the back of the dressing to simulate pressure produced by compression bandages, but this has the undesirable effect of occluding the back of the dressing and preventing the transpiration of moisture vapour - potentially an important function of the dressing. This problem was overcome in this model in a novel way by combining in one piece of apparatus, the functions of strike-through plate, moisture absorbing unit, and pressure plate. A stainless steel box one surface of which consists of a coarse stainless mesh supported internally by pillars attached to the inner face of the other surface to impart structural rigidity, can be filled with silica gel and when placed upon the test sample with the mesh surface downwards it fulfils three functions:

- Permits the application of pressure to the dressing without occluding the outer surface
- Provides a humidity gradient across the dressing to facilitate passage of moisture vapour
- Acts as an electrical contact to detect strike-through

Recording strike-through

A method of recording strike through method was devised which involved the use a Psion Organiser II (Model XP) fitted with a Digitron Model SF10 Data logger unit. The SF10 unit plugs into the top of the Psion II, and is a four channel unit capable of taking up to four external probes to measure temperature, pressure, relative humidity or voltage. For this application, a voltage probe was used capable of recording from 0 - 2500mV. A 1.5-volt (AA sized) alkaline cell was used to supply the necessary electromotive force. Initial experience with this equipment suggested that the combination provided a simple and reproducible technique for measuring strike-through, recording values that changed instantly from 0 mV to 1000 mV when strike-through occurred. At this point, the contribution made by the loss of moisture vapour to the fluid handling properties of the sheet dressings may be determined by measuring the change in weight of the silica gel in the strike-through plate. Further work is required to validate this part of the test.

Lateral strike-through detectors

The possibility for attaching lateral strike-through detectors also exists. Typically these consist of four brass strips connected together with short lengths of flexible cable. The under-surface of each strip is covered with a layer of insulating tape to prevent it from making electrical contact with the stainless steel plate. In use the strips, which are connected to the strike-through detector, can be pushed gently against the exposed edges of the dressing to detect any moisture that appears at the edge of the dressing.

Examples of results obtained with the WRAP apparatus

Any observed increase in the balance reading when using the WRAP apparatus is actually due to the accumulation of liquid in the reservoir which has *not* be taken up by the dressing under test.

To determine the absorbency of the sample it is necessary to undertake a simple, easily automated, manipulation of these based upon the flow rate of the test solution delivered by the syringe pump which has been carefully calibrated beforehand.

For the purpose of illustration, Figure 20 shows a series of graphs produced from four different hydrocolloid dressings which show marked differences in their fluid handling properties. Actual results generated using this test system, are quoted in detail elsewhere in this book.

Figure 20: Examples of test results obtained using the WRAP rig

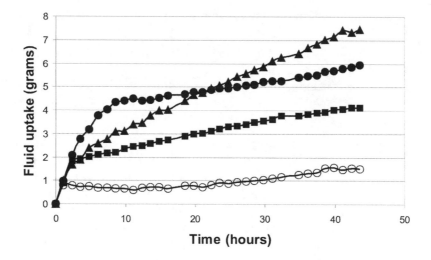

Clinical relevance of laboratory fluid handling studies

Any laboratory-based study can do no more than provide a broad indication of the ability of a dressing to cope with wound exudate *in vivo* as numerous other factors will undoubtedly impact upon the product's clinical performance. Some of these factors will tend to overestimate the fluid handling capacity of the dressing, whilst others will have the opposite effect.

For example, the previously described and commonly quoted 'Fluid Handling Capacity' is simply a theoretical value which is useful for comparing the performance of different dressings under similar test conditions. It is derived using the Paddington Cup method, in which results are obtained using a circular piece of dressing approximately 3.5 cm in diameter with an effective area of 10 cm^2.

In clinical practice, however, a small wound with an area of 10 cm^2 would normally be dressed with an island dressing or absorbent pad with an area of around 100 cm^2. If wound fluid were to be distributed uniformly throughout this pad, the intact dressing could theoretically absorb 5 - 10 times the weight of fluid predicted experimentally. Similarly the area of film available for evaporation would also be 5 - 10 times greater, which would further increase the fluid handling properties of the dressing. This suggests that the laboratory results quoted here will tend to significantly *underestimate* the fluid handling ability of a standard 10 × 10 cm dressing when applied to a relatively small wound. If, however, the same size pad were to be applied to a larger wound, perhaps 8 - 9 cm in diameter, the fluid handling capacity of the intact dressing would approximate more closely to predicted values.

In the case of extensive leg ulcers or pressure ulcers, the area of dressing not directly in contact with the wound is likely to be substantially less in percentage terms. This means that the laboratory test data will be less likely to underestimate the fluid handling properties of a large dressing applied to an extensive wound.

Laboratory results also take no account of the effects of gravity and patient position. In the case of a dressing applied to a large leg ulcer, for example, fluid will always tend to move towards the lowest point of the dressing with the result that the upper part may not be fully utilised.

Another potential source of error is the fact that laboratory data is normally generated with an aqueous solution containing only inorganic ions whereas wound fluid consists of a complex mixture containing proteins and cellular debris. As the aqueous component evaporates, the concentration of all these solutes will increase with the result that they may be deposited on the under surface of the film, thereby partially occluding it and reducing its permeability over time.

Perhaps most importantly, the rate at which water vapour passes across a film dressing is proportional to the difference in partial pressures (simplistically the amount of moisture vapour in the air) on both sides of the membrane. In the standard laboratory test, the relative humidity inside the Paddington Cup is 100%, but within the test chamber it is maintained below 20% thus producing a concentration gradient that will facilitate the passage of moisture through the membrane.

In clinical practice although the humidity beneath a dressing will be very high, the humidity outside will vary. In most instances, however, it will be considerably higher than 20%, - perhaps 50 - 65%. This means that clinically, the passage of moisture vapour through the dressing will be substantially reduced compared with experimental values. The temperature outside the dressing is also likely to be lower than 37°C and this will further influence the passage of moisture vapour across the film. These changes in environmental conditions will markedly affect a dressing's performance, something which is not generally recognised as few clinicians take account of the weather when selecting dressings! The exact reduction in permeability will depend upon the ambient conditions but some fairly basic calculations suggest that clinically relevant values could easily be half those determined experimentally.

FLUID AFFINITY TESTING

Some dressings such as hydrogels, are not primarily intended to absorb large quantities of exudate, but are applied to increase the moisture content of a wound. Some hydrogels, available in both sheet and amorphous form, have the ability to absorb or donate liquid according to the condition of the underlying tissue. This means that they can absorb fluid from a heavily exuding wound or donate moisture to dry or devitalized tissue to promote autolytic debridement. A technique was developed to assess this ability with formed the basis of three early publications.[20-22]

In summary, the material in question is placed in contact with other gels made from varying concentrations of agar or gelatin representing a spectrum of tissue types and the transfer of liquid to or from the test sample to the standard gels is measured by recording any change in weight of the sample. This test, which was gradually refined and used as the basis of a standard method described in BS EN 13726-1, is described in more detail in the hydrogel chapter.

LOW-ADHERENCE

Importance of low-adherence

The results of a international survey,[23] identified that pain and trauma were ranked as the most important factors to consider when changing dressings. A total of 3918 clinicians who responded to a written questionnaire, considered that pain was most commonly associated with dressings drying out or adhering to the wound bed, factors that were also considered to be responsible for wound trauma. Some products like alginates, hydrogels or silicone products show little propensity to adhere to granulating wounds whilst other such simple gauze or non-woven fabrics perform particularly badly in this context.

It is generally believed that at least two mechanisms are responsible for adherence. The first is the inherent 'stickiness' of serum which acts like a simple adhesive that forms a bond between two opposing surfaces. The second mechanism is a little more complex, involving the penetration into the dressing of serous fluid containing cellular debris which dries to form a solid 'scab' on the wound surface but which also incorporates some of the structure of the dressing. As a result when the dressing is removed the scab, together with underlying new epithelium, is ripped away, leading to rewounding and delayed healing.

Many dressings have therefore been developed with a wound-contact surface that is designed specifically to reduce adherence, (see chapter on low-adherent dressings).

Assessment of adherence potential

Predicting the way in which dressings will perform clinically in terms of adherence has proved unexpectedly difficult, and no laboratory test has yet been devised which is universally accepted for this purpose. In 1982 a method was described by SMTL,[3] which involved the application of a cold cure silicone material to the dressing which penetrated into the structure of the fabric before hardening, thus simulating the drying of wound exudate or serum (Figure 21).

No formal limits could be applied to this test, but the system was used to rank products in order of their adherence potential as determined by the magnitude of the peel force, the degree of disruption to the silicone block and the amount of dressing material that had become incorporated into it.

Although this test has some clinical relevance, in that it simulates the penetration and subsequent drying or hardening of serum or wound fluid within a dressing, it takes no account of the intrinsic 'stickiness' of serum and the contribution this makes to the problems of adherence. In a later modification to this test, an aqueous solution of gelatin was used in place of the silicone as this is more allied to the materials present within a wound.

Figure 21: Assessing adherence potential

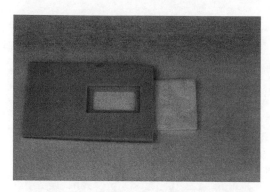

A suitably-sized sample of dressing is placed upon a flat surface and a plastic former positioned on top. The former is used to prevent excessive spreading of the silicone and ensure a consistent area of contact.

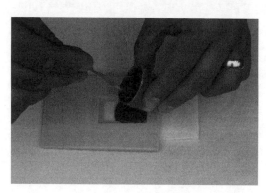

A suitable quantity of the cold cure silicone material is mixed with a small volume of light silicone oil to reduce the viscosity of the mixture and after the addition of the catalyst the mixture is stirred thoroughly before being added to the former.

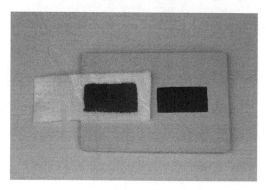

Once the rubber has cured, a tensiometer is used to record the force required to remove the dressing from the silicone block using a 180° peel.

Figure 22: Typical results of an adherency test

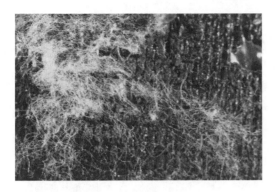 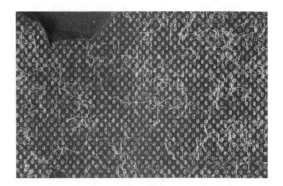

CONFORMABILITY

Dressings that are applied around joints or to other areas of tissue subject to movement or distortion must, to some degree, accommodate this without causing excess pressure, or in the case of adhesive products, shearing forces that can cause skin trauma.

Whilst products such as bandages tend to accommodate changes in body geometry fairly readily, products such as hydrocolloids, semipermeable film dressings and self-adhesive island dressings can sometimes cause clinical problems.[24] A test designed to assess the extensibility and permanent set conformability of primary wound dressings by measuring its extensibility and permanent set is described in BS EN 13726-4. In this test strips of dressing 25 mm wide with an effective test length of 100 mm are extended by 20% in a constant rate of traverse machine at 300 mm/min. The maximum load is recorded and the sample is held in this position for one minute. The sample is then allowed to relax for 300 seconds before being remeasured. Further samples taken from a direction perpendicular to the first are also tested in a similar way to account for any 'directionality' in the structure of the material. The standard requires that the test report records the maximum load, the extensibility and the permanent set which are calculated using the formulae provided

An alternative test method, which eliminates the problems of directionality by extending a sample in all directions at once, has been developed using a modification of the *Apparatus for the Measurement of Waterproofness* described in the British Pharmacopoeia 1993.

This consists of a chamber, open at one end, bearing a flange with an internal diameter of 50 mm. A retaining ring with the same internal diameter as the hole in the flange is mounted over the open end of the cylinder which can be lowered down onto the flange by means of a screw thread. A sample of the dressing under examination is placed on the flange and held firmly in place by means of the retaining ring.

During the course of this test, air is slowly forced into the chamber by means of a large syringe. The resultant rise in the pressure within the chamber causes the dressing to expand and form a hemisphere which gradually increases in size until the upper surface of the dressing comes into contact with a marker placed 20 mm above the dressing surface at the start of the test. This value is then recorded by means of a transducer.

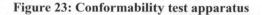

Figure 23: Conformability test apparatus

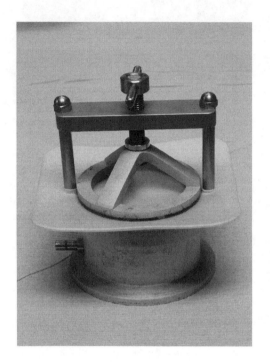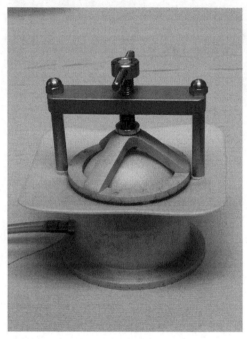

Photographs courtesy of P.Fram SMTL

In this test the conformability of a dressing is considered to be inversely proportional to the pressure required to deform it by a predetermined amount and is represented by the mean inflation pressure of the samples examined.

MICROBIOLOGICAL TESTS

Bacterial barrier tests

Wounds of all types represent a potential source of cross infection, particularly if they are infected with antibiotic resistant organisms such as MRSA. It is therefore important to ensure that, in so far as is possible, they are isolated from the environment to prevent the ingress or egress of pathogenic microorganisms.

Many dressings therefore consist of, or include in their construction, a layer which prevents the transmission of microorganisms into or out of a wound. Most commonly this layer consists of a piece of cast polyurethane film but sometimes closed cell foam is used for this purpose.

The ability of a bacterium to pass through a dressing depends upon the presence of a liquid pathway. For dry wounds a thick layer of absorbent cotton or gauze may be sufficient to prevent contamination but as soon as this becomes wet the barrier properties are lost and the dressing becomes useless in this regard. This property and its clinical significance were both demonstrated practically and discussed by Colebrook and Hood in 1947,[25] although they acknowledged that in a previous study conducted in 1943, Owens had shown it was possible to draw organisms through 64 layers of gauze. They proposed that this effect was responsible for episodes of cross-infection commonly encountered in hospitals around that time. They further suggested that the inclusion of a sheet of cellophane within the dressing should reduce or eliminate this problem.

It follows, therefore, that a test system is required for dressings designed to provide an effective bacterial barrier. Once again a method that has gained widespread acceptance was devised by SMTL which provides a stringent challenge to the material under test and thus represents the 'worst-case' scenario for the dressing.

In this test system, a sterile dressing is aseptically clamped between two sterile flanged hemispheres (closures of reactions vessels are typically used) such that the dressing is maintained in the vertical plane. A liquid microbiological medium is introduced into both chambers one side of which contains a heavy inoculum of a suitable test organism.

Figure 24: Bacterial barrier test

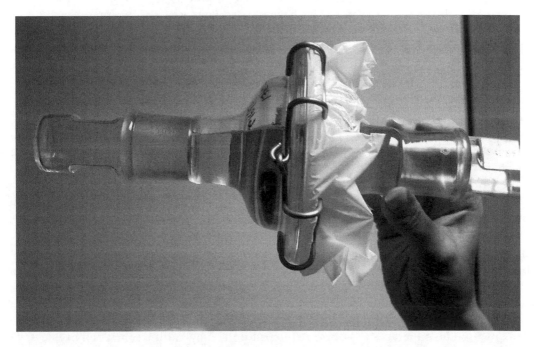

The apparatus is then incubated for an appropriate period after which the chamber containing the previously sterile nutrient solution is examined for evidence of growth. If no growth (turbidity) is detected, the test sample is considered to represent an effective bacterial barrier, but if signs of growth are present an aliquot of the solution is plated out to confirm that it is due to the test organism not extraneous environmental contamination or a failure of aseptic technique. This test is also currently being evaluated by the industry before being formally proposed as a new European Standard.

Antibacterial properties

Some dressings contain agents that have intrinsic antimicrobial activity such as antibiotics, antiseptics, silver ions or materials which posses a significant osmotic pressure capable of inhibiting bacterial growth. In clinical practice these materials are released from the dressing to exert an antibacterial effect. Such dressings are often recommended or promoted for the treatment or prevention of soft tissue infections.

Other products contain antimicrobials that are immobilised or fixed within the structure or the wound contact surface of the dressing, i.e. not released into the local wound environment. These materials are claimed simply to prevent the proliferation of microorganisms within the dressing itself. They have no direct upon the wound and as such are more suited for preventing cross infection than treating existing wound infections.

Tests for immobilised antimicrobial agents

A number of methods have been described for evaluating the antimicrobial properties of immobilized antimicrobial agents. A quantitative procedure for the evaluation of the degree of antibacterial activity of finishes on textile material has been published by the American Association of Textile Chemists and Colorists.[26] According to this method, swatches of test and control material are inoculated with the test organisms using sufficient test material to absorb the total volume of inoculum (1 ± 0.1 ml) leaving no free liquid. After incubation the samples are eluted with a suitable extractant containing a neutralizing agent and the number of viable organisms present in this solution determined using standard microbiological techniques.

Whilst this method may be appropriate for testing a homogeneous mass of material, it is not suitable for evaluating a structured product such as a dressing that has several different components of which only one, the wound contact layer for example, may have antimicrobial activity. Any bacterial suspension that is taken up by the non-medicated part of the dressing will remain unaffected by the antibacterial finish on the medicated portion thus greatly reducing the value of the procedure.

This deficiency in the method is noted in a standard test published by ASTM International,[27] which describes an alternative method which ensures good contact between the bacteria and treated substrate. It involves constant agitation of the test specimen in a bacterial suspension for a specified contact time after which the suspension is serially diluted and the number of remaining viable organism determined and compared with values obtained using an appropriate control or untreated sample. This method also includes a procedure to ensure that any antimicrobial activity detected is not caused by leaching of the active ingredient. An extract of the dressing is placed into an 8 mm hole in an agar plate inoculated with a test organism and the formation of a zone of inhibition around the well indicates the presence of leaching rendering the test invalid.

An alternative test, devised within the SMTL, graphically demonstrates the ability of a dressing to kill or inhibit the growth of microorganisms that come into contact with it and thereby prevent the transfer of contaminated material into or out of a wound.

In this test an agar plate has two channels cut out of it which effectively forms two separate agar blocks areas in the Petri dish. One of the agar blocks is sterile; the other is inoculated with the test organism. A strip of dressing under examination is placed on top of the two blocks forming a bridge across the intervening channel. Sterile water is place in the channel on the outer side of the contaminated agar to increase the water content of the gel and provide a 'driving force' to encourage the movement of moisture from the contaminated agar along or through the dressing to the sterile agar on the other side of the second channel. The Petri dish is incubated as normal with the dressings in place after which it is examined to detect the presence of growth around the margin of the test sample on the sterile agar surface.

Figure 25: Bacterial transfer test

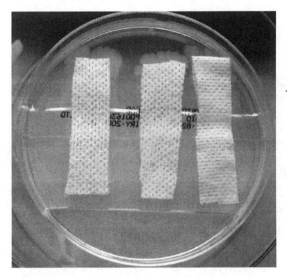

In the picture opposite it is possible to see how microorganisms have moved from the lower agar block, previously inoculated with he test bacteria, across the clear channel onto the surface of the sterile agar upper block. If the test samples have antimicrobial properties, the transfer of microorganism in this way is prevented.

A positive result in this test suggests that it is possible that microorganisms could be transported laterally out of a contaminated wound onto the surrounding skin, or potentially move in the opposite direction from the intact skin into the wound itself. No growth on the sterile agar suggests that the dressing does indeed have the ability to kill or prevent the growth of bacteria that come into contact with it.

Tests for antimicrobial agents released from dressings

For products that are designed to kill bacteria within the wound alternative test systems are required based upon the following considerations. The ability of an antimicrobial dressing to exert a beneficial clinical effect is dependent upon three factors:

- The nature and spectrum of activity of the agent concerned
- The concentration of the material present in the dressing
- The release characteristics (does the material actually get into the wound)

In its simplest form the test can consist of the application of a piece of dressing applied to an agar plate that has previously been seeded with the test organism. Antibacterial activity is indicated by the presence of a halo or zone of inhibition around the sample the size of which is determined at least in part by the concentration and solubility of the active ingredient. Such tests are easy to perform and can involve the use of different test organisms.[28-30]

Figure 26: Zone of inhibition, surface method

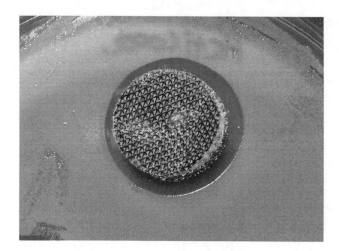

A well defined zone of inhibition of inhibition produced by a silver coated dressing confirms that silver ions have migrated out of the test sample.

A possible criticism of this type of simple test is that the moisture content of the agar may be insufficient to facilitate extraction of the active agent from the dressing, or that the affinity of the dressing for moisture may be such it effectively retains the moisture within its structure and thus limits the amount that is released onto the agar to exert an inhibitory effect. It is also possible that the active may require the presence of sodium or calcium ions normally present in exudate or serous fluid to release or activate the biocidal agent within the dressing. Both of these problems may be overcome by a modification to the method in which a well is cut in the agar plate into which the dressing sample is inserted. The residual volume within the well is then filled an appropriate test solution such as water, Solution A (as used in absorbency testing) or, for research purposes, calf or horse serum. Alternatively it is possible to make an extract of the dressing sample using an appropriate solution and place this into the well.

Figure 27: Zone of inhibition, well method

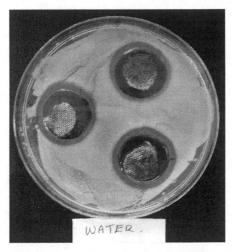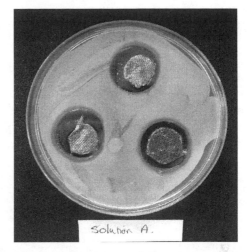

The test results shown in Figure 27 illustrate the importance of the choice of test solution. A markedly larger zone is present when water is used as the extractant compared with solution A. This point is discussed in detail in the chapter on silver dressings.

An alternative to the simple well method involves the production of a channel cut in an agar plate, previously seeded with the chosen test organism. A piece of the dressing under examination is laid across the channel onto the surface of the agar making sure that the test material is pushed down into the base of the channel which is then carefully filled with the chosen test solution. In this way the channel forms a reservoir which should prevent the dressing from drying out. Antimicrobial activity is indicated by a zone of inhibition as before.

Figure 28: Zone of inhibition, channel method

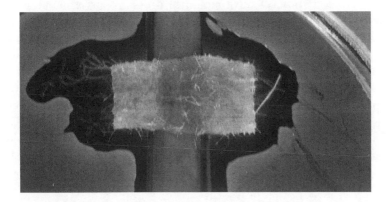

A further test involves the incubation of a piece of dressing with a suitable volume of a bacterial suspension containing a known number of microorganisms.

Following incubation, the dressing sample is extracted with an appropriate recovery medium and a total viable count performed on the extractant to determine the decrease in the number of viable organisms present. This test has the advantages that it can be conducted over various time intervals, and that it also provides a quantitative result. The tests have been described in detail previously, in laboratory-based comparisons of silver containing dressings.[31-32]

Unlike previous test systems, which gained fairly rapid acceptance by the industry enabling them to become adopted as official standards, it is more difficult to reach a consensus on tests for antimicrobial activity. Whilst there is a reasonable prospect of achieving agreement on the experimental techniques which can be used, there remains a problem in the interpretation of the results, the levels of activity that required clinically and therefore the limits which should be attached to each method.[33-36]

ODOUR CONTROL

Certain types of wounds such as pressure ulcers, leg ulcers and fungating (cancerous) lesions produce noxious odours caused by a cocktail of volatile agents produced by microorganisms. Numerous dressings have been developed to help address this problem, most of which contain activated charcoal in some form. The causes and treatment of wound odour are discussed in more detail in Chapter 17.

Despite the relatively widespread use of odour absorbing dressings, however, little objective comparative data is available on their odour and fluid handling characteristics. A number of possible test systems have been described,[37-39] but some of these have only considered the efficacy of the dressing in the dry state, the fluid handling properties of the dressing being considered separately.[40] This may be important because the presence of liquids particularly those containing organic solutes, may have implications for the performance of the activated charcoal, competing for active sites with the molecules responsible for the odour and thus reducing its effectiveness.

Previous workers have used both chemical,[37-39] and biological materials[41-42] to test the efficacy of odour adsorbing dressings. The former technique is often favoured as the efficiency of the dressing can be determined using standard analytical techniques such as gas liquid chromatography. Determination of dressing performance using biological materials is currently restricted to more subjective methods of assessment such as the use of a human test panel. Lawrence et al,[42] adopted this second approach when they compared the odour absorbing properties of five dressings containing activated charcoal with that of a cotton gauze swab, acting as a control.

A more objective test system that could be used to compare the ability of different dressings to prevent the passage of a volatile amine when applied to a wound model under simulated 'in-use' conditions was devised by SMTL. This apparatus consists of a stainless steel plate bearing a central recess 50 mm diameter about three mm deep into which is inset a removable perforated stainless steel disc and a disposable Millipore pre-filter. Fitted to the stainless steel plate is an airtight Perspex chamber with inlet and outlet ports. The dressing under examination is placed over the recess and sealed around the edges with impermeable plastic adhesive tape.

The test solution consists of Solution A to which is added 2% diethylamine and 10% newborn bovine serum

This test solution is applied to the dressing through the perforated plate at a rate of 30 ml/h by means of a syringe pump and the concentration of diethylamine in the air in the Perspex chamber is constantly monitored using a portable ambient infrared analyser linked to a data logger. The test is continued until the concentration of diethylamine present in the air above the dressing has risen to approximately 15 ppm. By relating the flow rate of test solution to the rate at which wounds normally exude, it is possible to use the apparatus to estimate the useful life of a dressing in the clinical environment.

Figure 29: Apparatus for testing odour absorbing dressings

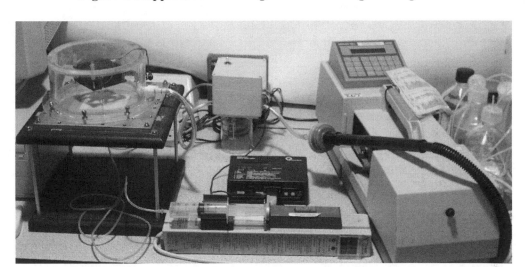

The test system was evaluated in an independent study which compare the odour absorbing properties of eight different dressings.[43] The authors concluded that although there were still shortcomings associated with the use of the technique related to the application and orientation of the test sample, it appears to be the best way of objectively ascertaining quantitative comparable data on the odour absorbing properties different dressing products.

BIOLOGICAL TESTS

Because dressings come into intimate contact with damaged tissue, blood or body fluids, it is important to ensure that they are free from any agents that can adversely effect wound healing or otherwise cause an adverse reaction within the wound. Detailed discussion of these test systems falls outside the scope of this book but some of the key parameter are summarized below.

Formal standards

The standard approach to testing medical devices is described in a formal standard BS EN ISO 10993. This standard is divided into 18 parts, each of which describes a particular type of test or procedure that may be relevant to specific types of medical devices. For topical wound dressings the most relevant parts are as follows.

Tests for 'in vitro' cytotoxicity

Part 5 of the standard,[44] describes test methods to assess the *in vitro* cytotoxicity of materials using techniques in which cultured cells (typically L-929 mouse fibroblasts) are either exposed to an extract of the test sample, or brought into intimate contact with the sample itself using an agar diffusion or filter diffusion method. Cytotoxicity is graded on a four point scale from non-toxic to severely cytotoxic according to the damage occasioned to the cell system used.

Tests for irritation and sensitization

Part 10 of the standard,[45] describes a technique in which extracts of the dressing are injected subcutaneously into multiple sites on the backs of rabbits following which the injection sites are examined visually for evidence of irritation (erythema and oedema) immediately and after 24, 48 and 72 hours.

The sensitization potential is determined by intradermally injecting and occlusively patch testing multiple sites on ten guinea pigs. The treated sites are examined visually for evidence of a skin reaction after 24, 48 and 72 hours.

REFERENCES

1. Lawrence JC. What materials for dressings? *Injury* 1982;13(6):500-12.
2. Piskozub ZT. The efficiency of wound dressing materials as a barrier to secondary bacterial contamination. *Br J Plast Surg* 1968;21(4):387-401.
3. Thomas S, Dawes C, Hay NP. Wound dressing materials - testing and control. *Pharmaceutical Journal* 1982;228:576-578.
4. Sprung P, Hou Z, Ladin DA. Hydrogels and hydrocolloids: an objective product comparison. *Ostomy Wound Manage* 1998;44(1):36-42, 44, 46 passim.
5. Thomas S. Observations on the fluid handling properties of alginate dressings. *Pharmaceutical Journal* 1992;248:850-851.
6. EN13726-2:2002 ES. Test methods for primary wound dressings. Moisture vapour transmission rate of permeable film dressings,.
7. Thomas S. Fluid handling properties of Allevyn foam dressing. *http://www.medetec.co.uk/Documents/Fluid%20handling%20properties%20of%20Allevyn%20foam%20dressing24-4-07.pdf* 2007.
8. Thomas S, Loveless P. A comparative study of the properties of twelve hydrocolloid dressings. *World Wide Wounds* 1998;247(17-Mar-1998).
9. Thomas S, Loveless P. Moisture vapour permeability of hydrocolloid dressings. *Pharmaceutical Journal* 1988;241:806.
10. Williams AA. Proficiency of contempory wound dressings. In: Turner TD, Brain KR, editors. *Surgical dressings in the hospital environment*. Cardiff: Surgical Dressings Research Unit, UWIST, Cardiff, 1975:163-179.
11. Anand SC, editor. An apparatus to measure the water absorption properties of fabrics and fibre assemblies. Medical Textile 96; 1997; Bolton. Woodhead Publishing Ltd Cambridge.
12. Ferrari F, Bertoni M, Carmella C, Maring MJ, Aulton ME. The hydration and transmission properties of hydrocolloid dressings over extended periods. *Pharmaceutical Technology Europe* 1993;November:28-32.
13. Ferrari F, Bertoni M, Caramella C, Waring MJ. Comparative evaluation of hydrocolloid dressings by means of water uptake and swelling force measurements:I. *International Journal of Pharmaceutics* 1994;112(1):29-36.
14. Ferrari F, Bertoni M, Bonferoni MC, Rossi S, Caramella C, Waring MJ. Comparative evaluation of hydrocolloid dressings by means of water uptake and swelling force measurements: II. *International Journal of Pharmaceutics* 1995;117(1):49-55.
15. Ferrari F, Bertoni M, Rossi S, Bonferoni MC, Caramella C, Waring MJ, et al. Comparative rheomechanical and adhesive properties of two hydrocolloid dressings: Dependence on the degree of hydration. *Drug Development and Industrial Pharmacy* 1996;22(12):1223-1230.
16. Lanel B, Barthes-Biesel D, Regnier C, Chauve T. Swelling of hydrocolloid dressings. *Biorheology* 1997;34(2):139-53.
17. Thomas S, Fram P. The development of a novel technique for predicting the exudate handling properties of modern wound dressings. *Journal of Tissue Viability* 2001;11(4):145-160.
18. Lamke LO, Nilsson GE, Reithner HL. The evaporative water loss from burns and water vapour permeability of grafts and artificial membranes used in the treatment of burns. *Burns* 1977;3:159-165.

19. Thomas S, Fear M, Humphreys J, Disley L, Waring MJ. The effect of dressings on the production of exudate from venous leg ulcers. *Wounds* 1996;8(5):145-149.

20. Thomas S, Hay NP. Assessing the hydro-affinity of hydrogel dressings. *Journal of Wound Care* 1994;3(2):89-92.

21. Thomas S, Hay P. Fluid handling properties of hydrogel dressings. *Ostomy Wound Manage* 1995;41(3):54-6, 58-9.

22. Thomas S, Hay NP. In vitro investigations of a new hydrogel dressing. *Journal of Wound Care* 1996;5(3):130-131.

23. Moffatt C. The principles of assessment prior to compression therapy. *Journal of Wound Care* 1998;7(7):suppl 6-9.

24. Ravenscroft MJ, Harker J, Buch KA. A prospective, randomised, controlled trial comparing wound dressings used in hip and knee surgery: Aquacel and Tegaderm versus Cutiplast. *Ann R Coll Surg Engl* 2006;88(1):18-22.

25. Colebrook L, Hood AM. Infection through soaked dressings. *Lancet* 1948;2(6531):682.

26. AATCC Test Method 100 - 2004 Antibacterial Finishes on Textile Materials: Assessment of. North Carolina: American Association of Textile Chemists and Colorists, 1999.

27. ASTM E 2149-101 Standard Test Method for determining the antimicrobial activity of immobilised antimicrobial agents under dynamic contact conditions. Pennsylvania: ASTM International, 2001.

28. Thomas S, Russell AD. An in vitro evaluation of Bactigras, a tulle dressing containing chlorhexidine. *Microbios Letters* 1976;2:169-177.

29. Thomas S. An experimental evaluation of a chlorhexidine medicated tulle gras dressing, (letter). *J. Hosp. Infect.* 1982;3:399-400.

30. Thomas S, Dawes C, Hay NP. Improvements in medicated tulle dressings. *J. Hospital Infection* 1983;4:391-398.

31. Thomas S, McCubbin P. A comparison of the antimicrobial effects of four silver-containing dressings on three organisms. *Journal of Wound Care* 2003;12(3):101-107.

32. Thomas S, McCubbin P. An in vitro analysis of the antimicrobial properties of 10 silver-containing dressings. *Journal of Wound Care* 2003;12(8):305-8.

33. Lansdown AB, Jensen K, Jensen MQ. Contreet Foam and Contreet Hydrocolloid: an insight into two new silver-containing dressings. *Journal of Wound Care* 2003;12(6):205-10.

34. Lansdown AB. Silver-containing dressings: have we got the full picture? *Journal of Wound Care* 2003;12(8):317; author reply 317-8.

35. Thomas S, McCubbin P. Silver dressings: the debate continues. *Journal of Wound Care* 2003;12(10):420.

36. Thomas S, Ashman P. *In-vitro* testing of silver containing dressings. *Journal of Wound Care* 2004;13(9):392-393.

37. Schmidt RJ, Shrestha T, Turner TD. An assay procedure to compare sorptive capacities of activated carbon dressings: the detection of impregnation with silver. *J. Pharm. Pharmacol* 1988;40:662-664.

38. A test method for quantifying absorbtive capacities of intact charcoal-containing wound management products. Proceedings of the 7th European Conference on Advances in Wound Management
1997; Harrogate UK.

39. Determination of malodour reduction performance in various charcoal containing dressings. Proceedings of the 7th European Conference on Advances in Wound Management, Harrogate, U.K.; 1997; Harrogate, U.K.

40. Investigation into the fluid handling characteristics of various charcoal containing dressings. Proceedings of the 7th European Conference on Advances in Wound Management, Harrogate, U.K.; 1997; Harrogate, U.K.

41. An investigation into the selective adsorption of malodour molecules onto charcoal containing dressings. Proceedings of the 7th European Conference on Advances in Wound Management, Harrogate, U.K.; 1997; Harrogate, U.K.

42. Harding KG, Cherry G, Dealey C, Turner TD, editors. Malodour and dressings containing active charcoal,. Proceedings of the 2nd European Conference on Advances in Wound Management; 1992; Harrogate, U.K. Macmillan magazines Ltd.

43. Lee G, Anand SC, Rajendran S, Walker I. Efficacy of commercial dressings in managing malodorous wounds. *Br J Nurs* 2007;16(6):S14, S16, S18-20.

44. BS EN ISO 10993-5:2003 Biological evaluation of medical devices - Test methods for primary wound dressings - Part 5: Tests for in vitro cytotoxicity. London: BSI, 1999.

45. BS EN ISO 10993-10:2003 Biological evaluation of medical devices - Part 10:Tests for irritation and sensitization. London: BSI, 1999.

8. Low-adherent dressings

IMPREGNATED FABRIC DRESSINGS

Early impregnated fabric dressings

As previously described, the application of simple fabric dressings, such as gauze, to a lightly exuding wound can lead to problems of adherence. Historically this problem was addressed by the production of various types of fabrics impregnated with oils or waxes to create a greasy dressing which was less likely to stick to the surface of an open wound. This hydrophobic coating also imparted a secondary benefit, helping to retain moisture within the wound. An early medical text,[1] published in 1766, describes the technique for producing one such preparation thus.

> 'Melt four Ounces of white Wax; add to it, if made in Winter, two Spoonfuls of oil; if in Summer none at all, or at most, not above a Spoonful. Dip in this Slips of Linen Cloth not worn too thin, and let them dry: or spread it thin and evenly over them.'

In 1915, during World War I, the prolific inventor, Lumière, developed 'Tulle gras ', gauze fabric impregnated with paraffin and Balsalm of Peru, and in 1916, an article in the British Medical Journal entitled 'Fried Wound Dressings' described a similar impregnated dressing which was produced by immersing gauze in a pail of lard heated to 300 - 400°F. Dressings impregnated with paraffin gauze dressings were later manufactured commercially, packed in flat tins and sterilized by dry heat.

Balsalm of Peru was originally included in the formulation as an antiseptic but was later omitted when it was shown to be responsible for marked skin reactions in about 0.25% of patients.[2]

Elliot,[3] in an interesting account of the history of tulle gras, described how many hospital pharmacies prepared their own from net curtain, which was washed, dried, cut into pieces, and packed in flat 50-cigarette tins, prior to the application of the paraffin base and eventual sterilization.

By the 1930s, Tulle gras had become very popular, and in 1949 it became the subject of a monograph in the British Pharmaceutical Codex. The original form of the dressing contained not less than 175 grams of paraffin base per square metre of cloth, but this was found to be occlusive, sometimes causing maceration of the wound or the periwound skin. An alternative preparation was therefore developed with a lower loading, bearing between 90-130 g/m^2 of paraffin. This preparation is usually presented individually wrapped, and is the version most commonly used for routine wound management. The fabric with the higher loading of paraffin is sometimes presented in bulk and is often used during plastic surgery for transferring skin grafts from donor to recipient sites. Both formulations formed the subject of monographs in the British Pharmacopoeia.

Winter was not a great advocate for the use of paraffin gauze dressings.[4] He reported that; 'The impregnated greasy mass is too mobile at wound surface temperature with the result that the coarsely woven fabric tends to sink into the exposed tissue. The epidermis migrating across the wound surface immediately beneath the dressing wanders into the interstices of the fabric and in consequence some adhesion results through growth of tissue into the dressing. Epidermal regeneration is uneven.' (Figure 30) He also stated that; 'Particles of cotton tend to detach from the dressing and become embedded in the epidermis and the sub-epidermal connective tissue where they provoke a foreign body giant cell and macrophage reaction.'

Figure 30: A shallow pig wound treated with paraffin gauze dressing for three days

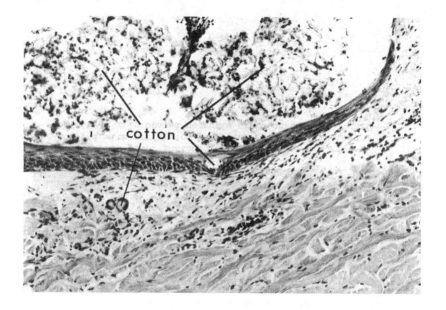

Note the epidermis migrating upwards around the bundles of cotton fibres.[6]

---

[6] Reproduced from Winter 1975 with permission

The 'official' tulles are made from gauze of leno weave which is said to impart stability to the fabric but other 'non-official' versions of paraffin gauze are produced using a fabric of plain weave some of which are finer and potentially less likely to cause problems of adherence. Examples of paraffin gauze dressings that comply with the BP monograph include:

- Cuticell Classic (high loading)
- Jelonet (high loading)
- Neotulle (high loading)
- Paranet (light loading)
- Paragauze (loading not known)

Examples of other 'non-official' types of paraffin gauze include:

- Lomatuell
- Branolind
- Vaseline Petrolatum Gauze

The popularity of the standard paraffin gauze dressings is declining and few wound care practitioners, with the possible exception of burns and plastics units, use them routinely for the management of extensive or problem wounds. Nevertheless, numerous papers have been published describing their use as comparators or controls in clinical studies involving other products such as alginates or hydrogels. Many of the publications are described in the following chapters.

Second-generation impregnated fabrics

In addition to the simple paraffin-impregnated fabrics, a number of dressings have been developed that consist of an open fabric impregnated with a more complex ointment base.

Adaptic consists of an apertured cellulose acetate fabric coated with a petrolatum emulsion. Primarily intended for use as a treatment for superficial wounds, it is also available in strip form for packing boils abscesses, fistulae and other draining wounds. The use of this formulation has also been described for packing following nasal surgery.[5]

Further examples of modified paraffin gauze-type dressings include three products from Hartmann. Grassolind comprises white Vaseline, fatty acid diglycerol esters of carbonate and bicarbonate, and synthetic wax. Atrauman contains an ester mixture of natural or vegetable fatty acids, bound as di- and triglycerides and Hydrotul consists of an ester mixture of natural or vegetable fatty acids, bound as di- and triglycerides containing hydrocolloid (CMC) particles.

Urgotul consists of a polyester textile mesh coated with a combination of a hydrocolloid mass, petroleum jelly and cohesion polymers. On contact with wound exudate, the hydrocolloid particles gel and interact with the petroleum jelly component to form a so called 'lipido-colloid' contact layer which creates conditions claimed to favour the healing process.

Initial clinical experience with new impregnated fabric dressings

Efficacy and safety of Urgotul was investigated in a multicentre non-comparative trial involving 92 patients with a variety of wound types who were treated for a maximum of four weeks.[6] During this period, 11/34 (32.4%) of the acute wounds, 3/24 (12.5%) leg ulcers and 2/14 (14.3%) of other chronic wounds healed completely. The wound areas decreased on average by 76.4%, 63.5% and 44.2% at study endpoint respectively. When applied to burns, 19 (95%) of wounds healed within 5-19 days. A total of 771 dressing changes were performed during the course of the study which were rated as 'easy' or 'very easy' in 90% of cases. Safety and patient acceptability were considered good; with five reports of a transitory local adverse event assumed to be dressing related being observed. Two patients (2.2%) prematurely stopped treatment because of moderate periwound erythema.

A second qualitative, descriptive, non-comparative study involving 27 hospital patients supported these initial findings with regard to ease of application, conformability and non-adherence, absence of trauma pain and bleeding on removal, with minimal maceration of the surrounding skin and odour.[7]

In plastic surgery

The use of Urgotul in the management of burns and skin graft donor sites was evaluated in a more formal manner in a prospective clinical study in 25 patients.[8] Two separate burn or donor sites on each patient were dressed with Urgotul or paraffin gauze dressing (PG) as a control, and covered with standard secondary dressings.

Wounds were assessed objectively by two reviewers, and patients' subjective assessments were also recorded. Mean time to complete epithelialization was 9.6 and 11.9 days for the Urgotul and PG sites respectively ($p < 0.05$). At first dressing change, bleeding was noted in 52% of Urgotul dressed wounds compared with 100% of wounds dressed with paraffin gauze ($p < 0.05$). Dressing changes were also significantly less painful with Urgotul. Patients reported 'moderate pain' in 22% and 57% of changes with Urgotul and paraffin gauze respectively ($p < 0.05$); with 35% of paraffin gauze treated wounds described as 'very painful' requiring extra analgesia.

In paediatrics

The low adherence and pain free nature of Urgotul make it a potentially useful treatment for paediatric patients. This was investigated in two non-comparative multicentre prospective studies conducted in France and Germany.[9]

A total of 100 patients were recruited from 16 centres and followed up for four weeks. Seventy wounds (55 burns and 15 other wounds) from France and 30 from Germany (22 burns and eight other wounds) were evaluated by nursing staff at every dressing change and by the medical investigator on a weekly basis. In the French study population, 86% of the burns (superficial and deep partial-thickness) and 53% of the other wounds healed completely within the four weeks. Figures for the German study population were 100% and 88% respectively. Pain was evaluated using pain scales adapted to the patient's age (objective pain scale, faces scale for pain and a visual analogue scale) at each dressing change. In each case dressing removal was non-traumatic, inducing very limited pain. Minor local adverse events were reported in four children. The authors concluded that Urgotul is not only efficacious, but also well-tolerated and accepted by children with acute and chronic wounds.

For epidermolysis bullosa

Equally positive results were obtained when Urgotul was assessed in the management of 20 patients (11 adults and nine children) with epidermolysis bullosa.[10]

Patients were eligible for inclusion if they presented with at least one skin lesion requiring management with a non-adherent wound dressing. Lesions were treated with the study dressing for a maximum of four weeks. Wound parameters, pain and effect on quality of life were recorded at each dressing change. All patients completed the trial and during the treatment period 19/20 wounds healed within 8.7 ± 8.5 days. The use of the dressing was considered to have improved the quality of life of 11 patients. It was said to be pain free and 'very easy' or 'easy' to remove at most dressing changes.

In traumatic wounds

The role of Urgotul in the treatment of traumatic digital wounds was described by Ma et al.,[11] following a randomized controlled trial involving 28 patients (16 treated with Urgotul and 12 with gauze), who had injuries to their fingers resulting in loss of tissue. Patients in the experimental group experienced faster healing than those in the control group ($p = 0.024$).

In leg ulcers

The value of Urgotul in the treatment of leg ulcers was reported in two studies. In the first,[12] 36 subjects with venous ulcers were treated with Urgotul and the K-Four multilayer compression bandaging system for a maximum of 12 weeks.

During this time 50% of wounds healed and those which did not, achieved almost 50% reduction in area during this period. As before the dressing was judged to be easy to apply and remove, and largely pain-free and non-adherent in use.

In the second ulcer study, the first reported randomized control trial involving Urgotul, the efficacy, tolerance and acceptability of the dressing was compared with that of Duoderm in the management of venous or mixed-aetiology leg ulcers in a prospective multicentre randomized phase IV study.[13] In total, 91 patients were recruited in 20 centres. Subjects presenting with non-infected, non-malignant leg ulcers which were predominantly venous in origin (ABPI > 0.8) with a surface area of between 4 cm^2 and 40 cm^2 were admitted to the study. Ulcer duration ranged from three to 18 months. Of the 91 patients, 47 were randomized to treatment with Urgotul and 44 to Duoderm. Baseline patient demographic data and wound characteristics were comparable in the two groups. After eight weeks of treatment wound area had reduced by a mean of 61.3% in the Urgotul group and 52.1% in the Duoderm group. This difference was not significant. Dressings were changed more frequently with the hydrocolloid (2.54 ± 0.57 times per week, *vs* 2.31 ± 0.45 in the Urgotul group, (p = 0.047). Thirty-three local adverse events were recorded in 27 patients: ten in the Urgotul group and 23 in the control (p = 0.039). Pain on removal, maceration and odour were significantly better in the Urgotul group (p < 0.0001).

In negative pressure treatment

Urgotul was also evaluated as an interface layer in patients receiving topical negative pressure (TNP) therapy in a prospective multicentre non-comparative open-label trial. It was judged that the use of the interface dressing in combination with TNP substantially reduced the pain caused by dressing changes.[14]

Results of *in vitro* studies

In an in vitro study,[15] the effect of Urgotul: vs Mepitel in vitro studies on normal human dermal fibroblast proliferation was compared with that of Mepitel and Tulle gras in a cell culture system in which cell proliferation was measured by the extent of thymidine incorporation into the replicating DNA of fibroblasts in contact with the complete dressing.

The morphology and ultrastructure of the cells was also investigated by immuno-labelling and confocal laser microscopy. It was reported that only Urgotul significantly stimulated thymidine incorporation, with a maximal proliferative effect after a contact time of 48 hours. This observation was confirmed by the presence of a greater number of dividing cells (mitotic cells) than in the control cultures. No cytotoxicity was observed following treatment with this dressing and the cells exhibited normal structural and ultrastructural features. It was suggested that these findings might at least partially explain the beneficial effects reported in previous clinical studies.

In a more recent development, the Urgotul low adhesive matrix has been supplemented by the addition of a so-called nano-oligosaccharide factor (NOSF), a compound with a structure derived from the oligosaccharide family which are known to inhibit metalloproteinase (MMP) activity. These agents, when present in excess, are known to cause degradation of the extracellular matrix, thereby delaying healing. Furthermore, laboratory studies suggest that the NOSF significantly stimulates fibroblast proliferation thereby potentially accelerating wound healing. The new version of Urgotul which contains the modified formulation is called Urgotul Start and the same wound contact layer is also applied to a semipermeable absorbent polyurethane foam dressing called Urgocell Start.[16]

Medicated impregnated fabric dressings

It was recognized very early on that the ointment applied to a dressing fabric could act as a carrier for a range of medicaments. Early examples included a penicillin impregnated tulle and 'M&M' Tulle which contained cod liver oil BP 23% w/w, purified honey BPC 23% w/w, and hexachlorophane BP 0.05% w/w.

Local anaesthetic agents, sulphonamides, or other chemicals were also incorporated into dressings to promote healing, or control or prevent infection. However, when it was realised that the topical use of antibiotics for the treatment of trivial conditions could lead to the emergence of resistant strains of microorganisms, and also cause sensitivity reactions in some patients, the use of tulle dressings containing these materials declined.

Framycetin tulle dressing

As a general guide, it was recommended that antibiotics that were used systemically should not be applied to the skin,[17] although those that were too toxic or unsuitable for systemic administration continued to be produced. One such product was Framycetin Gauze Dressing BP, known as Sofra-Tulle, a white soft paraffin basis containing 10% anhydrous lanolin and framycetin sulphate 1%.

Framycetin is a broad-spectrum antibiotic which is active against both Gram-positive and Gram-negative bacteria, including common skin pathogens such as *S. aureus*, *Escherichia coli* and *P. aeruginosa*. Framycetin, which consists mainly of neomycin B, was first isolated in 1947 and was used primarily in ophthalmology, where it was found to be particularly effective against staphylococcal infections.

The tulle preparation was developed some time later; its use in the treatment of wounds was first investigated in the early 1960s,[18-20] when it was claimed to reduce the risk of sepsis and promote healing. Similar beneficial results were reported after its use in the treatment of superficial and deep dermal burns,[21-22] and a variety of minor wounds in general practice.[23] The development of Sofra-Tulle was been described in detail by Wicks and Peterson.[24] Although many of the early reports on the use of framycetin stated that the material did not cause hypersensitivity reactions, Kirton and Munro-Ashman[25] reported that they had encountered 70 cases of contact dermatitis due to neomycin or framycetin over a two year-period, and argued that neither of these materials should be used without definite indications and, even then, not for extended periods.

Fucidin tulle dressing

Fucidin-Intertulle consists of a cotton gauze fabric impregnated with white soft paraffin and lanolin containing 2% sodium fusidate, an antibiotic which is highly active against *S. aureus* (including strains that are resistant to other antibiotics). Sodium fusidate is unusual in that it is able to penetrate intact skin; in the form of a dressing, it has been recommended for the treatment of ulcers, skin grafts and burns infected with susceptible organisms.

Unlike Sofra-Tulle, Fucidin-Intertulle does not appear to cause skin sensitization,[26-27] but it was suggested that the topical use of sodium fusidate on its own may lead to the development of bacterial resistance which could be very important in view of its value in the systemic treatment of serious infections, including osteomyelitis and intracranial abscesses. For this reason this preparation was discontinued in the United Kingdom in 2001 although it still remains available elsewhere.

Because of the problems of skin sensitivity and bacterial resistance associated with the topical use of antibiotics, some manufacturers produced dressings containing other well proven antimicrobial agents.

Chlorhexidine tulle dressing

Bactigras consists of a gauze fabric impregnated with yellow soft paraffin containing 0.5% chlorhexidine acetate, a potent antimicrobial agent which is active against a wide range of microorganisms.[28]

Chlorhexidine does not appear to readily induce bacterial resistance in normal use and has a low reported incidence of skin sensitization.[29] It is strongly bound to cellulose materials, such as cotton or viscose, and its antimicrobial activity is reduced in the presence of blood and pus.[30]

Despite the apparent advantages of chlorhexidine, the likely clinical effectiveness of Bactigras was questioned, following a series of in-vitro tests which suggested that chlorhexidine acetate, present in the basis as a dispersed powder, is not easily extracted from the dressing by serum or wound exudate and is therefore not readily available to exert an antimicrobial effect.[31-32] Other workers claimed that, despite these unsatisfactory laboratory test results, the dressing does appear to be effective in preventing the colonization of experimental burns,[33] although the issue remained the subject of some debate.[33-34]

Clinical experience with Bactigras suggested that the dressing may be of some value in the treatment of non-infected minor burns as a prophylactic agent against the growth of bacteria.[35] The dressing forms the subject a monograph in the British Pharmacopoeia entitled Chlorhexidine Gauze Dressing.

Other medicated tulle-type dressings

Dressings containing other antimicrobial agents have also been developed. Inadine consists of a knitted viscose fabric impregnated with polyethylene glycol (PEG) containing 10% povidone-iodine, equivalent to 1% available iodine. The use of a hydrophilic basis facilitates the extraction of povidone-iodine by serum or exudate, which imparts pronounced, though short-term, antibacterial activity to the dressing.[32] The use of PEG has the additional advantage that, should the dressing adhere to the wound, it may be removed by irrigation with sterile water or normal saline.

Other medicated dressings include Xeroform, which contains 3% bismuth tribromophenate in a paraffin ointment base and Xeroflow which also contains 3% bismuth tribromophenate in a bland oil emulsion.

In one American study, epithelial cell proliferation in donor sites was determined by measuring the uptake of tritium-labelled thymidine by regenerating epithelial cell DNA. They found that healing rates of wounds dressed with Xeroform and Scarlet red dressing (o -tolylazo-o-tolylazo-2-naphthol in a blend of lanolin, olive oil and soft paraffin), a formulation that was said to promote the growth of epithelium, were statistically superior at 48 hours to those obtained with more conventional treatments such as Betadine, fine mesh gauze and air exposure.[36] In contrast, the authors of a second study, which also included both Xeroform and Scarlet Red Ointment Dressing, and which was similarly designed to determine the clinical effectiveness of a range of impregnated dressings on the healing rate of donor sites, concluded that the rate and quality of healing of all wounds were virtually the same, regardless of the type of dressing used.[37]

Silver-containing tulle-type dressings

More recent developments include impregnated fabrics containing silver. Like the basic Urgotul, Urgotul SSD comprises a polyester mesh impregnated with hydrocolloid particles dispersed in a petroleum jelly matrix to which has been added silver sulphadiazine. This preparation was evaluated in a national multicentre phase III non-comparative open-label prospective study involving ten burns units. Forty one adults with second-degree thermal burn $< 500 \text{ cm}^2$ in area and under 24 hours old for whom SSD treatment was considered appropriate, were followed for four weeks. Of the 41 patients, 24 healed within a mean of 10.8 days and 13 had a skin graft on the study burn within a mean of 11.5 days. There were four premature study withdrawals. Mean dressing wear time was 1.73 days and none of the subjects acquired a secondary infection. *S. aureus* was isolated from one patient. The authors concluded that the dressing was well accepted by patients and clinicians alike and produced a good clinical outcome.

The cytotoxicity of Urgotul SSD was compared with that of other silver containing dressings (see later) using a monolayer cell culture technique, a tissue explant culture model, and a mouse excisional wound model. Under the conditions of test, Urgotul SSD demonstrated the least cytotoxicity in the cell culture model which correlated with the silver released from the dressings as measured by silver concentration in the culture medium. In the tissue explant culture model, in which the epidermal cell proliferation was evaluated, all silver dressings resulted in a significant delay of reepithelialization and in the mouse excisional wound model, inhibition of wound reepithelialization on the seventh day post wounding was noted with two of the comparator dressings.

ALTERNATIVE FORMS OF LOW-ADHERENT DRESSINGS

In the United Kingdom in the early part of the 20th Century, impregnated gauze rapidly replaced ordinary gauze as the primary wound dressing of choice for relatively shallow wounds, but plain gauze or ribbon gauze continued to be employed for packing cavity wounds and sinuses – an indication for which paraffin gauze and the other alternative types of low-adherent dressings was not appropriate.

Although formulations based upon paraffin-impregnated gauze dressings were generally considered to be of low adherence (particularly by surgeons), it was not uncommon for patients to experience considerable pain when these were removed. In some instances, this was severe enough to require the use of narcotic analgesics such as pethidine or morphine.[38] Often removal of a dressing led to additional trauma to the surface of the wound causing bleeding or removal of new epidermal tissue.

Nevertheless, paraffin gauze dressings continued to be used in very significant numbers until the latter part of the 20th Century when they were largely replaced as the product of choice by more effective 'low-adherent' wound contact materials including, in the 1980s, gel-forming products made from alginate fibre which could be easily removed from wounds by irrigation with saline solution (see later). These new low-adherent materials which came in many forms as described below could either be used as 'stand alone' dressings or as facing layers for absorbent dressing pads.

Plastic film-faced dressings

These included heat-calendared non-woven fabrics containing hydrophobic fibres which fuse together during heat treatment to form a discontinuous plastic layer but the most familiar products of this type have a simple fibrous absorbent layer covered on one or two sides with a perforated plastic film.

In most products, such as Melolin, shown on the left, the perforated plastic film is clearly identifiable as such, but in the case of Release, on the right, the film is textured to make it resemble a woven fabric.

Figure 31: Examples of perforated plastic film dressings

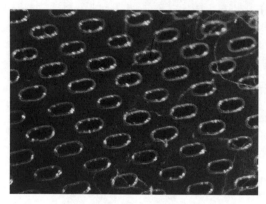 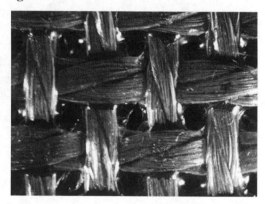

Careful control over the manufacturing process is required during the manufacture of these plastic films to ensure product consistency. At one time, during routine monitoring of dressing supplied to the NHS in the UK, one product was identified which showed an unacceptable degree of batch variation in the pore sizes (Figure 32).

**Figure 32: Batch variation in a perforated
film dressing**

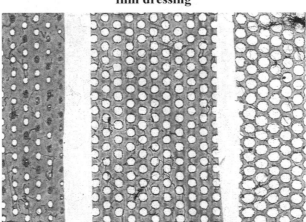

The perforated film dressings are usually indicated for the management of minor injuries and superficial lightly exuding wounds. They are not generally applied to leg ulcers or other lesions producing quantities of viscous exudate, as this may be unable to pass through the pores in the dressing - leading to maceration of the skin or, occasionally, the production of an inflammatory reaction. Examples include:

- Askina Pad
- Drisorb
- Interpose
- Release
- Skintact
- Solvaline N
- Melolin
- Telfa

Sometimes the plastic wound contact layer is provided without an integral absorbent layer. Telfa Clear is a thin polyester (polyethylene terephthalate) film perforated with holes that are claimed to permit the passage of exudate but prevent the ingress of larger epithelial buds. Dermanet from Deroyal is manufactured from a sheet of high density polyethylene which is extruded, patterned and then stretched causing the film to rupture in a predetermined way forming a series of polymer 'dots' connected by fine polymer strands with multiple small apertures, giving the dressing a lace-like appearance.

Both of these materials provide the clinician with the opportunity to use a secondary absorbent layer of their choice. They also allow this secondary layer to be changed without necessarily disturbing the wound contact layer. According to Edwards,[39] Telfa Clear may also be used with a variety of creams and ointments and can be of value in the treatment of burns, offering advantages over more commonly used treatments such as Jelonet and Flamazine. Examples of the some of various types of perforated film dressings are shown below.

Winter,[4] demonstrated in his pig work that even these so called low-adherent dressings can stick to a wound under certain conditions and that the length of time that the dressing is left on the wound is critical in this regard. He found 'Melolin to be non-adherent on the third day but strongly adherent by the seventh day', concluding that 'This happens when the columns of exudate connecting the dressing to the wound surface become dry, Removal at this stage causes fresh bleeding and disrupts the newly regenerated epidermis.

Histological studies (Figure 33) show that the wound surface is protected under the film but there are regular patches of secondary damage to the dermis caused by dehydration opposite the perforations.'

Figure 33: A shallow wound treated with a perforated plastic film dressing for three days.

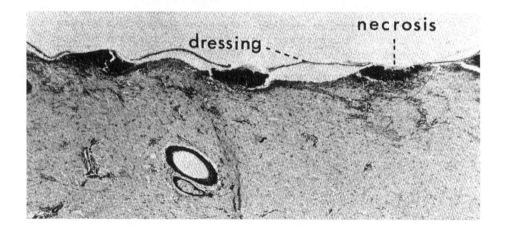

Note regularly spaced necrotic areas on the wound surface[7]

The early use of Melolin for the treatment of donor sites was described in an early study by Robb,[40] and Schumacher *et al.*,[41] who used it with sterile Bepanthen ointment as a postoperative dressing following urethral reconstruction in 30 male patients. The dressing was cut individually for each patient and retained with a cohesive elastic bandage and three cutaneous stitches. The dressings were left it in place for nine days. The authors reported that complete removal of the wound dressing was possible with no problems, although a chamomile-water bath was necessary in two cases.

---

[7] Reproduced from Winter 1975 with permission

Despite these early favourable reports, most practitioners would not now use these types of products for such indications, but restrict their use to the management of minor injuries and sutured wounds. For these applications they are often used to form the absorbent pad of self adhesive island dressings.

Knitted viscose primary dressing

Recognizing that impregnated dressings can sometimes cause maceration of the wound or surrounding skin due their occlusive nature, a simple knitted fabric was introduced which was designed to eliminate this problem.

Figure 34: Knitted viscose primary dressing

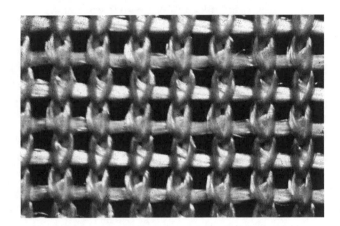

The construction of the fabric is such that the resultant dressing has a three dimensional structure which, the manufacturers claimed, helped to prevent it becoming incorporated into a wound or scab. This material was soon characterized by a monograph in the BP and numerous brands became available which include;

- Cestra Primary
- N-A Dressing
- Paratex
- Setoprime
- Tricotex

Relatively few clinical studies have been performed on these dressings *per se*, but they are sometimes used as comparators in clinical trials of newer or more advanced dressings. In one well known study,[42] N-A Dressing was compared with a hydrocolloid dressing in the treatment of 56 patients with chronic venous ulcers.

The authors reported no difference between the two groups, with complete healing in 21 out of 28 (75%) of occlusive dressing patients and 22 out of 28 (78%) with N-A dressings by 12 weeks leading them to conclude that; 'Careful graduated compression bandaging achieves healing even in the majority of so-called resistant chronic venous ulcers; there was no additional benefit from applying occlusive dressings which tend to be expensive.' This study was influential in the development of the 'Four Layer Bandaging System' in which the Knitted Viscose Primary Dressing forms the first layer.

Similar finding were obtained when Tricotex was compared with a hydrogel dressing (Intrasite) to compare the time to healing of moist desquamation after radiotherapy to the head-and-neck, breast, or anorectal areas in 357 patients.[43] The fabric dressing was either used alone or applied with the gel. Of the 357 patients, 100 (28%) developed moist desquamation. The time to healing was significantly prolonged in patients assigned to gel dressings and no evidence was found that gel dressings had a significant impact on subjectively reported skin symptoms.

The use of these simple knitted dressings as comparators in clinical studies will be discussed in more detail in the relevant chapters which follow.

Viscose silk

Ete has a wound contact layer of fine smooth rayon (viscose) silk stitched with a non absorbent polyester thread to an absorbent core of soft viscose wadding. The smooth surface of the fabric is claimed to reduce adherence whilst facilitating the transfer of exudate into the inner core of the dressing.

Foam dressings

In an attempt to overcome some of perceived problems associated with gauze and other fibrous materials, some manufacturers began to investigate the use of foam as a wound contact layer with mixed success. A more detailed account of the development of foam dressings is given in a later chapter.

Nylon mesh

Tegaderm Contact, formerly Tegapore, consists of a woven polyamide (nylon) net which is hot rolled to produce a uniform material with a precisely defined fibre diameter forming pores 90 microns across. These pores are large enough to permit the passage of exudate but too small to allow the ingress of granulation tissue. The dressing acts as a low adherence wound contact layer, allowing the passage of exudate from the wound to a secondary absorbent placed upon the outer surface. This secondary layer may be changed as often as required, but when applied correctly, in intimate contact with the wound surface, the primary dressing can be left in place for extended periods. Available in large pieces, Tegaderm Contact is used to dress full or partial thickness wounds of all types which may also be treated with topical preparations without first removing the nylon mesh.

Figure 35: Tegaderm Contact

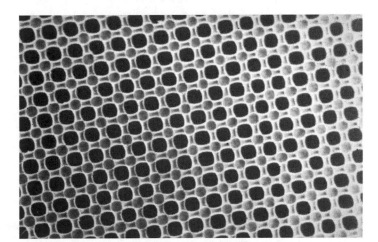

Aluminium-coated dressings

The use of aluminium foil as a wound dressing was first described in the late 1940s, and a few papers made reference to its use through the 1970s.[44-51] One early publication even described the use of aluminium powder as a treatment for burns.[52] The use of foil was very uncomfortable, so an attempt was made to overcome this problem by applying a thin coating of metallic aluminium to textile fibres which were then used to make up the wound contact surface of a dressing. Metalline, developed in 1957, consists of an absorbent pad faced with a layer of non-woven tissue onto which is vacuum deposited a thin layer of aluminium.

Figure 36: Metalline tracheostomy dressing

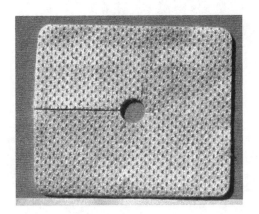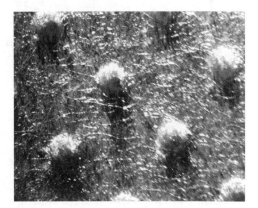

The dressing is available in a range of sizes and is sometimes used as a bed sheet for patients who have suffered extensive burns. Laboratory studies carried out by the author suggest that, in some production batches at least, there is a possibility that some of the aluminium coated fabric may be lost from the dressing during normal use which may enter the wound. The clinical significance of this observation is not known. Although not widely used in the UK, Metalline is used extensively in Europe. The Aluderm range from Söhngen contains many different products all of which have an aluminium wound contact layer. The company claims that the aluminized wound cover promotes and accelerates epithelization and the growth of granulation tissue but a review of the literature has not revealed any evidence to support this claim.

Silicone-impregnated dressings

In an attempt to enhance the low-adherent properties of the simple knitted viscose dressings, a silicone impregnated version was developed. Originally introduced as Silicone NA, and now called N-A Ultra, this was generally regarded as an improvement over the plain fabric dressing for indications where dressing adherence was a particular problem, such as in the treatment of epidermolysis bullosa.

Figure 37: Comparison of NA and NA Ultra

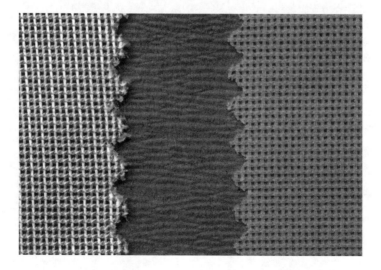

This material was subsequently eclipsed by the development of a new family of dressings which made a very significant impact upon the market. The first product of this type was Mepitel, a porous, semi-transparent wound contact layer consisting of a flexible polyamide net coated with soft silicone. Although Mepitel is non-absorbent, it contains 14 pores/cm^2, each nominally 1.2 mm in diameter; these allow the passage of exudate from the wound into a secondary absorbent dressing.

Figure 38: Mepitel showing nylon net encased in silicone

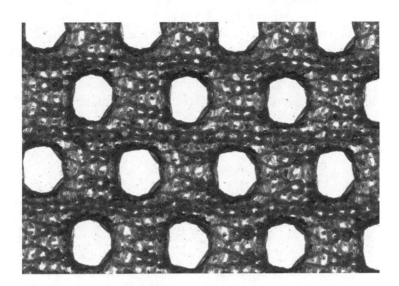

The effect of Mepitel upon healing rates in a experimental animal model was investigated by Troshev *et al.,*[53] who compared the dressing with cotton gauze in the treatment of full thickness burns in 200 rats. Wounds were either left alone to heal spontaneously, were surgically debrided then allowed to heal, or surgically debrided and grafted with an allotransplant. Microbiological and histological examinations were undertaken 3, 7, 14, 21 and 28 days after wounding as appropriate. The authors found that, when applied immediately to a burn, or to a wound that had been surgically debrided, Mepitel suppressed the development of normal microbiological flora and stimulated the normal healing process. However, when applied to the allotransplant it promoted the rapid and early rejection of the graft.

Development of soft-silicone products

Further developments in the silicone dressing field soon followed, as a result of which a new range of dressings was introduced which were coated with an adhesive based upon silicone technology. These were claimed to address the twin problems of adherence to the wound and damage to the surrounding skin.

Mepilex is an absorbent dressing made from polyurethane foam, the outer surface of which is bonded to a vapour-permeable polyurethane membrane that acts as a barrier to liquid and microorganisms. This membrane, which has a wrinkled appearance, is applied in this way to accommodate the slight swelling that occurs as the dressing absorbs exudate. The inner surface of the foam is coated with a layer of soft silicone that helps to hold the dressing in place without sticking to the surface of the wound or causing trauma to delicate new tissue on removal.

Mepilex Border is an absorbent, self-adhesive island dressing with a perforated soft silicone adhesive wound contact layer. The absorbent core of the dressing consists of three components: a thin sheet of polyurethane foam, a piece of non-woven fabric, and a layer of super-absorbent polyacrylate fibres. The core is located centrally upon a larger piece of polyurethane film and is held in place by the perforated soft silicone adhesive layer that extends to the outer margins of the dressing. This gentle adhesion also tends to prevent maceration by inhibiting the lateral movement of exudate from the wound on to the surrounding skin. Although Mepilex is generally held in place with tape or a bandage, Mepilex Border requires no additional retention aids.

Mepilex Transfer is a thin, conformable, soft silicone dressing that conforms closely to the wound and the surrounding skin, even where the surface is uneven. The seal that is formed between the dressing and the intact skin ensures that exudate moves vertically through the dressing into a secondary absorbent pad.

Both Mepilex and Mepilex Border are promoted for use on many types of exuding wounds including leg and pressure ulcers, and traumatic wounds with resulting skin loss. They may also be used under compression bandaging.

All the dressings in this range will, to some degree, maintain a moist wound environment while minimising the risk of maceration, although in the case of Mepitel and Mepilex Transfer, the moisture content of the wound will be greatly influenced by the choice of secondary dressing. Mepilex and Mepilex Border having an intrinsic absorbent layer, require no secondary dressings.

Adhesive and adherent: explanation of terms

Soft silicone is a material that adheres readily to intact dry skin but does not stick to the surface of a moist wound and does not cause damage upon removal.[54]

In a wound management context, the terms 'adherent' and 'adhesive' are sometimes incorrectly used interchangeably. This causes confusion and can lead to a misunderstanding of the properties of the products concerned. The term 'adherence', describe the interaction between a dressing and the wound, whilst the description 'adhesive' should be used to describe the interaction that takes place between the dressing and the intact periwound skin. Some products, such as island dressings, have a low-adherent pad located in the centre of an adhesive retention layer, and can therefore be described as both low-adherent and adhesive.

Atraumatic dressings

To overcome the confusion sometimes caused by the inappropriate use of the two terms, a new category of dressings was proposed to describe products, which, on removal, do not cause trauma either to newly formed tissue or to the periwound skin. It was suggested that such dressings be described as 'atraumatic dressings', a term that can be applied both to adhesive and non-adhesive dressings and one that more accurately reflects the overall characteristics of this product group.[55]

The gentle adhesion formed between the dressing and the intact periwound skin inhibits the movement of exudate from the wound on to the surrounding area and helps to prevent maceration.

The 'Eclipse' range of dressings also incorporates a soft silicone contact layer. Once again it is claimed that this selectively clings to the surrounding skin without adhering to the fragile wound bed and allows atraumatic removal. It can also be lifted easily for adjustment or wound inspection and replaced without losing adhesion.

Effect of soft silicone dressings on the skin: results of experimental studies

The effect on the structural integrity and function of the skin of dressings bearing a soft silicone adhesive compared with those bearing a more traditional adhesive system was described by Dykes and colleagues in a series of publications.

In the first, the force required to detach samples of different dressings from the skin and the degree of damage that resulted was assessed in a two part study.[54] The first part compared the effects of applying Duoderm Extra Thin, Mepiform Safetac and Tielle to the forearm of 12 normal volunteers aged 19-53 years whose skin was prestained with methylene blue. Treatments were applied either for a single 24 hour period or on three consecutive occasions each of 24 hours duration. Following dressing removal the dye left on the skin was sampled using a skin surface biopsy method and measured spectrophotometrically. The results revealed that after one and three applications the Mepiform Safetac skin sites had a higher level of dye than those on which the other dressings had been applied ($p < 0.05$ after three applications). Assuming that the amount of dye remaining is inversely proportion to the degree of stripping, the results suggest that Mepiform Safetac is less damaging to the skin surface than the other products tested.

In the second part of the same study, the peel force needed to remove adhesive dressings from prestained skin in 20 normal volunteers aged 23-64 years was measured and related to the amount of stratum corneum removed as before. The dressings used on this occasion were Allevyn Adhesive, Biatain Adhesive, Duoderm Extra Thin, Mepilex Border Safetac and Tielle. Three consecutive 24-hour applications of each product were made, and peel force readings recorded after each. The amount of dye remaining on the skin at 72 hours was assessed by the surface biopsy method. Statistically significant differences between products were observed in terms of both peak force and steady state force of removal. Differences in the level of damage to the superficial stratum corneum were also detected. However, a low peel force was not always associated with low damage and, therefore, other factors must contribute to stratum corneum removal in this model.

This work was repeated in a modified form some years later when the discomfort occasioned by removal of six dressings was investigated in 24 volunteers.[56] Allevyn, Biatain, Duoderm Extra Thin, Mepilex Border, Tielle and Versiva were applied to the lower back according to a randomization schedule and the force required to remove the dressings 24 hours later was recorded using a device which ensured the samples were removed at a constant speed and angle to the skin surface. The degree of discomfort experienced at each removal was assessed by the subjects themselves using an electronic visual analogue scale. Mepilex Border was given a significantly lower discomfort score ($p \leq 0.01$) by the subjects than the other dressings. There were no clear differences between the five other products tested. Tielle and Allevyn Adhesive developed a significantly higher (p ≤ 0.05) peel force than the other products.

Mepilex Border caused less discomfort on removal than Duoderm Extra Thin, Biatain and Versiva, even though the peel force was similar. Tielle and Allevyn had higher peel force, but the levels of discomfort were not significantly higher for these products. The authors concluded that the degree of discomfort experienced by subjects on removal of an adhesive dressing is not entirely dependent on the magnitude of the peel force and that other aspects of the interaction between the skin surface and the adhesive play a role.

In a final study,[57] the effect of repeated application and removal of samples of the adhesive edges from the same range of dressings on cutaneous irritancy and barrier function in 30 normal volunteer subjects was investigated using a repeat-insult patch test. Samples were applied continuously to the same site (six applications over a 14-day period. The test sites were assessed clinically before product reapplication using established ranking scales for cutaneous erythema. The cumulative irritancy score (CIS) for each test site was determined by adding the erythema scores at days 3, 5, 8, 10, 12 and 15. The barrier function of each test site was assessed at the end of the study by measuring transepidermal water loss (TEWL). The CIS results revealed showed that the products fall into two distinct groups. Allevyn, Mepilex Border and Tielle produced low scores and Biatain, Comfeel and Duoderm higher scores. Statistical analysis confirmed significant differences (p < 0.05) between Mepilex and Biatain, Mepilex and Comfeel, Mepilex and Duoderm, Tielle and Biatain, Allevyn and Biatain. The mean TEWL values also indicated that the products fall into two distinct groups: Statistical analysis indicated that Allevyn, Mepilex and Tielle were not significantly different from normal skin (p < 0.05), but Biatain, Comfeel and Duoderm were significantly higher than normal skin and the other products tested. These results might perhaps have been predicted as the higher scoring products are hydrocolloid-type dressing which are much more occlusive in their intact state. This would inevitably have the effect of increasing the moisture content of the skin which would then return to normal once the dressings were removed.

Zillmer et al,[58] also investigated effect of repeated removal of four different adhesive dressings on peri-ulcer skin using quantitative non-invasive techniques. Forty-five leg ulcers patients were included and peri-ulcer skin was treated for 14 days with patches of two different hydrocolloid-based adhesive dressings, one polyurethane adhesive and one soft silicone adhesive dressing. Normal skin on the patients' ventral forearm was similarly treated. The patches were replaced every second day and the skin barrier function was assessed by measuring transepidermal water loss and stratum corneum hydration by measuring electrical conductance. Thirty-nine patients completed the study. The hydrocolloid adhesives increased transepidermal water loss and conductance while the polyurethane and soft silicone adhesives did not influence these parameters significantly compared with adjacent non-treated peri-ulcer skin. For normal forearm skin, similar relative effects among the four adhesives were found. Repetitive treatment with hydrocolloid-based adhesive dressings induced major functional alterations of the stratum corneum. In contrast, a polyurethane adhesive and a soft silicone adhesive dressing did not alter transepidermal water loss or conductance of peri-ulcer skin. Once again, these results might have been predicted as hydrocolloids have a much lower moisture vapour transmission rate than the foams. This would almost inevitably result in an increase in the moisture content of the skin.

Clinical experience with soft silicone dressings

Some indication of the clinical relevance of the work of Dykes may be obtained from the results of two studies reported by Viamontes et al.[59-60] They first compared Allevyn Adhesive and Mepilex Border in a retrospective review of data collected in 'real time' in a database containing treatment details of nursing homes patients over a one year period in order to determine the incidence of skin stripping of periwound skin, wound healing rates and pain.

Data collected from 403 evaluable wounds in 206 patients was analysed. Evidence of skin stripping was detected following the use of both products, in 5% (5/106) patients dressed with Allevyn and 4% (4/100) in patients dressed with Mepilex Border. Closure rates achieved with the two dressings were similar. Independent nurse evaluations highlighted the failure of the self-adherent soft silicone foam dressing to either initially adhere to the wound area, or to remain in contact for more than a few days, as the dressing frequently needed the application of additional tape to ensure adhesion. They reported that the failure of the self-adhesive soft silicone foam dressing to adhere effectively to the periwound area was a significant disadvantage and a disincentive to use this type of dressing routinely.

In their second study, using the same methodology they review clinical data, collected over a 5-year period (1997-2002) which identified 1,891 residents with 4,200 wounds who had been treated with the products in question in 30 nursing homes in the state of Florida. The data collection period was chosen to capture a change in wound dressing regimens in these nursing homes which occurred in 2001. Patient demographic and wound assessment variables, including evidence of surrounding skin stripping, were abstracted from the database.

Of the 4200 relevant wounds, 3795 (90%) were treated with Allevyn Adhesive, 352 (8%) with Mepilex Border and 53 (1%) were treated with both dressings at some points. Of the 3,795 wound treated with the Allevyn Adhesive, 3,579 (94%) were pressure ulcers (mainly Grade II of Grade III), as were 339 of 352 wounds dressed with Mepilex Border and 51 wounds managed with both dressings. Wounds in the Allevyn group were larger, (7.53 vs 5.5 cm^2) and took longer to heal than those in the Mepilex group, (70.1 vs 39.2 days) but the proportion of ulcers healed was the same in both groups, (63%). Skin stripping was rare with either dressing occurring in less than 1% of wounds. Problems with infection occurred more frequently in the Mepilex Border group (9%) than in the Allevyn Adhesive group (3%). The authors, whilst acknowledging the limitations of retrospective studies, once again concluded that periwound skin stripping is uncommon and that differences between the two products are minimal. As in the previous study it was reported that the dressings using soft silicone technology tended to adhere less well, requiring the use of tape to retain the dressing firmly in place. This failure was considered a significant deterrent to staff to use this type of dressing routinely

Soft silicone dressings in paediatrics

The reduction in pain commonly attributed to the use of silicone dressings suggests that they could play a valuable role in paediatric wound management.

Two published studies have compared Mepitel with silver sulphadiazine (SSD) in treatment of burns and scalds and a third in the treatment of fingertip injuries. Gotschall et al.[61] performed a randomized clinical trial in children with partial-thickness burns caused by hot non-viscous fluids involving less than 15% total body surface area. Sixty-three children were assigned treatment with either Mepitel or SSD. Data were collected on time to wound healing, pain at dressing change, infection, and resource use. Wounds treated with Mepitel healed significantly faster than the controls and patients required 75% fewer dressing changes. Time to 25% epithelialization was 3.5 days for Mepitel dressed wounds and 6.7 days for the control, a reduction of 48%. The median time for complete healing for Mepitel-treated wounds was 10.5 days and for SSD-treated wounds 27.6 days. Wounds dressed with Mepitel exhibited less eschar formation, and patients experienced less pain during dressing changes. There were also financial savings associated with the use of Mepitel. Although no significant difference in wound infection rates was recorded between the two treatment groups, wounds dressed with Mepitel yielded higher levels of bacteria and a wider variety of species on microbiological examination. The authors concluded that 'the use of Mepitel represents a significant advance in the treatment of partial-thickness burns in children', but recommended that 'additional effort is required to determine treatment protocols that optimise efficacy while providing opportunities to adequately monitor wound healing and infection.'

In the second study Bugmann et al.[62] described a prospective randomized pilot investigation involving 76 children with previously untreated burns less than 24 hours old. After randomization 41 children were treated with Mepitel: vs SSD in paediatrics and 35 with SSD. Five children were subsequently withdrawn from both groups because they underwent tangential skin excisions and skin graft. Initial debridement and cleansing were the same for both treatment groups. In the Mepitel group, one or more sheets of the dressing were then applied directly to the burn in a single layer that overlapped onto the intact skin and covered with gauze soaked in chlorhexidine solution. Wounds in the control group were covered with a thick layer of SSD covered by a piece of paraffin gauze followed by a layer of absorbent gauze. Wounds in both treatment groups were redressed every two to three days until complete healing was achieved. As in the previous study, removal of Mepitel was easy and atraumatic. It also produced a significantly reduced healing time compared to SSD-treated wounds: 7.6 days and 11.3 days respectively. The authors suggested that the faster healing time found in the Mepitel group may be related to a direct effect of silicone on epithelial growth or to a decrease in surface-cell damage compared to the SSD group.

Hand injuries are common in children and can be a source of considerable pain and stress to the patient. In a prospective randomized trial, O'Donovan et al.[63] compared Mepitel with paraffin gauze in the treatment of 45 children with isolated fingertip injuries. Following randomization, 20 children received Mepitel and 25-paraffin gauze. Although no differences were found in healing rates, important statistically significant differences were recorded in both adherence of the dressing and the stress exhibited by the patient over the first three weeks of treatment, leading the authors to conclude that Mepitel dressings offers a less painful and easier alternative to traditional dressings for this indication.

In a second paper involving the management of hand wounds, Mepitel was compared with paraffin gauze and Adaptic.[64] A total of 108 patients undergoing hand surgery were recruited to the study and randomly assigned to treatment with one of the three products under examination. The selected primary dressing was covered with gauze and a crepe bandage together with a plaster of Paris splint as appropriate. The dressing was left intact until the first follow-up appointment. The performance of each dressing was judged in terms of ease of application and removal, amount of blood on secondary dressing, appearance and condition of the wound and pain experienced during dressing removal. Removal of Adaptic and Mepitel was reported to be 'very easy' for 88% and 84% of wounds respectively, compared to 57% of wounds dressed with paraffin gauze. This difference achieved significance for Adaptic but not Mepitel. Pain scores were also lower for Adaptic-treated patients, 75% of whom experienced no pain compared to 56% for Mepitel and 51% for paraffin gauze. All dressings were more difficult to remove from raw tissue and although Mepitel appeared to perform better than the other products in this situation, insufficient numbers of subjects with this type of wound prevented further analysis. The reason for the relatively poor pain scores achieved with Mepitel was discussed by the authors who suggested that this was probably due to the dressing adhering to the intact but bruised or injured skin around the wound. The authors concluded that of the three dressings, Adaptic had significant advantages over the other products examined in terms of performance and cost, and recommended it as the dressing of choice for this particular application. Mepitel, they suggested, could be used with advantage on wounds such as raw nail beds, as reported some years earlier by Williams,[65] who also described its use following traumatic amputation of the fingers, and in the treatment of a dehisced abdominal wound.

Vloemans and Kreis,[66] in an open prospective study, evaluated Mepitel as an alternative to conventional treatments including paraffin gauze, for the fixation of skin grafts in children. With Mepitel they found that changing the outer absorbent dressing was painless, as was the final removal of the dressing itself, requiring no analgesia or anaesthesia. Graft take rates were good; in 42 out 45 cases the take was almost complete (> 95%). Because the dressing requires a margin of healthy skin, its use was limited to minor skin grafts (maximum 6% of the total body area) and the authors suggested that it could only be used on flat or convex areas; on concave areas firm fixation is either difficult or impossible.

Platt et al.[67] also compared Mepitel with paraffin gauze as the first dressing layer applied to 38 newly grafted wounds in a prospective randomized trial. At the first postoperative dressing change all patients in the paraffin gauze group experienced some degree of pain on dressing removal. In contrast, 53% of patients dressed with Mepitel experienced no pain.

Soft silicone dressings following radiotherapy

Adamietz et al.[68] in a prospective study involving 21 patients evaluated Mepitel as a method of protecting skin during radiotherapy for malignant disease. In seven of the patients treated the skin was intact, but five patients had epithiliolysis, and nine patients had ulcers, seven of which were malignant.

The silicone-coated net was shown to cause no additional irritation of irradiated skin and it was suitable for the treatment of both dry desquamation and the moist desquamation that occurs with high doses of radiation. This latter condition is particularly difficult to manage with conventional dressings as the skin is very fragile and easily damaged by the removal of dressings that can adhere to the drying serous fluid on the skin surface. When applied over ulcerative wounds, the dressing was easy to remove and did not cause damage to the newly formed epithelium.

MacBride et al.,[69] used a silicone dressing, Mepilex Lite, to treat areas of dry and moist desquamation in 16 patients following radiotherapy. Some patients found that the dressing minimised pain during dressing changes and was easily lifted and adjusted without loss of adherent properties. Its use was also reported to produce a soothing or cooling effect in some patients and a number reported a more normal sleep pattern. No negative effect on wound healing were observed leading the authors to conclude that the dressing offers a useful alternative to existing therapies which is worthy of further research.

Soft silicone dressings: miscellaneous applications

The use of Mepitel in more extensive wounds resulting from wide local excision of skin tumours was investigated by Dahlstrøm.[70] Mepitel was compared with paraffin gauze as a temporary dressing before split skin grafting in a prospective randomized controlled trial involving 64 patients. After excision of the tumour, the wound was dressed according to the randomization schedule and covered with a saline-soaked absorbent secondary dressing. All dressings were removed on the following day and an unmeshed split skin graft applied, which was left exposed. The principal outcome variables of the study, determined upon removal of the primary dressing, were adherence, bleeding, pain and the time taken for removal. Highly significant differences were detected between the two treatments in favour of Mepitel for all parameters examined. The author concluded that Mepitel was 'an optimum temporary dressing for delayed split skin grafting'.

Taylor,[71] recorded how the dressing improved the quality of life in a patient with severe mycosis fungoides, a progressive skin tumour, which resulted in the formation of extensive ulceration over her scalp, neck and back. Gates,[72] similarly described how the dressing reduced the pain from an extensive arterial leg ulcer and improved the condition of the surrounding skin.

The genetic skin disorder, epidermolysis bullosa (EB) is particularly difficult to manage. Mepitel is said to be particularly useful for this indication, both for the treatment of intact blisters and areas where the epidermis has been lost. This is because it stays in place and prevents the type of frictional damage that can occur as a result of dressing slippage.

Other reported applications for the use of silicone dressings include urethral erosions in the male patient, a known but poorly documented sequelae of catheter injury,[73] and in skin tears.[74]

Where clinically indicated, topical steroids or antimicrobial agents can be applied either over or under Mepitel. Depending on the nature and condition of the wound, Mepitel may be left in place for extended periods, up to 7-10 days in some instances, but the outer absorbent layer should be changed more frequently as required. When Mepitel is used for the fixation of skin grafts and protection of blisters, it is recommended that the dressing should not be changed before the fifth day post-application. As with all types of dressings, wounds should be regularly monitored for signs of infection or deterioration. When used on bleeding wounds, or wounds producing high viscosity exudate, Mepitel should be covered with a moist absorbent dressing pad. If Mepitel is used on burns treated with meshed grafts, or applied after facial resurfacing, imprints can occur if excess pressure is placed upon the dressing. Following facial resurfacing it is recommended that the dressing be lifted and repositioned at least every second day. It has also been suggested that its use can lead to pigmentation abnormalities in black children.[75]

'Adherent' wound contact layers

A novel approach to the problems of dressing adherence is to use a dressing or wound contact material which, once applied, remains in position for an extended period or until the wound is healed. One such product is BreakAway Wound Dressing, Winfield Laboratories which has a facing layer (N-Terface) which separates easily from the absorbent layer and so remains on the wound when the outer adhesive component is removed. The N-Terface layer is also available as a stand alone dressing which like Telfa Clear and Tegaderm Contact can be used with a variety of topical applications and secondary dressings.

References

1. Tissot. *Advice to the People in General with Regard to their Health*. London: Becket and De Hondt, 1766.
2. Trevethick RA. Sensitization to tulle gras dressings, (letter). *Br. med. J.* 1957;2:883-884.
3. Elliott IMZ. *A Short History of Surgical Dressings*. London: The Pharmaceutical Press, 1964.
4. Winter GD. Methods for the biological evaluation of dressings. In: Turner TD, Brain KR, editors. *Surgical dressings in the hospital environment*. Cardiff: Surgical Dressings Research Unit, UWIST, Cardiff, 1975:47-81.
5. Leone CR, Jr., Van Gemert JV, Underwood L. Dacryocystorhinostomy: a modification of the Dupuy-Dutemps operation. *Ophthalmic Surg* 1979;10(5):35-8.
6. Meaume S, Senet P, Dumas R, Carsin H, Pannier M, Bohbot S. Urgotul: a novel non-adherent lipidocolloid dressing. *Br J Nurs* 2002;11(16 Suppl):S42-3, S46-50.
7. Benbow M, Iosson G. A clinical evaluation of Urgotul to treat acute and chronic wounds. *Br J Nurs* 2004;13(2):105-9.
8. Tan PW, Ho WC, Song C. The use of Urgotul in the treatment of partial thickness burns and split-thickness skin graft donor sites: a prospective control study. *Int Wound J* 2009;6(4):295-300.

9. Letouze A, Voinchet V, Hoecht B, Muenter KC, Vives R, Bohbot S. Using a new lipidocolloid dressing in paediatric wounds: results of French and German clinical studies. *Journal of Wound Care* 2004;13(6):221-5.

10. Blanchet-Bardon C, Bohbot S. Using Urgotul dressing for the management of epidermolysis bullosa skin lesions. *J Wound Care* 2005;14(10):490-1, 494-6.

11. Ma KK, Chan MF, Pang SM. The effectiveness of using a lipido-colloid dressing for patients with traumatic digital wounds. *Clin Nurs Res* 2006;15(2):119-34.

12. Smith J, Hill J, Barrett S, Hayes W, Kirby P, Walsh S, et al. Evaluation of Urgotol plus K-Four compression for venous leg ulcers. *Br J Nurs* 2004;13(6 Suppl):S20-8.

13. Meaume S, Ourabah Z, Cartier H, Granel-Brocard F, Combemale P, Bressieux JM, et al. Evaluation of a lipidocolloid wound dressing in the local management of leg ulcers. *J Wound Care* 2005;14(7):329-34.

14. Teot L, Lambert L, Ourabah Z, Bey E, Steenman C, Wierzbiecka E, et al. Use of topical negative pressure with a lipidocolloid dressing: results of a clinical evaluation. *J Wound Care* 2006;15(8):355-8.

15. Bernard FX, Barrault C, Juchaux F, Laurensou C, Apert L. Stimulation of the proliferation of human dermal fibroblasts in vitro by a lipidocolloid dressing. *J Wound Care* 2005;14(5):215-20.

16. Powell G. The new Start dressing range--Urgotul Start, UrgoCell Start. *Br J Nurs* 2009;18(6):S30, S32-6.

17. D'Arcy PF. Drugs on the skin: a clinical and pharmaceutical problem. *Pharm. J.* 1972;209:491-492.

18. Lunn JA. Controlled trial of a wound dressing: Sofra-Tulle. *Practitioner* 1962;188:527-528.

19. Jackson PW. Sofra-Tulle in the treatment of minor wounds. *Practitioner* 1962;189:675-678.

20. Currie JPS, D.M. Framycetin in the treatment of cutaneous injuries. *Practitioner* 1963;190:112-113.

21. Ramirez AT. Topical framycetin in the treatment of burns. *Philippine J. surg. Special.* 1969;24:Jan-14.

22. Smith RA. The treatment of burns: a clinical evaluation of Sofra-Tulle. *Clin. Trials J.* 1972;9:37-40.

23. Milwidsky J. Soframycin unitulle in general practice. *Medical Proceedings* 1971;17(3):42-43.

24. Wicks CJ, Peterson HI. Medicated wound dressings - a historical review. *Opusc. med.* 1972;17:90-95.

25. Kirton V, Munro-Ashman D. Contact dermatitis from neomycin and framycetin. *Lancet* 1965;2:138-139.

26. McCormack BL, Nathan MS, Fernandez A. Practical evaluation of a new sodium fusidate (Fucidin) wound dressing. *J. Ir. med. Ass.* 1968;61:137-141.

27. Ritchie IC. Clinical and bacteriological studies of a new antibiotic tulle. *Br. J. clin. Pract.* 1968;22:15-16.

28. Davies GE. 1:6-Dichlorophenyldiguanidohexane (`Hibitane'): laboratory investigation of a new antibacterial agent of high potency. *Br. J. Pharmac. Chemother.* 1954;9:192-196.

29. Senior N. Some observations on the formulation and properties of chlorhexidine. *J. Soc. cosmet. Chem.* 1972;11:Jan-19.

30. Lowbury EJL. Chlorhexidine. *Curr. Ther.* 1957;179:489-493.

31. Thomas S, Russell AD. An in vitro evaluation of Bactigras, a tulle dressing containing chlorhexidine. *Microbios Letters* 1976;2:169-177.

32. Thomas S, Dawes C, Hay NP. Improvements in medicated tulle dressings. *J. Hospital Infection* 1983;4:391-398.

33. Andrews JK. An experimental evaluation of a chlorhexidine medicated tulle gras dressing, (letter). *J. Hosp. Infect.* 1982;3:401.

34. Thomas S. An experimental evaluation of a chlorhexidine medicated tulle gras dressing, (letter). *J. Hosp. Infect.* 1982;3:399-400.

35. Lawrence JC. Minor burns. *Nurs Mirror Midwives J* 1977;144(17):58-60.

36. Salomon JC. Effect of dressings on donor site epithelialization. *Surg. Forum* 1974;25:516-517.

37. Gemberling RM, Miller TA, Caffee H, Zawacki BE. Dressing comparison in the healing of donor sites. *J Trauma* 1976;16(10):812-4.

38. Thomas S. Pain and wound management. *Nurs. Times Community Outlook Suppl.* 1989;85:Nov-15.

39. Edwards J. Telfa Clear. *Journal of Community Nursing* 2002;16(5):36-37.

40. Robb WA. Clinical trial of melolin: a new non-adherent dressing. *Br J Plast Surg* 1961;14:47-9.

41. Schumacher S, Fisch M, Schurig E, Hohenfellner R. Properties and acceptance of Melolin wound dressing in postoperative management of male urethral reconstruction. *Urologe A* 1996;35(1):14-7.

42. Backhouse CM, Blair SD, Savage AP, Walton J, McCollum CN. Controlled trial of occlusive dressings in healing chronic venous ulcers. *Br J Surg* 1987;74(7):626-7.

43. Macmillan MS, Wells M, MacBride S, Raab GM, Munro A, MacDougall H. Randomized comparison of dry dressings versus hydrogel in management of radiation-induced moist desquamation. *Int J Radiat Oncol Biol Phys* 2007;68(3):864-72.

44. Johns WA. Aluminum foil as a dressing for burns. *Va Med Mon (1918)* 1949;76(12):640, illust.

45. Fuchs HK, Lutzeyer W. [Clinical results of aluminium therapy in burns.]. *Arztl Wochensch* 1951;6(19):447-9.

46. Steinhardt O. [A new bandage of metal foil.]. *Klin Med Osterr Z Wiss Prakt Med* 1955;10(10):460-1.

47. Hambury HJ. Aluminium foil dressing. *Med World* 1957;87(5):416-20.

48. Volnohradsky R. Aluminium foil manufactured in Czechoslovakia in the treatment of chronic skin defects and ulcerations. Evaluation of mechanical properties. *Cesk Dermatol* 1974;49(5):325-7.

49. Fox JWh, Golden GT, Rodeheaver G, Edgerton MT, Edlich RF. Nonoperative management of fingertip pulp amputation by occlusive dressings. *Am J Surg* 1977;133(2):255-6.

50. McAvoy J, Charles DM, Moore GE. A meshed aluminum foil wound dressing system. *Ann Plast Surg* 1979;3(5):469-73.

51. Poole MD, Kalus AM, von Domarus H. Aluminium foil as a wound dressing. *Br J Plast Surg* 1979;32(2):145-6.

52. Farmer AW, Maxmen MD, Chasmar LR, Franks WR. Aluminum powder as a dry dressing in exposure treatment of thermal burns. *Plast Reconstr Surg (1946)* 1954;14(3):171-7.

53. Troshev K, Kolev Z, Zlateva A, Shishkov S, Pashaliev N, Raycheva-Mutafova E. Bacteriostatic and biological stimulation effect of Mepitel on experimental burns on the skin of rats. *Acta Chir Plast* 1997;39(3):97-102.

54. Dykes PJ, Heggie R, Hill SA. Effects of adhesive dressings on the stratum corneum of the skin. *Journal of Wound Care* 2001;10(2):7-10.

55. Thomas S. Atraumatic Dressings. *World Wide Wounds* 2003.

56. Dykes PJ, Heggie R. The link between the peel force of adhesive dressings and subjective discomfort in volunteer subjects. *Journal of Wound Care* 2003;12(7):260-2.

57. Dykes PJ. The effect of adhesive dressing edges on cutaneous irritancy and skin barrier function. *J Wound Care* 2007;16(3):97-100.

58. Zillmer R, Agren MS, Gottrup F, Karlsmark T. Biophysical effects of repetitive removal of adhesive dressings on peri-ulcer skin. *J Wound Care* 2006;15(5):187-91.

59. Viamontes L, Jones AM. Evaluation study of the properties of two adhesive foam dressings. *Br J Nurs* 2003;12(11 Suppl):S43-4, S46-9.

60. Viamontes L, Temple D, Wytall D, Walker A. An evaluation of an adhesive hydrocellular foam dressing and a self-adherent soft silicone foam dressing in a nursing home setting. *Ostomy Wound Manage* 2003;49(8):48-52, 54-6, 58.

61. Gotschall CS, Morrison MI, Eichelberger MR. Prospective, randomized study of the efficacy of Mepitel on children with partial-thickness scalds. *J Burn Care Rehabil* 1998;19(4):279-83.

62. Bugmann P, Taylor S, Gyger D, Lironi A, Genin B, Vunda A, et al. A silicone-coated nylon dressing reduces healing time in burned paediatric patients in comparison with standard sulfadiazine treatment: a prospective randomized trial. *Burns* 1998;24(7):609-12.

63. O'Donovan DA, Mehdi SY, Eadie PA. The role of Mepitel silicone net dressings in the management of fingertip injuries in children. *J Hand Surg [Br]* 1999;24(6):727-30.

64. Terrill PJ, Varughese G. A comparison of three primary non-adherent dressings applied to hand surgery wounds. *Journal of Wound Care* 2000;9(8):359-363.

65. Williams C. Mepitel: a non-adherent soft silicone wound dressing. *Br J Nurs* 1995;4(1):51-2, 54-5.

66. Vloemans AF, Kreis RW. Fixation of skin grafts with a new silicone rubber dressing (Mepitel). *Scand J Plast Reconstr Surg Hand Surg* 1994;28(1):75-6.

67. Platt AJ, Phipps A, Judkins K. A comparative study of silicone net dressing and paraffin gauze dressing in skin-grafted sites. *Burns* 1996;22(7):543-5.

68. Adamietz IA, Mose S, Haberl A, Saran FH, Thilmann C, Bottcher HD. Effect of self-adhesive, silicone-coated polyamide net dressing on irradiated human skin. *Radiation Oncology Investigations* 1995;2:277-282.

69. MacBride SK, Wells ME, Hornsby C, Sharp L, Finnila K, Downie L. A case study to evaluate a new soft silicone dressing, Mepilex Lite, for patients with radiation skin reactions. *Cancer Nurs* 2008;31(1):E8-14.

70. Dahlstrøm KK. A new silicone rubber dressing used as a temporary dressing before delayed split skin grafting. A prospective randomised study. *Scand J Plast Reconstr Surg Hand Surg* 1995;29(4):325-7.

71. Taylor R. Use of a silicone net dressing in severe mycosis fungoides. *Journal of Wound Care* 1999;8(9):429-30.

72. Gates A. The use of a non-adherent silicone dressing in arterial leg ulceration. *Journal of Wound Care* 2000;9(2):79-81.

73. LeBlanc K, Christensen D. Addressing the challenge of providing nursing care for elderly men suffering from urethral erosion. *J Wound Ostomy Continence Nurs* 2005;32(2):131-4.

74. Meuleneire F. Using a soft silicone-coated net dressing to manage skin tears. *Journal of Wound Care* 2002;11(10):365-9.

75. Williams G, Withey S, Walker CC. Longstanding pigmentary changes in paediatric scalds dressed with a non- adherent siliconised dressing. *Burns* 2001;27(2):200-2.

9. Film dressings

INTRODUCTION

The history of film dressings

The first transparent film dressings were probably those manufactured in the 18th Century from isinglass prepared from the dried prepared swim bladders of sturgeon or cod. This, together with other ingredients, was spread, in the form of a solution, onto layers of ribbon, linen, or oiled silk, to form a plaster. The resulting materials were so thin and translucent that the wound was visible underneath. Any fluid that accumulated beneath the dressing could be easily seen and if this became excessive, it could be drained off through a small hole cut in the fabric.

Robert Liston (1846), quoted by Elliot,[1] said that isinglass plaster was not irritating to wounds and - unlike the common adhesive plasters - it did not become loose or give rise to erythema. It was therefore considered to represent a great advance over other dressings in current use which generally did no real good and often hindered wound healing. In 1880, isinglass plaster was used successfully as a dressing after skin grafting, an indication for which it was thought to be particularly well suited.

Another early film dressing was manufactured from pyroxylin or gun cotton, which was prepared by nitrating cotton fibre with equal parts of nitric and sulphuric acid. After purification and drying, the highly inflammable residue was dissolved in a mixture of ether and rectified spirit to form a clear colourless solution known as collodion. When poured onto the skin, the solvent evaporated leaving a thin transparent plastic film which contracted on drying. In 1848 collodion was used in America for dressing suture lines, and later formed the subject of a monograph in the first edition of the British Pharmacopoeia in 1864. In the 1867 edition, it was joined by a second formulation - containing Canada balsam and castor oil - which was known as Flexible Collodion, and was used as a dressing for burns, ulcers and abrasions of the skin. Squire's Companion to the British Pharmacopoeia of 1874 described both of these materials, together with two non-official preparations: Dr Richardson's Styptic Colloid, containing tannic acid, and Dr Pavisi's Haemostatic Collodion, which contained carbolic acid, tannic acid and benzoic acid. In 1903, it was said that the thin film that formed when a solution of collodion was allowed to dry on a sheet of glass made a valuable dressing for open wounds.

Collodion proved to be a very popular material and the British Pharmaceutical Codex of 1934 contained thirteen monographs for various medicated preparations, some of which contained ether and benzene. The use of collodion in its various forms has declined over the years because of the toxic and inflammable properties of some of the solvents used, although modified formulations are still available for use as wart removers.

Modern versions of these solvent-based film dressings have been developed, using different solvent systems and synthetic polymers. Opsite Transparent Film Dressing

Spray consists of an ethoxyethyl methacrylate-methoxyethyl methacrylate copolymer ('Hydron') dissolved in a mixture of ethyl acetate and acetone. Once applied to the skin and allowed to dry, it forms a tough protective film, which is said to be impervious to bacteria. The dressing is used for application to minor injuries and suture lines following surgery.

Cavilon No Sting Barrier Film is an alcohol-free liquid barrier film that dries quickly to form a breathable, transparent coating on the skin which is designed to protect intact, damaged or 'at-risk' skin from urine, faeces, other body fluids, adhesive trauma and friction. As its name suggests, it does not sting even when applied to broken skin. This new material was evaluated in a hospital study involving 33 patients in the geriatric and spinal cord rehabilitation units.[2] The authors reported that the dressing reduced skin redness in 96% of at risk patients and maceration in 94% of subjects. Dressing adhesion improved significantly in 90% of subjects and no incidence of skin stripping was found in any trial patient.

Cellulose films

Over the years, the development of synthetic or hemisynthetic polymers has led to the production of a range of plastic films, a number of which have been used for medical applications. The first such product was cellophane, produced from cellulose derived from modified wood pulp. A method for producing regenerated cellulose on a commercial scale was first described in the latter part of the 19th Century by the English scientists Cross, Bevan and Beadly who discovered that cellulose, treated with sodium hydroxide (caustic soda) and carbon disulphide, transforms into soluble sodium - cellulose - xanthogenate. This viscous solution could be coagulated in an ammonium sulphate bath then converted back to pure cellulose with dilute sulphuric acid. A continuous process for producing this in the form of a transparent film was patented by the Swiss expatriate Dr. J.E. Brandenberger in 1908. He named the new product 'cellophane', derived from 'cello' from cellulose, and from the Greek word "diaphanis" meaning transparent.

According to one fascinating review,[3] cellophane was first used in wound care in a field hospital during the First World War under the direction of Alexis Carrel, who used cellophane sheets to make daily tracings of wounds in order to measure their progress towards healing. The first use of Cellophane as a dressing may possibly be attributed to Dr Helmut Schmidt in 1927 who was able to demonstrate that the use of this material in place of standard bandages reduced infections rates and healing times, thereby anticipating the work of Winter by nearly 40 years.

Elder, a surgeon commander in the British Navy, used cellophane in 1933 to treat a burn on his own leg caused by a hot water bottle bursting with produced an acute burn over two thirds of the shin. In an attempt to reduce the pain he was experiencing with conventional dressings 'every dressing applied caused a state of semi-shock', he turned to cellophane. He was so impressed with the results, he subsequently used the material routinely to dress the wounds of his patients until his retirement when he published an account of his experiences.[4] Although he encountered some initial objections from patients due to the unusual nature of the treatment, he reported that once applied 'satisfaction was universal'.

He used the film in a number of different ways. To exclude the air in the treatment of superficial burns and scalds he sealed the film to the skin along the edges, but where ventilation of the wound was required as in the treatment of ulcers, the film was first perforated, sometimes using a paper punch.

A year later Howes, an American doctor, independently rediscovered the advantages of cellophane as a dressing for clean wounds and published an article in *Surgery* in 1939 in which he described its use in 70 wounds including hernioplasties, abdominal incisions and wounds on the extemities.[5] He recommended that the film, which should be 0.0017 inches thick, be sterilised by autoclaving, placed over the wound and stuck down around all four edges with adhesive plaster. If fluid accumulated under the dressing he recommended a small air vent be formed in one corner and subsequently covered with a gauze swab. He also made passing reference to the use of the film over wet dressings, claiming it to be less expensive than oiled silk.

During the Second World War, three clinicians, a Dr M. Ellis, Major John Farr, M.D. and Lieutenant Commander Kimbrough began to use cellophane apparently with excellent results.[6-7] Ellis, of the Colonial Medical Service in Lagos, Nigeria, initially obtained cellophane (Rayophane) from packets of cigarettes sold by the local Forces canteen, but subsequently he obtain scrap material directly from the cigarette factory which he applied directly to tropical ulcers, sometimes in conjunction with sulphanilamide or urea powder. The film was found to adhere lightly to the skin and was commonly left undisturbed for about a week.

Farr used a similar technique in the treatment of burns but applied a layer of 'unguentum sulphanilamidi' (sulphanilamide ointment) to the film before application. A layer of perforated oiled silk was then applied covered by wool, to facilitate even compression, and the entire dressing was held in place with a firm bandage.

Lieutenant Commander Kimbrough of the US navy,[8] recognised that cellophane was of particular value in 'industrial surgery' where dressings are subject to soiling with grease or oil. He may also have been the first to develop a 'self-adhesive' film dressing which he produced himself by dissolving the adhesive off packaging tape with ether and applying this solution to sheets of previously prepared cellulose film.

He reported that wounds dressed with cellulose appeared to heal 1-5 days faster, and with less scarring, than those dressed with conventional materials. Microbiological investigations of the exudate from beneath the film applied to two chronic heavily exuding wound revealed the presence of staphylococci, but both wounds healed well, with no sign of clinical infection, leading the author to conclude that the natural 'bacteriostatic substances present in the secretion are able to keep in check any ordinary infection present'.

These three clinicians were fortunate in that they were able to process the film appropriately prior to use. Rather less fortunate was Capt. H. Bloom of the Royal Army Medical Corps who was captured in the North African campaign. In the terrible conditions under which he worked, within a prison camp with severely limited supplies of medicines and surgical equipment, he began to use cellophane from cigarette packets to dress the wounds of 55 of his injured comrades. He published an account of his findings in 1945,[9] when once again he reported that wounds treated with the film healed rapidly, claiming that even infected wounds healed normally, under a thin layer of 'inspissated purulent serum'. He also claimed that patients found that the application of the material resulted in an immediate relief of pain. After the War, however, interest in the use of cellophane declined, not least because other synthetic polymers were being developed.

Development of modern film dressings

In 1948 Bull et al.,[10] described the development of a dressing in which a semipermeable window, manufactured from a nylon derivative, was supported in an adhesive polyvinyl frame. The nylon film formed an effective bacterial barrier and was claimed to be sufficiently permeable to prevent maceration of the underlying skin. The results of a clinical trial into the use of this dressing were reported some two years later by Schilling et al.[11]

Despite the promising results achieved with film-dressed wounds during the 1940s, these materials failed to impact significantly upon clinical practice. It was not until after the publication of the work of Winter and Hinman in the 1960s that the industry became interested in producing and marketing film dressings commercially.

The early films were of limited permeability and although some were employed successfully as incise drapes, to cover the area around an operation site, it was found that their extended use on large wounds frequently led to bacterial proliferation and skin maceration, making them unsuitable for use as dressings.

In 1971 Smith & Nephew introduced Opsite, a film dressing that effectively overcame the problems of skin maceration. Originally produced as an incise drape, the film was manufactured from a Type 1 polyurethane, coated with a vinyl ether adhesive system. In 1974 this was changed to Type 2 polyurethane, and the product was marketed as a dressing.

Because of the success that Opsite enjoyed in the market-place, film dressings were soon developed and produced by other manufacturers, subject to licences given by Smith & Nephew. As the potential for significant improvement to the basic film was somewhat limited, Smith & Nephew's competitors were forced to identify aspects of the performance of the dressing that they could develop or improve and use as the basis of their marketing strategy. One obvious area for improvement lay in the method of application, as the original presentation of Opsite had one well-recognised disadvantage.

Prior to use, the adhesive film had to be removed completely from its backing sheet and once free, it had a marked tendency to curl up and stick firmly to itself. If this happened, the dressing had to be discarded, which was wasteful in terms of both time and material costs.[12]

Considerable attention was paid to this problem; as a result, a number of interesting new application systems were developed, which the manufacturers claimed, made their dressings much easier to apply. The problems with the early presentation of Opsite were referred to by Haessler,[13] when reporting a study in which she compared Opsite with Tegaderm and gauze for catheter sites. Although the two films were found to be broadly equivalent, and superior to gauze in most respects, Tegaderm was preferred to Opsite because of its ease of application. As a result of these commercial pressures, Smith & Nephew eventually introduced an improved presentation of Opsite called Opsite Flexigrid. This incorporates a carrier support film which keeps the primary film rigid during application following which it easily removed. The carrier film also has a second function in that it is printed with a grid and can be used to form tracings of the wound which can be retained to monitor progress to healing. This new presentation was enthusiastically described by Bedford and Craven in 1991.[14]

In a further short-lived product development, two layers of film, one larger than the other, were stuck together to form an island 'pouch'. The inner film was perforated and it was intended that exudate would pass from the wound into the void.[15] Called the 'Tegaderm Pouch Dressing', this new presentation was not particularly well received and so was soon discontinued.

The other area in which it was thought that improvements could be made was the type of adhesive system applied to the film. Opsite was originally coated with a poly (vinyl ethyl ether) high resin and zinc resinate, formed by the interaction of zinc oxides with the resin acids in partially dimerised colophony. As will be described later, the zinc component of this adhesive was assumed to be responsible for producing marked toxic effects on test results in laboratory studies, and although the use of this material was never shown to produce problems in patients, it was subsequently changed to an acrylic-based system, similar to that used on most other film dressings.

Since Opsite was originally developed, further improvements have taken place in he manufacture of polyurethane dressings and products are now available that are many times more permeable to moisture vapour than the original preparation, and at least one product, Episil, has a soft-silicone adhesive which is claimed to facilitate removal of the dressing.

A non-adhesive film dressing, Omiderm, was developed in 1982. Described by the inventor as a thin synthetic temporary skin substitute, it consists of an elastic membrane of polyurethane film with grafted monomers such as acrylamide and hydroxyethylmethacrylate.[16] The film is inelastic when dry, but highly flexible when wet with a permeability of about 5000 $g/m^2/24$ h. Omiderm adheres to a moist wound surface but peels off easily when soaked or separates spontaneous as the wound heals.

Telfa Clear, is sometimes described as a film dressing, but actually consists of a piece of non-adhesive, plain perforated polyester film of the type used to form the Telfa dressing pad range. This material does not form a bacterial barrier or provide effective moisture control. It is simply intended for use as a low adherent interface layer.

EXAMPLES OF MODERN FILM DRESSINGS

Examples of plain unmedicated adhesive film dressings include:

- Activheal Film
- Askina Derm
- Bioclusive
- C-View
- Cutifilm
- Dermafilm
- Ensure
- Episil
- Hydrofilm
- Leukomed
- Mepore Film
- Opsite Flexigrid
- Polyskin
- Suprasorb F
- Tegaderm
- Vacuskin (polyethylene not polyurethane)

PROPERTIES OF FILM DRESSINGS

General properties

A film dressing should be lightweight, transparent and easy to apply and remove. It should also stick firmly to periwound skin without adhering to the surface of the wound itself and be sufficiently extensible to permit the free movement of a joint or swelling of soft tissue without causing secondary damage from lateral shearing forces.

The film should also form an effective bacterial barrier, and both the film and the adhesive applied to it should be 'skin friendly' and contain no extractable agents capable of producing a cytotoxic response within the healing wound.

Finally the dressing should be sufficiently permeable to water vapour to prevent moisture, formed by transepidermal water loss through the periwound skin, from accumulating beneath the film as at best this might lead to failure of the adhesive bond, or at worst maceration and bacterial proliferation resulting in infection.

Permeability of the film to oxygen has also been claimed to be an advantage for some clinical indications.

Performance requirements of film dressing

Based upon the general requirements of a film dressing identified above, it is possible to characterize their performance by a number of inter-related physical parameters which include:

- Thickness
- Extensibility
- Moisture vapour permeability
- Gaseous permeability
- Tissue compatibility
- Bacterial barrier properties

In 1988, a laboratory-based comparison was undertaken of the properties of six film dressings available at that time.[17] Since the study was published, many new products have been introduced and numerous product developments have taken place. As a result some of the results quoted below may no longer be applicable.

Thickness

The thickness of a dressing affects both its permeability and extensibility, which in term influences its conformability. The thickness of the six films with the adhesive in place was found to range from 0.045 - 0.75 mm. Following removal of the adhesive by solvent extraction, the thickness of the films was found to vary from 0.01 - 0.04 mm.

Extensibility

An elastic film that requires a relatively high force to bring about a small change in extension may, when placed over a joint, restrict movement or cause tissue damage by a shearing effect. A more extensible product will tend to stretch or move with the joint, allowing maximum mobility whilst reducing the possibility of skin damage. From the study cited previously, the force required to extend the dressings by 10% ranged from 85g/2.5cm width to 233g/2.5cm width, a not inconsiderable difference which was judged to have possible clinical implications.

Moisture vapour permeability

Within the published literature, there exists considerable variation in the values quoted for the moisture vapour transmission rates (MVTR) of film dressings. For one product, Tegaderm, for example, the results quoted in separate studies ranged from 268 $g/m^2/24/h$ to around 950 $g/m^2/24$ h.[17-19]

This variability is due to differences in the way in which MVTR is measured, but unfortunately in clinical papers that quote these values, experimental details are often omitted. Of particular importance are the temperature and humidity gradient across the film, and whether the permeability of the film is determined in contact with liquid water or simply moisture vapour.

When tested at 37°C in accordance with the method described in the British Pharmacopoeia 1980, Addendum 1986 (SDM IX Method B), the basis of a new British and European Standard,[20] the MVTR of Opsite was found to 862 ± 13 g/m^2/24 h and Tegaderm 846 ± 13 g/m^2/24 h, values which are approximately six times that of normal skin.

The ability of a film dressing to cope with the moisture which is continually lost through normal skin is a major factor in determining its clinical performance. As previously identified, measured values for transepidermal water loss (TEWL) of intact skin commonly range from around 150 to 200 g/m^2/24 h in healthy young adults but in elderly patients or those with inflammatory skin disorders, values can vary between 100 and 800 g/m^2/24 h.

Similar variability has been recorded in measurements of evaporative loss from damaged skin or wounds. Lamke et al.,[21] measured the evaporative loss from intact skin and a variety of wound types and found it to be as follows:

Table 9: Moisture loss from wounds and skin

Wound type	No of measurements	Evaporative loss (g/m^2/24 h)
Normal skin	60	204 ± 12
First degree burn	12	268 ± 26
Second degree burn	30	4274 ± 132
Third degree burn	20	3437 ± 108
Granulating wound	21	5138 ± 202
Donor site	35	3590 ± 180

The values for evaporative loss from granulating wounds reported by Lamke are consistent with those of Thomas et al,[22] who showed that leg ulcers commonly produce around 5000 g/m^2/24 h, a value that could double in the presence of infection, (see Chapter 5).

In addition to water, skin secretions from sweat glands also contain dissolved solids and hydrophobic agents which may accumulate beneath a film dressing and thereby reduce its permeability – eventually leading to failure of the adhesive bond. An adhesive semipermeable film must therefore be able to accommodate significant degradation in performance before it is reduced to the point at which the effectiveness of the dressing becomes seriously compromised.

Advances in polyurethane film technology have resulted in products that are significantly more permeable than the original materials. In some cases the permeability of the new films change in response to changes in the local environment. In the presence of liquid, the permeability of the film increases but reverts to lower levels as the entrapped moisture is dissipated.

The development of such a film, designed for use as a catheter dressing, was described by Richardson,[23] who also showed the effect that the adhesive had upon permeability. When the MVTR of the standard uncoated film (called Reactic) was measured using the standard technique it was found be 10,200 $g/m^2/24$ h when in contact with liquid. If the film was coated with adhesive in the normal way this was reduced to 880 $g/m^2/24$ h but if the adhesive was applied as a discontinuous film, so that 20-30% of the area remained exposed to liquid, the permeability of the resultant dressing was found to be in excess of 2900 $g/m^2/24$ h.

Films which have the ability to vary their MVTR in this way clearly offer potential advantages in the treatment of wounds in which exudate production reduces over time. Such products are sometimes referred to as 'smart' or 'intelligent' dressings. Palamand[19] measured the change in permeability that occurred in one product when the film was brought into contact with liquid. Under the conditions of test the MVTR increased from 1,425 to 12,730 $g/m^2/24$ h.

When used as backing layers for polyurethane foam dressings, these highly permeable or intelligent films greatly increase the fluid handling capacity of the product and thus greatly increase its wear time.[24]

Values for the MVTR of a number of film dressings drawn from published sources are shown in Table 10, although it should be stressed that these values apply to test conditions which may be very different from those encountered clinically.

Table 10: Permeability of film dressings

Dressing	MVTR $g/m^2/24$ h	
	Upright	Inverted
Opsite	829[23]	847[23]
	839[17]	862[17]
Opsite IV 3000	982[23]	2930[23]
Opsite IV 3000*	2612[25]	11791[25]
Tegaderm	794[23]	846[23]
	794[17]	846[17]
	702[25]	666[25]
Tegaderm IV	693[25]	776[25]
Tegaderm HP	973[25]	1100[25]
Tegaderm Plus	722[23]	780[23]
Bioclusive	547[17]	605[17]
	515[25]	528[25]
Ensure	436[17]	436[17]
Polyskin	221[25]	209[25]
Polyskin MR	1152[25]	2598[25]

Following formulation change in January 2003

It might seem, therefore, that as film dressings appear able to cope with all the moisture lost through the intact epidermis, they should be able to stay in place indefinitely. This, however, is clearly not the case for as the normal process of skin replacement occurs and the outer epidermal layer is shed, the dressing will inevitably become displaced at some point.

Because the permeability of the standard films is substantially less than the rate at which fluid is produced by exuding wounds, they are now generally not used as primary dressings for these indications.

Tissue compatibility

No dressing should liberate any agent into a wound that may be toxic or otherwise adversely affect the healing process. Cell culture techniques offer a rapid, sensitive screening method for potentially toxic dressing components that can be easily performed in the laboratory. It is assumed that products that show no evidence of toxicity when examined in this way are unlikely to produce adverse effects upon healing *in vivo*.

A convenient method for comparing the tissue compatibility of film dressings was described previously,[17] in a study which showed considerable variability in the tissue compatibility of the products and formulations that existed at that time. The original formulation of Opsite performed particularly badly in this test because of the presence of the zinc in the adhesive formulation.

Similar findings were reported by Van Luyen *et al.*,[26] who used transformed fibroblasts in methylcellulose gels to assess the cytotoxicity of 16 different wound dressings comprising conventional wound dressings, polyurethane-based films, composites, hydrocolloids and a collagen-based dressing. Using light and transmission electron microscopy, they found that only five out of 16 wound dressings did not induce cytotoxic effects. All five hydrocolloids were found to inhibit cell growth by greater than 70%, and the cells had strongly deviant morphologies. The remaining wound dressings showed medium cytotoxic effects, with cell growth inhibition, which varied from low (± 15%), medium-low (± 25%) to medium-high (± 50%). Two films were examined in this study; Tegaderm appeared free of any cytotoxic effects but old formulation of Opsite caused a marked reduction in cell proliferation.

Sieber *et al.*,[27] used a more complex test based on the Bell model[28] of cultured composite skin equivalents to assess the effect of different wound dressing materials, including Opsite and Tegaderm, on DNA synthesis. In this technique the material under examination is applied to a fibroblast-impregnated collagen gel overlain with keratinocytes which is regarded as a useful *in vitro* model for human skin. Small pieces of different dressings were placed upon individual gels and incubated for seven days after which DNA synthesis within the gels was assessed using immunocytochemistry. Although a number of the products tested, including Opsite, resulted in the production of a damaged or incomplete epidermal layer and decreased DNA production, the morphology of Tegaderm treated cells was similar to the controls and DNA production appeared to be enhanced.

Gaseous permeability

The role of atmospheric oxygen in wound healing is extremely complex. Epidermal cells have been shown experimentally to grow faster with increasing pO_2[29] and therefore it might be expected that the use of a dressing with a high oxygen permeability would contribute positively to wound healing.

This was investigated by Winter,[30] who confirmed that the rate of epidermal wound healing in his experimental model varied with the oxygen permeability of the film. Under polyethylene film 90% of the wound surface was covered by new epidermis in three days; under polypropylene film, which has 60% of the permeability of polyethylene, only 70% wound cover was achieved in the same time; under polyester, which has only 1% of the permeability of polyethylene, 52% of the wound surface was covered with new epithelium.

Silver,[31] measured the partial pressures of oxygen beneath different types of dressings in the treatment of superficial wounds and found that under polyethylene film the oxygen concentration was relatively high (123 mmHg) but under polyester it was very low (21 mmHg). He subsequently reported that in wounds that were moist and relatively free of exudate, the rate of migration of epidermal cells under occlusive dressings was related to the oxygen permeability of the film: the greater the permeability, the faster the rate of epithelial growth.[32]

In the laboratory study referred to previously,[17] under the conditions of test, the permeability of the six dressings ranged from $0.54 \, \text{L/m}^2/24 \, \text{h}$ to $2.0 \, \text{L/m}^2/24 \, \text{h}$. A sample of polyethylene film tested by the same method had a permeability of $1.8 \, \text{L/m}^2/24 \, \text{h}$, suggesting that, in terms of oxygen permeability, the permeability of some of the films at least was probably equal to or better than polyethylene film used by Winter and Silver, and therefore likely to have beneficial effects upon epithelial growth.

In heavily exuding wounds such as leg ulcers, however, oxygen is rapidly removed from the surface of the lesion; taken up, it is supposed, by bacteria and inflammatory cells. Under such conditions the permeability of the film has little direct effect upon healing rates.[33] In animal studies it has been shown that hypoxia is a stimulus to angiogenesis and when the hypoxic gradient is destroyed, capillary growth ceases.[34] If oxygen permeability of film dressings offers any clinical benefit, it is therefore likely to be restricted to the latter stages of healing.

According to some authors, the permeability of film dressings to carbon dioxide may also be clinically important. Sirvio and Grussing[35] examined the effect of thin film dressings with varying oxygen and carbon dioxide permeability on the pO_2, pCO_2, and pH of wound exudate and the rate of epithelialization in shallow wounds on domestic pigs. They compared three films, Saran Wrap, (Dow Chemical Company), made from polyvinylidine chloride which is of low permeability to gas; a highly gas permeable medical Grade silicone film formed from poly (dimethyl silicone), and Tegaderm, the gaseous permeability of which was intermediate between the two.

As expected the highest pO_2 and the lowest pCO_2 was recorded under the silicone film. Exudate under the polyvinylidine chloride had the lowest pO_2 and highest pCO_2 with intermediate vales for both parameters recorded beneath the polyurethane film. Despite the massive differences in the absolute transmission rates of the three films determined experimentally, the magnitude of the difference in the values determined *in vivo* was small. The pO_2 levels beneath the three films were in the approximate ratio of 1:2:3 and the pCO_2 levels in the ratio 1:3:5. This relatively small difference in clinical values compared with the large difference in the permeability values of the films determined experimentally (1:100:700 for oxygen and for 1:300:900 for CO_2), had previously been noted by Silver.[31] An inverse correlation was noted between the pH of wound fluid and permeability of the film to CO_2 (7.02, 7.25 and 7.73).

The authors reported that although reepithelialization of wounds dressed with the silicone film was significantly less than that of wounds dressed with polyvinylidine chloride and polyurethane, there was no statistical difference between these two films. Whilst the difference between the two less permeable films may not have reached statistical significance there was a small (4%) difference in favour of the polyvinylidine chloride film.

Morphological differences were noted during histological examination of the silicone dressed wounds that were not present in the wounds dressed with the other types of films. The authors suggested that the delayed closure of the wounds treated with the highly gas permeable silicone dressings may be associated with the elevated pH of these wounds caused by the loss of CO_2. It is possible, however, that there may be some other explanation for these observed effects which is not related to gaseous permeability. When Sieber *et al.*[27] compared the cytotoxicity of a range of dressings using a cell culture method; they found that a silicone gel sheet had marked adverse effects upon the viability of keratinocytes. The possibility that this was due to the high permeability of the gel to CO_2 can be discounted because in this study they used uncovered gels as controls. The conclusions of the Sirvio paper about the significance of CO_2 permeability must therefore be regarded with some caution.

Permeability to pharmaceutical preparations

Some dressings have been shown to be permeable to antibacterial agents both in aqueous solution and in various pharmaceutical preparations such as creams and ointments. Behar,[36] compared the permeability of Omiderm with that of Biobrane and found Omiderm to be two to three orders of magnitude greater. The permeability of Omiderm was such that it permitted sufficient antimicrobial agent to pass through to produce a pronounced effect in both laboratory tests and an infected animal wound model.

Ease of application and removal

No dressing, no matter how effective it might be appear to be in laboratory or clinical studies, will gain widespread use unless it is acceptable to patients and clinicians. For this reason most film dressings now incorporate relatively sophisticated application systems to overcome the problems encountered with the early presentation.[12]

Removal of film dressings is relatively easy, although it has to be done carefully to avoid damaging fragile skin. The film is first lifted slightly at a corner and stretched parallel to the skin while supporting the rest of the dressing. As the thin film stretches the adhesive breaks and the dressing lifts off without causing any pain or trauma.

Removing in the same direction of the hair growth is also said to make removal more comfortable.[37]

Film dressings coated with a silicone adhesive system, such as Episil, have also been developed which are claimed to further reduce the possibility of pain or trauma when the dressing is removed.

EXPERIMENTAL STUDIES

Healing of experimental wounds

Shelanski *et al.*,[18] in a two part study, compared the effects of films with different moisture vapour permeability on the healing rate of superficial skin wounds, and bacterial proliferation in wounds of volunteers (see below).

In the first part of the study, an adhesive polyurethane film dressing with a quoted MVTR of 352 $g/m^2/24$ h was compared with a more permeable non-adhesive product with a quoted MVTR of 820 $g/m^2/24$ h to assess healing rates of dermatome wounds on the arms of healthy volunteers. (No information was provided on the method used to determine the permeability of these films but from other published work it is believed that the MVTR value quoted for the polyurethane material is less than half that normally obtained when the film is tested in accordance with the European Standard).

The dressings were removed on days 3,6,9,13,16 and 21, when the wounds were examined and redressed. No difference in the healing rates of the two groups was detected but the more permeable product resulted in the formations of crusts and debris that obscured the wound surface and made assessment difficult. The PUF dressing produced a moister environment which prevented crust formation, but the adhesive nature of the film resulted in damage to newly formed tissue when the dressing was repeatedly removed (although this would not happen in normal clinical practice).

A useful indicator of healing progress is the restoration of the barrier function of the skin to transepidermal water loss (TEWL). The effects of semipermeable films on human skin following the production a standardised wound (tape stripping) were evaluated using measurements of TEWL, skin hydration, rate of moisture accumulation, and erythema.[38] Wounds treated with semipermeable films regained their barrier function more rapidly than either unoccluded wounds or those under complete occlusion, suggesting that semipermeable wound dressings augment barrier repair and skin quality by providing an optimised water vapour gradient during the wound healing process.

The importance of the time at which film dressings are applied and removed relative to wounding was investigated by Eaglestein *et al.*,[39] who allocated excised wounds in pigs to groups which were treated as follows:

- air exposed
- dressed applied immediately after left in place until wounds were evaluated
- dressed immediately after wounding and removed at 6, 24, or 48 hours
- dressed 2, 6, and 24 hours after wounding

Wounds were excised on days three through seven and specimens were considered healed if no defect was present. Based upon their observations, the authors concluded that in order to promote optimal resurfacing in superficial wounds, polyurethane dressings need to be applied within two hours of wounding and should be kept in place for at least a 24-hour period.

Biochemical properties of wound fluid beneath film dressings

Although as previously indicated, polyurethane film dressings are sufficiently permeable to prevent the accumulation of moisture lost through intact skin, in the presence of an open wound, particularly in the early stages of healing, it is not uncommon to see wound fluid (WF) trapped beneath the membrane. The composition, biochemical properties and antimicrobial activity of this fluid have been investigated by numerous workers.

Buchan et al.,[40] first studied the cell population, neutrophil bactericidal activity, protein type and the content of human wound exudate harvested from split skin graft donor sites dressed with a semipermeable film dressing. At all times throughout the study, the total white cell counts (TWC), percentage of neutrophils and absolute neutrophil numbers in the exudate were significantly higher than those present in blood samples collected at the same time. Microbiological studies undertaken on the neutrophils showed them to be actively bactericidal for up to 24 hours postoperatively. Elevated levels of lysozyme were also detected in WF compared with the patients' own blood at each time point measured over a period of 72 hours. The protein content of the wound fluid remained constant, similar to that of blood, despite the loss of water through the film dressing leading the authors to propose that the maintenance of this concentration is due to a dynamic exchange with the blood, or an osmotic effect whereby water is drawn from the blood to compensate for the increased concentration beneath the membrane.

Buchan and his colleagues,[41] then repeated this work using partial thickness wounds on the pig as an experimental model. They showed that, other than a few minor differences which could be explained by the differences in wound types and skin physiology, the composition and properties of the pig wound exudate was very similar to human WF, leading them to conclude that this animal model was suitable for *in vivo* studies of the bactericidal activity of wound exudate.

Alper et al.,[42] collected wound fluid from beneath dressings on seven different patients and added it to growth medium applied to synchronised fibroblast cultures *in vitro* using human serum as a diluent and a control. They showed that the wound fluid stimulated fibroblast cell division and produced an altered pattern of fibroblast growth.

Ono et al.,[43] also investigated the stimulatory activity of wound fluid collected from beneath film dressings applied to donor-site and showed that platelet derived growth factor (PDGF), interleukin-6 (IL-6), transforming growth factor-alpha (TGF-alpha) and TGF-beta were present in relatively large amounts.

Effect of film dressings upon wound and skin microbiology

The antimicrobial properties of Opsite and Tegaderm were challenged Holland *et al.*,[44] with three bacteria, *S. aureus*, *E. coli* and *S. pyogenes*. Both dressings appeared to inhibit the growth of *E. coli*, *S. Pyogenes* and *S. aureus*, but Tegaderm was less active than Opsite in this regard. Opsite was also active against *P. aeruginosa* but Tegaderm showed no significant inhibitory effects against this organism. Once again this difference in activity between the dressings in this and the previously described biochemical studies may be at least partially attributed to the presence of zinc ions in the vinyl ether adhesive applied to Opsite at that time.

In a second study Holland *et al.*[45] examined the effect of three film dressings Opsite, Ensure and Tegaderm, on the bacterial population of the skin of volunteers using a piece of occlusive film as a control. They reported that occlusion greatly increased the bioburden of the skin and that although Ensure and Opsite yield bacterial numbers similar to that of the occlusive film, those on skin dressed with Opsite remained comparable with normal skin. This activity is once again assumed to be due to the presence of the zinc ions.

Although the inherent antimicrobial activity of wound fluid may initially be sufficient to prevent the proliferation of bacteria in socially clean wounds, over time or in the presence of a large inoculum of microorganisms, these defences are likely to become overwhelmed. Metz *et al.*,[46] using a pig model, showed an increase in the number and types of microorganisms present in superficial wounds dressed with a polyurethane film dressing compared with air exposed wounds.

Katz[47] inoculated a series of standard wounds on human volunteers with heavy cultures of *S. aureus*, *P. aeruginosa*, *S. epidermidis* and *S. pyogenes*. The wounds were covered with different types of 'occlusive' dressings and quantitative cultures taken after 6, 24 and 48 hours. The results were expressed relative to Saran Wrap, which acted as a control. The authors concluded that, in the test system used, there was no significant difference in the healing rates recorded beneath any of the materials examined, including the control. However, the number of microorganisms recovered from beneath the dressings varied according to species and the time of sampling.

In the second part of the study referred to previously, Shelanski[18] determined the number of bacteria that could be recovered from the surfaces of chemically-induced superficial skin wounds on the arms of volunteers dressed with four different films. Each wound was inoculated with 1.4×10^6 of a non-pathogenic strain of *S. epidermidis* and covered with one of the dressings under examination. Two adhesive polyurethane films dressings, Opsite, and Tegaderm, were compared with a non-adhesive polyurethane film, Blister Film, and the impermeable Saran Wrap. Two days after inoculation the dressings were removed and the volume of liquid that had accumulated beneath the dressing and number of organisms present in each determined. It was found that both the volume of fluid and the number of organisms recovered were inversely related to the MVTR of the applied film.

The effects of prolonged occlusion on the physiology and microbial skin flora were studied by Aly *et al.*[48] who measured pH, transepidermal water loss (TEWL) and carbon dioxide emission rate (CDER). The average bacterial count which, before occlusion was $1.8 \times 10^2/cm^2$, increased to 9.8×10^7 on Day four, dropping back to 4.5×10^6 on Day 5.

The pH of the skin increased from 4.38 to 7.05 over five days, and after five days of occlusion, TEWL increased from 0.56 mg/cm^2/h to 1.87 mg/cm^2/h and CO_2 emission increased from 25 nl/cm^2/min to 118 nl/cm^2/min, equivalent to 360-1700 ml/m^2/24 h.

Film dressings also find application as incise drapes where they are used to provide a sterile field and immobilise bacteria in order to prevent them from entering the wounds. A film that is commonly used for this purpose is Steridrape

Bacterial barrier properties of film dressings

The results of stringent laboratory tests indicate that most film dressings form an effective barrier to bacteria. It may therefore be assumed that an intact polyurethane film, which remains firmly adhered to intact periwound skin, should also prevent the ingress or egress of microorganisms into or out of a wound and thus help to prevent the spread of infection.

The ability of a film dressing to function in this way was investigated in an animal model, in which standard wounds on a pig were dressed with a film dressing (Opsite), a hydrogel dressing, Vigilon, and a hydrocolloid dressing,[49] Duoderm. Both the dressing itself and the skin immediately around the perimeter were challenged with suspensions of bacteria S. aureus and P. aeruginosa on one, two or three occasions and following removal of the dressings, the wounds were examined for the presence of the test organisms. Although the hydrocolloid dressing prevented the ingress of both organisms in all the tests, the film dressing and the hydrogel failed to prevent contamination of 50% of the wounds challenged with S. aureus and all the wounds challenged with P. aeruginosa. This failure was considered to be due to bacteria gaining access from the edge of the dressing (through wrinkles or channels formed beneath the film), rather than by direct penetration through the film itself.

CLINICAL EXPERIENCE WITH FILM DRESSINGS

Films as wound dressings

Film dressings have been used successfully in the treatment of many types of wounds. Historically, before the development of other more absorbent, products designed to maintain a moist healing environment, films were frequently used for indications for which they would probably now be considered less than ideally suited. Alper,[50] for example, reported good results following a small study involving 18 patients with leg ulcers in which he compared a film dressing, Opsite, with a debriding ointment and 10% benzyl peroxide. More recently, however, the introduction of new families of dressings such as the alginates and foams has meant that the role of the films has been re-evaluated. They now tend to be used for more lightly exuding wounds or as secondary dressings where their moisture vapour permeability enhances the fluid handling properties of absorbent primary wound contact agents.

Burns

Burns are one of the most devastating conditions encountered in medicine and represent an assault on all aspects of the patient, from the physical to the psychological.[51] In the United Kingdom about 250,000 people are burnt each year. Of these, 175,000 attend accident and emergency departments, and 13,000 are admitted to hospital. Burns affect all ages, from babies to elderly people and are a source of severe pain.

Excessive heating of the skin destroys the semipermeable membrane associated with the lipo-protein layer in the stratum corneum which normally controls moisture loss through the skin.[21] In the absence of this regulatory control, second degree burns can lose around 4000 g/m^2/24 h. This fluid loss can lead to localised devitalization of damaged tissue causing the wound to extend or become deeper,[52] but in more extensive wounds it can also have serious consequences for the patient's fluid balance. According to Lamke,[21] the application of a film dressing can reduce the fluid loss from burns by 73%.

From the time of the First World War to the end of the 20th Century, most partial thickness burns were dressed with paraffin gauze covered with a secondary absorbent layer such as Gamgee tissue. Such dressings are bulky and difficult to remove, sometimes causing such pain that the patient may require an anaesthetic to have their dressings changed. The introduction of film dressings therefore provided an alternative form of treatment which is more convenient for the patient and less likely to cause pain upon removal.

An early account of the use of Opsite in burn management was provided by Conkle in 1981.[53] In the same year the dressing was evaluated in a trial involving 51 patients with partial thickness burns.[54] Wounds dressed with the film healed significantly faster than comparable wounds dressed with a paraffin gauze dressing containing chlorhexidine (10 ± 5 vs 14.1 ± 7 days). One patient treated with film and two treated conventionally developed a proven infection. Patients dressed with the film reported significantly less pain than those dressed with conventional dressings. The authors speculated that this was either because of reduced tissue damage due to decreased evaporation, or because there was less trauma at dressing changes.

A film dressing was evaluated in a prospective study involving 150 patients with partial thickness burns ranging from < 5% to 25% of the total body area.[55] The film was applied to all anatomical sites with the exception of the head and face. The authors reported that 80% of patients did well, but the remainder had to have the dressing discontinued for various reasons, the most common being infection. The advantages of the dressing were reported to be the ease of wound observation, patient comfort, early mobilization and relative economy. It was concluded that a film dressing is a suitable treatment for partial thickness burns, especially of the trunk and limbs, and is very useful in children. The complications were judged to be relatively few and minor.

In an outpatient study, a semipermeable film dressing was compared with silver sulphadiazine cream in the treatment of minor burns.[56] The treatment groups were closely matched in age, sex, and the extent of their burns. Compared with the silver sulphadiazine group, patients dressed with the film experienced a 39% greater reduction in pain following the application of their dressing. Patients in the film group also reported fewer problems with their wounds interfering with their normal activities. The clinical infection rate and time to healing were similar in both groups. The authors concluded that for the management of outpatient burns a film dressing was superior to silver sulphadiazine.

Clinical experience with film dressings in the treatment of burns was supported by the results of an animal study in which healing time, infection rate, and residual scar formation were compared in carbon dioxide laser burns in rats.[57] Experimental wounds were dressed with a semipermeable polyurethane film, Petrolatum Gauze (USP), a prototype gel or left exposed to the air. There were no infections and no differences in scar formation among the treatment groups. The mean healing times were ten days for the polyurethane dressings and the prototype material, 13 days for Petrolatum Gauze, and 16 days for the untreated group. The authors concluded that synthetic gas-permeable dressings promote healing after cutaneous carbon dioxide laser surgery more effectively than conventional treatments or leaving the wound exposed to the air.

More favourable results for the use of gauze were reported following a further prospective, randomized clinical study,[58] in which Opsite was compared with paraffin gauze dressing in the treatment of outpatients with partial-thickness burns. Thirty patients were treated with the polyurethane film and twenty five with the conventional dressing. The patients were followed until the wounds had fully healed and they were also assessed three months later for evaluation of residual scars and pigmentation. The burns treated with polyurethane films healed with a median of ten days as in previous studies, but the conventionally treated burns were reported to have healed in a median time of seven days. Residual scars were noted in 21% of the patients treated with polyurethane films and in eight percent treated conventionally. Neither difference achieved statistical significance. Despite these apparently poor results for the film dressing, 96% of patients treated in this way stated that they were satisfied with the treatment compared with 20% of those in the gauze treated group.

Donor sites

As with burns, until the introduction of film dressings, split-skin grafts were traditionally treated either by simple exposure or the application of bulky dressings which frequently consisted of paraffin gauze covered with layers of absorbent material held in place with a crepe bandage. Both treatments were extremely painful, and it was not uncommon for patients to complain more about the pain from the donor site than the original injury.

One of the earliest accounts of the use of Opsite for this indication was published in 1975,[59] when 53 patients with donor sites on thighs, buttocks, arms and backs had their wounds treated in this way. In all the early cases it was reported that sero-sanguineous fluid which collected under the dressing often leaked or ruptured the film, necessitating the application of an outer padding layer in the immediate post operative period. Initially the film dressing was removed when epithelialization appeared to be complete but this was found to cause stripping leaving a fresh wound that was slow to heal. Subsequently the film was left in place until it separated spontaneously. When used in this manner the film dressing was found to cause less pain than conventional treatments and was judged to result in accelerated healing. Four of the fifty three patients developed wound infections thought to be associated with a poor aseptic technique when changing a leaking dressing.

Bergman in 1977,[60] and Dinner *et al.* in 1979,[61] similarly reported that in uncontrolled studies the application of a film dressing resulted in improved healing rates and greatly reduced pain.

The first prospective randomized control trial involving the use of film dressings on donor sites was reported by Barnett *et al.* in 1983.[62] Sixty donor sites on 24 patients were randomized to treatment with either fine mesh gauze, Opsite or Tegaderm and the mean time to heal was 10.5 *vs* 6.8 days respectively. An analogue scale of 0-10 was used to assess wound related pain which was found to be 'almost nonexistent' when film dressings were used, resulting in a score of 1.6 ± 0.8 compared with 4.7 ± 2.2 for fine mesh gauze. Two patients in each film group developed wound infections caused by *P. aeruginosa*. Three of these occurred on one patient known to be colonised with this organism. No differences were detected between the films used in this study.

Barnett *et al.* published a second paper in 1983,[63] in which they reanalysed their earlier data to compare the healing rates of scalp wounds used as donor sites compared with sites elsewhere on the body. Overall healing times were 4.9 days and nine days respectively. Scalp sites treated with fine mesh gauze healed in 6.3 days whilst other sites treated in this way took 11.9 days. With film dressings the healing time was 4.7 days for scalp wounds and 8.9 days for other sites. The authors concluded that the combination of a scalp donor site and a film dressing produce the optimal donor site/dressing combination.

Morita *et al.*,[64] also used film dressings for scalp donor sites but experienced difficulties in retaining the dressings in place, a problem they overcame by the use of skin staples. Eight donor sites in four patients were dressed in this way. Three had their scalps re-harvested several times and all wounds healed uneventfully with a mean healing time of 6.8 days.

Early studies on the use of semipermeable films on split-skin donor sites involved mainly Caucasian patients. Iregbulem,[65] undertook a study to assess the value of the technique in the black population of a developing country where donor sites were reported to be notoriously slow to heal. Fifty Nigerians of varying age groups had split-skin grafts of identical thickness taken from both thighs by the same surgeon. All patients had one thigh dressed with Sofratulle, a paraffin gauze dressing containing soframycin, and the other with Opsite. Of the donor sites treated with the antibiotic containing tulle, 25 (53.4%) were healed by the 13th postoperative day compared with 30 (62.5%) treated with film dressing that were healed by the 7th postoperative day. All film dressed wounds were completely healed by the 11th day but it took nearly four weeks for the paraffin gauze treated thighs to heal. Minimal discomfort was experienced by 10% of the patients treated with film dressings but about 80% of those treated with paraffin gauze required mild analgesics on ambulation during the first 48 hours. The author concluded that film dressings are easy to use, reduce healing time, eliminate pain and well tolerated by patients.

More quantitative information on the pain associated with donor sites covered with a polyurethane film dressing was collected in a further study using a modified visual analogue scale (VAS) which was analysed to determine differences between pain levels under conditions of rest and activity.[66] When applied correctly, film-covered donor sites could be maintained relatively pain free, but if applied incorrectly they could cause the patient to experience donor-site pain comparable to concurrent burn-wound pain. Pain was also increased during ambulation.

Because donor site healing can be delayed in elderly patients, Blight *et al.*[67] undertook a study to evaluate the potential value of a cultured allogenic epithelial graft (CAG) for this indication, comparing it with paraffin gauze and a semipermeable film dressing, Opsite. Compared with the paraffin gauze dressing, both the CAG and the film significantly reduced the number of patients with delayed healing but no significant difference was detected between the film and the CAG.

The use of film dressings in the treatment of donor sites can result in the accumulation of fluid beneath the film in the immediate postoperative period. This can be addressed by the aspiration of fluid from beneath the dressing using a syringe, or the application of an absorbent covering to take up fluid that escapes from around the margin of the dressing. Following a controlled trial involving fifty patients with donor sites,[68] it was reported that the administration of one gram of ethamsylate immediately prior to surgery significantly reduced the number of interventions required to deal with this problem; ethamsylate is a haemostatic agent that increases platelet adhesiveness decreasing capillary fragility and bleeding time.

A semipermeable film dressing, Tegaderm, was compared with three other products in a prospective randomized study involving 80 patients undergoing elective split thickness skin grafting.[69] The dressings used were paraffin gauze, Lyofoam, a thin hydrophobic polyurethane foam dressing with an absorbent wound contact layer and a polyethane film dressing with a low MVTR normally used as an incise drape (Steri-Drape). All wounds were assessed for healing on the 14th day after surgery at which time there were no dressing-dependent differences in healing rates detected; had an early assessment of healing been made, perhaps at day seven or day 10, it is likely that differences in healing rates would have been detected. Polyurethane film was shown to be more comfortable in use and easier to remove. As a result of this investigation it was selected as the dressing of choice for this application within the department concerned.

Surgical wounds

Film dressings have been widely used in surgical practice as a dressing following primary closure by suturing or some other means when their properties have been appreciated by surgeons and patients alike.

An early account of the use of Opsite in the management of some 1600 surgical patients was provided by Tinckler.[70] He considered it to be of particular value in situations where cosmetic considerations are especially desirable and concluded that the use of such material represented a significant advance in surgical technique, not least because it enabled patients to bathe throughout the postoperative period.

This view was supported by Drake,[71] who reported upon the use of the film to achieve wound closure in some 400 children aged one week to 12 years with widely different wounds over an eighteen month period, and Rubio[72] who used three different film dressing as a protective cover for 3637 surgical incisions over an eight year period. He concluded that the film resulted in faster wound healing, decreased pain and less scarring. It also permitted visual assessment of wound healing, as well as promoting patient mobility and hygiene.

In a comparative study which compared the use of Tegaderm and gauze following breast surgery in 120 patients,[73] staff and patients found that Tegaderm was easier to apply and more comfortable to wear. Visual inspection of the wound was possible at all times and patients could bath or wash with no adverse effects upon the dressing. The appearance of the healed wound was also improved by the use of the film. It was estimated that the cost of the dressing treatment was less than one-third of the cost of using gauze.

The effect of dressings upon postoperative incisional pain was investigated in a prospective randomized controlled trial involving 30 patients undergoing total abdominal hysterectomy.[74] One group of patients were treated with a film dressing, Opsite Flexigrid, left intact until suture removal; patients in the control group were treated with Primapore, an adhesive island dressing which was removed after 48 hours. Incisional wound pain was assessed using a VAS and the McGill Pain Questionnaire, recorded daily for four days until discharge. Although the pain scores were not significantly different between the groups one or two days postoperatively, on day three when the wounds in the dry dressing group were exposed, there was a statistically significant difference in 24-hour average pain. Patients whose wounds were covered with the film dressing experienced less pain and requested fewer non-steroidal anti-inflammatory drugs on Day 3. The authors concluded that maintaining a cover over a surgical wound until suture removal appeared to reduce incisional pain compared to air exposure. The film dressing also had the advantage that it permitted inspection of the wound without removing the dressing.

The effect of film dressings on incisional pain following removal of the saphenous vein for a coronary artery bypass graft was examined in a controlled trial in which patients were randomly allocated to have their wounds dressed with a film dressing, dry sterile gauze or left exposed to the air.[75] Treatments were allocated on the first postoperative day. Patients were requested to complete a pain and distress VAS on postoperative days one, three and five, and a cosmetic result VAS upon discharge. Film treated patients reported decreasing pain from days one to three, whilst those whose wounds were air-exposed or treated with gauze reported increasing pain from days one to three ($p < 0.05$).

Film dressings have also been used successfully to form a protective, moisture retaining cover for wounds left to heal by secondary intention. In these situations they may be applied either alone or in combination with another primary dressing.

A semipermeable film dressing, Bioclusive, was compared with a conventional dressing which consisted of dry gauze and an antibiotic ointment, Polysporin, in 58 patients with fresh skin wounds following Mohs micrographic surgery for removal of skin basal and squamous cell carcinomas.[76] All the lesions were on the head, most commonly on the nose and forehead. The group dressed with the film showed a faster rate of wound contraction and reepithelialization and a shorter total healing time than the other two groups. It was also rated better with regard to comfort, ease of use, and ease of dressing removal. At six-month follow-up, the film-dressed group had scars that were softer, smoother, and showed less thickening and anatomic deformities. Better cosmetic appearance and greater patient acceptance were also noted with the film dressing.

The clinical benefits of products that provide moist wound healing were evaluated in patients with open abdominal incisions. An amorphous hydrogel dressing, Intrasite, or a foam wound cavity filler, Allevyn Cavity, were used in conjunction with a semipermeable film, Bioclusive, and compared with traditional wet-to-dry dressings. Patients treated with the modern dressings experienced less pain, and reduced healing times resulting in a significant cost savings.[77]

In the management of intra-abdominal sepsis, the abdomen is often left open after the first laparotomy which represents a major wound management problem. One technique that has been used in the management of this condition involves the application of a large film dressing over the entire wound. Suction catheters positioned under the film are connected to a low-vacuum suction system (1 - 2kPa) to facilitate wound drainage. The effectiveness of this method was evaluated in 12 patients.[78] It was reported that the dressings were changed every six days and that the majority of problems related to the traditional method of managing this problem were overcome by the use of the film.

Orthopaedic wounds

Film dressings also have a role in orthopaedic surgery. Hip and knee replacements are performed in very large numbers each year and provided wounds do not become infected, these operations result in a significant improvement in the quality of life for the individuals concerned. Antibiotic prophylaxis and the use of laminar air-flow operating theatres have reduced deep infections rates to less than one percent,[79] but effective postoperative wound management is still necessary to prevent complications developing later.

Orthopaedic wounds closed with tapes or adhesive dressings sometimes develop blisters around the wound margin,[80] a not uncommon problem that has been particularly associated with the use of some types of self-adhesive nonwoven fabric post-operative dressings.[81] This blistering is believed to be caused by firm bonding of the dressing to the epidermis and the development of superficial shear forces (possibly caused by swelling), which result in weakening of the epidermal and dermal junction, thereby allowing the two layers of skin to separate. This severity of this effect is thought to be inversely related to the extensibility of the dressing.

Dressing related problems following arthroplasty were reviewed in a clinical study involving patients undergoing total knee or hip arthroplasty who were treated with either standard dressing, consisting of an adhesive dressing and absorbent pad secured by tape and adhesive net (n = 22), or Aquacel, an absorbent gel forming fibrous dressing, made from carboxymethylcellulose covered by an adhesive semipermeable polyurethane film (CMC/film dressing) (n = 36).[82]

The principal aim of the study was to determine whether the novel dressing would delay the first dressing change and reduce the frequency of changes thereafter, factors which might be expected to reduce postoperative infections caused by the loss of a bacterial barrier. Patients undergoing a total hip arthroplasty whose wounds were dressed with a film/absorbent fibre combination had a mean of 2.4 dressing changes but those treated with the standard dressing required 6.2 changes. Patients who had undergone a total knee arthroplasty required 2.3 and 4.7 changes respectively. Leakage of blood and exudate was also reduced for the film/fibre dressing combination, as was the incidence of skin problems including blistering.

In a further study involving 100 patients undergoing arthroplasty patients were randomized to treatment which consisted of the CMC/film or a conventional wound pad dressing with tape fixation.[83] At the first dressing change, 59% of patients dressed with CMC/film had skin reactions (blister, erythema, oedema, skin injury and haematoma) compared with 81% in the control group (p = 0.02).

A CMC/Tegaderm film combination was compared with a nonwoven fabric-backed self adhesive island dressing[84] in a study in which 200 patients were randomized to treatment following elective and non-elective surgery to the hip and the knee in order to compare the incidence of adverse events such as skin blistering or signs of infection. The number of dressing changes was also recorded. Results were obtained for 183 patients. Taking blisters alone, 22.5% of patients dressed with the nonwoven fabric island dressing group developed blisters compared to only 2.4% of the group dressed with CMC/film. Overall wounds dressed with the nonwoven fabric dressing were 5.8 times more likely to experience complications compared with those dressed with CMC/film (p < 0.00001). Pain scores were also significantly lower for the patients receiving the CMC/film dressing (p = 0.001).

In a modified version of this technique twenty consecutive patients who underwent total hip or knee arthroplasty received a simple gauze dressing covered with Tegaderm. A cumulative sum technique (cusum) was used to assess the dressing with regards to skin blistering which showed that this simple dressing met specified standards with regards to postoperative wound blistering.[85]

Cosker et al.,[86] evaluated three types of postoperative dressings in the treatment of 300 orthopaedic wounds. These were; Opsite Post-Op, a film-based post operative dressing with a moisture vapour permeability in excess of 3000 $g/m^2/h$, Tegaderm + Pad (a Tegaderm semipermeable transparent film with an integral absorbent pad) and a nonwoven fabric backed post-operative dressing. The incidence of blistering, which occurred mostly on the 5th or 6th postoperative day, was 6%, 16% and 24% within the three groups respectively. Problems relating to the accumulation of a serosanguinous discharge beneath the dressings also varied between the treatment groups, 7%, 21% and 26% respectively.

The authors suggested the difference in the performance of the two film based dressings was possibly due in part to the difference in permeability, as excessive moisture reduces the ability of the epidermal tissue to withstand frictional forces, but the difference in the extensibility of the two films was probably also an important factor. Values quoted were 0.04 kgf/cm extension for the plain film, compared with 0.09 kgf/cm for the Tegaderm + Pad dressing.

The use of film dressings has also been reported in the treatment of other types of orthopaedic wounds.[87] Fifteen patients, including those with rheumatoid arthritis or systemic sclerosis, who had wounds with exposed bones were treated either with a standard procedure, consisting of local wound care involving debridement with a scalpel, bed rest and parenteral antibiotics (n = 8), or with an alternative new technique (n = 7) in which the affected bone was initially exposed by debridement with a scalpel, followed by partial excision with a bone scraper until bleeding was observed from the exposed bone. The lesions were immediately covered with Tegaderm Plus for 3-8 days to trap the coagulated clots within the marrow, and were eventually treated with epidermal grafts obtained from suction blisters. Although the time needed for wound healing was similar in the two treatment groups, the more aggressive therapy reduced the risk of amputation (p = 0.020).

A film dressing was used in conjunction with Tobramycin-PMMA beads to dress 381 severe compound fractures in 335 patients using the antibiotic bead pouch technique.[88] The fractures were managed with early administration of broad spectrum antibiotics, copious wound irrigation, serial debridement, and external skeletal stabilization. Tobramycin-PMMA beads were placed in the wound, and a film dressing applied to cover the soft tissue defect. This dressing was changed every 48 to 72 hours until wound coverage/closure could be obtained. Fractures that did not develop an infection were closed at a mean time of 7.6 days; those that developed an infection were closed at a mean time of 17.9 days. The difference was statistically significant (p < 0.001).

Film dressings (Opsite or Tegaderm) were used in a combination with suction drainage to treat 20 orthopaedic patients without any wound complication and with satisfactory comfort to the patient.[89] Although the authors claimed this to be a novel form of treatment it is essentially the same as vacuum assisted closure first described several years earlier.

Pressure ulcers

Semipermeable film dressings can protect wounds and damaged skin from contamination with urine and faeces. They also reduce frictional forces,[90] which may in turn help to reduce skin damage caused by shearing forces generated between the patient and the bed linen. Films are therefore useful in the management of patients with existing superficial pressure ulcers or those at risk of developing such wounds.

An early account of the use of film dressings in the treatment and prevention of pressure ulcers was provided in 1979 by Hammond,[91] who described the practical benefits associated with the successful use of Opsite in four patients with active sores and 20 patients who were treated prophylactically.

In an early clinical trial, Braverman et al.[92] in 1981 described how thirty elderly patients with pressure damage were treated with Opsite or a non specified control. Twenty patients completed the study and in a four week period, the wounds of 10/12 patients in the film dressing group were healed compared with 5/12 in the control group. After 12 weeks the numbers of healed wounds in the two groups were 10/12 and 8/12 respectively. The authors concluded that although preliminary unpublished work had demonstrated that film dressings were not helpful in the management of deep ulcers, the application of a film to superficial wounds may reduce infection and provide an environment which is conducive to healing.

In a prospective randomized study, Tegaderm dressings were compared with respect to healing rates and costs of treatment in patients with Grade II or III pressure ulcers. In an eight week period, 64% of Grade II ulcers dressed with the film healed, but none of the patients in the control group healed within this time. The median improvement for the Grade II group was 100% for the film (n = 22) and 52% for gauze (n = 12), (P < 0.05, Wilcoxon rank sum test). The healing rates for Grade III ulcers were not significantly different in the two dressing groups but there was a trend towards a greater decrease in area when the film dressing was used. The mean eight-week labour and supply cost per ulcer using the MVP was $845, while that for gauze treatments was $1359, (p < 0.05, Wilcoxon rank sum test). The cost difference for Grade III ulcers was not significant in the two dressing groups.[93]

Films as secondary dressings

 Much has been written on the selection and use of dressings for the management of different types of wounds, but as previously described,[94] this has largely been devoted to primary wound dressings, products such as hydrogels, alginates and hydrocolloids, which are placed in intimate contact with damaged tissue. Although the choice of an appropriate primary wound dressing is undoubtedly a major factor in promoting rapid wound healing, these materials cannot be used in isolation.

With the exception of compression bandages, which play a key role in the management of venous leg ulcers, relatively little attention has been given to the importance of secondary dressings. This is an important oversight because the choice of secondary dressings has an influence on hydrodynamics (the control of the moisture content of the wound), the spread of bacteria from the wound, and the prevention and/or containment of malodour. The contribution made by a secondary dressing to treatment outcomes in published clinical studies designed to compare the effectiveness of different primary dressings is often either not recognised or ignored.

It is the strongly held belief of the author that the failure of many clinical investigators to understand the importance of the correct choice of secondary dressing has greatly reduced the value of numerous clinical trials which have sought to compare healing rates achieved with different types of primary dressings.

Banks et al.,[95] compared a film dressing, used as a secondary over an N-A Dressing, with a self adhesive foam dressing, Lyofoam A in the treatment of Grade II and III pressure ulcers in 50 patients, no statistical difference was detected between the two dressings.

Cannavo et al.,[96] published the results of a study involving 39 patients with large abdominal wounds in which they compared an alginate dressing with swabs soaked in 0.05% solution of sodium hypochlorite covered with a simple absorbent dressing pad, all of which were covered with a semipermeable film, Tegaderm, as a secondary dressing. Treatment outcomes assessed included healing rates, both area and volume, patient comfort, and cost. The simple dressing pad protocol performed well when compared with the calcium alginate in terms of healing time, patient comfort and cost but maximum pain was significantly greater ($p = 0.011$) and satisfaction significantly lower among patients treated with sodium hypochlorite soaks. The cost of the hypochlorite treatment was also substantially higher. The authors proposed that the trial results supported the proposition that the use of the sodium hypochlorite dressing should be abandoned

The ability of film dressings to act as bacterial barrier and provide some control over moisture loss from the wound and the surrounding area makes them in many ways the ideal secondary dressing. In the majority of the orthopaedic studies identified above, for example, the film was used in this way in conjunction with an absorbent pad.[82-85]

Perhaps because of the lack of understanding of the important contribution made by secondary dressings, few randomized controlled clinical trials have been conducted that are specifically concerned with this aspect of treatment One such study was undertaken by Thomas et al.,[97] specifically to compare the performance of two films when used as secondary dressings. Tegaderm and Duoderm Extra Thin, a polyurethane film coated with a hydrocolloid adhesive, were compared with respect to their ability to resist wrinkling and prevent maceration defined as the primary outcome variables. A total of 100 patients were stratified and randomized to treatment with the film applied over an alginate or hydrogel depending upon the condition of the wound. Although the Tegaderm was found to be significantly easier to apply, the stratification to different wound types and treatments meant that, in some of groups, the numbers involved were too small to allow the results to achieve statistical significance, despite the relatively large number of patients included in the trial. It was concluded that the study failed to demonstrate a difference between the two secondary dressings.

Paediatric wound care

The reduction in wound pain that is frequently achieved by the application of semipermeable film dressings makes these materials particularly useful for treating wounds in children. This was recognized at an early stage by Lobe et al.[98] who applied film dressings to fifty children with skin graft donor sites, partial thickness burns, traumatic abrasions and a variety of other potentially painful wound types. The authors reported that although the exudate that accumulated beneath the exudate had a 'purulent' appearance this was not associated with clinical infection. The use of the film resulted in less pain, greater freedom of movement of the affected part, fewer dressing changes and apparently faster healing in many cases. Because of these benefits the dressing gained rapid acceptance by nurses, patients and parents.

Tegaderm has been used with advantage in the treatment of certain birth defects. In one study, following surgery to correct hypospadias,[99] a penile nerve block and the application of a film dressing facilitated early postoperative mobilization. But, in a second study,[100] when 100 children with hypospadias were randomized either to receive no dressing or a transparent film dressing for two days, no particular complication was more common in either group. Of 49 patients 44 (90%) had successful results in the film-dressed and control groups. Although postoperative calls were more common in the undressed group ($p = 0.02$) no particular complication was more common in either group ($p < 0.05$). The authors considered that in terms of clinical outcomes the success rate for hypospadias surgery that preserves the urethral plate is independent of dressing usage and suggested that dressings may not be indicated for all hypospadias repairs.

Film dressings were used successfully in the treatment of eight children with ulcerative haemangiomas,[101] the most common tumours occurring in young children. In all eight infants, prompt pain relief and healing within 1-2 months were observed. An increased regression was also noted within 2 - 4 months, when the haemangiomas were in the normal proliferative phase. Although the reason for the observed clinical benefits associated with the use of the film was not fully understood, the authors recommended that the application of a polyurethane film should be considered as the treatment of choice for this condition.

Gastroschisis is a congenital anomaly of the anterior abdominal wall that results in the abdominal contents protruding through a defect usually located to the right side of the umbilicus. Sandler et al.,[102] described a technique called 'plastic closure' in which the bowel was decompressed and reduced, and the defect covered with the umbilical cord tailored to fit the opening. Two Tegaderm dressings were subsequently applied to reinforce the defect. Ten children were treated using this method which the authors described as 'simple, safe, and cosmetically appealing'.

In a somewhat unique application, the fluid regulating properties of film dressings were utilised in the management of infants with extremely low birth weight (< 1.0 kg).[103] In such infants significant fluid and electrolyte disturbances occur during the first few days of life. Tegaderm dressings were applied to the skin of 30 babies shortly after birth and information on fluid and electrolyte status was collected and compared with historical data collected from the records of 39 infants not treated in this way. Throughout the first week of life, serum Na^+ levels, daily fluid intake and daily weight loss were significantly higher in the infants who were not dressed with the film ($p < 0.05$). Hypernatremia ($Na^+ > 150$ mEq/l) developed in 51% of untreated infants compared to 17% of film-covered babies ($p = 0.0005$). Survival was significantly higher in babies who received the film, 90% vs 64% ($p = 0.02$). The authors concluded that the application of a semipermeable polyurethane membrane to the skin of ELBW infants shortly after birth decreased postnatal fluid and electrolyte disturbances and significantly improved their outcome by reducing severity of lung disease and decreasing mortality.

Radiotherapy wounds

A semipermeable film dressing, Tegaderm, was compared with gauze coated with lanolin for the treatment of skin reactions following radiotherapy in 16 patients with moderate or severe desquamation injuries.[104] Although the authors only detected a non-significant trend towards a decrease in healing time in wounds dressed with the film (19 days compared with 24 days), it was considered that there were also other benefits to be obtained from its use. The film dressing required less frequent replacement and did not need to be removed prior to therapy. It was also said to be less bulky, and cause less pain upon removal than the lanolin-impregnated gauze.

Cryotherapy

The effect of different types of dressings upon the efficiency of cryotherapy was determined in a volunteer study involving eighteen individuals divided equally into three groups.[105] Each group had one knee dressed with either a Tegaderm, a 'wool and crepe' bandage or had no dressing applied. Cryotherapy was applied to one knee with the other serving as control. Skin temperature was measured bilaterally every five min for two hours. The mean decrease in skin temperature after two hours was 17°C in the volunteers with a film dressing or no dressing, but an average of only 5 °C degrees in those with a 'wool and crepe' bandage. This difference was highly significant ($p < 0.001$). The authors concluded that the application of a traditional bandage following knee surgery would prevent effective cryotherapy but a film dressing would not.

Diabetic neuropathy

A total of 33 patients with chronic diabetic neuropathy were dressed with Opsite or received no treatment.[106] After a run-in period of two weeks, the film was applied to one of the painful legs for four weeks. This was followed by another period of four weeks when the film was switched to the opposite leg. Pain was assessed by VAS and the primary analysis variable was within patient difference in pain between the film dressed leg and the control leg at week four corrected for baseline. The consumption of analgesic and quality of life measures, sleep, mobility, contact discomfort, appetite, and mood were also monitored. There was a significantly greater reduction in pain in the film treated limbs than the control limbs ($p < 0.001$). By week four analgesic use had declined significantly ($p = 0.034$) and patients experienced a significant improvement in contact discomfort, sleep, mood, appetite, and mobility ($p < 0.002$) for all five variables. The authors concluded that the use of the film appeared to alleviate the pain associated with diabetic painful neuropathy and thus improved patients' quality of life but were unable to provide a definitive explanation for the mechanism of this observed effect. They suggested that the presence of the film over the skin might protect the sensitive skin from extraneous normally innocuous stimuli (allodynia) or that the film might have stimulated light touch afferent fibres which in turn inhibit transmission in small unmyelinated C fibres that are thought to be responsible for pain in diabetic neuropathy in accordance with the spinal gate control theory. Given the lack of side effects the authors recommended that this technique should be considered before resorting to the use of pharmacological treatments.

Exposure keratopathy

Chronic exposure keratopathy, damage to the cornea, the surface of the eye, can be caused by increased evaporation of tears and increased corneal exposure. This may be caused by abnormal protrusion of the eyeball known as proptosis or exophthalmos.

Airiani[107] described how a proptotic eye caused by the intraorbital extension of a basal cell carcinoma was successfully treated with Tegaderm and appropriate topical treatments over an extended period. The application of the film reduced loss of water vapour and facilitated reepithelialization of the corneal surface within six weeks.

Further applications over a 15 month period kept the patient comfortable with an intact epithelial surface, a vascularised cornea, and non-irritated surrounding skin.

Electrode fixation

Wantanabe *et al.*[108] described how a Tegaderm dressing was successfully used to provide a secure method of fixation for recording electrodes on non-shaved scalp for intra-operative electrophysiological monitoring. The needle electrodes were held in place by the film which was then stapled in position.

Fingertip injuries

Chronic Mennen *et al.*[109] devised a technique for the treatment of fingertip injuries involving Opsite which was easy to apply and required infrequent replacement, which resulted in the development of a healed digit of near normal shape. This technique was used to treat 200 such injuries which closed within an average of 20 days.

Films as catheter site dressings

All types of intravascular devices (IVD), widely used for vascular access, are associated with substantial risk of development of IVD-related bloodstream infection. The risk varies according to the type of device, but more than 90% of all intravascular device-related septicaemias are due to central venous or arterial catheters.[110]

A significant proportion of all infections are caused by skin organisms which gain access to the extra-luminal or intra-luminal surface of the device during insertion or subsequently.[111] It is therefore postulated that the use of topical antiseptics and dressings that inhibit the growth and/or migration of microorganisms could help to reduce infection rates, and a number of studies have been undertaken to test this hypothesis.

Film dressings appear to be ideally suited for this application because, being transparent, they permit frequent examination of the site without the need to disturb the dressing, however, their occlusive nature was initially regarded by some as potential cause for concern as it was felt that they might encourage the growth of microorganisms - a potentially serious or even life threatening event in such a situation.

Numerous studies have been undertaken to compare the on the effect of film dressings on IVD-related infections to resolve this issue, with conflicting outcomes. Interpretation of the results is also difficult because of the wide range of infection rates reported by the various centres.

A very early account of the use of Opsite for catheter care was presented in a conference by Jarrard in February 1980.[112] She described how 30 patients with jugular or subclavian catheters were successfully dressed with the film for a total of 938 catheter days. She stated that the dressing was comfortable with a degree of elasticity which accommodated movement. It adhered well to the skin and facilitated hair washing and bathing, and she concluded that it had useful a role in the maintenance of central venous catheters.

Palidar *et al.*,[113] compared Opsite with gauze for dressing hyperalimentation catheter sites. Twenty one patients dressed with the film were followed for a total of 319 patient days during which time there were two catheter related infections, a rate of 0.6% per patient-day. In a group of eleven patients dressed with sterile gauze, who were followed for 196 patient-days, there were also two catheter-related infections, a rate of 1%. The number of dressing changes was also less in the sites dressed with the semipermeable film, 2.7 *vs* 9.1, from which the authors calculated that the use of the film dressing saved in excess of $26 per patient without producing any increase in the rate of wound infection.

Vazquez *et al.*,[114] reported low levels of infection following a non-comparative study involving 100 patients with intravenous catheters. Dressing life averaged 5.3 days with silicone rubber catheters and 4.3 days for polyvinyl chloride catheters. One patient developed catheter induced sepsis (incidence 1%) which they suggested compared favourably with a 3 - 7% reported incidence when sterile gauze and tape was used. The authors concluded that the film dressing was useful for central venous catheters, permitting continuous inspection of the insertion site whilst reducing nursing time.

Peterson and Freeman,[115] compared treatment outcomes in 40 patients whose catheter sites were dressed with transparent polyurethane dressing with those of 38 retrospective controls whose sites were dressed with gauze. Phlebitis was recorded in 14.3% of patients treated with the polyurethane film compared with 26.3% of patients treated with gauze, and extravasations occurred in 10% and 21% respectively. The mean number of days that the I.V. remained in place was 2.46 with the film dressing and 1.97 with the gauze. Despite these apparently major differences in performance, only the difference in the length of time that the catheters remained place achieved statistical significance by the analytical method employed.

Four dressings regimens for 2088 Teflon peripheral venous catheters were studied in a prospective randomized clinical trial described by Maki *et al.*[116] The sites were dressed with either (a) sterile gauze, replaced every other day, or one of three dressings which left on for the lifetime of the catheter. These dressing treatments were (b) gauze, (c) a standard film dressing; and (d) a film dressing containing an iodophor. Overall no statistically significant differences were detected in skin colonization rates or catheter-related infections which ranged from 4.6% to 5.9% but moisture was found to have accumulated more frequently under the transparent dressings (26% to 28% *vs* 20% to 21%). Multivariate analysis showed moisture under the dressing to be significant risk factors for catheter-related infection. The authors concluded that it is not cost-effective to redress peripheral venous catheters at periodic intervals; for most patients, either sterile gauze or a transparent dressing can be used and left on until the catheter is removed.

The effect upon infection rates of changing film dressings on a regular basis was further investigated by Young *et al.*,[117] in 168 patients receiving parenteral nutrition via an infraclavicular central venous catheter. Four protocols were compared: 36 patients received gauze dressings changed three times per week, 31 received Opsite dressings changed every 7th day (Ops-7), 32 received Opsite changed every 10th day (Ops-10), and 69 received Opsite changed twice weekly (Ops-ICU). The mean duration of parenteral nutrition was approximately two weeks and all groups were well matched except that Ops-ICU patients suffered more frequently from an acute illness.

Catheter-related sepsis rates were low in all groups: 1/36 for gauze, 0/31 for Ops-7, 1/32 for Ops-10, and 2/69 for Ops-ICU. Bacterial colonization of skin beneath Opsite was no more common in the Ops-10 than in the other groups. Signs of inflammation at catheter insertion sites were common in all groups but did not relate closely to skin colonization. The authors suggested that Opsite can be left in place for seven days with a margin of safety lasting to ten days, thus saving on cost of materials and nursing time.

Hoffmann et al.[118] compared a polyurethane film dressing (Bioclusive) with a cotton gauze dressing on peripheral intravenous access sites in a case controlled, prospective, randomized trial involving 598 hospitalised patients over a period of four months. Patients were monitored for the incidence of phlebitis, catheter tip colonization, skin colonization, and catheter-related bacteraemia. The phlebitis rate for film and standard dressings was 9.8% and 7.6% respectively but this difference was not significant. Catheter tip colonization rates for the two treatments, which was defined as greater than 15 colony forming units per catheter, were determined by a semi-quantitative technique and found to be 5.7% and 4.4% respectively. Cultures of specimens from the skin and catheter tips of the majority of patients (91%) showed no growth. An association was found between those patients with greater than 15 CFU isolated from catheter tips and those with phlebitis. ($p = 0.022$). No incidence of catheter-related bacteraemia occurred in either study group.

Aly et al.[119] monitored cutaneous flora of the skin of 50 healthy volunteers and 49 long-term inpatients covered with three film dressings Opsite, Tegaderm, Uniflex and a traditional dressing of gauze and tape after iodine and alcohol disinfection of the skin. Dressings also were evaluated clinically for adhesion and the presence of skin reactions including erythema, pruritis, hyperpigmentation, vesiculitis, and tenderness.

Each volunteer, 25 of whom were receiving antibiotic therapy, simultaneously received on their volar forearm, patches of each dressing under examination. Two control areas were also established, one exposed skin site and one covered with occlusive moisture-retaining Saran Wrap. Although after three days, all three commercial dressings prevented indigenous flora from returning to normal population densities, no significant quantitative differences were found between them and the gauze-and-tape dressing. All dressings maintained normal flora at one tenth the population of the uncovered site but under the occlusive Saran the number of organisms present increased 100-fold compared to the exposed site.

Conflicting results concerning the safety of film dressings in patients with central venous catheters was presented by Conly et al.[120] Patients catheterised for three or more days were prospectively randomized to receive a film dressing (n = 58) or gauze (n = 57) dressing to compare the incidence of insertion site colonization, local catheter-related infection, and catheter-related sepsis. Quantitative cultures of the catheter insertion site (25 cm^2) revealed significantly greater colonization ($p \leq 0.009$) after 48 h in the transparent versus the gauze dressing group. Local catheter-related infection occurred significantly more often ($p = 0.002$) in the film treated group (62%) than in the gauze group (24%). Seven episodes of catheter-related bacteraemia occurred in the transparent group (16.6%) and none in the gauze group ($p = 0.015$). Stepwise logistic regression analysis revealed that cutaneous colonization at the insertion site of greater than or equal to 10^3 cfu/mL was a significant factor for catheter-related infection. The authors suggested that their data suggest that transparent dressings are associated with significantly increased rates of insertion site colonization, local catheter-related infection, and systemic catheter-related sepsis in patients with long-term central venous catheters.

Given the fact that the increased moisture that accumulated beneath an impermeable film (Saran Wrap) caused a large increase in the bioburden of the skin, it might be expected that a dressing which is very permeable to moisture might have beneficial properties compared to a standard film.

One such product is Opsite IV3000 which has the ability to increase its permeability to moisture vapour in the presence of liquid. The development of this new product was described by Richardson in 1991[23] who quoted permeability values for the film of 982 $g/m^2/24$ h and 2930 $g/m^2/24$ h (dry and wet respectively).

In a second paper, published at the same time, Richardson[121] also described the results of volunteer study in which they placed samples of four dressings, Opsite, Opsite IV3000, Tegaderm and Tegaderm Plus, (a film dressing containing an iodophor) on the back of 12 volunteers. A small volume of serum, 1.5 ml, was placed under each dressing and the sites were monitored over a 24 hour period. At the end of this time the dressings were examined and the number of organisms present at each site determined using a standard microbiological technique.

At the end of the test about half the original volume of serum was still present beneath Opsite, Tegaderm and Tegaderm Plus but all the serum beneath the Opsite IV3000 had dried up after 12-14 hours.

The microbiological results showed that on the skin exposed the serum, the total counts were around two logs higher (100-fold) under the Opsite dressing than the normal skin while with Tegaderm and Tegaderm Plus the counts were about three logs higher (1000-fold) With Opsite IV3000 the counts were comparable to normal skin. The iodophor in Tegaderm Plus appeared to provide no particular benefit in terms of reducing bacterial proliferation.

When Tegaderm and Opsite IV3000 were compared in two small studies involving 39 and 72 patients, Opsite IV3000 was found to be easier to apply, provided better security of fixation and was associated with less pooling of moisture.[122-123]

Opsite IV3000 was compared with the standard version of Opsite in a randomized controlled trial in 1993.[124] One hundred and one patients with subclavian and jugular single-lumen venous catheters provided two well-matched populations receiving a total of 153 dressings for a total of 780 catheter-days. In total three patients treated with the standard material developed an episode of catheter-related sepsis compared with one in the Opsite IV3000. Because of the low infection rate in both groups this difference, although interesting and in line with expectations, did not achieve statistical significant.

Opsite IV3000 was compared with a standard film dressing in a second randomized control trial involving 39 patients that was designed to compare the products in terms of security of fixation, skin condition and moisture accumulation beneath the dressings.[125] The result, which were not subjected to statistical analysis, appear to suggest that the skin of patients dressed with Opsite IV3000 was less likely to become 'very moist/sweaty' than patients dressed with a standard film, (11% compared with 20% respectively). There was also a slight trend for Opsite IV3000 to provide more secure catheter fixation and be less subject to lifting.

Maki et al.,[126] also compared Opsite IV3000 with a standard film, Tegaderm, and gauze and tape as site dressings for pulmonary artery catheters. A total of 442 adult patients with pulmonary artery catheters were randomized at the time of catheter insertion to have one of three dressing regimens: sterile gauze and tape, replaced every two days (n = 133), a conventional polyurethane dressing (n = 127), or a highly permeable film dressing (n = 185), both of which were replaced every five days. Microbiological investigations were undertaken to identify the source of any catheter-associated bloodstream infections by quantitatively culturing the skin of the insertion site and all potential sources on the catheter. Patients and catheters in the three dressing groups were very comparable. Ninety-six (21.7%) of the 442 catheters studied showed colonization of the introducer sheath or the pulmonary artery catheter, and five (1.1%) catheters caused bloodstream infection. All pulmonary artery catheter-related bloodstream infections occurred with catheters (introducers) in place for five or more days ($p < 0.001$)

Catheter-related bloodstream infections were associated with concordant cutaneous colonization of the insertion site (n = 2), a contaminated catheter hub or infusate (n = 3), contamination of the extravascular segment of a repositioned catheter beneath the external protective plastic sleeve (n = 1), or haematogenous colonization of the catheter (n = 1). Cutaneous colonization under the dressing at catheter removal was lowest with gauze ($10^{1.3}$ cfu), intermediate with the new highly permeable polyurethane dressing ($10^{1.8}$ cfu; $p < 0.01$), and highest with the conventional polyurethane dressing (10^2 cfu; $p < 0.001$).

The authors concluded that in terms of protection provided to the skin, the more permeable Opsite IV3000 was closer to standard gauze and tape than was the standard film but also suggested that neither film was associated with increased risk of catheter-related infection. They further stated that their results were consistent with those of earlier studies which suggested that dressings for vascular catheters should be designed to keep the site as dry as possible and to this end the goal for a polyurethane film should be a high moisture vapour transmission rate.

A retrospective analysis of infection rates in a 550 bed teaching hospital over a four year period during which time three different cannula dressings systems had been used revealed catheter-related infection rates for tape and gauze, standard film dressing and Opsite IV3000 to be 8.5%, 5.5% and 3.3% respectively.[127] The difference between standard film and Opsite IV3000 was highly significant ($p < 0.002$) as was the difference between tape and gauze and standard film ($p < 0.001$) Informal interviews with staff confirmed an enhanced level of satisfaction with Opsite IV3000 compared with gauze and tape. Whilst recognising the limitations of a retrospective study the authors considered that the dramatic reduction in catheter-related infection rates appeared to be associated with the switch to the more permeable Opsite IV3000 as no other changes had taken place in procedures during this period.

An alternative approach to the prevention of infection is the inclusion within the dressing of some form of antimicrobial agent. One such product, Arglaes containing silver ions, was compared with a standard film dressing, Tegaderm by Madeo et al.[128] Thirty-one patients admitted to the intensive care unit and requiring the insertion of an arterial line or central venous catheter were recruited into a randomized trial. Skin swabs were taken from the insertion sites prior to catheterization and on removal of the intravascular device to measure skin colonization rate between the two dressings. The catheter tips were also cultured on removal to establish if there was a difference between the two groups. No statistical differences were found in bacterial growth between the two dressings.

The importance of pre-treatment of the skin prior to dressing application in the prevention of prevent catheter-associated infection was investigated by Maki et al.[110] Three antiseptics were compared during the preparation and maintenance of patients' central venous and arterial catheter insertion sites in a surgical intensive care unit. A total of 668 catheters were randomized to treatment with 10% povidone-iodine, 70% alcohol, or 2% aqueous chlorhexidine disinfection of the site before insertion and for site treatment every other day thereafter. Local catheter-related infection rates per 100 catheters for the three treatments were 2.3 vs 7.1 and 9.3, for chlorhexidine, alcohol and povidone-iodine, respectively, (p = 0.02). Catheter-related bacteraemias were 0.5 vs 2.3 and 2.6. Of the 14 infusion-related bacteraemias one was in the chlorhexidine group and 13 were in the other two groups. (p = 0.04). The authors concluded that use of 2% chlorhexidine, rather than 10% povidone-iodine or 70% alcohol, for cutaneous disinfection before insertion of an intravascular device and for post-insertion site care can substantially reduce the incidence of device-related infection.

The practical advantages associated with the use of a film dressing (Tegaderm) compared with gauze and a 'silk' tape in the management of central venous catheter sites in children were described by Kellam et al.,[129] following a clinical trial involving thirty two infants. The film dressing was changed weekly, and the tape three times each week. The results clearly showed a statistically significant difference in favour of the film for the condition of the skin and a non-significant but marked difference in adverse events including purulence, catheter displacement and possible catheter-acquired infection in favour of the film.

Similar benefits were noted when film dressings were used to cover peritoneal dialysis and gastrojejunostomy catheters in infants,[130] as the use of the film prevented contamination whilst minimizing restriction of their activity, particularly in pre-toilet trained children.

In January 2003 the film used in the manufacture of Opsite IV3000 was changed to a much more permeable version. A report published by Smith and Nephew in 2005,[25] quoted MVTR values for this new dressing which were about four times those of the original preparation, (2,612 vs 11,791g/m^2/24 h) when tested dry and wet respectively. At this time the dressing became known simply as 'IV3000'.

Given the importance of dressing permeability in determining the moisture content of the skin surface and its consequent effect upon the proliferation of microorganisms in the experimental studies described previously, it is reasonable to assume that such as dramatic change in permeability will have important consequences, potentially reducing the incidence of catheter-related infections below the levels previously encountered with the original Opsite IV3000. Further clinical research is required to confirm this supposition.

The differences in infection rates recorded between various types of dressings used to secure central venous catheters have formed the subject of a number of systematic reviews. In one, published by Hoffmann et al. in 1992,[131] the authors identified 15 studies in which film dressings were used to dress central venous catheters and 12 studies in which they were used in peripheral catheter sites. Seven studies in each group met the inclusion criteria and were therefore included in the meta-analysis using three outcome measures, catheter-tip infections, and bacteraemia and catheter sepsis. For central venous catheters the relative risk was statistically higher for all three parameters. This was statistically significant ($p < 0.001$) for catheter tip infections but failed to reach significance for the other parameters examined. ($p = 0.2$ and $p = 0.06$). For peripheral lines there was a marked statistically significant increased risk of a catheter tip infection with the film dressing ($p = 0.002$) but there was no difference in other parameters examined.

On the basis of these results, one centre reported that they had began to use gauze dressings in place of film, but this had resulted in practical problems associated with the observation of the insertion site and an impression that cannulae were less securely anchored than before.[132] They therefore undertook a study to compare the two types of dressing systems which involved 229 patients who were randomized to receive either gauze (n = 121) or transparent polyurethane (n = 108) dressings.

The frequency of catheter dislodgment by the patient was significantly higher ($p < 0.05$) in patients with the gauze dressing than in patients with the transparent polyurethane dressing (15% vs 6%). A trend toward lower frequencies of phlebitis (1.8% vs 3.3%) and infiltration (17.6% vs 20.7%) was also noted in the patients with the transparent polyurethane dressings. The authors concluded that clinical advantages of the transparent polyurethane dressings lie in the ease of direct visualization of the insertion site and the securement of the catheter. For this reason the decision was made at their institution, to revert to the use of transparent polyurethane rather than gauze dressings for peripheral intravenous catheters.

In a second systematic review published by Gillies et al.[133] A total of 23 studies were reviewed of which 15 were excluded from the analysis. Of the remaining eight, data were available for meta-analysis from six studies. Of the six included studies, two compared gauze and tape with Opsite IV3000, two compared Opsite with Opsite IV3000, one compared Tegaderm with Opsite IV3000, and one compared Tegaderm with Opsite. The authors concluded that was no evidence of any difference in the incidence of infectious complications between any of the dressing types compared in this review.

It will be recognised, that at the time at which the first review was undertaken,[131] only the original formulation of Opsite was available. Whilst the second review[133] included studies involving Opsite IV 3000, these related to the original version not the new highly permeable material launched in January 2003.This means that while both reviews were of some relevance at the time at which they were published the results have no relevance to the current formulation of IV3000 which is effectively a totally different product.

The importance of taking account of the changes that have taken place in dressing design when reading systematic reviews was noted by Jones[134] in a useful and detailed review. She concluded that the development of highly permeable film dressings has been a significant advance for the management of catheter sites

An overview of the different types of IV cannula dressings available on the UK market, including film products, was published by Campbell in 1999,[135] who discussed the advantages and disadvantages of each.

REFERENCES

1. Elliott IMZ. *A Short History of Surgical Dressings*. London: The Pharmaceutical Press, 1964.
2. Campbell K, Woodbury MG, Whittle H, Labate T, Hoskin A. A clinical evaluation of 3M no sting barrier film. *Ostomy Wound Manage* 2000;46(1):24-30.
3. Root-Bernstein R, Root-Bernstein M. *Honey, Mud,Maggots*. London: Macmillan, 1999.
4. Elder AV. Cellophane as a surgical dressing. *Journal of the Royal Navy Medical Service* 1938;24:154-155.
5. Howes EL. Cellophane as a wound dressing. *Surgery* 1939;6:426-427.
6. Ellis M. Transparent wrapping material for dressing open wounds and ulcers. *British Medical Journal* 1943:697.
7. Farr J. Cellophane for the treatment of burns. *British Medical Journal* 1944:749-750.
8. Kimbrough EL. New Cellophane dressing. *United States Naval Medical Bulletin* 1942;40:432-435.
9. Bloom H. Cellophane dressing for second degree burns. *Lancet* 1945;2:559.
10. Bull JP, Squire JR, Topley E. Experiments with occlusive dressings of a new plastic. *Lancet* 1948;2:213-215.
11. Schilling RSF, Roberts M. Clinical trial of occlusive plastic dressings. *Lancet* 1950;1:293-296.
12. Myers JA. Ease of use of two semipermeable adhesive membranes compared. *Pharm. J.* 1984;233:685-686.
13. Haessler RM. Transparent IV dressing vs. traditional dressings. *J. natn. intraven. Ther. Ass.* 1983;6:169-171.
14. Bedford A. Dressed to map. *Journal of District Nursing* 1991;January 1991:5-6.
15. Barnes E, Malone-Lee J. Pressure sores: Tegaderm pouch dressings. *Nurs Times* 1985;81(48):45-6.
16. Golan J, Eldad A, Rudensky B, Tuchman Y, Sterenberg N, Ben-Hur N, et al. A new temporary synthetic skin substitute. *Burns Incl Therm Inj* 1985;11(4):274-80.
17. Thomas S, Loveless P, Hay NP. Comparative review of the properties of six semipermeable film dressings. *Pharm. J.* 1988;240:785-789.
18. Shelanski MV, Nicholson JE, Shelanski JB, Constantine BE. The influence of moisture vapor transmission rates of polymer dressings on the rate of wound healing and bacterial proliferation on wound surfaces. *Wounds* 1989;1(2):115-531.
19. Palamand S, Brenden RA, Reed AM. Intelligent wound dressings and their physical characteristics. *Wounds: A Compendium of Clinical Research and Practice* 1992;3(4):149-156.
20. EN13726-2:2002 ES. Test methods for primary wound dressings. Moisture vapour transmission rate of permeable film dressings,.

21. Lamke LO, Nilsson GE, Reithner HL. The evaporative water loss from burns and water vapour permeability of grafts and artificial membranes used in the treatment of burns. *Burns* 1977;3:159-165.
22. Thomas S, Fear M, Humphreys J, Disley L, Waring MJ. The effect of dressings on the production of exudate from venous leg ulcers. *Wounds* 1996;8(5):145-149.
23. Richardson MC. I. The research and development of a new transparent film dressing for intravenous catheter care In: Maki DG, editor. *Improving Catheter Site Care*. London: Royal Society of Medicine, 1991:29-31.
24. Thomas S, Young S. Exudate-handling mechanisms of two foam-film dressings. *Journal of Wound Care* 2008;17(7):309-315.
25. Jung W. IV 3000 1-Hand competitor analysis, Data on File Report 0505005: Smith and Nephew Wound Management, 2005.
26. van Luyn MJ, van Wachem PB, Nieuwenhuis P, Jonkman MF. Cytotoxicity testing of wound dressings using methylcellulose cell culture. *Biomaterials* 1992;13(5):267-75.
27. Sieber VK, Otto WR, Riches DJ. Cytotoxicity of wound dressing materials assessed using cultured skin equivalents see comments. *Burns* 1995;21(4):249-54.
28. Bell E, Sher S, Hull B, Merrill C, Rosen S, Chamson A, et al. The Reconstitution of Living Skin. 1983;81(s1):2s-10s.
29. Hunt TK. Oxygen and skin wound healing. In: Rovee DT, Maibach HI, editors. *The Epidermis in Wound Healing*. Boca Raton: CRC Press, 2004:183-197.
30. Winter GD. Epidermal regeneration studied in the domestic pig. In: Maibach HI, Rovee DT, editors. *Epidermal Wound Healing*. Chicago: Year Book Medical Publishers, 1974.
31. Silver IA. Oxygen tension and wound healing. In: Maibach H, Rovee TD, editors. *Epidermal Wound Healing*. Chicago: Medical Publishers, 1972:291-304.
32. Silver IA. Oxygen and tissue repair. In: Ryan TJ, editor. *An Environment for Healing: The Role of Occlusion,*. London: Royal Society of Medicine, 1985:15-19.
33. Varghese MC, Balin AK, Carter DM, Caldwell D. Local environment of chronic wounds under synthetic dressings. *Arch Dermatol* 1986;122(1):52-7.
34. Knighton DR, Silver IA, Hunt TK. Regulation of wound-healing angiogenesis - effect of oxygen gradints and inspired oxygen concentration. *Surgery* 1981;90(2):262-171.
35. Sirvio LM, Grussing DM. The effect of gas permeability of film dressings on wound environment and healing. *J Invest Dermatol* 1989;93(4):528-31.
36. Behar D, Juszynski M, Ben Hur N, Golan J, Eldad A, Tuchman Y, et al. Omiderm, a new synthetic wound covering: physical properties and drug permeability studies. *J Biomed Mater Res* 1986;20(6):731-8.
37. Benbow M. Best Practice - appliance of dressing products. *Journal of Comunity Nursing Online* 2009;23(03):32-36.
38. Visscher M, Hoath SB, Conroy E, Wickett RR. Effect of semipermeable membranes on skin barrier repair following tape stripping. *Arch Dermatol Res* 2001;293(10):491-9.
39. Eaglstein WH, Davis SC, Mehle AL, Mertz PM. Optimal use of an occlusive dressing to enhance healing. Effect of delayed application and early removal on wound healing. *Arch Dermatol* 1988;124(3):392-5.
40. Buchan IA, Andrews JK, Lang SM, Boorman JG, Harvey Kemble JV, Lamberty BGH. Clinical and laboratory investigation of the composition and properties of human skin wound exudate under semi-permeable dressings. *Burns* 1981;7:326-334.
41. Buchan IA, Andrews JK, Lang SM. Laboratory investigation of the composition and properties of pig skin wound exudate under Opsite. *Burns* 1981;8:39-46.
42. Alper JC, Tibbetts LL, Sarazen AA. The in vitro response of fibroblasts to the fluid that accumulates under a vapor-permeable membrane. *J. invest. Derm.* 1985;84:513-515.

43. Ono I, Gunji H, Zhang JZ, Maruyama K, Kaneko F. Studies on cytokines related to wound healing in donor site wound fluid. *J Dermatol Sci* 1995;10(3):241-5.
44. Holland KT, Davis W, Ingham E, Gowland G. A comparison of the in-vitro antibacterial and complement activating effect of Opsite and Tegaderm dressings. *J. Hosp. Infect.* 1984;5:323-328.
45. Holland KT, Harnby D, Peel B. A comparison of the in vivo antibacterial effects of 'OpSite', 'Tegaderm' and 'Ensure' dressings. *J Hosp Infect* 1985;6(3):299-303.
46. Mertz PM, Eaglstein WH. The effect of a semiocclusive dressing on the microbial population in superficial wounds. *Arch Surg* 1984;119(3):287-9.
47. Katz S, McGinley K, Leyden JJ. Semipermeable occlusive dressings. Effects on growth of pathogenic bacteria and reepithelialization of superficial wounds. *Arch Dermatol* 1986;122(1):58-62.
48. Aly R, Shirley C, Cunico B, Maibach HI. Effect of prolonged occlusion on the microbial flora, pH, carbon dioxide and transepidermal water loss on human skin. *J Invest Dermatol* 1978;71(6):378-81.
49. Mertz PM, Marshall DA, Eaglstein WH. Occlusive wound dressings to prevent bacterial invasion and wound infection. *J Am Acad Dermatol* 1985;12(4):662-8.
50. Alper JC, Welch EA, Ginsberg M, Bogaars H, Maguire P. Moist wound healing under a vapor permeable membrane. *Journal of the American Academy of Dermatolgy* 1983;8(3):347353.
51. Hettiaratchy S, Dziewulski P. ABC of burns. Introduction. *Bmj* 2004;328(7452):1366-8.
52. Zawacki BE. Reversal of capillary stasis and prevention of necrosis in burns. *Ann Surg* 1974;180(1):98-102.
53. Conkle W. Op-Site dressing: new approach to burn care. *J Emerg Nurs* 1981;7(4):148-52.
54. Neal DE, Whalley PC, Flowers MW, Wilson DH. The effects of an adherent polyurethane film and conventional absorbent dressing in patients with small partial thickness burns. *Br J Clin Pract* 1981;35(7-8):254-7.
55. Fong PH, Wong KL. Opsite, a synthetic burns dressing. *Ann Acad Med Singapore* 1985;14(2):387-90.
56. Waffle C, Simon RR, Joslin C. Moisture-vapour-permeable film as an outpatient burn dressing. *Burns Incl Therm Inj* 1988;14(1):66-70.
57. Chan P, Vincent JW, Wangemann RT. Accelerated healing of carbon dioxide laser burns in rats treated with composite polyurethane dressings. *Arch Dermatol* 1987;123(8):1042-5.
58. Poulsen TD, Freund KG, Arendrup K, Nyhuus P, Pedersen OD. Polyurethane film (Opsite) vs. impregnated gauze (Jelonet) in the treatment of outpatient burns: a prospective, randomized study. *Burns* 1991;17(1):59-61.
59. James JH, Watson ACH. The use of Opsite, a vapour permeable dressing, on skin graft donor sites. *Br. J. plast. Surg.* 1975;28:107-110.
60. Bergman RB. A new treatment of split-skin graft donor sites. *Arch Chir Neerl* 1977;29(1):69-72.
61. Dinner MI, Peters CR, Sherer J. Use of semipermeable polyurethane membrane as a dressing for split-skin graft donor sites. *Plast. reconstr. Surg.* 1979;64:112-114.
62. Barnett A, Berkowitz RL, Mills R, Vistnes LM. Comparison of synthetic adhesive moisture vapor permeable and fine mesh gauze dressings for split-thickness skin graft Donor sites. *Am J Surg* 1983;145(3):379-81.
63. Barnett A, Berkowitz RL, Mills R, Vistnes LM. Scalp as skin graft donor site: rapid reuse with synthetic adhesive moisture vapor permeable dressings. *J Trauma* 1983;23(2):148-51.
64. Morita R, Ishikura N, Kawakami S, Heshiki T, Shimada K, Kurosawa T. Use of skin staples to fix film dressings on scalp donor wounds in patients with burns. *Burns* 2002;28(3):267-9.

65. Iregbulem LM. Use of a semi-permeable membrane dressing in Donor sites in Nigerians. *Ann Acad Med Singapore* 1983;12(2 Suppl):425-9.

66. Ehleben CM, May SR, Still JM, Jr. Pain associated with an adherent polyurethane wound dressing. *Burns Incl Therm Inj* 1985;12(2):122-6.

67. Blight A, Fatah MF, Datubo-Brown DD, Mountford EM, Cheshire IM. The treatment of Donor sites with cultured epithelial grafts. *Br J Plast Surg* 1991;44(1):12-4.

68. Richmond JD, Sutherland AB. A new approach to the problems encountered with Opsite as a donor site dressing: systemic ethamsylate. *Br. J. plast. Surg.* 1986;39:516-518.

69. Persson K, Salemark L. How to dress donor sites of split thickness skin grafts: a prospective, randomised study of four dressings. *Scand J Plast Reconstr Surg Hand Surg* 2000;34(1):55-9.

70. Tinckler L. Surgical wound management with Op-site - a new and preferred method. *Natnews* 1982;19(5):14-6.

71. Drake D. Surgical wound management with adhesive polyurethane membrane. *Ann. R. Coll. Surg.* 1984;66:74-75.

72. Rubio PA. Use of semiocclusive, transparent film dressings for surgical wound protection: experience in 3637 cases. *Int Surg* 1991;76(4):253-4.

73. Moshakis V, Fordyce MJ, Griffiths JD, McKinna JA. Tegaderm versus gauze dressing in breast surgery. *Br J Clin Pract* 1984;38(4):149-52.

74. Briggs M. Surgical wound pain: a trial of two treatments. *Journal of Wound Care* 1996;5(10):456-60.

75. Wipke-Tevis DD, Stotts NA. Effect of dressings on saphenous vein harvest incision pain, distress and cosmetic result. *Prog Cardiovasc Nurs* 1998;13(3):3-13.

76. Hien NT, Prawer SE, Katz HI. Facilitated wound healing using transparent film dressing following Mohs micrographic surgery. *Arch Dermatol* 1988;124(6):903-6.

77. Gates JL, Holloway GA. A comparison of wound environments. *Ostomy Wound Manage* 1992;38(8):34-7.

78. Westrate JT. Care of the open wound in abdominal sepsis. *Journal of Wound Care* 1996;5(7):325-8.

79. Taylor D. Improving Outcomes-The role of Modern Dressings in Orthopaedic Wound Care. London: Proffesional Select Committee.

80. Blaylock B, Murray M, O'Connell K, Rex J. Tape injury in the patient with total hip replacement. *Orthop Nurs* 1995;14(3):25-8.

81. Aindow D, Butcher M. Films or fabrics: is it time to re-appraise postoperative dressings? *Br J Nurs* 2005;14(19):S15-6, S18, S20.

82. Folestad A. The management of wounds following orthopaedic surgery: The Molndal dressing. *European Product News* 2002;March/April.

83. Harle S, Korhonen A, Kettunen JA, Seitsalo S. A randomised clinical trial of two different wound dressing materials for hip replacement patients. *Journal of Orthopaedic Nursing* 2005;9:205-210.

84. Ravenscroft MJ, Harker J, Buch KA. A prospective, randomised, controlled trial comparing wound dressings used in hip and knee surgery: Aquacel and Tegaderm versus Cutiplast. *Ann R Coll Surg Engl* 2006;88(1):18-22.

85. Chang WR, McLean IP. CUSUM: a tool for early feedback about performance? *BMC Med Res Methodol* 2006;6:8.

86. Cosker T, Elsayed S, Gupta S, Mendonca AD, Tayton KJ. Choice of dressing has a major impact on blistering and healing outcomes in orthopaedic patients. *J Wound Care* 2005;14(1):27-9.

87. Yamaguchi Y, Sumikawa Y, Yoshida S, Kubo T, Yoshikawa K, Itami S. Prevention of amputation caused by rheumatic diseases following a novel therapy of exposing bone

marrow, occlusive dressing and subsequent epidermal grafting. *Br J Dermatol* 2005;152(4):664-72.

88. Ostermann PA, Ekkernkamp A, Henry SL, Seligson D. Optimal timing of wound closure in severe open fractures with temporary coverage by skin substitute. *Unfallchirurgie* 1994;20(3):157-61.

89. Strover AE, Thorpe R. Suction dressings: a new surgical dressing technique. *J R Coll Surg Edinb* 1997;42(2):119-21.

90. Suzumura N, Hagisawa S. Effect of polyurethane film dressing applied to the skin of healthy older subjects on frictional forces. *Jpn J PU* 2006;8(2):153-159.

91. Hammond MA. Moist wound healing: breaking down the dry barrier. *Nurs Mirror* 1979;149(18):38-40.

92. Braverman AM, Nasar MA. The treatment of superficial decubitus ulcers. *Practitioner* 1981;225:1842-1843.

93. Sebern MD. Pressure ulcer management in home health care: efficacy and cost effectiveness of moisture vapor permeable dressing. *Arch Phys Med Rehabil* 1986;67(10):726-9.

94. Thomas S. The importance of secondary dressings in wound care. *Journal of Wound Care* 1998;7(4):189-192.

95. Banks V, Bale S, Harding KG. Superficial pressure sores: comparing two regimes. *Journal of Wound Care* 1994;3(1):8-10.

96. Cannavo M, Fairbrother G, Owen D, Ingle J, Lumley T. A comparison of dressings in the management of surgical abdominal wounds. *Journal of Wound Care* 1998;7(2):57-62.

97. Thomas S, Banks V, Fear M, Hagelstein S, Bale S, Harding K. A study to compare two film dressings used as secondary dressings. *Journal of Wound Care* 1997;6(7):333-336.

98. Lobe TE, Anderson GF, King DR, Boles ET, Jr. An improved method of wound management for pediatric patients. *J Pediatr Surg* 1980;15(6):886-9.

99. Retik AB, Bauer SB, Mandell J, Peters CA, Colodny A, Atala A. Management of severe hypospadias with a 2-stage repair. *J Urol* 1994;152(2 Pt 2):749-51.

100. Van Savage JG, Palanca LG, Slaughenhoupt BL. A prospective randomized trial of dressings versus no dressings for hypospadias repair. *J Urol* 2000;164(3 Pt 2):981-3.

101. Oranje AP, de Waard-van der Spek FB, Devillers AC, de Laat PC, Madern GC. Treatment and pain relief of ulcerative hemangiomas with a polyurethane film. *Dermatology* 2000;200(1):31-4.

102. Sandler A, Lawrence J, Meehan J, Phearman L, Soper R. A "plastic" sutureless abdominal wall closure in gastroschisis. *J Pediatr Surg* 2004;39(5):738-41.

103. Bhandari V, Brodsky N, Porat R. Improved outcome of extremely low birth weight infants with Tegaderm application to skin. *J Perinatol* 2005;25(4):276-81.

104. Shell JA, Stanutz F, Grimm J. Comparison of moisture vapor permeable (MVP) dressings to conventional dressings for management of radiation skin reactions. *Oncol Nurs Forum* 1986;13(1):11-6.

105. Ibrahim T, Ong SM, Saint Clair Taylor GJ. The effects of different dressings on the skin temperature of the knee during cryotherapy. *Knee* 2005;12(1):21-3.

106. Foster AV, Eaton C, McConville DO, Edmonds ME. Application of OpSite film: a new and effective treatment of painful diabetic neuropathy. *Diabet Med* 1994;11(8):768-72.

107. Airiani S, Braunstein RE, Kazim M, Schrier A, Auran JD, Srinivasan BD. Tegaderm transparent dressing (3M) for the treatment of chronic exposure keratopathy. *Ophthal Plast Reconstr Surg* 2003;19(1):75-6.

108. Watanabe K, Watanabe T, Takahashi A, Hirato M, Saito N, Sasaki T. Reliable and convenient method for the fixation of recording electrodes on nonshaved scalp for intraoperative electrophysiological monitoring: technical note. *Surg Neurol* 2003;60(3):267-9.

109. Mennen U, Wiese A. Fingertip injuries management with semi-occlusive dressing see comments. *J Hand Surg Br* 1993;18(4):416-22.
110. Maki DG, Ringer M, Alvarado CJ. Prospective randomised trial of povidone-iodine, alcohol, and chlorhexidine for prevention of infection associated with central venous and arterial catheters. *Lancet* 1991;338(8763):339-43.
111. Crnich CJ, Maki DG. The promise of novel technology for the prevention of intravascular device-related bloodstream infection. I. Pathogenesis and short-term devices. *Clin Infect Dis* 2002;34(9):1232-42.
112. Jarrard M. Use of transparent polyurethane dressing (Opsite) for central venous catheter care. *4th Clinical Congress, The Art and Science of Nutrition*. Chicago, 1980.
113. Palidar PJ, Simonowitz DA, Oreskovich MR, Dellinger EP, Edwards WA, Adams S, et al. Use of Op Site as an occlusive dressing for total parenteral nutrition catheters. *J. parent. ent. Nutr.* 1982;6:150-151.
114. Vazquez RM, Jarrard MM. Care of the central venous catheterization site: the use of a transparent polyurethane film. *JPEN J Parenter Enteral Nutr* 1984;8(2):181-6.
115. Peterson PJ, Freeman PT. Use of a transparent polyurethane dressing for peripheral intravenous catheter care. *National intraven. Ther. Ass.* 1982;5:387-390.
116. Maki DG, Ringer M. Evaluation of dressing regimens for prevention of infection with peripheral intravenous catheters. Gauze, a transparent polyurethane dressing, and an iodophor-transparent dressing. *JAMA* 1987;258(17):2396-403.
117. Young GP, Alexeyeff M, Russell DM, Thomas RJ. Catheter sepsis during parenteral nutrition: the safety of long-term OpSite dressings. *JPEN J Parenter Enteral Nutr* 1988;12(4):365-70.
118. Hoffmann KK, Western SA, Kaiser DL, Wenzel RP, Groschel DH. Bacterial colonization and phlebitis-associated risk with transparent polyurethane film for peripheral intravenous site dressings. *Am J Infect Control* 1988;16(3):101-6.
119. Aly R, Bayles C, Maibach H. Restriction of bacterial growth under commercial catheter dressings. *Am J Infect Control* 1988;16(3):95-100.
120. Conly JM, Grieves K, Peters B. A prospective, randomized study comparing transparent and dry gauze dressings for central venous catheters. *J Infect Dis* 1989;159(2):310-9.
121. Richardson MC. II. An *in vivo* assessment of the microbial proliferation beneath transparent film dressings. In: Maki DG, editor. *Improving Catheter Site Care*. London: Royal Society of Medicine, 1991:31-33.
122. Keenlyside D. Central venous catheters - a randomized comparative study of Opsite IV3000 and Tegaderm. In: Maki DG, editor. *Improving Catheter Site Care*. London: Royal Society of Medicine, 1991:47-51.
123. Joyeux B. Opsite IV3000 versus Tegaderm on peripheral venous catheters. In: Maki DG, editor. *Improving Catheter Site Care*. London: Royal Society of Medicine, 1991:53-55.
124. Wille JC, Blusse van Oud Albas A, Thewessen EA. A comparison of two transparent film-type dressings in central venous therapy. *J Hosp Infect* 1993;23(2):113-21.
125. Keenlyside D. Avoiding an unnecessary outcome. A comparative trial between IV3000 and a conventional film dressing to assess rates of catheter-related sepsis. *Prof Nurse* 1993;8(5):288-91.
126. Maki DG, Stolz SS, Wheeler S, Mermel LA. A prospective, randomized trial of gauze and two polyurethane dressings for site care of pulmonary artery catheters: implications for catheter management. *Crit Care Med* 1994;22(11):1729-37.
127. Treston-Aurand J, Olmsted RN, Allen-Bridson K, Craig CP. Impact of dressing materials on central venous catheter infection rates. *J Intraven Nurs* 1997;20(4):201-6.

128. Madeo M, Martin CR, Turner C, Kirkby V, Thompson DR. A randomized trial comparing Arglaes (a transparent dressing containing silver ions) to Tegaderm (a transparent polyurethane dressing) for dressing peripheral arterial catheters and central vascular catheters. *Intensive Crit Care Nurs* 1998;14(4):187-91.

129. Kellam B, Fraze DE, Kanarek KS. Central line dressing material and neonatal skin integrity. *Nutr Clin Pract* 1988;3(2):65-8.

130. Plante B, Amadei M, Herbert E, O'Regan S. Tegaderm dressings for peritoneal dialysis and gastrojejunostomy catheters in children. *Adv Perit Dial* 1990;6:279-80.

131. Hoffmann KH, Weber DJ, Samsa GP, Rutala WA. Transparent polyurethane film as an intravenous catheter dressings A Meta-analysis of the infection risks. *Journal of the American Medical Association* 1992;267(15):2072-076.

132. Tripepi-Bova KA, Woods KD, Loach MC. A comparison of transparent polyurethane and dry gauze dressings for peripheral i.v. catheter sites: rates of phlebitis, infiltration, and dislodgment by patients. *Am J Crit Care* 1997;6(5):377-81.

133. Gillies D, O'Riordan E, Carr D, O'Brien I, Frost J, Gunning R. Central venous catheter dressings: a systematic review. *Journal of Advanced Nursing* 2003;44(6):623-632.

134. Jones.A. Dressings for the Management of Catheter Sites: A Review. *JAVA* 2004; 9(1):26-33(8).

135. Campbell H, Carrington M. Peripheral i.v. cannula dressings: advantages and disadvantages. *Br J Nurs* 1999;8(21):1420-2, 1424-7.

10. Foam dressings

INTRODUCTION

Foam in various forms has a long history in wound management. Current materials, mainly made from polyurethane, appear to satisfy most of the requirements of the 'ideal dressing' and as a result have become the treatment of choice for many types of wounds. Unlike hydrocolloid sheets (Chapter 12), foam dressings tend not to facilitate autolytic debridement of very dry wounds, and are therefore most commonly indicated for exuding lesions.

A variety of products are available, designed for treating both superficial and deep cavity wounds. Some versions have an adhesive wound contact layer to facilitate placement, others are available in the form of self-adhesive island dressings.

Most foam dressings designed for the treatment of surface wounds incorporate a semipermeable outer surface to act as a bacterial barrier and provide an element of environmental control. This surface is frequently, but not invariably, made from a polyurethane film or membrane or a closed-cell polyurethane foam sheet.

A considerable amount of clinical data has been published describing the use of foams in a diverse range of wound types. Most of this literature suggests that the dressings are easy to apply, relatively painless to remove and therefore well liked by patients and healthcare professionals alike. They are also generally considered to be cost effective in use.

By their very nature, foam dressings offer opportunities to act as carriers for medicaments, most commonly antimicrobial agents, and a number of foam dressings are available that contain silver salts or other bactericidal compounds.

HISTORY OF FOAM DRESSINGS

The first cellular or foam-like materials to be utilized in medicine were naturally occurring marine sponges, small pieces of which were impregnated with extracts of opium, nightshade, hemlock, mandragora, ivy and lettuce seed and inserted into the nostrils of patients as anaesthetic devices to induce sleep prior to surgery. These 'soporific sponges' were widely employed in European and Arabic culture during the Middle Ages.[1]

Sponges were also used during surgical procedures as absorbents, haemostats and simple cleansing aids, a practice which continued until the end of the 19th Century when experience showed that despite attempts to disinfect or sterilise them, being natural organic materials they remained a potent source of infection. They also had a marked tendency to adhere badly to the surface of wounds and so their popularity gradually declined.[2] A fascinating account of the collection, preparation, sterilization and use of sponges was published by Maylard in 1891.[3]

Alternative surgical absorbents were therefore sought, and one such product was described in 1884 by Joseph Gamgee. This consisted of an 'artificial antiseptic absorbent sponge' composed of gauze, cotton and coconut fibre, in the centre of which was placed a capsule of glass or gelatin which was broken to release the antiseptic content immediately prior to use.[4]

Despite some interest in the development of artificial sponges in the 1950s, primarily for use in surgery, dressings made from foam were not introduced into wound management until the 1970s. Epigard, a reticulated polyurethane foam sheet laminated to a microporous film was developed in 1973 as a temporary skin substitute prior to grafting. Originally the backing layer was made from microporous polypropylene, but in a later publication it was said to consist of Teflon.[5] Information provided by the manufacturer now indicates that the film is made from polyurethane. Any effects that these structural changes may have had on the clinical performance of the dressing are unknown.

The first foam product to be used in general wound management was Silastic Foam, principally used for the management of cavity wounds, which was formed *in situ* from two liquid components mixed at the patient's bedside.

Figure 39: Silastic Foam kit

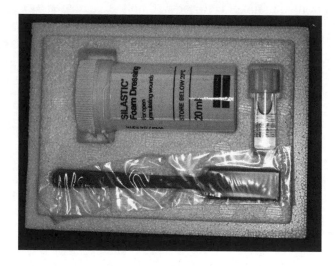

This was followed by the development of preformed 'foam membranes', thin sheets of foam produced with and without an adhesive coating.

Although some of these early dressings achieved a degree of commercial success, their use was limited by relatively poor absorbency. It was not until products made from hydrophilic polyurethane were developed that foam dressings began to gain widespread acceptance.

As previously indicated, in many of these dressings the absorbent foam is bonded to a semipermeable polyurethane film, or a second thin sheet of closed cell foam. This backing layer frequently extends past the margins of the absorbent pad to form an island or bordered dressing.

After a relatively slow start, the popularity of foams grew rapidly as different presentations were developed. Some were shaped to fit particular anatomical sites; others incorporated gel forming agents within their structure to enhance fluid retention

CLASSIFICATION OF FOAM DRESSINGS

Cavity dressings

Silastic Foam, developed by Dow Corning in the 1950s, consisted of two components, a viscous medical-grade poly(dimethylsiloxane) base and a stannous octoate catalyst which were mixed together immediately prior to use. The resultant chemical reaction released hydrogen which caused the viscous mixture to expand to approximately four times its original volume before setting to form soft, resilient, open-cell foam.

Silastic Foam was first used medically in 1962 as a diagnostic aid in the detection of sigmoid cancer.[6] For this application the liquid catalysed base was inserted into the colon as an enema where it expanded and set, taking up the shape and surface characteristics of the gut wall. This somewhat unusual procedure was superseded when improved radiological techniques and more sophisticated instruments were developed.

When used as a dressing, the two components were mixed as before, and then introduced directly into the lesion to form a 'stent' that precisely adopted the contours of the wound. The stent usually remained in position in a deep wound without the need for bandages or secondary dressings, but as healing progressed and the wound became shallower, the use of surgical tape or some other form of retention was sometimes required.

A stent could often be used for a week or more if a simple routine of wound toilet was adopted. To this end, it was recommended that the dressing be removed from the wound twice a day and soaked in a solution of a suitable antiseptic agent, such as chlorhexidine gluconate 0.5%, for a minimum of 10-15 minutes.[7] Other antiseptics were subsequently evaluated for this purpose, including cetrimide and povidone iodine, but these performed less well than chlorhexidine for this application.[8]

During the time the dressing was soaking, the patient could wash the wound or take a bath as appropriate. Once the dressing had been adequately disinfected, it was rinsed very thoroughly under a running tap, with repeated gentle squeezing, to remove all traces of antiseptic. After a final squeeze to express any remaining water, the dressing was replaced in the wound. Removal of antiseptic agents was important, as residual traces of some antiseptics were capable of causing irritation to the wound and surrounding skin.

Although there were few reports of infections resulting from the use of Silastic Foam, one paper recorded that a rare pigment-producing strain of *Serratia rubideae* was isolated from one dressing on several occasions.

In 1987 a report in the scientific press questioned the biological safety of some chemicals used in the manufacture of certain plastics.[9] Although these chemicals were not found in Silastic Foam, one of them was related to a theoretical breakdown product produced during the catalytic reaction during which the foam is formed. The US Environmental Protection Agency requested further pre-clinical testing of these chemicals and the manufacturers of Silastic Foam in the USA therefore decided, for industrial and commercial reasons, that they would suspend production of the dressing until this information became available. Further toxicological studies and an in-depth review of all available scientific data revealed no evidence of any adverse effects resulting from the use of Silastic Foam and as a result, manufacture of the foam was recommenced.

A major advantage of Silastic Foam was its versatility; it could be used to form a covering over very large or awkward wounds which were difficult to dress with conventional materials as illustrated below.

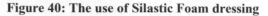

Figure 40: The use of Silastic Foam dressing

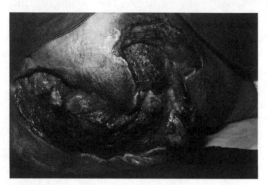

A hemiplegic elderly lady who had undergone a hindquarter amputation presented with a massive area of pressure damage involving both buttocks. After trying a number of different treatments, a Silastic Foam dressing was made to provide protection, absorb exudate, assist with pressure distribution and facilitate dressing changes.

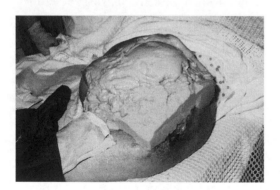
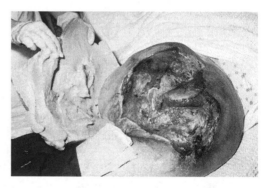

In the mid 1990s Silastic Foam was reformulated, at which ownership transferred to Smith and Nephew and its name changed to Cavi-Care. Like Silastic Foam, Cavi-Care consists of two components presented in dual aluminium sachets. One ten gram sachet contains polydimethylsiloxane polymer together with a platinum catalyst, inhibitor and ethanol. The second contains polymers, cross-linkers (copolysiloxanes), inhibitor and ethanol. In use the contents of the two sachets are mixed vigorously for 5-15 seconds then, within 30 seconds, they are poured into the wound. The mixture becomes opaque and increases in volume by about four times as it sets to form a soft foam which must be left to cure for 3 - 5 minutes. The resultant stent is managed in the same way as Silastic Foam and the indications and precautions relating to the two products are broadly similar.

The disinfection procedure for the new dressing was reviewed by Cooper and Harding who, in a trial involving 20 patients,[10] investigated the possibility of extending the interval between cleansing from the 12 hours previously recommended to 48 hours. Changes in wound microbiology were examined and it was found that in both treatment groups the number and range of organisms increased over time as the wounds became colonised with a variety of different bacterial species. Extending the interval to 48 hours appeared to lead to increased numbers of bacteria but this was not associated with an increase in clinical infection rates. The authors therefore concluded that the possibility existed to reduce the frequency of dressing changes, but that further investigations were required. Cavity wound dressings have also been developed from pre-formed forms which are supplied as simple foam sheets which may be rolled up prior to insertion in the wound. One specialist product, Allevyn Cavity Wound Dressing, consists of a bag made from a soft, perforated, polymeric film, containing small chips of hydrophilic polyurethane foam. Available in a range of sizes, these dressings can be easily inserted (and removed) from a cavity wound.

Figure 41: Allevyn Cavity Wound Dressings

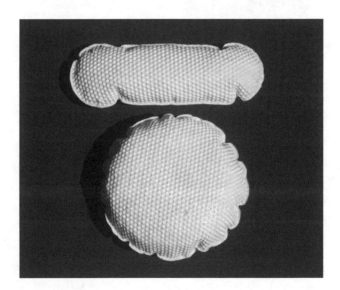

Foam membranes

The first commercially successful 'preformed' foam dressing for the treatment of surface wounds was Lyofoam. Made from a sheet of soft, hydrophobic, open-cell polyurethane foam approximately eight millimetres thick, Lyofoam was originally marketed by Ultra Laboratories which was later acquired by Seton Healthcare, subsequently SSL International. It is now marketed by Mölnlycke in Europe, and Convatec in the USA.

Lyofoam evolved from an unsuccessful product called 'Sterafoam' manufactured by Bowater Scott. Sterafoam had a large open-cell structure into which granulation tissue rapidly became incorporated, causing the dressing to adhere strongly to the wound.[11] To overcome this problem, the wound-contact surface of Lyofoam is modified by the application of heat to collapse the outermost foam cells to produce an absorbent layer about one millimetre thick which takes up liquid by capillary action whilst preventing the ingress of tissue.

The external layer of the dressing remains highly hydrophobic and so does not permit the uptake of exudate but the aqueous component of wound fluid evaporates though this outer layer as moisture vapour. This causes absorbed fluid to become increasingly more concentrated within the collapsed foam cells of the interface layer and eventually solutes precipitate out within these cells, effectively preventing any further uptake of fluid and reducing the permeability of the system. This in turn can lead to the accumulation of unabsorbed exudate beneath the dressing, increasing the risk of maceration or infection. For this reason standard Lyofoam is indicated only for the treatment of lightly exuding wounds.

Figure 42: Section through Lyofoam dressing

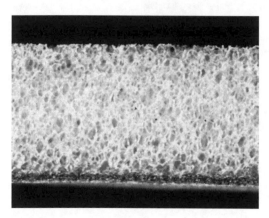

A section through a Lyofoam dressing that has been placed in contact with blood in a laboratory test. Cellular debris is clearly visible trapped in wound contact layer of dressing and had not been transported into backing layer.

Lyofoam T (T for tracheotomy) is a simple variation of the basic dressing which contains a cross-cut in the centre, forming an aperture designed to enable the dressing to fit closely around the tubes, cannulae or pins used in invasive medical procedures.

Synthaderm, now discontinued, was similar to Lyofoam in that it consisted of a thin sheet of polyurethane foam with two surfaces that were structurally different. The wound contact surface was formed from a layer of open cells, whilst the upper or outer surface was composed of closed cells. When Synthaderm was placed on an exuding wound, tissue fluid and exudate taken up by the inner hydrophilic layer was prevented from passing right through the dressing by the closed cells of the upper surface. The solid components of the exudate were retained within the foam but the aqueous component was lost by evaporation as with Lyofoam. In the early stages of use, an increase in exudate production was sometimes noted; possibly associated with a slight increase in wound size, as necrotic material present was removed by autolysis. This was not a cause for concern provided the dressing was changed frequently (daily or on alternate days). As the wound became cleaner, the frequency of dressing changes was reduced, so that in the final stages of healing, weekly changes were sufficient.

Synthaderm had several practical disadvantages in use, including poor conformability and loss of tensile strength when wet. In addition, it had a marked tendency to curl up and wrinkle when it came into contact with moisture, and so had to be bandaged firmly in position to prevent this occurring. This was caused by the fact that the dressing increased in surface area by almost 20% when hydrated. When the lower hydrophilic surface took up moisture, its ability to expand was inhibited by the more hydrophobic outer surface, and this constraint was responsible for the dressing rolling up. The expansion of the foam was accompanied by a seven-fold increase in its moisture vapour permeability; thus, to some extent, the permeability of the dressing was related to the moisture content of the wound, Synthaderm therefore could perhaps be described as an early 'intelligent' wound dressing. Nevertheless, it failed to make a significant impact in the market place and so was discontinued. Some of the practical problems with Synthaderm were claimed to have been addressed in the second generation product, Coraderm, also discontinued, and marketed as Epi-lock in the USA.

Activheal Flexipore, now marketed by Medlogic Global, a subsidiary of the manufacturers, Advanced Medical Solutions (previously Innovative Technologies), is the same product as Spyroflex, previously marketed by Britcair, which is now produced in the USA by Innovative Technologies (US).

Acivheal Flexipore was originally sold as Flexipore 6000 by Beam Tech Ltd, and like Synthaderm and Coraderm it consists of a polyurethane membrane about one millimetre thick. It is produced in a similar way by casting the polymer solution onto a belt but instead of allowing the solvent to evaporate, as in film production, the belt is plunged into a series of water baths which cause the polyurethane to precipitate immediately as the solvent is washed away. Gas bubbles released during this procedure form bubbles in the polymer giving it a 'cellular' structure. These bubbles vary in size from quite large, where the polymer first makes contact with the water, to extremely small where the polymer is in contact with the belt. At the interface between the foam and the belt a 'skin' is produced which is permeable to air and water vapour, but provides a reasonable barrier to water and bacteria. A discontinuous layer of adhesive is subsequently applied to the wound contact surface in a cross-hatched fashion. The dressing is intended for light to moderately exuding wounds such as superficial pressure sores and leg ulcers, IV sites, abrasions, lacerations and donor sites. It is not recommended for application to full thickness or heavily exuding wounds.

Flexzan is similar to the above, consisting of thin, highly conformable, open cell foam with a closed cell outer surface.

Another early foam dressing which was not made from polyurethane, was Release produced by Johnson and Johnson. Now discontinued, it consisted of a carboxylated styrene-butadiene rubber latex foam, bonded to a non woven fabric coated with a ruptured polyethylene film which formed a low-adherent wound contact layer. A surface active agent was included within the foam to facilitate fluid uptake. The dressing had limited absorbent capacity but could be used as a wound contact layer beneath a secondary absorbent. The properties of some of the early foam dressings were described previously.[12-13]

Also available are foam-like dressings made from collagen used alone or in combination with other agents. Examples include Collatek, a bovine collagen matrix bonded to a polyurethane foam sheet, CollaWound sponge, a primary dressing consisting of 97% porcine collagen and Suprasorb C, a primary dressing made from non cross-linked bovine collagen.

Multilayer foam dressings

In contrast to the hydrophobic polyurethane foam used in the Lyofoam range, hydrophilic polyurethane prepolymers facilitate the production of more absorbent dressings with much greater affinity for aqueous solutions. Some of these dressings have been given pseudoscientific names such as 'hydrocellular' (Allevyn) and 'hydropolymer' (Tielle), terms which convey little to most clinicians.

The foam used in the construction of some of these new dressings is able to retain in excess of ten times its own weight of exudate. Consequently they therefore offer considerable advantages over the earlier products in terms of fluid handling but potentially suffer from two major disadvantages.

Firstly, absorbed fluid is rapidly distributed throughout the foam with the result that a moist pathway quickly forms between the wound and the external environment along which bacteria may pass in either direction. Secondly as healing progresses and exudate production diminishes, the highly permeable foam will dry out, potentially leading to problems of desiccation and adherence.

These problems may be overcome by laminating the foam to a semipermeable polyurethane film which reduces evaporative loss and provides an effective bacterial barrier. Sometimes a thin sheet of closed cell polyurethane foam is used in place of the film which fulfils a similar function.

Among the most commercially successful foam dressings are the Allevyn range marketed by Smith and Nephew. A non-adhesive form of Allevyn was launched in 1987 followed in 1995 by the adhesive version. In 2006 the dressings were improved by the introduction of a more permeable outer film which increased their fluid handling capacity.

A family of dressings, the Cutinova range, developed by Beiersdorf AG, but later marketed by Smith and Nephew, consist of a polyurethane matrix containing particles of a sodium polyacrylate superabsorbent. Following the change in ownership, Cutinova Foam was rebranded as Allevyn Compression, Cutinova Thin as Allevyn Thin, and Cutinova Cavity as Allevyn Plus Cavity. Cutinova Hydro and Cutinova Hydro Border remain unchanged.

In Allevyn Compression, Thin, and Plus Cavity Dressing, the polyurethane matrix is foamed, but this is not the case in Cutinova Hydro. As a result this dressing more resembles the hydrocolloid sheets although it differs from them in chemical composition.

With the exception of Allevyn Cavity Plus, all the dressings in this range are designed for application to relatively superficial exuding wounds and ulcers and incorporate a polyurethane film backing layer to act as a bacterial barrier. Exudate taken up by the superabsorbent particles forms a gel within the cross-linked polyurethane matrix and leaves no residue upon the wound surface after removal of the dressing.

Foam dressings have been developed in a variety of forms. Some are coated with acrylic or hydrocolloid-based adhesives, but more recently adhesives based upon silicone technology have been devised which are claimed to facilitate removal without causing pain or trauma. Sometimes the adhesive bond formed between the dressing and the skin is very weak, intended only to retain the dressing in place temporarily, whilst a secondary retention layer is being applied.

An early example of an adhesive film-foam combination, now discontinued, was Spyrosorb originally marketed by Britcair (later CV Laboratories). According to Williams,[14] the foam sheet was coated with acrylic adhesive and bonded to a 'moisture responsive' polyurethane membrane.

Many dressings share this simple bi-component structure but others have additional features which make them unique. The foam used in the Polymem range, for example, contains a non-ionic surfactant thought to be a block copolymer of ethylene oxide and propylene oxide which is activated by moisture and claimed to facilitate wound cleansing. These non-ionic surfactants were tested by Rodeheaver[15] and shown to have no adverse effects upon wound healing in an experimental model. The dressing also contains a humectant (glycerol) which prevents the dressing from drying out and adhering to the wound bed, and a starch copolymer to enhance its fluid handling properties.

One feature of Polymem foam which has attracted some interest is the finding that application of the dressing appears to reduce the sensitivity of the subject or patient to painful stimuli.

This so-called antinociceptive effect was demonstrated in an animal study using a hind limb penetrating stab wound model.[16] Two small wounds were made in the calf muscles of previously shaved adult rats whilst under anaesthesia. These wounds were then dressed with Polymem Plus or gauze dressings held in place with elastic tape. Each animal's response to mechanical and thermal stimuli applied to the hind paw remote to the injury was recorded. Application of Polymem Plus, but not gauze dressing, significantly reduced the development of both mechanical and thermal hyperalgesia induced by the penetrating stab wounds.

To eliminate the possibility that inhibition of limb movement caused by the application of the dressing was influencing the test results both legs were shaved and wrapped with dressings as appropriate but only the left limb received the surgical incision. Animals with stab wounds also showed a significant decrease in cage activity, but this decrease was reversed by the application of Polymem Plus dressing.

The authors concluded that these observations clearly indicated that the application of Polymem Plus, but not gauze, markedly reversed the increased pain behavioural responses exhibited by the animals who had received surgical stab wounds. Interestingly the application of Polymem Plus, but not gauze, appeared to reduce the sensitivity of limbs that had not received stab wounds, suggesting that the dressing produces a local anaesthetic effect when applied to the skin.

In the second part of the study the authors quantified the number of Fos-positive neurones in the lumbar spinal cord after incisional stab wounds and dressing application. The C-Fos protein is the product of c-fos mRNA, a member of a family of immediate early gene (IEG) transcription factors. The basal expression of c-fos and other IEGs is typically low but increases relatively quickly and often dramatically in response to changes in cellular activity typically caused by external stimuli, such as metabolic stress or neuronal activation. For this reason Fos protein is routinely used as a marker of neuronal activation.

The results indicated that Polymem, but not gauze dressing, significantly decreased stab wound-induced Fos expression within the spinal cord. Surprisingly, application of the foam, but not the gauze dressing, to the limbs of untreated animals elicited a significant increase in spinal Fos neurons suggesting that the dressing itself causes spinal cord activation, a finding that was consistent with the earlier observation that the dressing appeared to reduce the sensitivity of untreated limbs to external stimuli.

In the third part of the study, histological sections were made through the stab wounds to examine the number and distribution of neutrophils and macrophages present. Compared with untreated controls, both dressings reduced the number of inflammatory cells but Polymem Plus greatly reduced the spread of these cells into surrounding tissue. In untreated wounds, or those dressed with gauze, the inflammation spread into the periosteum of the tibia or fibula but periosteal involvement did not occur in animals whose wounds were wrapped with Polymem Plus. Other studies, not reported here, suggest that the application of the dressing can also effectively prevent or reduce bruising follow traumatic injuries if applied at an early stage.

The mechanism(s) by which the foam produces this antinociceptive effect is unclear. It is possible that the a local effect is responsible for limiting the extent of the inflammatory process within the wound but the observed effect of the dressing on animal who had not be subjected to surgery indicates that an alterative mechanism must also be involved which is mediated both peripherally and centrally.

One possible explanation advanced by the authors was that the dressing might absorb sodium ions from the skin and subcutaneous tissue which would result in reduced nerve conductance and a local anaesthetic effect which in turn reduces the development of secondary hyperalgesia. What is not known, however, is the identity of agent or agents within the foam responsible for this activity, and whether this effect is unique to Polymem foam or if it is shared by other foam products. Further research is clearly required in this area.

Other multi-component foam dressings include Mepilex and Mepilex Border, the structure of which has been described previously.

Tielle, like Mepilex Border, also contains a 'spreader layer' between the foam and the backing layer: Tielle Plus is similar but also contains a superabsorbent powder dispersed in the spreader layer. An overview of the Tielle range was produced by Carter in 2003.[17]

Foam dressings are produced in a variety of shapes and sizes, some of which are specifically designed to fit hard-to-dress anatomical sites including the elbow, heel or sacrum, whilst others have preformed apertures to enable them to be used around tracheostomy or pin sites.

Figure 43: Examples of shaped foam dressings

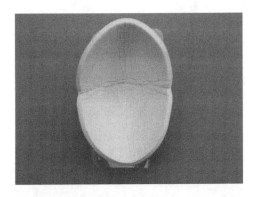

Allevyn heel dressing

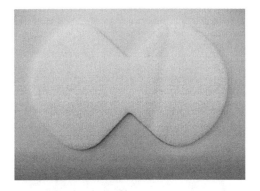

Mepilex heel dressing

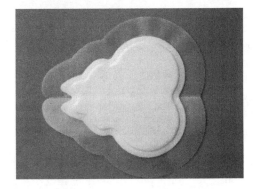

Allevyn sacral dressing

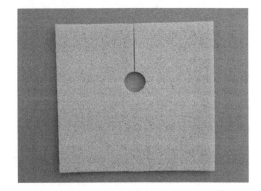

Polytube dressing

Some dressings incorporate a low-adherent wound contact layer such as an apertured plastic film, but the Restore range from Hollister bears a fine polyester mesh impregnated with petrolatum containing hydrocolloid particles, the same material used in Urgotulle described in the chapter on low-adherent dressings.

Lyofoam Extra, the most absorbent product in the Lyofoam range is unique, in that it is constructed from three different types of foam. The wound contact layer, which is identical to that used in standard Lyofoam, is bonded to a hydrophilic foam layer which in turn is attached to a high density polyurethane foam backing layer. Lyofoam Extra dressing works in a very similar way to the standard dressing. The collapsed cells of the hydrophobic inner layer take up fluid from the wound surface which is then transferred into the more absorbent secondary layer. The outer layer prevents this absorbed fluid from seeping out of the back of the dressing.

Lyofoam C consists of a piece of Lyofoam that is heat-bonded around the perimeter to a sheet of plain polyurethane foam. A layer of a non-woven fabric impregnated with activated carbon granules is sandwiched between the two polyurethane sheets.

Lyofoam C is claimed to provide the wound-management benefits of the standard dressing whilst absorbing the noxious odours associated with certain types of wounds. The substances that are responsible for the formation of odour appear to be partly retained within the foam itself, but the principal odour-absorbing ability of the dressing are due to the presence of the activated carbon.

The properties of foam are such that potentially it makes a useful carrier for topical antimicrobial agents and other agents which are to be delivered into a wound. AMD Antimicrobial Foam Dressing from Covidien contains 0.5% polyhexanide, polyhexamethylene biguanide (PHMB) - an antimicrobial agent with a broad spectrum of activity.

Given the current enthusiasm for the use of silver in wound management, it is not surprising that several manufacturers have developed foam dressings containing a variety of silver salts: these are discussed in more detail in the chapter on silver dressings.

Despite the fact that foam dressings are widely used for the management of a variety of exuding wounds, clinical experience suggests that, for some indications at least, their fluid handling capacity is less than optimal, necessitating more frequent dressing changes than might otherwise be considered desirable. Although it is theoretically possible to improve their performance by increasing the thickness of the foam or the content of gel-forming agents to improve fluid retention, such modifications would also increase the weight of the exudate-soaked dressing causing it to sag or separate away from the wound surface, greatly reducing its efficiency and patient acceptability. An alternative, more acceptable strategy is to increase the permeability of the backing layer to facilitate evaporation and thereby enhance its fluid handling capacity.

The key properties of the foam dressings in current use are summarised in a series of tables in which they are grouped together by structure. Table 11 describes the foam-based cavity wound dressings, Table 12 to Table 14 contains details of simple absorbent foam sheets, and Table 15 and Table 16 the self-adhesive island dressings.

Table 11: Foam Cavity Dressings

Dressing	Manufacturer
Allevyn Cavity Wound Dressing	SN
Allevyn Plus Cavity	SN
Askina Foam Cavity	BB
Cutimed Cavity	BSN
Medifoam B	BIO

Table 12: Foam Dressings Sheets

Dressing	Manufacturer	Codes
Non-adhesive film-backed		
Activheal Foam Heel	ACT	H, WCL
Activheal Non-adhesive foam	ACT	H, WCL
Allevyn Ag Non-adhesive	SN	H, WCL, Ag
Allevyn Heel	SN	H, WCL
Allevyn Non-adhesive	SN	H, WCL, FEN
AMD Antimicrobial Dressing	COV	H
Askina Foam	BB	H, Heel
Biatain IBU	COL	H
Comfifoam	SYN	H
Copa Plus	COV	H
Medifoam	BIO	H, FEN
Optifoam Ag Non-adhesive	MED	H, Ag
Optifoam Non-adhesive	MED	H, FEN
Polymem	FE	L, SA
Polymem Max	FE	H, SA
Polymem Silver	FE	L, SA, Ag
Polymem tube	FE	L, SA
Sof-Foam	JJ	H
Suprasorb P	LR	H
Tegaderm Foam	3M	H

'H' Heavily exuding wounds, 'L' Lightly exuding wounds, 'FEN' Fenestrated dressing, 'Ag' Silver,' SA' Superabsorbent, 'WCL' Low-adherent or silicone wound contact layer

Table 13: Foam Dressings Sheets (cont)

Dressing	Manufacturer	Codes
Non-adhesive foam-backed		
Lyofoam Extra	MOL	H, FEN
Restore Foam Dressing	HOL	H, SA
Restore Foam Dressing with silver	HOL	H, SA
Tielle Extra	JJ	H, SA
Trufoam NA	UNO	H
Non-adhesive unbacked		
Allevyn Lite Non-adhesive	SN	L, WCL
AMD Antimicrobial Dressing	COV	H
Copa	COV	H, FEN
Lyofoam	MOL	L, FEN
Permafoam	P H.	H
Polymem Rhinopak	FE	L, SA
Polymem WIC	FE	H, SA
Polymem WIC Silver	FE	H, SA, AG
Suprasorb M	LR	L
Low-tack adhesive unbacked		
Mepilex Transfer	MOL	H

'H' Heavily exuding wounds, 'L' Lightly exuding wounds, 'FEN' Fenestrated dressing, 'Ag' Silver,' SA' Superabsorbent, 'WCL' Low-adherent or silicone wound contact layer

Table 14: Foam Dressings Sheets (cont)

Dressing	Manufacturer	Codes
Low-tack adhesive film-backed		
Allevyn Gentle	SN	H, WCL
Biatain-IBU Soft-Hold	COL	H, WCL
Biatain Soft Hold	COL	WCL, H
Cutimed Siltec	BSN	WCL, H, SA
Cutimed Siltec L	BSN	L, SA
Mepilex	MOL	H
Mepilex Ag	MOL	H
Urgocell Non adhesive	URG	H
Urgocell Start Non adhesive	URG	H
Adhesive film-backed		
Advazorb Plus	ADV	H
Allevyn Compression	SN	H, SA
Allevyn Thin	SN	L
Biatain Adhesive Heel	COL	H
Medifoam A	BIO	L
Adhesive unbacked		
ActivHeal Flexipore	AMS	L
Flexzan	UDL	H
Optifoam Thin, Self-adhesive	MED	L

'H' Heavily exuding wounds, 'L' Lightly exuding wounds, 'FEN' Fenestrated dressing, 'Ag' Silver,' SA' Superabsorbent, 'WCL' Low-adherent or silicone wound contact layer

Table 15: Foam Island Dressings

Dressing	Manufacturer	Code
Film backed		
Activheal Foam Island	ACT	H,
Advazorb Border	ADV	H, SIL
Allevyn Adhesive	SN	H, WCL, S
Allevyn Ag Adhesive	SN	H,WCL, AG
Allevyn Gentle Border	SN	H, WCL, SIL
Allevyn Plus Adhesive	SN	H, WCL, SA
AMD Antimicrobial Dressing	COV	L, S
Biatain Adhesive	COL	H
Biatain Adhesive Contour	COL	H, S
Comfifoam Adhesive	SYN	H
Copa Island	COV	L
Cutimed Siltec B	BSN	L, WCL, SIL, SA
Episil	ADV	L,SIL
Medifoam F	BIO	H
Mepilex Border	MOL	H, WCL, SIL, SA
Mepilex Border Lite	MOL	L, WCL, SIL
Optifoam Self-adhesive	MED	H, S
Optifoam Ag Self-adhesive	MED	H, AG
Polymem Shapes	FE	L, S, SA
Polymem Shapes Silver	FE	L, S, SA, AG
Suprasorb P Adhesive	LR	H, S
Tegaderm Foam Adhesive Dressing	3M	H
Urgocell Self adhesive	URG	L, WCL

'H' Heavily exuding wounds, 'L' Lightly exuding wounds, 'FEN' Fenestrated dressing
'Ag' Silver,' SA' Superabsorbent, 'WCL' Low-adherent wound contact layer,
'SIL' Silicone coated, 'S' Shaped

Table 16: Foam Island Dressings (cont)

Dressing	Manufacturer	Codes
Foam backed		
Permafoam Comfort	P H.	H
Lyofoam Extra Adhesive	MOL	H, WCL
Activheal Foam Island	AMS	H
Restore Foam Dressing Adhesive	HOL	H, WCL,SA
Restore Foam Dressing with Silver	HOL	H, WCL, SA, AG
Tielle	JJ	L, S
Tielle Lite	JJ	L, WCL
Tielle Plus	JJ	H, S, SA
Trufoam SA	UNO	H
Fabric backed		
Optifoam Site Self-adhesive	MED	L

'H' Heavily exuding wounds, 'L' Lightly exuding wounds, 'FEN' Fenestrated dressing
'Ag' Silver,' SA' Superabsorbent, 'WCL' Low-adherent wound contact layer,
'SIL' Silicone coated, 'S' Shaped

KEY PROPERTIES OF FOAM DRESSINGS

Foam dressings were amongst the first 'modern' dressings to become widely adopted by the international wound management community as they possess a number of the important characteristics of the ideal dressing. Specifically, they provide thermal insulation, do not shed fibres or particles, are easily cut or shaped, and help to maintain a moist environment at the surface of the wound. They are also gas-permeable, non-adherent, light, and comfortable to wear, and can be medicated with antimicrobials or other biologically active agents.

Their most important function, however, is that of exudate management. Unlike hydrocolloids such as Granuflex, which are virtually impermeable to moisture vapour in their intact state, the foams are intrinsically permeable and therefore do not readily conserve moisture or facilitate the promotion of autolysis in dry wounds. They are therefore best suited for the management of exuding lesions and are regarded by many as the products of choice for moderate to heavily exuding wounds, although as will be seen later the variation in permeability between different brands means that products are available to suit most clinical requirements

Fluid handling

The principal function of foam dressings is the management of exudate from wounds such as leg ulcers, pressure ulcers burns and donor sites.

The fluid handling properties of foam dressing may be determined, as described in Chapter 7, by means of a Paddington Cup to measure the absorbency and permeability of the dressing in order to calculate its Fluid Handling Capacity (FHC). This test can be performed either with the dressing in contact with test solution, simulating an exuding wound, or with the Paddington cups inverted, so that the dressing is only in contact with water vapour, thus simulating a dry wound.

Test results for different dressings have been collated from a variety of sources including independent laboratory test reports, technical publications,[18] and manufacturers' literature.[19-20] Where data sets relating to a specific product have been obtained from more than one source, these have been averaged to construct the graphs shown in Figure 44 to Figure 46. In each case these indicate the combined absorbency and MVTR results expressed as grams/10cm^2. It should be recognized, however, that he permeability values derived experimentally will be much higher than those achieved clinically, thus overestimating the performance of each of the dressings.

Whilst every attempt has been made to ensure that these results are correct and relate to current production materials, the possibility that recent design or manufacturing changes have resulted in products with that exhibit different performance figures from those quoted cannot be excluded.

Figure 44: Fluid handling of non-adhesive foam dressings

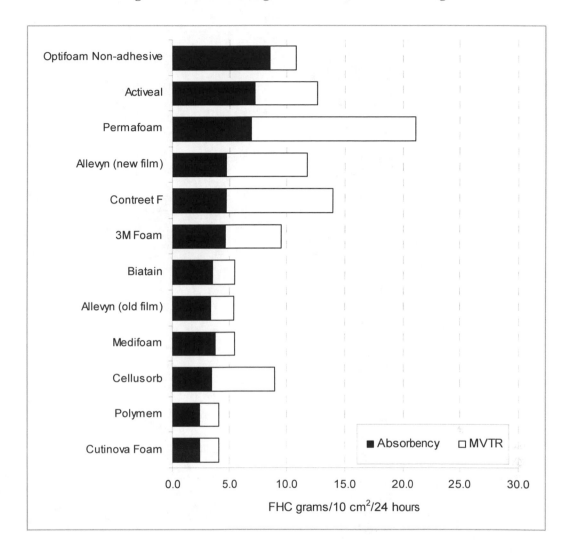

Figure 45: Fluid handling of adhesive foam dressings

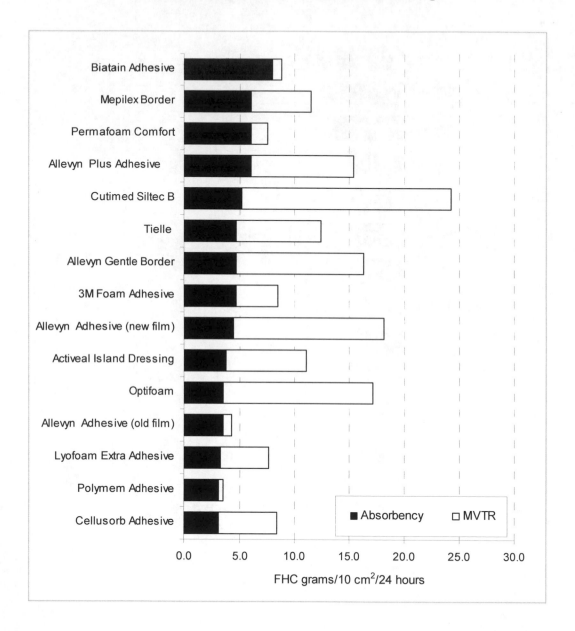

Figure 46: Fluid handling of 'tacky' foam dressings

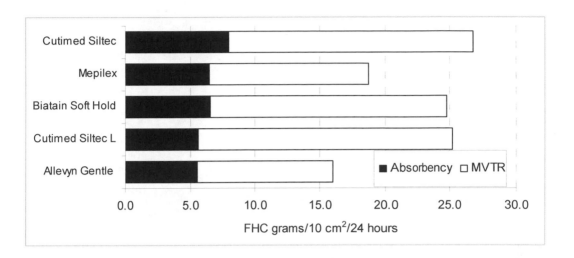

The graphs indicate that some products, notably some of those in the Allevyn and Siltec range, are markedly more permeable than the majority of the other dressings examined.

Whilst this degree of permeability might be desirable in the treatment of heavily exuding wounds, it suggests that these dressings could be of less value in the management of lightly exuding wounds as they might permit excessive moisture loss leading to desiccation and adherence. In fact this is prevented in both dressings by the use of an 'intelligent' semipermeable film backing layer, the permeability of which changes in contact with aqueous solutions.

This was demonstrated in detail in an earlier publication in which Allevyn was compared with a foam dressing bearing a standard film backing layer.[21] The switching effect in Allevyn was illustrated graphically by placing a sample of dressing in a Paddington cup on a top pan balance in a controlled environment chamber in the inverted position so that the fluid was not in contact with the dressing. The change in weight of the cup was logged electronically for six hours, then, without stopping the logging process, the cup was inverted so that the test fluid came into contact with the dressing. Logging was continued for a further 18 hours at which time the balance readings were downloaded and used to construct the graphs shown in Figure 47. The marked change in the permeability of the dressing is clearly illustrated by the change in the slope of the curve at the time of inversion.

Figure 47: Effect of hydration on permeability of Allevyn

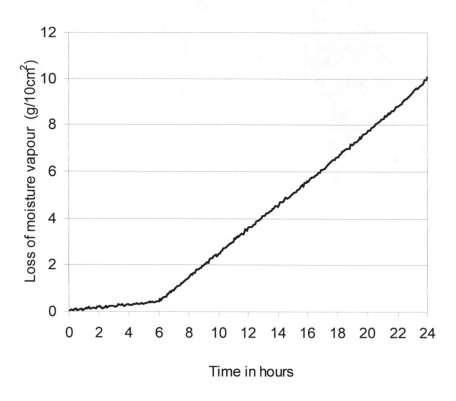

Note change in slope of graph at six hours indicating change in permeability

In a further independent laboratory study also conducted by SMTL, the effect of liquid upon the permeability of a small number of other dressings designed for more lightly exuding wounds was determined. Some of these dressings exhibited a switching effect whilst other did not. The results are summarized in Figure 48.

Figure 48: Effect of hydration of permeability of film backing

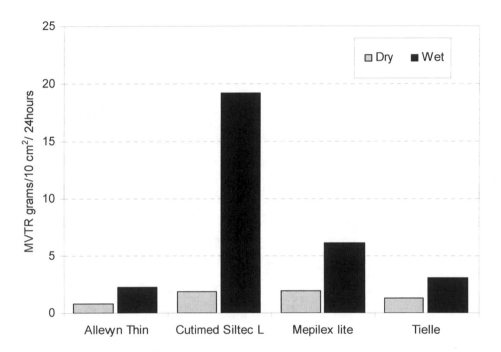

Clinical relevance of fluid handling data

Using published values for exudate production from different wound types reported in an earlier chapter,[21] a graph has been constructed to represent the cumulative amount of fluid produced by each wound type over a seven day period (Figure 49).

Overlaid on this graph are the limits for the fluid handling capacity of the Allevyn dressing derived from the laboratory study. The upper boundary of the area filled in grey represents the maximum amount of fluid that the dressing might be expected to handle determined from the absorbency and permeability test data. The lower boundary represents the moisture vapour permeability of the dressings in the absence of wound fluid which provides an indication of the ability of the dressings to retain low levels of moisture within the wound in order to maintain a moist wound healing environment.

Figure 49: Predicted ability of Allevyn to cope with exudate from different wound types

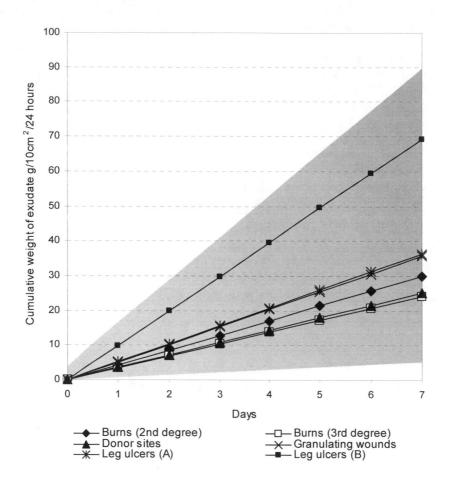

Within the graph, the projected volume of exudate produced by all the wound types fell between the upper and lower boundaries of the marked area, suggesting that the dressing should be able to cope with even the most heavily exuding wounds for an extended period because of the high permeability of the polyurethane film backing.

In the absence of liquid, the dressing appears capable of forming an effective barrier to moisture vapour loss and is thus able to facilitate moist wound healing. In clinical practice, however, there are many factors not addressed by this test procedure. These have been discussed in more detail in an earlier chapter.

Although the fluid handling tests provide useful quantitative data which facilitates comparisons between different dressings, they provide little information on the way in which fluid it is transported throughout their structure during normal clinical use.

Young *et al.*[22] in a novel study used high frequency ultrasound and a probe with an axial resolution of 60 microns to image the inside of four adhesive foam dressings in order to assess their degree of hydration following the application of a bolus of test fluid.

Four dressings were examined in this way ActivHeal Foam Island, Allevyn Adhesive, Biatain Adhesive, and Mepilex Border. Allevyn hydrated the dressing most rapidly followed by Activheal, Biatain and Mepilex. It was also shown that Allevyn dehydrated most rapidly followed by Mepilex, Activheal and Biatain.

This initial study was followed by a second in which ultrasound was used to monitor the movement of exudate within an Allevyn dressing applied to an exuding wound.[21] Initially as fluid was absorbed it appeared to be distributed fairly evenly throughout the thickness of the foam, but as the amount of exudate present in the dressing progressively increased there was clear evidence to suggest that liquid accumulated just beneath the outer membrane, not as perhaps might have been expected, at the wound contact interface.

The explanation proposed to explain this observation was that as moisture vapour from wound fluid is transpired through the back of the dressing it has the effect of increasing the concentration of dissolved solutes immediately behind the membrane. It is proposed that as this process continues the viscosity of the exudate increases due to its high protein content and this tends to prevent it from dispersing back throughout the main body of the foam. This increase in concentration also helps to establish an osmotic gradient which would effectively draw still more fluid up through the dressing away from the wound contact surface. This mechanism, which requires further investigation, was tentatively described as a form of active 'osmotic pump' preventing pooling of fluid on the wound surface.

Some support for this theory may be found in the ultrasound scans, which clearly show that exudate taken up by the dressing is moves upward in a columnar fashion with apparently little tendency to spread laterally to form a uniform distribution of fluid through the body of the foam. These columns are assumed to be formed initially by the perforated plastic wound contact layer of the dressing preventing uniform uptake of liquid by the lower surface of the dressing. In the absence of an osmotic effect drawing the liquid upwards, it might be expected that absorbed fluid would spread more uniformly throughout the dressing's structure.

Barrier properties

Foam dressings, particularly those backed with a semipermeable film membrane are assumed to provide an effective barrier to microorganisms. When Ameen *et al.*[23] challenged a number of dressings over an 11-day period with bacterial cultures; they found that three dressings, Allevyn, Combiderm and Tegaderm, were able to resist penetration by a range of organisms. A fourth, Tielle showed evidence of bacterial penetration within three to five days. The reason for this is that Allevyn and Combiderm incorporate a semipermeable film in their structure which is known to form an effective bacterial barrier, Tielle does not and depends instead upon the small pore size of its polyurethane backing layer to prevent bacterial penetration.

Both the methodology and finding findings of this study were subsequently seriously criticised by Harvey,[24] who pointed out that there have been no cases of infection associated with the use of Tielle even though by that time 50 million pieces had been used worldwide. Harvey's criticism of the methodology is not unreasonable as the technique described places the test sample under sustained hydrostatic pressure, far greater than is ever likely to be encountered clinically, which can lead to disruption of the cellular structure of the foam, and potentially, the passage of microorganisms.

CLINICAL EXPERIENCE WITH FOAM DRESSINGS

A summary of publications which describe the use of various types of foam dressings is provided below.

Liquid foam and cavity wound dressings

In 1972-3, Silastic Foam was used to treat 40 patients with open wounds following excision of a pilonidal sinus.[25] Conventionally, gauze packs, sometimes moistened with Eusol, were used for this application. These had to be changed once or twice daily, a very painful and time consuming procedure which often led to re-wounding as capillary loops were torn from new tissues. In contrast, wounds dressed with foam were found to heal faster with less trauma, thus enabling patients to leave hospital earlier.

This initial study was followed by a second which involved 250 patients with a variety of granulating wounds including sacral pressure areas, perineal wounds and extensive lesions resulting from post-surgical abdominal wall breakdown.[26] Once again it was found that the use of Silastic Foam increased patient comfort and reduced the time required for routine nursing care. The authors concluded that the foam formed 'an ideal dressing, maintaining constant drainage'

Macfie et al.[27] described the use of Silastic Foam in a variety of open abdominal and perineal wounds including a pressure sore, and in 1980 in a second publication,[28] they reported the results of the first prospective randomized control trial involving this material. Fifty patients with open perineal wounds were randomized to receive either conventional gauze packing or treatment with the foam. Wounds were reviewed weekly until healing occurred. Healing times were shorter in patients who received foam, but not significantly so, however, statistically less analgesia and fewer district nurse visits were required by patients in the foam-treated group. The authors concluded that the foam dressing was not only a more comfortable alternative to gauze in the management of perineal wounds it also substantially reduced the amount of nursing supervision required, leading them to recommend its routine use for this application. Their data later formed the subject a further paper,[29] in which they suggested that the foam was also less costly both in terms of material and labour time.

Silastic Foam was also compared with gauze packing following pilonidal sinus excision in a multicentre study reported by Williams et al. in 1981.[30] Eighty patients were followed to healing and although healing times, duration of hospital stay and time lost from work were similar, perceived pain and nursing time were much reduced in patients dressed with Silastic Foam.

When Silastic Foam was compared with the dextranomer beads, Debrisan, now discontinued, in the treatment of 50 patients following surgical wound breakdown, the two treatments were judged equivalent in terms of healing time and patient comfort although the cost of Debrisan treatment was significantly greater than that of the foam.[31]

The global success of Silastic Foam was confirmed by reports from around the world which highlighted its superiority over products such as gauze, particularly in relation to its low-adherent properties.[32]

In 1977 in the USA its use reduced the treatment times of nine individuals with enterocutaneous fistulae or problem stomas, and enabled them to be treated as outpatients.[33] In Australia, in 1981, 55 patients with wounds following excision of a pilonidal sinus, or infected abdominal wounds and perineal wounds following abdo-perineal resection of the rectum, were successfully treated as outpatients using the foam.[34]

Gledhill[35] recorded its use in Canada in 1983, and the French experience was reported by Balique in 1984.[36] Frobel,[37] Linke,[38] and Muller,[39] described the use of foam in Germany during the period 1984-86.

Silastic Foam dressing also found early application in a variety of other wound types including the management of a below knee amputation stump with delayed healing,[40] and the extensive wounds formed following surgical treatment for advanced hidradenitis suppurativa.[41-44] Others reported its successful use as an ear dressing,[45-46] a dressing for cancerous wounds of the head, neck, face and breast,[47-51] a graft fixation material,[52-53] a dressing for the orbital cavity following removal of the eye,[54] and as a postoperative penile dressing following hypospadias repair and other related surgical procedures.[55-63] One paper described its value as an aid to applying pressure to newly formed scar tissue to prevent deforming scars and contractures, particularly in areas such as the axillae, clavicle and hands.[64]

Harding,[65] in a preliminary report, described a modified application technique for Silastic Foam in the treatment of donor sites. For these patients the material was precast into sheets about one centimetre thick before being applied to the wound. Using Silastic Foam for this indication was said to reduce healing times and increase patient comfort.

The vast majority of wounds treated with Silastic Foam cited in these publications were acute or post-surgical, the indications for which it was best suited. Experience with chronic wounds, however, was less convincing.

The principal advantages of Silastic Foam were its versatility, and a high degree of patient acceptability.[36,66] Many patients were able to manage their own wounds and thus the dressing facilitated an early discharged from hospital or allowed patients to make an earlier return to work than might otherwise have been the case.[67]

Only a limited number of clinical papers have been published describing the use of Cavi-Care, Silastic Foam's successor, but a few have been identified which make reference to its use in hypospadias repair,[68] pressure damage to the ear,[69] as dressing for an infected groin wound after distal bypass surgery,[70] and following syndactyly correction.[71] Given the similar nature of the two dressings, it is likely that the observations and experiences recorded with Silastic Foam should also apply to Cavi-Care.

Standard foam dressings

The significant fluid handling properties of polyurethane foam/film laminates, suggests that these dressing should be of value in the treatment of all types of exuding wounds such as leg ulcers, burns and donor sites. However, given their affinity for liquid and/or their considerable permeability to moisture vapour, some products may be less appropriate for the treatment of lightly exuding wounds which could become excessively dry.

A summary of published accounts of clinical experience with a variety of different foam dressings is given below. Where these studies have compared foam with some other type of dressing, the summaries are collated by the brand name of the foam dressing but if two or more foam dressings have been compared with each other, the studies are described in a separate section.

Allevyn

An early reference to the use of Allevyn was published in Germany in 1988 by Friederich,[72] but the first clinical study to be identified was not published until some years later when Allevyn was compared with petrolatum gauze dressing in a prospective randomized controlled trial involving patients with donor sites.[73] Wounds were examined 14 days after surgery when the degree of epithelialization was recorded. Of the 68 patients recruited, 14/38 (37%) *vs* 5/30 (17%) achieved full closure in the Allevyn and petrolatum gauze treated groups respectively. This difference just failed to reach significance (p = 0.06). Donor site and operative site pain were also assessed using a visual numeric scale which revealed that the mean maximum pain intensity scores were statistically lower for Allevyn on postoperative days one to three (p < 05). Pain levels were elevated in larger donor site dressed with petrolatum gauze but not in wounds dressed with Allevyn. These results do not compare favourably with healing rates reported for donor sites in other studies where, using modern wound dressings, healing times in the order of 7 - 10 days are commonly recorded (see Chapters 11 and 12) but this is probably due to the poor the design of this study dictating that wounds should not be examined until day 14.

Rather more positive findings reported with Allevyn when the adhesive version was compared with paraffin gauze in 50 patients with donor site wounds which ranged from 20 cm^2 to 71 cm^2. Half of each wound was dressed with one of the products under examination and thus each patient acted as his/her own control. In necessary, the foam was changed after four days, the paraffin gauze after seven days according to normal practice. Outcome measures were time to complete epithelialization, ease of dressing removal, pain on removal and appearance of the wound bed. After four days, the wounds of 52% of 44 evaluable patients dressed with foam had completely reepithelialized and by seven days this figure had risen to 93%. By the tenth day all wounds dressed with the foam were completely healed. After seven days, the first assessment point for the control group, only 36% of wounds had healed, rising to 59% by Day 10. The difference in healing rates was statistically significant. Patients reported slight or no pain on removal of the trial dressing but 'unbearable pain' with the paraffin gauze. The results of this study were published twice.[74-75]

Similarly positive healing rates were achieved with Allevyn for the same indication when the dressing was compared with a silver coated product.[76] Fifteen patients with burns who had undergone excision and grafting with pairs of identical side-by-side split thickness donor site wounds were dressed with Allevyn and Acticoat. Healing was directly assessed daily by a single observer from post-operative day six onward, and by four independent observers who rated the extent of reepithelialization by viewing standardised digital images of the wounds that had been obtained on post-operative days 6, 8, 10 and 12.

Donor sites dressed with Allevyn were judged to have a greater degree of epithelial cover than those dressed with Acticoat at each time point, achieving > 90% coverage in a mean of 9.1 ± 1.6 days compared with 14.5 ± 6.7 days with Acticoat. This difference was statistically significant (p = 0.004). Swabs taken from the donor sites on days 3, 6, and nine revealed no significant differences in the incidence of positive bacterial cultures between the dressings.

Each healed wound was rated by a blinded observer using the Vancouver Scar Scale at one, two and three months. Donor sites dressed with Acticoat had significantly worse scars at one and two months but this difference resolved by three months. The authors concluded that while healing rates achieved with Allevyn were comparable with those reported for other types of modern dressings, Acticoat appeared to actively delay healing in this type of wound.

Somewhat contradictory results were reported following a second study in which Allevyn was compared with Acticoat in the treatment of donor sites in 27 patients with burns with particular regard to healing rates, infection, pain and cost effectiveness.[77] Fifteen sites were treated with Acticoat, and 12 with Allevyn. All healed sites were evaluated using the Vancouver Scar Scale after four, eight, and twelve weeks. Compared with Allevyn, the authors reported statistically significant faster epithelization with Acticoat on postoperative Day eight (p = 0.012) and Day ten (p = 0.008). The Acticoat was also found to be more comfortable and less adherent to the wound (p < 0.05). No statistically significant differences were detected in infection rates, treatment costs, or the final quality of healing.

The most important difference between this and the previous study was the method of managing the Acticoat dressed wounds. In the earlier study the Acticoat was covered with a damp swab, dry gauze and bandages. In the second study the authors covered the primary dressing with four layers of wet gauze, four layers of dry gauze and then wrapped the area in polyethylene film to retain moisture. The moist environment produced under this second dressing might be expected to be promote healing and help to prevent adherence. This was confirmed by the results. In this study 90% coverage with Acticoat was achieved in 8.27 ± 0.70 days compared with the 14.5 ± 6.7 days in the previous study, reinforcing once again the considerable importance of the choice of secondary dressing. The Allevyn dressing was applied and held in place with an adhesive retention sheet and the authors noted that the foam tended to adhere to the wound, presumably in the later stages of treatment as the wound began to dry, which increased the risk of damaging the new epithelium upon removal. Time to achieve 90% coverage was 10.0 ± 1.21 days compared with 9.1 ± 1.6 days previously.

The performance and safety of Allevyn was compared with that of Granuflex, in a prospective, multicentre randomized clinical trial involving 61 patients with Grade II or Grade III pressure ulcers.[78] Dressings were changed in accordance with the manufacturers' instructions and at each change assessments were made of the condition of the wound and surrounding skin, comfort, ease of use and leakage from the dressing. Treatment continued for a maximum of 30 days or until the wounds healed. Ease of application of the two dressings was comparable, but the foam dressing was found to be significantly easier to remove with superior fluid handling properties.

Allevyn was similarly compared with an alginate dressing, Kaltostat, in the treatment of 20 consecutive patients with split-thickness skin-graft donor sites following removal of grafts 0.4 mm thick.[79] The dressings were applied to equal halves of each wound and a secondary dressing of gauze, cotton wool and crepe bandage was applied over both products, it not being possible to dress them individually. Wounds were examined and dressing changed weekly in accordance with normal practice. Four patients were lost to follow up. In the remaining patients Allevyn showed a tendency to earlier healing, 12 patients healed at two weeks compared with ten dressed with alginate, but this difference was not statistically significant. However, Allevyn was found to be significantly more comfortable than Kaltostat, leading the authors to recommend it as a donor site dressing because of increased patient comfort, lower cost and reduced time to healing.

These results should have been anticipated, however, for alginates require a moist environment to form a gel and maintain this state in order to provide favourable conditions for wound healing. The application of a thick dry bandage, although appropriate in the early stages of healing, could easily cause the alginate to dry out towards the end of this process which could delay healing or cause problems of adherence during removal. This is less likely to occur with film-backed foam dressings which tend to provide a more moist environment. Also monitoring the wounds on a weekly basis meant that the significant differences in healing rates identified in a previous investigation might be missed.

Allevyn has also been used as a graft site tie-over dressing, a form of application used to encourage skin graft take by minimising dead space, reducing seroma and haematoma formation by graft immobilization. In a prospective study, 66 patients were randomized to treatment with Allevyn or the standard technique which consisted of paraffin gauze (Jelonet) supported by a bolster of proflavine-soaked cotton wool. Outcome measures included percentage take, pain on dressing removal and infection. No statistical difference in graft take was recorded between the two groups at day five but Allevyn dressed wounds were statistically more comfortable (p = 0.018).[80]

The management of leg ulcers is potentially a major indication for all modern dressings. The non-adhesive form of Allevyn was evaluated for the treatment of this condition in an open, observational multicentre study in 24 patients.[81] In the 22 patients who completed the study, 17 (77.3%) had ulcers caused by venous disease, one leg ulcer was of mixed aetiology, and one followed an amputation. In three instances the cause of the ulcer was not specified. Seven wounds healed completely and the remainder reduced in area. The dressing was found to be easy to use and was well tolerated by patient with no evidence of any adverse events.

The largest study ever published on Allevyn was that described by Verdu Soriano et al.,[82] which involved 441 elderly patients 63% of whom had pressure ulcers, 27.2% leg ulcers of venous origin and 9.8% wounds of some other aetiology. Each wound was subjected to a maximum of 20 dressing changes unless closure was achieved during the treatment period. The wounds, which had been present for 6.1 months, had an average area of 30.4 cm^2 at the start of the study. During the study period 126 wounds (28.8%) healed in an average of 47.3 days. Of the 315 lesions which remained open at the end of the study, 90.5% showed evidence of improvement. Whist the numbers included in this investigation are impressive and the results appear positive, as with the previous study, the absence of a control group greatly limits the value of this publication.

Allevyn Adhesive was compared with Versiva, in the management of venous leg ulcers in a multicentre randomized, controlled 12-week study involving 15 centres in the US, Canada, France, Germany, and the UK.[83] Within this publication Versiva is described as a 'foam composite' but this is probably something of a misnomer. The absorbent core of the dressing consists of a layer of sodium carboxymethylcellulose fibres which is located centrally upon a larger piece of a thin sheet consisting of a polyurethane foam/film laminate which is present as a backing layer. The dressing may be more accurately described as an absorbent gel-forming island dressing rather than a foam dressing.

Patients with venous ulcers ≥ 2.0 cm^2 but no larger that 11×15 cm^2 were randomized to treatment for 12 weeks with Allevyn (n = 52) or Versiva (n = 55). Dressings were changed and compression bandages applied in accordance with the manufacturers' recommendations. Dressing performance was assessed at every dressing change and at the final evaluation. Healing rates in the two groups were not statistically different, 36% in a mean of 66 days for Versiva and 39% in a mean of 73 days for Allevyn Adhesive. However, the Versiva performed significantly better than Allevyn with regard to improvement in the condition of the periwound skin, 55% vs 37% respectively, (p = 0.03). Versiva was also more conformable than Allevyn, rated 'very good' to 'excellent' in 87% vs 75% of instances (p = 0.05). It was also more highly rated in terms of ease of application, 93% vs 81% (p = 0.01). The authors concluded that Versiva offers significant improvements in the quality of life of patients with venous leg ulcers as well as for their caregivers.

A more unusual application for Allevyn was suggested by Abela et al.[84] who employed it as a penile dressing following grafting to treat a full thickness alkali (sodium hydroxide solution) burn. The dressing was applied over a piece of perforated plastic film, Telfa Clear, and formed into a tube held in place with staples until healing was achieved.

One presentation of Allevyn is made from a standard foam sheet, preformed into a cup-shape to accommodate a heel or elbow to treat or prevent the development of pressure damage or dress pre-existing wounds on these areas.

The ability of this shaped dressing to prevent pressure damage was compared with that of a standard treatment in a comparative, multicentre study over an eight week period.[85] A total of 130 patients were recruited, half of whom were treated with the foam and the remainder with an orthopaedic wadding bandage, Soffban, held in place with a bandage. Of those in the bandage group, 50/65 completed the study compared with 61/65 in the Allevyn group. Pressure damage developed in 44% of patients dressed with the bandage compared with 3.3% of those dressed with Allevyn. This difference was highly significant (p < 0.001). Despite the higher unit cost of Allevyn, the dressing was more cost effective in use, producing savings both in material costs and staff time (average cost 84 *vs* 38 Euros).

The value of Allevyn Heel Dressing as a treatment for existing wounds was investigated in a small uncontrolled study involving 22 patients, 13 with heel pressure ulcers, four with diabetic heel ulcers, four with arterial heel ulcers and one other.[86] Ulcers were assessed before treatment, at weeks two and four, and at the end of the study. Patients were treated for a mean of 47.2 days, and dressings were left in place for an average of 2.2 days before being changed. By the end of treatment, 32% of the ulcers had completely or almost healed, and a further 27% showed evidence of granulation. Application was considered easy in 98% of instances, and 91% of the patients reported that Allevyn Heel was comfortable to wear.

The Allevyn Cavity Wound Dressing was first described by Cutting and Harding in 1990,[87] who described the practical application of the dressing in a small number of wounds. This dressing was later was compared with a calcium/sodium alginate dressing, Kaltostat, in the treatment of twenty patients following excision of pilonidal excision wounds.[88] Patients were randomized to receive the cavity wound dressing, followed by a standard piece of Allevyn when the wound was sufficiently reduced in depth, or alginate packing followed by Lyofoam as the wound progressed towards healing. The mean time to heal in the two groups was 56.7 days (range 36 - 78 days) and 65.5 days (range 43 - 106 days) for the foam and alginate dressings respectively. This difference was not statistically significant.

Biopsy were taken weekly from each wound which showed a normal healing profile in the foam-treated wounds, but in the alginate treated wounds fibres were found to have become incorporated in the tissue and these were surrounded by a giant cell foreign body reaction, although these fibres disappeared over time. Although patients' diary records appeared to indicate that the alginate dressing was easier to use, this difference was not statistically significant, leading the authors to conclude that both dressings are equally suitable for this particular indication.

Sometime dressings are used with no expectation of achieving wound closure. Young[89] described how Allevyn Adhesive was used to cover a severe meningocele in a terminally ill infant and, by so doing, enabled the parents' focus of care to be diverted away from the problems of the wound during the baby's short life.

Within the wound care community, there exists an interest in tissue engineering of skin and the use of cultured cells to promote healing, although this technique has yet to be generally adopted. The success of such treatments is influenced significantly by the techniques and materials used to apply and maintain these cultured cells on the recipient site. The choice of wound dressing is particularly important as the cultured cells may be poorly attached initially and thus easily disrupted by adherent dressings. This issue was addressed by Price *et al.,*[90] who used a porcine acute wound chamber model in a prospective randomized trial to compare four different wound dressings with reference to the amount of epidermal cover gained and the histological quality of the regenerated skin after three weeks. Of the four materials evaluated, polyurethane foam (Allevyn) was superior histologically, although equal in take rate with paraffin gauze, whilst a polyurethane sheet (Opsite) and silicone sheet were found to be substantially inferior.

Allevyn Thin (then called Cutinova Thin) and dry gauze were compared in a randomized, controlled trial on 60 patients with acute facial lacerations.[91] The wounds were assessed clinically and microbiologically prior to closure, then after 5, 28 and 56 days. Each dressing, which was removed at day 5, was sent for microbiological culture and total of 518 isolates were recovered from the patients during the study. A similar range of microorganisms were obtained from both treatment groups with no clear difference in organism colonization. Wounds treated with the polyurethane dressing showed improved comfort and contour (p < 0.04), less erythema (p < 0.03) and less potential for scarring (p < 0.01) at day 5.

At day 28 and day 56, however, there were no significant differences between the test and control groups. The authors concluded that although short-term clinical benefits could result from the use of occlusive dressings, these differences were not detectable in the long term and recommended that, in the management of acute wounds, studies of scarring should extend over at least three months post-injury to allow for spontaneous improvement to occur.

The ability of Cutinova Thin to reduce hypertrophic scarring was investigated by Schmidt et al.,[92] who compared the relative effectiveness of the treatment applied continuously, or for 12 hour periods (overnight). Evaluation of the hypertrophic scars was by clinical assessment and measurement of colour difference to normal skin, elevation and elasticity. After eight weeks no significant differences could be detected between the scars in both treatment groups.

The cost of treatment with Allevyn Thin was compared with that using traditional saline-soaked gauze in a 4-week, prospective, multicentre randomized clinical trial involving 36 patients with a Stage II pressure ulcer.[93] Participants were randomized to treatment with a foam (n = 20) or saline-soaked gauze dressing (n = 16). No difference in time to wound closure was observed (P = 0.817). Patients in the foam group had fewer frequent dressing changes (P <0.001). Total cost over the study period was lower by $466 per patient (P = 0.055) and spending on dressings was lower by $92 per patient in the foam group (P = 0.025). Cost per ulcer healed was lower by $1,517 and cost per ulcer-free day was lower by $80 for patients in the foam group. The authors concluded that based upon these findings the foam dressing represents is a more cost-effective treatment than saline-soaked gauze for the treatment of Stage II pressure ulcers.

A novel application for the use of Allevyn, was published by Bjellerup[94] who described how a dressing printed with the expression lines of a human face could be used to train dermatologists in minor facial surgery for the removal of tumours. The foam was said to have good skin-like qualities when incised, extended and sutured, and also possessed numerous other qualities which offered advantages over pigs' feet conventionally used for this purpose.

Most Allevyn references cited above relate to the original formulation of the dressing, not the version with the moisture reactive film backing layer introduced in 2006. White et al.[18] reported the results of the clinical in-market evaluation of this new preparation which took the form of an on-going multinational study with a target treatment population of 250 individuals. At the time of publication of the review 82 patients had been treated with various presentation of the new form of the dressing the performance of which equalled or exceeded that of the original, particularly in terms of absorbency and durability.

Young[95] also reported the results of an uncontrolled assessment of the new form of Allevyn which involved 113 patients 94% of whom expressed a favourable opinion of the dressing relative to their impressions of the original formulation.

Biatain

Biatain, introduced in 1998, is available in both a plain and adhesive form. An assessment of the non-adherent dressing the treatment of established foot ulcers in patients with diabetes, was made by Lohmann in an open non-comparative, prospective study.[96] Thirty five of 37 patients completed the treatment, during which time their ulcers more than halved in size, decreasing from an average of $5.4\,cm^2$ to $2.5\,cm^2$. 'Wearing comfort' improved throughout the study and maceration remained stable or improved. No device related adverse events were recorded. The authors concluded that Biatain Non-adhesive Dressing was safe and effective in the management of these wounds.

Meaume *et al.*[97] used Biatain as a standard treatment in a study designed to identify possible prognostic indicators of healing in a non-selected patient population with leg ulcers for whom compression was considered appropriate. The study took the form of a prospective observational survey involving 151 physicians and 330 ambulatory patients. Based upon previously published data, a reduction in the largest wound dimension $\geq 40\%$ was selected as an indicator of a favourable healing outcome, for this had previously been shown to be an appropriate predictor of complete healing in 12-24 weeks. At follow-up after three to six weeks, 19% of ulcers had healed and 54% reduced in length by 40% or more. Predictors for not achieving this outcome were the presence of lower limb arterial disease, ulcer duration of more than three months and an initial dimension of 10 cm or more. Linear regression showed that old age and a high body mass index were independent predictors of a poor outcome.

In 2006 a new formulation of Biatain was introduced called Biatain Soft Hold, which has a discontinuous weak adhesive layer that covers less than 50% of the foam surface designed to facilitate accurate application of the dressing whilst permitting easy pain-free removal. This new formulation was favourably reviewed by Vogensen.[98]

Biatain-Ibu

Wound-related pain is a commonly reported problem with some acute wounds, such as burns and donor sites, as well as chronic wounds such as leg ulcers. In 2006 Biatain-Ibu was introduced as a novel way of addressing this problem. The foam contains ibuprofen a widely used non-steroidal anti-inflammatory drug (NSAID) which is released from the dressing into the wound bed when it comes into contact with wound fluid.

The efficacy and safety of Biatain-Ibu was examined by Jorgensen *et al.*,[99] in a single-blinded crossover study in which the dressing was compared with the original unmedicated version. Pain and quality of life was measured using standard techniques. In addition to the usual fluid-handling assessments, blood plasma samples were drawn from each patient and examined for the presence of the drug. Use of Biatain-Ibu correlated with a decrease in pain intensity scores from seven in the run-in period to approximately 2.5 in the treatment phase. The healing rates achieved with Biatain-Ibu were similar to those achieved with the standard dressing and ulcer size was reduced by 24% during the treatment period. No side effects were noted, and no measureable levels of ibuprofen were detected in blood plasma.

Biatain-Ibu was compared with local best practice in an open block-randomized comparative study involving 24 patients with chronic, painful exuding leg ulcers conducted in a Canadian wound clinic.[100] Twelve patients were randomized to ibuprofen-foam and 12 patients to local best practice. Patients rated the intensity of their wound pain at baseline and after the first dressing application. The ibuprofen-foam dressing was shown to be associated with diminished chronic pain between dressing changes, reduced acute pain at dressing change, increased healthy granulation tissue, decreased periwound erythema and excellent exudate handling capacity.

Jorgensen et al.[101] in a second study combined Biatain-Ibu with an ionised silver-releasing wound contact layer, Physiotulle Ag, in the treatment of 24 patients with painful, infected non-healing venous leg ulcers. Persistent pain and pain at dressing change were monitored. The appearance of the wound bed, the dressings' combined ability to absorb exudate and minimise leakage, the ibuprofen content in the exudate, the reduction in wound area and the occurrence of adverse effects were also recorded. During the study, the score for persistent wound pain decreased from a mean of 6.3 ± 2.2 to 3.0 ± 1.7 after 12 hours and remained low thereafter. Pain at dressing change also decreased and remained low. Forty-eight hours after the first dressing application, the mean concentration of ibuprofen in the wound exudate reached a constant level of 35 ± 21 µg/ml. After 31 days, the relative wound area had reduced by 42%, with an associated decrease in fibrin and an increase in granulation tissue. The number of patients with malodorous wounds fell from 37% to 4%. No serious adverse events were reported. The authors concluded that the combined use of the two dressings reduced wound pain and promoted healing without compromising safety.

The release characteristics of ibuprofen from Biatain-Ibu were characterized by Steffansen and Herping who used two wound models which simulated both low and high exudate wounds and correlated these with in vivo studies.[102] They showed that in heavily exuding wounds the release of the drug appears to be controlled by ibuprofen diffusion from the dressing, but in lightly exuding wounds fluid absorption is the rate-limiting factor. They concluded that when assessing the performance of Biatain-Ibu and any other similarly medicated products, it is necessary to simulate both types of wounds during this process.

Several studies have compared the ibuprofen containing dressing with best practice. The first was a multinational, randomized, double-blind clinical trial involving 122 patients, 62 of whom were randomized to Biatain-Ibu and 60 to the non adhesive foam without ibuprofen.[103] Pain relief was significantly greater in the ibuprofen-foam group on days 1-5, with a rapid onset of action ($p < 0.05$). The patients in the ibuprofen-foam group had a significantly greater reduction in the persistent wound pain from baseline than patients treated with the comparator, 40% vs 30% ($p < 0.05$). Wound healing was similar in both groups. No difference in adverse events between placebo and local sustained release of low-dose ibuprofen was observed in this study.

The second study involved 185 patients.[104]The primary endpoint was pain relief over seven days of treatment assessed daily using a 5-point verbal rating scale. Secondary endpoints included a total reduction in pain intensity for the whole study period. Compared with controls, patients in the ibuprofen foam group reported greater wound pain relief and lower wound pain intensity values after seven days (p < 0.0001 for both variables). Statistically greater pain relief was achieved in all wound types, i.e. venous, mixed-arterial, arterial, and vasculitic ulcers. In all groups, patients in the ibuprofen foam group also experienced lower pain intensities and these results were statistically significant for venous and arterial leg ulcers.

A potentially important indication for a pain-relieving dressing is in the management of donor sites. Cigna *et al.*[105] described the results of a prospective study involving 40 patients undergoing surgery for any reconstructive purposes which involved the production of a split thickness donor site. The patients were randomized to treatment with either Biatain-Ibu foam dressing or a standard dressing. Pain experienced by the patients was recorded using a visual analogue scale. They were also required to answer questions on the nature of their pain and the way in which it affected their normal daily activities. The results indicated that compared to fine-mesh gauze, the use of Biatain-Ibu accelerated wound healing and almost eliminated pain and discomfort in all patients treated. It also reduced itching.

In the largest study yet reported,[106] 853 patients were randomized to either ibuprofen-releasing foam (n = 467) or local best practice (n = 386). Primary endpoint was wound pain relief from day 1-7, assessed by the patients twice daily using a five-point verbal rating scale. Secondary endpoints were reduction in pain intensity from day 0 to day 7, quality of life and effect on health-related activities of daily living, and the incidence of adverse events. After seven days, significantly more patients in the experimental group experienced relief from temporary and persistent pain and a reduction in pain intensity, when compared with patients in the local best practice group (p < 0.0001). Subjects also experienced a greater improvement in quality of life. The number of adverse events in both groups was low.

All of these studies strongly suggest that Biatain-IBU is both safe and efficacious for addressing wound related pain associated with a variety of common wound types.

Coraderm / Epi-Lock

Epi-Lock was evaluated by Wayne in 1985,[107] who compared it with a tulle dressing in the treatment of partial thickness burns, deep abrasions, and selected lacerations. Following a 200 patient study, he concluded that, in terms of quality and rate of healing, and the patient's perception of pain, Epi-Lock appeared to offer significant benefits over the tulle dressing for all wound types.

Epi-Lock was also compared with silver sulfadiazine cream, Silvadene, in a prospective, randomized, cross-over-controlled study in which 50 patients alternated changing antibiotic cream daily with leaving the polyurethane sheet in place for a week.[108] Overall, patient and physician preference for Epi-Lock was statistically significant, based on reduced pain, easier care, and faster healing, but the pooling of fluid beneath the polyurethane dressing and the requirement to leave the wound covered for a week were less well accepted. Nevertheless, the authors concluded that Epi-Lock represented a major advance in wound dressing materials and predicted that it would eventually gain wide application in outpatient treatment of partial thickness burns and abrasions. In fact, this proved not to be the case and Coraderm/Epi-Lock, like Synthaderm before it, was soon discontinued.

Cutinova

Cutinova was compared with Comfeel and Granuflex in the management of venous leg ulcers.[109] Patients that met the study trial criteria were randomized to receive one of the three primary dressings and secondarily bandaged with a short-stretch compression bandage. The dressings were compared in terms of their ability to promote ulcer healing and their effects on the prevalence and severity of ulcer-associated pain over a 12-week period. The ease with which dressings could be used in a busy outpatient clinic setting was also considered. The three dressings were found to be equally effective at promoting ulcer healing (55% - 59% healed in 12 weeks). Patients in all three groups similarly showed an equivalent decrease in ulcer-related pain scores during this time.

Epigard

Epigard is not a conventional dressing as it is used principally to provide short-term protection to large areas of exposed tissue prior to surgery and a number of early publications reported how it could be used to prepare a wound bed for grafting by promoting granulation and vascularization.[110-116]

In 1979 Spitalny[5] used the dressing to provide long term coverage to avoid bacterial contamination during holding periods and to prepare for regrafting in 32 patients undergoing plastic surgery, including the formation of cross-leg-flaps. The dressing was also used as a temporary covering following eyelid surgery,[117] and following surgical removal of skin tumours prior to grafting.[118] In both these applications its ability to produce a regular lawn of granulation and prevent contracture was noted.

In an animal study it was shown that granulation tissue was able to infiltrate evenly throughout the entire area of the dressing, right up to the underside of the outer surface. Epithelium was also able to spreads evenly throughout the foam leading the authors to conclude that Epigard is suitable for long-term covering of large wounds.[119] However, the ability of new tissue to grow freely into the dressing must also be considered to be a disadvantage in some circumstances. The manufacturer recommends that the dressing is changed daily. This is necessary because according to Borowka et al.,[120] if it is left in place for more than three days, removal causes disruption of wound healing, and after eight days the foam became so firmly bound that sharp dissection is usually required to remove it. For this reason Epigard has found little application as a dressing in routine wound management.

Flexzan

Scurr et al.[121] in a randomized controlled trial involving 20 patients with leg ulcers, compared Flexzan with Opsite as secondary dressings applied over an alginate dressing, Sorbsan. Compared to the film, the use of the foam significantly reduced the number of dressing changes required, 87 vs 192 (p =0.0038). This was explained by the enhanced permeability of the foam membrane which allowed exudate to evaporate through the exudate at a greater rate than was possible with the film.

Flexipore/Spyroflex

When 46 patients with abrasions, burns or scalds were treated with Flexipore 6000 over a four-month period, good wound healing was recorded in all cases and patient acceptability was high.[122] The dressing was also used in place of sutures or clips in the management of 25 patients undergoing elective surgery, 15 for hernia repair and ten for high saphenous ligation.[123] All wounds healed normally with excellent cosmetic results. Nursing time was reduced as a result of the use of the dressing and patients' satisfaction was good, leading the authors to suggest that the foam membrane was 'a cost effective, patient favoured and cosmetically satisfactory alternative closure and dressing method for clean surgical wounds'.

Lyofoam

Lyofoam, was first evaluated by Winter,[124] who compared the healing rates of shallow cutaneous wounds in pigs dressed with the foam with those of similar wounds dressed with cotton gauze. After four days, wounds covered with the foam were almost completely healed, which the formation of a new uniform epithelial layer whilst those dressed with gauze were only 56% healed (see Figure 50).

An early account of the successful use of Lyofoam dressings in the management of ten patients with surgical wounds and burns was presented in a surgical conference in Padua in 1977.[125] The authors claimed that the use of the foam provided superior healing to the use of cotton gauze products previously employed. In the same year, Davenport et al.[126] compared Lyofoam with paraffin gauze on adjacent halves of split skin donor sites in 31 patients. No significant differences were noted in healing rates or pain but healed Lyofoam dressed wounds initially appeared smoother and less flaky than those dressed with paraffin gauze. The principal difference between the two treatments was cost, Lyofoam treatment was found to be approximately one third of that of paraffin gauze at £0.31p vs £0.89p.

Salisbury[127] compared Lyofoam with Xeroform, Telfa, scarlet red and fine mesh gauze in partial thickness wounds in pigs. Accelerated healing did not appear to result from the use of Lyofoam dressing; in fact there was evidence that wounds treated with scarlet red healed the fastest. During a subsequent clinical evaluation, Lyofoam separated earlier from the underlying wounds but there was no evidence to suggest that the wounds were more mature than those covered with fine-mesh gauze.

In 1985 Creevy provided an early account of the use of Lyofoam in the management of four patients with leg ulcers, claiming that the application of the dressing appeared to reduce wound pain.[128] A more detailed account of the use of Lyofoam for this condition was provided by Mayerhausen and Kreis.[129] When 30 patients were treated for a six-week period five patients healed and 21 others were considered to have made moderate to good progress. Two patients failed to respond favourably to treatment and four were withdrawn because of pain, intolerance or deterioration. The authors concluded that Lyofoam accompanied by compression produced very promising results in the treatment of leg ulcers but the uncontrolled nature of these studies seriously limited their value.

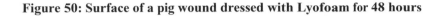

Figure 50: Surface of a pig wound dressed with Lyofoam for 48 hours

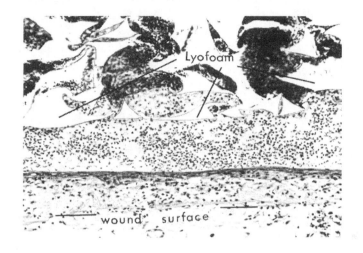

Note continuous layer of epidermis formed beneath the dressing and compare with Melolin results shown in Chapter 8.[8]

In 1989 a prospective comparative study was undertaken in which Lyofoam was compared with a simple low-adherent perforated plastic film dressing, Melolin, in 200 community patients with superficial granulating wounds less than five millimetres deep.[130] Lyofoam dressings were found to be significantly less painful in use, and less likely to adhere to the surface of the wound than the perforated plastic film dressing. Financial benefits also resulted from the use of the foam, as savings could be demonstrated in both materials and staffing costs.

In a well designed study involving 43 evaluable patients with venous leg ulcers, Pessenhofer and Stangl[131] convincingly demonstrated that the foam was far more effective at promoting healing than the conventional therapy in use at that time.

The highly permeable nature of Lyofoam suggests that it might be of value in the treatment of hypergranulation tissue, the formation of which is sometimes associated with the use of occlusive products such as hydrocolloid dressings. This possibility was investigated in a prospective uncontrolled study involving ten patients with 12 wounds over a two week period. The use of the foam resulted in a significant decrease,

---

[8] Reproduced from Winter 1975 with permission

(p < 0.01), in the height of the exuberant growth of two millimetres compared with initial measurements.[132]

Further papers which describe the use of Lyofoam in a variety of wound types have also been published.[133-137] When Banks compared Lyofoam A with N-A Dressing and Tegaderm in a small study involving 50 patients with Grade II or Grade III pressure ulcers,[138] the large withdrawal rate (nine patients) and the absence of a structured analysis of the resultant healing rates meant that the results were of limited value. The authors concluded that the study showed no statistical significance between the two treatment groups but a review of the data showed that after one week four patients dressed with Lyofoam had healed compared with 11 dressed with NA and Tegaderm. By two weeks this ratio had changed to 7 and 12. These results appear to suggest considerably faster healing in wounds in the control group but this possibility was not tested for significance in the publication.

In a randomized controlled trial of 56 patients with moderate to heavily exuding leg ulcers, Lyofoam Extra and Sorbsan were compared with particular attention to key parameters such absorbency, safety, condition of the wound and surrounding skin, and ease of use.[139] Little difference was detected in absorbency between the two dressings but Lyofoam Extra was considered superior to Sorbsan as there was fewer episodes of wound adherence, reduced wound odour and reduced leakage.

A novel application for Lyofoam was described in which it was used as a substrate for training junior hospital doctors the art of suturing.[140]

Mepilex

A 10-year-old boy with epidermolysis bullosa experienced a problem passing urine caused by blisters and erosions on the urethral meatus. He was advised to apply Mepilex after each micturition and leave it *in situ* until the next episode of micturition.[141] By following this simple procedure, he successfully prevented recurrence of the problem.

Permafoam

The use of Permafoam was evaluated in an open, multicentre observational study lasting a maximum of eight weeks which involved 53 patients with 56 moderate to heavily exuding wounds: 26 pressure ulcers, 11 venous ulcers, ten ulcers of mixed aetiology, and nine miscellaneous wounds. The average duration of the wounds prior to treatment was 270 days (median 85 days). During the treatment period, complete healing occurred in 21 wounds (37.5%), and the mean reduction in area was 61.31%[142]

Permafoam cavity dressing was assessed in a similar manner in a multicentre non-comparative study involving 47 patients with a variety of wound types.[143] Wounds were treated for an average of nine days during which time there was a marked reduction in the amount of slough and necrotic tissue present and a corresponding increase in granulation tissue. Use of the foam was also said to result in reduced wound-related pain and an improvement in the condition of periwound skin. Despite these positive outcomes, once again the lack of a control group limited the value of both of these studies.

Polymem

Polymem island dressing was assessed over a period of 70 days in an open uncontrolled study involving 18 lesions on 13 elderly subjects with Grade 1, Grade II or Grade III pressure ulcers.[144] Prior to commencement of treatment with Polymem, the mean length of time the ulcers had been present was 144 days with 50% of the ulcers (n = 9) present for 75 days or longer. During the treatment period over 60% of the wounds healed and all but one were considered to have improved. In the absence of a control group the authors compared these healing rates with published historical data and concluded that they were superior for all grades of ulcer treated.

Fowler and Papen[145] also undertook an early assessment of Polymem dressings in an open uncontrolled study involving a total of 31 patients with 41 partial or full thickness wounds of all types, irrespective of aetiology. Twelve subjects were outpatients, and 19 residents in a healthcare facility. Twenty-four of the patients recruited completed the study. The aim of the investigation was to collect data on the wound cleansing properties of the dressing and its effect upon the condition of the wound bed and the periwound skin, and monitor progress toward healing using standard data collection forms. Patients were followed for a maximum of 120 days during which time the wounds of 19 resolved completely, ten showed significant improvement and two showed minimal improvement. The dressing was found to promote debridement and the production of granulation tissue, and prevent maceration of the surrounding skin.

In a third, more formal study,[146] 19 subjects with foot ulcers associated with diabetes of greater than 20 weeks duration, and which were free of hard eschar, were randomly assigned to treatment with Polymem island dressing or to wet-to-dry saline gauze. At the end of two months, on average, the wounds of all the patients in this treatment group were reduced to $35 \pm 16\%$ of their size on admission to the study. In contrast conventionally-treated wounds were, on average, slightly larger at the end of the study, $105 \pm 28\%$ ($p < 0.03$).

When five subjects who failed to respond to treatment with wet-to-dry saline were crossed over to Polymem treatment after two months, their wounds also decreased in size to $35 \pm 11\%$ of their baseline values ($p < 0.02$) in the following two months.

Spyrosorb

Banks *et al.* compared Spyrosorb with a hydrocolloid dressing, Granuflex E, in the treatment of Grade II or Grade III pressure ulcers in two small studies. The first involved 29 hospital patients,[147] the second 40 patients in a community environment.[148] No statistically significant differences were detected in healing rates, but in the community study in particular there was a marked trend in favour of the foam, (18 *vs* 10 patients healed or improved in the foam and hydrocolloid groups respectively). In both studies, compared with the hydrocolloid, Spyrosorb was found to be significantly easier to remove ($p < 0.005$) and also caused less pain at dressing changes ($p < 0.005$) A trend was also detected in both studies for the hydrocolloid to leak or become detached more readily than the foam.

Suprasorb P

Andriessen et al.[149] compared Suprasorb P either used alone or applied over Suprasorb C, a collagen sponge primary dressing in the treatment of patients with non-healing venous ulcers. Paraffin gauze dressings were used as controls. All patients wore short-stretch high compression bandages. Ulcers were monitored to measure the effects of the various treatments on the microcirculation using $TcPO_2$ measurements and video laser Doppler measurements. A reduction in ulcer area and the formation of granulation tissue were taken as indicators of healing. Over a four week period significant increases in $TcPO_2$ values were recorded between baseline values for patients receiving the foam dressing only ($p < 0.008$) or the collagen plus foam dressing combination ($p < 0.003$). There was also a significant increase in the number of capillaries for the collagen plus foam treatment only ($p < 0.002$). The authors concluded that the moist wound environment provided by the foam stimulates perfusion of blood and oxygen to the wound tissue, thereby promoting angiogenesis. Still further improvements were obtained by the inclusion of the collagen matrix as the primary dressing.

Synthaderm

Early anecdotal accounts of the use of the now discontinued Synthaderm were presented in a conference in Finland in 1980.[150-152] These were followed by a published account of a formal trial involving 52 patients with pre-tibial lacerations in which the authors suggested that wounds dressed with Synthaderm healed more rapidly, and with reduced scarring, that those dressed conventionally.[153]

Synthaderm was subsequently compared with paraffin gauze in the treatment of 71 patients with leg ulcers in a controlled study reported by Banerjee et al.[154] Healing rates and the requirement for nursing involvement both favoured the paraffin gauze treatment and the authors concluded that the results showed little advantage to the use of Synthaderm for this indication. They also commented upon the poor standing of bandaging sometimes encountered during this study would could have adversely affected healing in both treatment groups.

Tegaderm Foam

Charles et al.[155] commented favourably upon Tegaderm Foam following an uncontrolled study involving six patients with leg or pressure ulcers.

Tielle

An early report of the use of Tielle was provided by Williams who described its use in a diabetic patient with a longstanding superficial venous leg ulcer. The wound healed uneventfully and the dressing appeared to perform well.[156]

In an early randomized controlled study the dressing was compared with Duoderm E in the treatment of 68 patients with 71 leg ulcers of varying aetiology.[157] Following randomisation 39 wounds were dressed with Tielle and 32 with the hydrocolloid; compression therapy was provided as appropriate. The principal parameters monitored during the investigation included ease of application and removal, wound condition and odour production. Healing rates were not compared, although changes in ulcer size were recorded. Statistically significant differences between the treatments in favour of Tielle were recorded for all subjective parameters ($p \geq 0.05$). Furthermore the condition of 74% of wounds dressed with Tielle was judged to have improved compared with 50% of those dressed with the hydrocolloid.

A more formal assessment of Tielle was made in a randomized controlled study in which the dressing was compared with Granuflex in the treatment of 100 patients with leg ulcers and 99 patients with pressure ulcers.[158] Both dressings were well received by patients and no statistically significant differences were recorded in healing rates of patients with leg ulcers, but 44/49 (90%) of pressure ulcers dressed with the foam reduced in area compared with 34/47 (72%) dressed with the hydrocolloid ($p = 0.028$). Statistically significant differences were also noted in favour of Tielle in terms of odour production and exudate leakage. The latter probably reflects the superior fluid handling properties of the foam.

The potential value of Tielle dressings for the treatment of chronic exuding wounds in primary care was investigated in three multicentre, open label, single arm, observational Phase IV studies undertaken in Germany as part of the normal regulatory process.[159] A total of 6,993 patients with pressure sores (26.6%), venous leg ulcers (59.8%), diabetic foot disease (9.5%) and other wounds (5.1%) were enrolled for a period of either four or twelve weeks. Within the four week study 43.3% of the wounds healed and 51.6% improved and wound area was reduced by 78.2%. In the twelve week study 59.1% of wounds healed and a further 36.9% improved in which the area was reduced by 85.1%. Exudate production was greatly reduced and as a result the frequency of dressing changes was reduced from five to three per week. Cosmetic outcomes were judged to be excellent or good in 96.3% of patients. Compared with previous treatments, efficacy and tolerability were assessed as 'better' or 'much better' in 92.5% and 70.4% of instances respectively and adverse events occurred in less than 3% of patients. The authors concluded that Tielle provides an effective and safe dressing in the management of chronic exuding wounds in primary care improving patient's comfort.

In a second German post-marketing study, the efficacy and safety of Tielle Plus was similarly assessed by 624 physicians in the treatment of 2121 patients with a variety of wound types which included: leg ulcers (59.1%), pressure ulcers (20.7%), diabetic foot ulcers (10.9%) or other chronic wounds (9.4%).[160] All wounds had been present for at least four weeks prior to treatment and many had been treated with other dressings previously. Within the 12 week observational period 43% of the wounds healed and 50.4% were considered as 'improved'. The frequency of side-effects was low at 4.8%. Over 90% of patients rated Tielle as 'much better' or 'better tolerated' than the previous treatment regime, and for the large majority of patients the quality of life was also judged to have improved. On the basis of the positive experiences with respect to effectiveness, safety and handling, 96.8% of the participating doctors indicated that they wished to continue to use Tielle Plus in their practice.

Tielle Plus was formally compared with an alginate dressing, Kaltostat, in a multicentre trial of 113 patients with exuding venous leg ulcers.[161] Wounds were stratified according to the degree of exudate production then randomized to treatment. Originally the trial protocol dictated that the alginate dressing be covered with a semipermeable film dressing, but following numerous problems with skin reactions the protocol was amended to include the use of nonwoven swabs instead. For this reason data were analysed in three treatment groups: Tielle Plus, alginate plus film, and alginate plus swabs (n = 54, 22, and 37 respectively). Within the three respective groups, six wounds healed (2, 3, 1), 41 remained unhealed after for weeks (25, 7, 9), 25 withdrew as exudate levels decreased (10, 1, 14) and 41 withdrew for other reasons including adverse events (17, 11, 13). Adverse events such as maceration erythema and infection were encountered in 20%, 45%, and 19% of the three groups respectively. This difference in the incidence of maceration could perhaps have been predicted from the differences in the fluid handling properties of the three dressings systems. A statistically significant difference between treatment groups was observed in mean wear time, 3.91 days for Tielle Plus compared with 3.09 days for the alginate treated wounds (p = 0.001). This difference was said to have implications for overall treatment costs which also marginally favoured Tielle Plus. Patient and user acceptability markedly favoured Tielle Plus. The principal criticism of this study is that it took no account of healing rates. It could be argued, for example, that despite the practical problems of maceration, healing rates appeared greater in the alginate plus film group, and had the study continued longer it is possible that more of the patients treated in this way would have healed which would have had a marked influence on outcomes - including treatment costs.

The fluid handling properties of Tielle Plus were utilised in the treatment of a large fungating breast wound for which indication it was found to be both clinically and cost effective, easy to use, and comfortable to wear, even under clothing.[162]

The performance of Tielle Lite, the member of the Tielle family intended for lightly exuding wounds was investigated in a multi-centre non-comparative clinical trial of four weeks' duration involving 74 patients with 75 wounds. Particular attention was given to the possibility that the dressing would cause problems of adherence, leading to pain or minor trauma upon removal from wounds in the final stages of healing. Fifty eight patient completed the study and 40 of the original 75 wounds healed during the four weeks A total of 244 wound assessments were made and in only four (1.6%) of these were problems of adherence noted. During the study 82% of patients described changes as painless and 10% reported minimal pain.[163]

Comparisons of foam dressings

Different types of foam dressings have been compared in numerous publications which are summarized below.

Allevyn vs Lyofoam Extra

Banks et al.[164] carried out an early assessment of Lyofoam Extra by comparing it with Allevyn in a prospective, stratified, randomized trial involving 61 patients with leg ulcers, pressure ulcers or other lesions grouped according to wound type. The condition of each wound and surrounding skin, comfort, ease of use, and the presence of leakage from the dressing were monitored at each dressing change. Treatment continued for six weeks or until the wound had become 'lightly exuding', arbitrarily defined as absence of leakage when the dressing remained in place for more than four days on two consecutive occasions. The two dressings were found to be similar in performance in that they could remain in place for approximately 2.5 days, irrespective of wound type. There were no statistically significant differences in surrounding skin condition, reduction in wound size, patient comfort or ease of application and removal.

Allevyn vs Biatain

Allevyn and Biatain were compared in a multicentre randomized control trial involving 118 patients with venous leg ulcers with dimensions less than 9×9 cm which were judged to be moderately or heavily exuding.[165] The use of secondary dressings, compression systems, and periulcer skin treatments were determined by the investigator.

Patients and their wounds were assessed every seven days until the ulcer was completely healed or eight weeks of treatment were completed. Dressings were changed once every seven days if leakage of exudate occurred or when an interim assessment was deemed necessary. Ulcer area was determined by tracing and planimetry, and the proportion of black, yellow and granulating tissue was also estimated. Estimates were made of dressing absorbency, periulcer skin condition, odour and pain using appropriate descriptors.

Of the 118 patients recruited, 99 completed the study. The number of wounds that healed in the two treatment groups was identical (39%). Additionally, 41/53 ulcers in the Biatain group and 30/46 ulcers in the Allevyn group (77% and 65%), respectively were covered with healthy granulating tissue by the end of the study period. This difference was not significant.

Statistically significant differences were detected between the products in terms of their fluid handling ability. Absorbency was rated as excellent during 124/163 (76%) Biatain dressing changes, compared with 12/170 (7%) of the Allevyn dressing changes. This difference was supported by the presence of leakage at weekly assessment (64% *vs* 48% respectively), and the requirement to use a secondary absorbent layer (72% *vs* 43% respectively). As a consequence of this difference in absorption, statistically fewer dressing changes per week were required in wounds dressed with Biatain 2.14 *vs* 3.34 which resulted in lower in treatment costs, $10.87 *vs* $18.99, in favour of the Biatain.

Allevyn vs Mepilex

Allevyn and Mepilex were compared in the treatment of venous leg ulcers in a multicenter prospective randomized clinical trial.[166] Patients were also randomized to compression therapy using either a 4-layer bandage system or a short stretch cohesive bandage in a factorial design. A total of 156 patients from 12 clinical centres were randomized to treatment, stratified according to ulcer size (greater or less than 10 cm^2). Initial ulcer size median (range) was 4.33 cm^2 (0.33 - 123.0). After 24 weeks 100 (64.1%) of ulcers had closed and nine wounds (5.8%) remained unhealed. One patient died and 46 (29.5%) withdrew from the trial.

Of the patients randomized to Mepilex, 50/75 (66.7%) achieved complete ulcer healing compared with 50/81 (61.7%) treated with Allevyn. Withdrawal rates were similar between the Allevyn and Mepilex treated groups, 28.4% *vs* 30.7% respectively. Pain improved following treatment with both dressings (p<0.001), but with no difference between dressings. No statistical difference was detected between the treatment groups in terms of wound healing.

Whilst adhesive dressings offer clear advantages over non-adhesive versions in terms of preventing exudate leakage, there exists the risk that removal of an adhesive material might, in some circumstances, cause damage to the *stratum corneum*. This possibility was investigated by Dykes and others in a series of publications in which they reviewed superficial skin damaged following repeated application and removal of different types of dressings.

Allevyn Adhesive, Mepilex Border, Tielle, Biatain, Comfeel, Duoderm

These publications, which have been reviewed previously in the chapter on low adherent dressings, suggested that the products examined tended to fall into two distinct groups, Allevyn, Mepilex Border and Tielle in one group, and Biatain, Comfeel and Duoderm in the other. As previously described, the authors concluded that the degree of discomfort experienced by subjects on removal of an adhesive dressing is not entirely dependent on the magnitude of the peel force and that other aspects of the interaction of the skin surface and adhesive play a role.

Allevyn Adhesive vs Mepilex Border

Viamontes and Jones[167] compared treatment outcomes with Mepilex Border and Allevyn in a retrospective review of data contained in a 'real time' outcomes database containing treatment details of nursing homes patients over a one year period in order to determine the incidence of skin stripping of periwound skin, wound healing rates and pain.

Data collected from 403 evaluable wounds in 206 patients was analysed. Evidence of skin stripping was detected following the use of both products, in 5% (5/106) patients dressed with Allevyn and 4% (4/100) in patients dressed with Mepilex Border. Closure rates achieved with the two dressings were similar. Independent nurse evaluations highlighted the failure of the self-adherent soft silicone foam dressing to either initially adhere to the wound area, or to remain in place for more than a few days; the dressing frequently needed the application of additional tape to ensure adhesion. They reported that the failure of the self-adhesive soft silicone foam dressing to adhere effectively to the periwound area was a significant disadvantage and a disincentive to use this type of dressing routinely.

A second study,[168] used the same methodology to review clinical data collected over a 5-year period (1997-2002) involving 1,891 residents and 4,200 wounds in 30 nursing homes in the state of Florida treated with the products in question. The data collection period was chosen to capture a change in wound dressing regimens in these nursing homes which occurred in 2001. As before, patient demographic and wound assessment variables, including evidence of surrounding skin stripping, were abstracted from the database.

Of the 4200 relevant wounds, 3795 (90%) were treated with Allevyn Adhesive, 352 (8%) with Mepilex Border and 53 (1%) were treated with both dressings at some points. Of the 3,795 wound treated with the Allevyn Adhesive, 3,579 (94%) were pressure ulcers (mainly Grade II or III), as were 339 of 352 wounds dressed with Mepilex Border and 51 wounds managed with both dressings. Wounds in the Allevyn group were larger (7.53 cm^2 *vs* 5.5 cm^2), and took longer to heal than those in the Mepilex group (70.1 days *vs* 39.2 days), but the proportion of ulcers that healed, 63%, was the same in both groups. Skin stripping was rare with either dressing, occurring in less than 1% of wounds. As in the previous study it was reported that the dressings using soft silicone technology tended to adhere less well, requiring the use of tape to retain the dressing firmly in place. Problems with infection occurred more frequently in the Mepilex Border group (9%) than in the Allevyn Adhesive group (3%). The authors, whilst acknowledging the limitations of retrospective studies, once again concluded that periwound skin stripping is uncommon and that differences between the two products are minimal.

Allevyn Adhesive vs Biatain Adhesive

Allevyn Adhesive and Biatain Adhesive were compared in a prospective multicentre study involving 32 patients with a Grade II or III pressure ulcers.[169] The principal aim of the study was to assess dressing delamination and the effect of residue remaining in the ulcer following foam breakdown. The performance of the dressings was assessed over seven dressing changes or a maximum of six weeks. The primary efficacy variable was the proportion of patients with at least one delaminated dressing, delamination being defined as the falling apart of a dressing during wear or removal, or the presence of residue from the dressing in the ulcer.

Allevyn Adhesive was found to be significantly less likely to delaminate than Biatain Adhesive, for of those patients dressed with Biatain Adhesive, 83% had a dressing that delaminated compared with 14% for those dressed with Allevyn Adhesive (p = 0.014). Furthermore, a greater proportion of the Biatain Adhesive dressings delaminated compared with the Allevyn Adhesive dressings: 50% *vs* 4% (p < 0.001). Allevyn Adhesive also performed significantly better in terms of handling, comfort, ease of application and removal, adherence to the skin during application and prior to removal. Three patients dressed with Allevyn Adhesive (21%) reported three adverse events compared with six patients with Biatain Adhesive (33%) who reported eight adverse events. The authors concluded that Allevyn Adhesive is well tolerated in the management of pressure ulcers and less likely to delaminate than Biatain Adhesive.

Allevyn Cavity Wound *vs* Silastic Foam

Allevyn Cavity Wound Dressing and Silastic Foam were compared in 80 patients who attended a specialized wound clinic with a cavity wound following abdominal surgery or surgical removal of a pilonidal sinus.[170]

Wound assessments were made on 111 occasions with the Allevyn in the clinic and on 693 occasions by the patient at home. The corresponding figures for Silastic Foam were 166 and 871 respectively. The results of the assessments showed little difference between the two dressings. Hospital staff considered that the Silastic Foam was the easier dressing to use but patients expressed an opposite view. Wounds managed with Silastic Foam took on average nine days longer to heal but this difference was not significant. Exudate management was better with Silastic Foam, 84% of patients reporting no, or only slight, discharge compared with 75% for Allevyn. Overall the results of this study support the proposition that the Allevyn Cavity Wound Dressing is comparable with Silastic Foam for most parameters and may offer some advantages in terms of its ease of use by patients.

Allevyn Cavity Wound, Granuflex Paste, Kaltostat, Sorbsan

Allevyn Cavity Wound Dressing was one of four dressings which were evaluated in the treatment of Grade IV pressure ulcers 1 - 4 cm deep, reported by Johnson.[171] The others were: Granuflex Paste covered with a Granuflex wafer, Kaltostat and Sorbsan.

Ten patients were allocated to each treatment group and all patients healed in an average of 44 days. Dressings were changed as required and a record was maintained of both the number of changes, the materials used as secondary dressings as well as ancillary materials used during the changing procedure. From this information the daily treatment costs for each product were calculated together with a figure for the average cost to achieve closure with each product. They were: £40.44 for Allevyn Cavity Wound Dressing, £44.17 for Granuflex, £45.69 for Kaltostat and £81.81 for Sorbsan.

The use of Allevyn Cavity Wound Dressing in a pressure sore was also described by Todd.[172]

REFERENCES

1. Muller WE, Batel R, Schroder HC, Muller IM. Traditional and Modern Biomedical Prospecting: Part I-the History: Sustainable Exploitation of Biodiversity (Sponges and Invertebrates) in the Adriatic Sea in Rovinj (Croatia). *Evid Based Complement Alternat Med* 2004;1(1):71-82.
2. Elliott IMZ. *A Short History of Surgical Dressings*. London: The Pharmaceutical Press, 1964.
3. Maylard AE. I. Sponges and Their Use in Surgery. *Ann Surg* 1891;13(5):321-32.
4. Gamgee S. A new sponge. *Lancet* 1884;1:795-796.
5. Spitalny HH, Lemperle G. Utilization of a synthetic skin substitute instead of split skin in cross-leg-flap and other pedicle flap grafting. *Fortschr Med* 1979;97(20):969-72.
6. Cook GB, Margulis AR. Silicone Enema Diagnostic Technique. *CA Cancer J Clin* 1963;13:11-16.
7. Thomas E, Hall BW, Bassan S. Silastic foam dressing - an evaluation of the disinfection procedure. *Br. J. pharm. Pract.* 1983;5:Dec-13.
8. Evans BK, Harding KG, Marks J, Ribeiro CD. The disinfection of silicone-foam dressings. *J. clin. Hosp. Pharm.* 1985;10:289-295.
9. Ritter EJ, Scott WJ, Randall JL, Ritter JM. Teratogenicity of di(2-ethylhexyl)phthalate, ethylhexanol, 2-ethylhexanoic acid, and valproic acid, and potentiation by caffeine. *Teratology* 1987;35:41-46.
10. Cooper R, Bale S, Harding KG. An improved cleansing regime for a modified foam cavity dressing. *Journal of Wound Care* 1995;4(1):13-6.
11. Winter GD. Methods for the biological evaluation of dressings. In: Turner TD, Brain KR, editors. *Surgical dressings in the hospital environment*. Cardiff: Surgical Dressings Research Unit, UWIST, Cardiff, 1975:47-81.

12. Thomas S. The role of foam dressings in wound management. In: Turner TD, Schmidt RJ, Harding KG, editors. *Advances in Wound Care*. Cardiff: John Wiley, 1985:23-29.

13. Thomas S. Foam dressings. *Journal of Wound Care* 1993;2(3):153-156.

14. Williams C. Spyrosorb and Spyroflex. *Br J Nurs* 1994;3(12):628-30.

15. Rodeheaver G. Controversies in topical wound management. *Ostomy and Wound Management* 1989;1(1):19-27.

16. Beitz AJ, Newman A, Kahn AR, Ruggles T, Eikmeier L. A polymeric membrane dressing with antinociceptive properties: analysis with a rodent model of stab wound secondary hyperalgesia. *J Pain* 2004;5(1):38-47.

17. Carter K. Hydropolymer dressings in the management of wound exudate. *Br J Community Nurs* 2003;8(9 Suppl):suppl 10-6.

18. White R, Hartwell S, Brown S. Interim report on a study to assess the effectiveness and improved fluid uptake of new Allevyn. *Wounds UK* 2007;3(4).

19. Painter S. Comparison of the fluid handling capabilities of absorbent adhesive dressings Smith and Nephew Wound Management 2006:1-6.

20. Painter S. Comparison of the fluid handling capabilities of absorbent non-adhesive dressings Smith and Nephew Wound Management 2006:1-6.

21. Thomas S, Young S. Exudate-handling mechanisms of two foam-film dressings. *Journal of Wound Care* 2008;17(7):309-315.

22. Young S, Bielby A, Milne J. Use of ultrasound to characterise the fluid-handling characteristics of four foam dressings. *J Wound Care* 2007;16(10):425-8, 430-1.

23. Ameen H, Moore K, Lawrence JC, Harding KG. Investigating the bacterial barrier properties of four contemporary wound dressings. *Journal of Wound Care* 2000;9(8):385-388.

24. Harvey RE. Clinical trials versus laboratory studies. *Journal of Wound Care* 2000;9(9):414.

25. Wood RA, Hughes LE. Silicone foam sponge for pilonidal sinus: a new technique for dressing open granulating wounds. *Br Med J* 1975;4(5989):131-3.

26. Wood RAB, Williams RHP, Hughes LE. Foam elastomer dressing in the management of open granulating wounds: experience with 250 patients. *Br. J. Surg.* 1977;64(8):554-557.

27. Macfie J, Cowell M, Pawsey G, Bancroft J, McMahon M. Foam elastomer dressing: a liquid alternative to gauze. *Nurs Mirror* 1979;149(5):30-2.

28. Macfie J, McMahon MJ. The management of the open perineal wound using a foam elastomer dressing: a prospective clinical trial. *Br J Surg* 1980;67(2):85-9.

29. Culyer AJ, MacFie J, Wagstaff A. Cost-effectiveness of foam elastomer and gauze dressings in the management of open perineal wounds. *Soc Sci Med* 1983;17(15):1047-53.

30. Williams RH, Wood RA, Mason MC, Edwards M, Goodall P. Multicentre prospective trial of Silastic foam dressing in management of open granulating wounds. *Br Med J (Clin Res Ed)* 1981;282(6257):21-2.

31. Young HL, Wheeler MH. Report of a prospective trial of dextranomer beads (Debrisan) and silicone foam elastomer (Silastic) dressings in surgical wounds. *Br J Surg* 1982;69(1):33-4.

32. Malone WD. Wound dressing adherence: a clinical comparative study. *Arch Emerg Med* 1987;4(2):101-5.

33. Streza GA, Laing BJ, Gilsdorf RB. Management of enterocutaneous fistulas and problem stomas with silicone casting of the abdominal wall defect. *Am. J. Surg.* 1977;134:772-776.

34. Smith RC, Flynn PW, Gillett DJ, Guinness MD, Levey JM. Treatment of granulating wounds with silastic foam dressings. *Aust N Z J Surg* 1981;51(4):354-7.

35. Gledhill T, Waterfall WE. Silastic Foam: a new material for dressing wounds. *Can Med Assoc J* 1983;128(6):685.

36. Balique JG, Espalieu P, Hugonnier G, Peyre C, Cuilleret J. A new concept of dressing: silastic foam. *J Chir (Paris)* 1984;121(11):685-9.

37. Frobel WJ, Kohnlein HE, Treusch J. Silicone rubber dressing in wound healing disorders. *Langenbecks Arch Chir* 1984;364:313-6.
38. Linke E, Kloss HP, Jung W. Wound management using a silicone foam dressing. Results of a multicenter study. *Fortschr Med* 1986;104(47-48):979-82.
39. Muller KH, Ekkernkamp A. Treatment of infected tissue defects--experiences with silicon foam dressings. *Unfallchirurg* 1986;89(3):101-16.
40. Stewart CP. Foam elastomer dressing in the management of a below-knee amputation stump with delayed healing. *Prosthet Orthot Int* 1985;9(3):157-9.
41. Morgan WP, Harding KG, Richardson G, Hughes LE. The use of silastic foam dressing in the treatment of advanced hidradenitis suppurativa. *Br J Surg* 1980;67(4):277-80.
42. Morgan WP, Harding KG, Hughes LE. A comparison of skin grafting and healing by granulation, following axillary excision for hidradenitis suppurativa. *Ann R Coll Surg Engl* 1983;65(4):235-6.
43. Miller L, Bale S. Surgical management of a patient with axillary hidradenitis. *Journal of Wound Care* 1993;2(1):16-20.
44. Cook PJ, Devlin HB. Boils, carbuncles and hidradenitis suppurativa. *Surgery* 1985;19:440-442.
45. Bandey SA, Atkins J, Neil WF. Silastic foam dressing in pinnaplasty. *J. Laryng. Otol.* 1986;100:201-202.
46. Ross JK, Matti B, Davies DM. A silastic foam dressing for the protection of the post-operative ear. *Br J Plast Surg* 1987;40(2):213-4.
47. Shukla HS. Silastic foam elastomer wound dressing in wound management. *Indian J Med Res* 1983;77:150-3.
48. Regnard CF, Meehan SE. The use of a silicone foam dressing in the management of malignant oral- cutaneous fistula. *Br J Clin Pract* 1982;36(6):243-5.
49. Deeg M, Maier H. Silastic foam: a new dressing in otorhinolaryngology. *Laryngol Rhinol Otol (Stuttg)* 1986;65(6):314-6.
50. Bale S, Harding K. Fungating breast wounds. *J. Distr. Nurs.* 1987;5:04-May.
51. Chambers PA, Worrall SF. Closure of large orocutaneous fistulas in end-stage malignant disease. *Br J Oral Maxillofac Surg* 1994;32(5):314-5.
52. Groves AR, Lawrence JC. Silastic foam dressing: an appraisal. *Ann. R. Coll. Surg.* 1985;67:116-118.
53. Watson SB, Miller JG. Optimizing skin graft take in children's hand burns--the use of silastic foam dressings. *Burns* 1993;19(6):519-21.
54. Benson MT, Gilmour H, Nelson ME, Rennie IG. Silastic foam dressing for healing exenteration cavities. *Ophthalmic Surg* 1990;21(12):849-51.
55. De Sy WA, Oosterlinck W. Silicone foam elastomer: a significant improvement in postoperative penile dressing. *J Urol* 1982;128(1):39-40.
56. Mattelaer JJ, Baert L, van Dorpe EJ. Silastic foam dressing--the ideal penile dressing. *Urology* 1983;22(1):68.
57. Aragona F, Artibani W, Milani C, Pegoraro V, Passerini Glazel G. Silicone foam dressing in the surgery of hypospadias. *Arch Esp Urol* 1984;37 Suppl 1:606-8.
58. Whitaker RH, Dennis MJ. Silastic foam dressing in hypospadias surgery. *Ann R Coll Surg Engl* 1987;69(2):59-60.
59. Mollard P. Penile dressings of C.M.H. silicone elastomer foam. *Chir Pediatr* 1984;25(2):117-9.
60. Zumbe J, Kierfeld G. Results of single-stage repair of distal hypospadias using the King modification. *Urologe A* 1988;27(4):246-9.

61. Weissbach L. Dressing technic with silastic foam following penis operations. *Urologe A* 1987;26(4):220-1.
62. Gaylis FD, Zaontz MR, Dalton D, Sugar EC, Maizels M. Silicone foam dressing for penis after reconstructive pediatric surgery. *Urology* 1989;33(4):296-9.
63. Guralnick ML, al-Shammari A, Williot PE, Leonard MP. Outcome of hypospadias repair using the tubularized, incised plate urethroplasty. *Can J Urol* 2000;7(2):986-91.
64. Malick MH, Carr JA. Flexible elastomer molds in burn scar control. *Am. J. occup. Ther.* 1980;34:603-608.
65. Harding KG, Richardson G, Hughes LE. Silastic foam dressing for skin graft Donor sites--a preliminary report. *Br J Plast Surg* 1980;33(4):418-21.
66. Brossy JJ. Foam elastomer dressings in surgery. *S Afr Med J* 1981;59(16):559-560.
67. Johnson SR, Jones DG. Silastic foam in injured patients. *Injury* 1988;19(2):121-3.
68. Davalbhakta A, Summerlad BC. Cavi-Care dressing for hypospadias repair [letter]. *Br J Plast Surg* 1999;52(4):325-6.
69. Staiano J, Richard B, Graham K. Pressure sore of the helical rim: a new problem, a novel treatment. *Plast Reconstr Surg* 2004;114(6):1655-7.
70. Chalmers RT, Turner AR. A silicone foam dressing used in treating an infected wound. *Journal of Wound Care* 1996;5(3):109-10.
71. Dillon CK, Iwuagwu F. Cavi-care dressings following syndactyly correction. *J Plast Reconstr Aesthet Surg* 2008.
72. Friederich HC. Wound coverage following dermabrasion. *Z Hautkr* 1988;63(10):853-7.
73. Weber RS, Hankins P, Limitone E, Callender D, Frankenthaler RM, Wolf P, et al. Split-thickness skin graft donor site management. A randomized prospective trial comparing a hydrophilic polyurethane absorbent foam dressing with a petrolatum gauze dressing. *Arch Otolaryngol Head Neck Surg* 1995;121(10):1145-9.
74. Martini L, Reali UM, Borgognoni L, Brandani P, Andriessen A. Comparison of two dressings in the management of partial-thickness donor sites. *Journal of Wound Care* 1999;8(9):457-60.
75. Reali UM, Martini L, Borgognoni L, Brandani P, Andriessen A. Advantages of an adhesive hydrocellular dressing in the treatment of partial-thickness skin graft donor sites *Annals of Burns and Fire Disasters* 2001;14 (1):18-21.
76. Innes ME, Umraw N, Fish JS, Gomez M, Cartotto RC. The use of silver coated dressings on donor site wounds: a prospective, controlled matched pair study. *Burns* 2001;27(6):621-7.
77. Argirova M, Hadjiski O, Victorova A. Acticoat versus Allevyn as a split-thickness skin graft donor-site dressing: a prospective comparative study. *Ann Plast Surg* 2007;59(4):415-22.
78. Bale S, Squires D, Varnon T, Walker A, Benbow M, Harding KG. A comparison of two dressings in pressure sore management. *Journal of Wound Care* 1997;6(10):463-6.
79. Vaingankar NV, Sylaidis P, Eagling V, King C, Elender F. Comparison of hydrocellular foam and calcium alginate in the healing and comfort of split-thickness skin-graft donor sites. *J Wound Care* 2001;10(7):289-91.
80. Atherton D, Sreetharan V, Mosahebi A, Prior S, Willis J, Bishop J, et al. A randomised controlled trial of a double layer of Allevyn compared to Jellonet and proflavin as a tie-over dressing for small skin grafts. *J Plast Reconstr Aesthet Surg* 2008;61(5):535-9.
81. Torra i Bou JE. [Clinical evaluation of a hydro-cellular dressing for the treatment of venous leg ulcers]. *Rev Enferm* 1999;22(7-8):531-6.
82. Verdu Soriano J, Nolasco Bonmati A, Lopez Casanova P, Torra i Bou JE. ["Auriga-04" study on the use of a range of Allevyn hydro-cellular dressings in the treatment of bed sores and leg ulcers by primary health care professionals]. *Rev Enferm* 2006;29(4):43-9.

83. Vanscheidt W, Sibbald RG, Eager CA. Comparing a foam composite to a hydrocellular foam dressing in the management of venous leg ulcers: a controlled clinical study. *Ostomy Wound Manage* 2004;50(11):42-55.
84. Abela C, Lucas N, McLeod I, Myers S. Protection of skin grafts to the penile shaft using a novel manipulation of Allevyn dressing--case report of an alkali burn. *Burns* 2006;32(7):925-6.
85. Torra i Bou JE, Rueda Lopez J, Camanes G, Herrero Narvaez E, Blanco Blanco J, Martinez-Esparza EH, et al. [Heel pressure ulcers. Comparative study between heel protective bandage and hydrocellular dressing with special form for the heel]. *Rev Enferm* 2002;25(5):50-6.
86. Kammerlander G, Eberlein T. Use of Allevyn heel in the management of heel ulcers. *Journal of Wound Care* 2003;12(8):313-5.
87. Cutting K, Harding K. Dressing cavities. *Nurs Times* 1990;86(50):62-4.
88. Berry DP, Bale S, Harding KG. Dressings for treating cavity wounds. *Journal of Wound Care* 1996;5(1):10-7.
89. Young T. Use of a hydrocellular adhesive dressing in a terminally ill baby. *Journal of Wound Care* 1997;6(6):264.
90. Price RD, Das-Gupta V, Frame JD, Navsaria HA. A study to evaluate primary dressings for the application of cultured keratinocytes. *Br J Plast Surg* 2001;54(8):687-96.
91. Thomas DW, Hill CM, Lewis MA, Stephens P, Walker R, Von Der Weth A. Randomized clinical trial of the effect of semi-occlusive dressings on the microflora and clinical outcome of acute facial wounds. *Wound Repair Regen* 2000;8(4):258-63.
92. Schmidt A, Gassmueller J, Hughes-Formella B, Bielfeldt S. Treating hypertrophic scars for 12 or 24 hours with a self-adhesive hydroactive polyurethane dressing. *J Wound Care* 2001;10(5):149-53.
93. Payne WG, Posnett J, Alvarez O, Brown-Etris M, Jameson G, Wolcott R, et al. A prospective, randomized clinical trial to assess the cost-effectiveness of a modern foam dressing versus a traditional saline gauze dressing in the treatment of stage II pressure ulcers. *Ostomy Wound Manage* 2009;55(2):50-5.
94. Bjellerup M. Novel method for training skin flap surgery: polyurethane foam dressing used as a skin equivalent. *Dermatol Surg* 2005;31(9 Pt 1):1107-11.
95. Young S. Does Allevyn foam's management system improve wound healing? *Br J Community Nurs* 2007;12(6):S31-4.
96. Lohmann M, Thomsen JK, Edmonds ME, Harding KG, Apelqvist J, Gottrup F. Safety and performance of a new non-adhesive foam dressing for the treatment of diabetic foot ulcers. *Journal of Wound Care* 2004;13(3):118-20.
97. Meaume S, Couilliet D, Vin F. Prognostic factors for venous ulcer healing in a non-selected population of ambulatory patients. *J Wound Care* 2005;14(1):31-4.
98. Vogensen H. Evaluation of Biatain Soft-Hold foam dressing. *Br J Nurs* 2006;15(21):1162-5.
99. Jorgensen B, Friis GJ, Gottrup F. Pain and quality of life for patients with venous leg ulcers: proof of concept of the efficacy of Biatain-Ibu, a new pain reducing wound dressing. *Wound Repair Regen* 2006;14(3):233-9.
100. Sibbald RG, Coutts P, Fierheller M, Woo K. A pilot (real-life) randomised clinical evaluation of a pain-relieving foam dressing: (ibuprofen-foam versus local best practice). *Int Wound J* 2007;4 Suppl 1:16-23.
101. Jorgensen B, Gottrup F, Karlsmark T, Bech-Thomsen N, Sibbald RG. Combined use of an ibuprofen-releasing foam dressing and silver dressing on infected leg ulcers. *J Wound Care* 2008;17(5):210-4.
102. Steffansen B, Herping SP. Novel wound models for characterizing ibuprofen release from foam dressings. *Int J Pharm* 2008;364(1):150-5.

103. Gottrup F, Jorgensen B, Karlsmark T, Sibbald RG, Rimdeika R, Harding K, et al. Reducing wound pain in venous leg ulcers with Biatain Ibu: a randomized, controlled double-blind clinical investigation on the performance and safety. *Wound Repair Regen* 2008;16(5):615-25.

104. Romanelli M, Dini V, Polignano R, Bonadeo P, Maggio G. Ibuprofen slow-release foam dressing reduces wound pain in painful exuding wounds: preliminary findings from an international real-life study. *J Dermatolog Treat* 2009;20(1):19-26.

105. Cigna E, Tarallo M, Bistoni G, Anniboletti T, Trignano E, Tortorelli G, et al. Evaluation of polyurethane dressing with ibuprofen in the management of split-thickness skin graft donor sites. *In Vivo* 2009;23(6):983-6.

106. Palao i Domenech R, Romanelli M, Tsiftsis DD, Slonkova V, Jortikka A, Johannesen N, et al. Effect of an ibuprofen-releasing foam dressing on wound pain: a real-life RCT. *J Wound Care* 2008;17(8):342, 344-8.

107. Wayne MA. Clinical evaluation of Epi-lock - a semiocclusive dressing. *Ann. emerg. Med.* 1985;14:65-69.

108. Stair TO, D'Orta J, Altieri MF, Lippe MS. Polyurethane and silver sulfadiazene dressings in treatment of partial- thickness burns and abrasions. *Am J Emerg Med* 1986;4(3):214-7.

109. Charles H, Callicot C, Mathurin D, Ballard K, Hart J. Randomised, comparative study of three primary dressings for the treatment of venous ulcers. *Br J Community Nurs* 2002;7(6 Suppl):48-54.

110. Bohmert H, Petzold D, Schmidtler F, Simon T, Schleuter B. [Experimental and clinical testing of polyurethane foam (Epigard) in burns]. *Langenbecks Arch Chir* 1974;Suppl:257-9.

111. Schmidtler F, Bohmert H. Experimental testing and clinical investigation of polyurethane foam (Epigard) for burn wounds pp. 309-13. *In: Hohler H, ed. Plastische und Wiederherstellungs-Chirurgie. Stuttgart, Schattauer,* 1975.

112. Kiffner E, Bohmert H. [Experiences with Epigard, a synthetic skin substitute, in the treatment of skin defects]. *Fortschr Med* 1976;94(15):861-4.

113. Bohmert H. Epigard as a temporary skin substitute in burns. *Med Welt* 1977;28(17):826-31.

114. Frese J, Kohaus H. Covering of skin defect wounds with a synthetic skin substitute. Conditioning of defect wounds of various origins with a synthetic skin substitute as a preparation for skin transplantation. *Fortschr Med* 1977;95(45):2687-90.

115. Palmer B. Clinical experience of Epigard. *Lakartidningen* 1977;74(32):2690-2.

116. Eriksson H, Mannheimer C. Treatment of ischemic ulcers using EPIGARD--a synthetic dressing proceedings. *Aktuelle Gerontol* 1978;8(10):555.

117. Roth RR, Winton GB. A synthetic skin substitute as a temporary dressing in Mohs surgery. *J Dermatol Surg Oncol* 1989;15(6):670-2.

118. Petres J, Muller RP. Temporary covering in the surgery of skin tumors. *Z Hautkr* 1985;60(1-2):185-96.

119. Kastner KH, Wunsch PH, Eckert P. Temporary skin replacement with lyophilized swine skin and foam substances--comparative experimental studies. *Langenbecks Arch Chir* 1988;373(5):287-97.

120. Borowka S, Gubisch W. Synthetic wound dressing (Epigard Syspur-derm). *European Journal of Plastic Surgery* 1982;7(1):83-86.

121. Scurr J, H. , Wilson LA, Coleridge -Smith PD. A Comparison of the Effects of Semipermeable Foam and Film Secondary Dressings over Alginate Dressings on the Healing and Management of Venous Ulcers. *Wounds* 1993;5(6):259-265.

122. Somers SS, Lyons C, Brown AF, Klein J, Sherriff HM. The Flexipore 6000 membrane as a wound dressing for use in the accident and emergency department. *Arch Emerg Med* 1992;9(2):246-8.

123. Whiteley MS, Domers.S.S., Eyres P. Sutureless closure of surgical wounds using the Flexipore 6000 Membrane dressing. . *First European Conference on Advances in Wound Management.*: Macmillan Ltd, 1992:103-104.

124. Winter GD. Epidermal wound healing under a new polyurethane foam dressing (Lyofoam). *Plast Reconstr Surg* 1975;56(5):531-7.

125. Baccari G, Boschetti E. Ferite, ustione e piaghe medicate con spugnoa di poliuretano,. *Sixth National Congress of the Societa Italiana di Chirurgia d, Urgenza e Pronto Soccorso*. Padua, 1977.

126. Davenport PJ, Dhooghe PL, Yiacoumettis A. A prospective comparison of two split-skin graft donor site dressings. *Burns* 1977;3:225-228.

127. Salisbury RE, Bevin AG, Dingeldein GP, Grisham J. A clinical and laboratory evaluation of a polyurethane foam: a new donor site dressing. *Arch Surg* 1979;114(10):1188-92.

128. Creevy J. Lyofoam - use in the treatment of leg ulcers In: Turner TD, Scmidt RJ, K.G. H, editors. *Advances in Wound Management*. London: John Wiley, 1985:39-40.

129. Mayerhausen W, Kreis M. Ulcus cruris. *Arzt. Prax.* 1987;5:2033-2035.

130. Hughes L. Wound management in the community - comparison of Lyofoam and Melolin. *Care Science and Practice* 1989;7:64-67.

131. Pessenhofer H, Stangl M. The effect on wound healing of venous leg ulcers of a two-layered polyurethane foam wound dressing. *Arzneimittelforschung* 1989;39(9):1173-7.

132. Harris A, Rolstad BS. Hypergranulation tissue: a nontraumatic method of management. *Ostomy Wound Manage* 1994;40(5):20-2, 24, 26-30.

133. Johnson A. Lyofoam in the treatment of open wounds. *Nurs Stand Spec Suppl* 1989(4):8-12.

134. Bayliss D. A secondary problem is cured. *Nursing mirror* 1979:May 17.

135. Riffel L, Smithson C. Selected case studies of wounds treated with Lyofoam: tracheostomies. *Ostomy Wound Manage* 1990;29:suppl 1-4.

136. Wenger RA. Clinical case updates. Selected case studies of wounds treated with Lyofoam. *Ostomy Wound Manage* 1990;26:suppl 1-4.

137. Rigby D. Treating tropical ulcers in a young patient. *Journal of Wound Care* 1994;3(3):122-126.

138. Banks V, Bale S, Harding KG. Superficial pressure sores: comparing two regimes. *Journal of Wound Care* 1994;3(1):8-10.

139. Dmochowska M, Prokop J, Bielecka S, Urasinska K, Krolicki A, Nagaj E, et al. A randomized, controlled, parallel group clinical trial of a polyurethane foam dressing versus a calcium alginate dressing in the treatment of moderately to heavily exuding venous leg ulcers. *Wounds-a Compendium of Clinical Research and Practice* 1999;11(1):21-28.

140. Platt AJ, Holt G, Caddy CM. A new method for the assessment of suturing ability. *J R Coll Surg Edinb* 1997;42(6):383-5.

141. Rubin AI, Moran K, Fine JD, Wargon O, Murrell DF. Urethral meatal stenosis in junctional epidermolysis bullosa: a rare complication effectively treated with a novel and simple modality. *Int J Dermatol* 2007;46(10):1076-7.

142. Martinez Cuervo F, Segovia Gomez T, Alonso Perez F, Verdu Soriano J, De Con Redondo J, Lahuerta Garcia T. [Evaluation of the clinical effectiveness of the dressing PermaFoam for the treatment of chronic ulcers]. *Rev Enferm* 2005;28(6):29-34.

143. Zoellner P, Kapp H, Smola H. A prospective, open-label study to assess the clinical performance of a foam dressing in the management of chronic wounds. *Ostomy Wound Manage* 2006;52(5):34-6, 38, 40-2 passim.

144. Carr RD, Lalagos DE. Clinical evaluation of a polymeric membrane dressing in the treatment of pressure ulcers. *Decubitus* 1990;3(3):38-42.

145. Fowler E, Papen JC. Clinical evaluation of a polymeric membrane dressing in the treatment of dermal ulcers. *Ostomy Wound Manage* 1991;35:35-8, 40-4.

146. Blackman JD, Senseng D, Quinn L, Mazzone T. Clinical evaluation of a semipermeable polymeric membrane dressing for the treatment of chronic diabetic foot ulcers. *Diabetes Care* 1994;17(4):322-5.

147. Banks V, Bale S, Harding KG. The use of two dressings for moderately exuding pressure sores. *Journal of Wound Care* 1994;3(3):132-134.

148. Banks V, Bale SE, Harding KG. Comparing two dressings for exuding pressure sores in community patients. *Journal of Wound Care* 1994;3(4):175-178.

149. Andriessen A, Polignano R, Abel M. Monitoring the microcirculation to evaluate dressing performance in patients with venous leg ulcers. *J Wound Care* 2009;18(4):145-50.

150. Bayliss DJ. A clinical application for Synthaderm a new plastic dressing material - a new treatment for an old problem. In: Sundell N, editor. *Proceedings of a Symposium on Wound Healing*. Espoo, Finland, 1980:189-200.

151. Lock PM, Riddle MD. The use of Synthaderm in the treatment of ischaemic leg ulcers. In: Sundell N, editor. *Proceedings of a Symposium on Wound Healing*. Espoo, Finland, 1980:135-141.

152. Dahle JS. Conservative treatment of leg ulcer *Tidsskr Nor Laegeforen* 1980;100(29):1731-3.

153. Martin A, Kirby NG, Tabone Vassallo M, Glucksman E. Synthaderm in the management of pre-tibial lacerations: a controlled clinical study. *Arch Emerg Med* 1987;4(3):179-86.

154. Banerjee AK, Levy DW, Rawlinson D. Leg ulcers - a comparative study of Synthaderm and conventional dressings. *Care of the elderly* 1990;2(3):123-125.

155. Charles H, Corser R, Varrow S, Hart J. A non-adhesive foam dressing for exuding venous leg ulcers and pressure ulcers: six case studies. *Journal of Wound Care* 2004;13(2):58-62.

156. Williams C. Treating a patient's venous ulcer with a foamed gel dressing. *Journal of Wound Care* 1993;2(5):264-265.

157. Collier J. A moist, odour-free environment. A multicentred trial of a foamed gel and a hydrocolloid dressing. *Prof Nurse* 1992;7(12):804, 806, 808.

158. Thomas S, Banks V, Bale S, Fear-Price M, Hagelstein S, Harding KG, et al. A comparison of two dressings in the management of chronic wounds. *Journal of Wound Care* 1997;6(8):383-386.

159. Diehm C, Lawall H. Evaluation of Tielle hydropolymer dressings in the management of chronic exuding wounds in primary care. *Int Wound J* 2005;2(1):26-35.

160. Schulze HJ. Clinical evaluation of TIELLE* Plus dressing in the management of exuding chronic wounds. *Br J Community Nurs* 2003;8(11 Suppl):18-22.

161. Schulze HJ, Lane C, Charles H, Ballard K, Hampton S, Moll I. Evaluating a superabsorbent hydropolymer dressing for exuding venous leg ulcers. *Journal of Wound Care* 2001;10(1):511-8.

162. Naylor W. Using a new foam dressing in the care of fungating wounds. *Br J Nurs* 2001;10(6 Suppl):S24-30.

163. Taylor A, Lane C, Walsh J, Whittaker S, Ballard K, Young SR. A non-comparative multi-centre clinical evaluation of a new hydropolymer adhesive dressing. *Journal of Wound Care* 1999;8(10):489-92.

164. Banks V, Bale S, Harding K, Harding EF. Evaluation of a new polyurethane foam dressing. *Journal of Wound Care* 1997;6(6):266-9.

165. Andersen KE, Franken CPM, Gad P, Larsen AM, Larsen JR, van N, A., et al. A randomized, controlled study to compare the effectiveness of two foam dressings in the management of lower leg ulcers. *Ostomy Wound Management* 2002;48(8):34-41.

166. Franks PJ, Moody M, Moffatt CJ, Hiskett G, Gatto P, Davies C, et al. Randomized trial of two foam dressings in the management of chronic venous ulceration. *Wound Repair Regen* 2007;15(2):197-202.

167. Viamontes L, Jones AM. Evaluation study of the properties of two adhesive foam dressings. *Br J Nurs* 2003;12(11 Suppl):S43-4, S46-9.

168. Viamontes L, Temple D, Wytall D, Walker A. An evaluation of an adhesive hydrocellular foam dressing and a self-adherent soft silicone foam dressing in a nursing home setting. *Ostomy Wound Manage* 2003;49(8):48-52, 54-6, 58.

169. Amione P, Ricci E, Topo F, Izzo L, Pirovano R, Rega V, et al. Comparison of Allevyn Adhesive and Biatain Adhesive in the management of pressure ulcers. *J Wound Care* 2005;14(8):365-70.

170. Butterworth RJ, Bale S, Harding K, Hughes LE. Comparing Allevyn cavity wound dressing and Silastic foam. *Journal of Wound Care* 1992;1(1):10-13.

171. Johnson A. Dressings for deep wounds. *Nurs Times* 1992;88(4):55-8.

172. Todd M. Treating a cavity wound in the community. *Journal of Wound Care* 1993;2(4):202-204.

11. Polysaccharide fibre dressings

INTRODUCTION

Dressings made from a variety of gel-forming polysaccharides are used in the management of exuding wounds. Alginates in particular have been employed in a fibrous form for many years as haemostats and surgical absorbents but freeze-dried preparations have also been developed. More recently, dressings made from chemically modified carboxymethylcellulose have also been produced in a fibrous form which bears a marked similarity to alginates in terms of their appearance, physical properties and indications for use. Dressings made from other polysaccharides such as hyaluronidase, chitin and chitosan are also available although many of these have yet to achieve significant commercial success. Some fibrous dressings are medicated with honey or silver, but these are described in separate chapters.

ALGINATE DRESSINGS

Large quantities of alginate dressings are used each year for the treatment of exuding wounds such as leg ulcers, pressures sores and infected surgical wounds. Originally these were presented in the form of a loose fleece, formed primarily from fibres of calcium alginate, but subsequently dressings have been developed in which the fibres are entangled to form a product with a more cohesive structure and enhanced strength when soaked with exudate or blood. Some products contain a significant proportion of sodium alginate to improve the gelling properties of the dressing and a few have been made by a freeze drying process and as a result have no fibrous structure at all.

Once in contact with an exuding wound, an ion exchange reaction takes place between the calcium ions in the dressing and sodium ions in serum or wound fluid. When a significant proportion of the calcium ions present in the fibres have been replaced by sodium, the fibres swell and partially dissolve forming a gel-like mass. The degree of swelling is governed principally by the chemical composition of the alginate which in turn is determined by its botanical source.

Although it is recognised that differences between the various brands of dressings may influence their handling characteristics - particularly when wet, it is generally assumed that these differences are of limited relevance to the performance of the dressings clinically or at a cellular level. There is some evidence to suggest, however, that these assumptions may not be correct and that alginates may influence wound healing in a number of ways not yet fully understood.

Discovery of alginates

Alginic acid and its salts were first described and partially characterized in 1883 by Stanford,[1] a British chemist who spent many years seeking a use for the large quantities of seaweed thrown up onto the Atlantic coast of the British Isles. He observed that the long flat fronds of one species, *Laminaria*, contained sacs of a near colourless solution which, on partial drying, formed a jelly-like substance that could be drawn out in long tenacious strings. This substance, which he called 'algin', he found to be freely soluble in alkali but coagulated by alcohol or mineral acids. In 1881 he patented a process to extract this material for commercial use.

The viscous nature of purified alginate solutions eventually led to their widespread use as thickening and stabilizing agents in the food and brewing industry where they have found application in products as diverse as ice cream and beer. A significant quantity of alginate is also used by the pharmaceutical industry in the production of controlled release agents, bio-adhesive systems, tablet disintergrants suspending agents and implants; it is estimated that in excess of 20,000 tons of alginate are consumed globally each year for these and other purposes.

According to Gacesa,[2] most alginate is obtained commercially from three of the 265 reported genera of the marine brown algae, *Phaeophyceae*. The majority is extracted from members of the genus *Macrocystis* that includes the giant kelp (*Macrocystis pyrifera*) harvested off the West Coast of the USA. In northern Europe alginates are extracted from horsetail kelp (*Laminaria digitata*) and sugar kelp (*Laminaria. saccharina*) collected from waters off the Outer Hebrides and the west coast of Ireland.

Although the extraction of alginates is a relatively recent process, seaweed has been used for centuries for a variety of purposes. Some reports suggest that in China it was used as early as 2700BC.[3] In Europe, in Greek and Roman times, seaweed was used as fodder and for the production of herbal medicine. In Ireland it has been exploited since at least the 12th Century, and where, from the early 1700s, ash made from seaweed heated in kelp kilns, was used in the manufacture of soap and glass and also as a fertiliser and a source of iodine.

The function of alginates within the algae is thought to be primarily skeletal,[4] with the gel conferring the strength and flexibility required to withstand tidal activity in the water in which the seaweed grows.

Certain species of bacteria, including *Azobacter vinelandii* and *P. aerugino*sa, produce alginates that form a protective coating around the organism but these are not used commercially.

Chemistry of alginates

Alginates occur naturally as mixed salts of alginic acid and are found primarily as the sodium form. The yield varies with the species but is typically in the order of 20 - 25%. Chemically alginates consist of a three-dimensional network of long-chain molecules held together at junctional sites. As no evidence of branching has been detected, the molecule is thought to be essentially linear.[2] The alginate molecule is a polysaccharide formed from homopolymeric regions of β-D-mannuronic acid, (M) and α-L-guluronic acid, (G), commonly called M-blocks and G-blocks, interspersed with regions of mixed sequence, (MG-blocks). Methods for characterizing the structure and molecular weight of alginates were published by Johnson et al.[4] who examined five different samples of alginate and found that their MG ratios ranged from 42 - 63.6% with molecular weights ranging from 12,000 to 180,000.

The relative proportions and arrangement of the M, G and MG blocks have a marked effect upon the chemical and physical characteristics of the alginate and therefore any fibre made from it. These properties are determined by the botanical source of the seaweed from which the alginate is extracted. Even within species, some seasonal variations have been reported, particularly in *Laminaria* sp. where alginates were found to have a higher proportion of mannuronic acid in the summer.[4]

Regions in which the M-blocks predominate form an extended ribbon-like molecule, analogous to cellulose, whereas regions rich in G-blocks form a 'buckled chain'.[2] All of the block structures are capable of forming ionic bonds with di or multivalent cations, but regions containing G-blocks are also able to chelate the metal ions because of the spatial arrangement of the ring and the hydroxyl oxygen atoms thus forming a much stronger interaction. It is this interaction between the polyguluronic acid blocks that is responsible for the nature and strength of the gel that is formed when solutions of sodium alginate come into contact with divalent metal ions such as calcium. The calcium ions cross-link the polymeric chains producing an 'egg-box' like structure in which the calcium ions represent the eggs within the convoluted polysaccharide chain.[5] The higher the content of guluronic acid in the alginate, the greater the interaction, and the more stable and harder the resultant gel.

The calcium ions present in high-M alginates are less firmly attached to the molecule and as a result are more easily replaced by sodium ions, resulting in increased fluid uptake and fibre swelling and faster gel formation. High-M alginates are therefore more absorbent on a gram for gram basis and form softer gels than those rich in high-G; they are also more readily soluble in saline solution.

The ability of alginates to bind divalent metal ions is also related to the ion-exchange coefficient between the divalent metal ion and the sodium ion and is calculated thus:

$$K = \frac{[\textit{Metal ion concentration in the gel}][\textit{Sodium ion concentration in the solution}]^2}{[\textit{Sodium ion concentration in the gel}]^2 \, [\textit{Metal ion concentration in solution}]}$$

The ion exchange coefficients of alginate extracted from two different types of seaweed are shown in Table 17. The data within this table are taken from Qin[6] who in turn has quoted the earlier work of Haug and Smidsrod originally published in 1965.

Table 17: Ion exchange coefficient of alginate extracted from two different species of seaweed

Metal ions	Ion exchange coefficients	
	L. digitata M/G ratio = 1.60	L. hyperborea M/G ratio = 0/45
Cu^{2+}- Na^+	230	340
Ba^{2+}- Na^+	21	52
Ca^{2+}- Na^+	7.5	20
Co^{2+}- Na^+	3.5	4

According to Haug and Smidsrod, as quoted by Qin, the binding abilities of metal ions for alginate are in the order:

$$Pb^{2+} > Cu^{2+} > Cd^{2+} > Ba^{2+} > Sr^{2+} > Ca^{2+} > Co^{2+} = Ni^{2+} = Zn^{2+} > Mg^{2+}$$

The relative weak bond that is produced between calcium and alginate is important as it readily permits ion exchange in the presence of sodium ions in solution. Clearly the use of alginate containing some other divalent metal ions would be less likely to gel as readily in the presence of sodium ions.

When alginate produced by the bacterium *P. aeruginosa* was purified and analysed, it was found to have an M/G ratio of 1.27 - 3.55, a much narrower range than is found in the brown seaweeds. It was also found to be present in the acetylated form. No evidence of any G-block structure was detected, suggesting that the alginate was not capable of forming the 'egg box' structures characteristic of the relatively rigid high-G seaweed gels.[7]

Alginate dressings function by interacting with exudate to form a gel on the wound surface. In this way they produce the moist wound healing conditions that Winter showed were able to reduce healing times of wounds in his animal model.[8]

In an unpublished laboratory study, the fibre swelling characteristics of a number of alginate dressings were determined by measuring the diameters of the fibres intact, then after two minutes contact with Solution A, a mixture of sodium and calcium chloride containing 142 millimoles of sodium ions and 2.5 millimoles of calcium. This ionic composition was chosen because it approximates to that of blood or serum and therefore probably provides the most clinically relevant data (Table 18).

Table 18: Swell characteristics of polysaccharide fibres

Dressing	Fibre diameter (mm) Mean (sd)		% increase
	Initial	Final	
Aquacel*	0.0136 (0.0015)	0.1477 (0.0132)	994 (157)
Kaltostat	0.0196 (0.0039)	0.0378 (0.0173)	211 (135)
Kaltogel	0.0166 (0.0032)	0.0714 (0.0067)	343 (77)
Sorbsan	0.0173 (0.0027)	0.1000 (0.0067)	491 (98)
Sorbalgon	0.0167 (0.0024)	0.0946 (0.0091)	472 (66)
Tegagen HG	0.0175 (0.0024)	0.0737 (0.0049)	329 (67)
Tegagen HI	0.0238 (0.0045)	0.0927 (0.0065)	309 (123)
Urgosorb**	0.019 (0.0031)	0.0727 (0.0051)	291 (64)

*Carboxymethylcellulose fibre** Carboxymethylcellulose/alginate blend*

The differences in gel structure and rheology caused by the differences in chemical structure have important implications for the clinical use of the products. The soft gel residues from products made from high-M alginates can be washed off the wound or irrigated out of sinuses or cavities with a jet of saline, but the fibres in dressings made from high-G alginates swell only slightly in the presence of wound fluid and may appear relatively unchanged even after an extended period. Such dressings are therefore usually removed in one piece using a forceps or gloved hand.

By carefully controlling the manufacturing process, it is possible to produce alginates in which some of the calcium ions are replaced by sodium in order to accelerate the gel forming process. These are known as calcium/sodium alginate[5] and can be produced both from alginates with a high guluronic acid content, e.g. Kaltostat, and high mannuronic acid content, e.g. Kaltogel.

Production of alginate dressings

Alginate is extracted from washed, milled seaweed using an aqueous alkali solution which results in the formation of alginate 'dope' a crude viscous colloidal solution of sodium alginate. This is clarified by filtration and the alginate subsequently precipitated by the addition of calcium chloride. The resultant gel is washed with acid before being redissolved in sodium carbonate solution from which sodium alginate is obtained by a drying and milling process.[5]

If a solution of sodium alginate is extruded under pressure through a fine orifice into a bath containing calcium ions, an ion-exchange reaction takes place resulting in the formation of fibres of insoluble calcium alginate. Although a method of manufacturing calcium alginate fibre was first disclosed in a patent in 1898, production of the material on a commercial scale only became possible after the publication of a further series of patents in the 1930s.

The fibre that was produced at that time was used principally in the textile industry as a soluble yarn that would dissolve in a scouring process, and which could therefore be used as a support during the manufacture of fine lace, or as draw threads in the production of hosiery.[9] Fabrics made from alginate fibre were also once produced commercially for their fire-resistant properties, (a feature of their high metallic content)[5] and for the manufacture of bags used to transport soiled hospital linen that were designed to dissolve in the wash. By the 1970s alginates were replaced for these applications by cheaper non-flammable and water-soluble alternatives.

At that time, the amount of alginate fibre that was used in surgery and wound management represented only about 10% of annual production and it therefore became uneconomic to continue to produce the relatively small quantity of fibre required for medical applications. Some years later, technological advances and improvements in production techniques in the textile industry, together with an increased understanding of the mechanisms of wound healing, reawakened interest in the potential value of alginate which enjoyed a renaissance in the early 1980s.

Modern alginate dressings

Most alginate dressings are produced as flat sheets, which are used to cover superficial wounds, or in the form of a ribbon or rope,[5] which is used for packing deeper wounds and cavities. The flat dressings are normally made in a nonwoven fabric process in which the fibres are carded to form a web that is then cross-lapped to form a felt. In some products, the felt is then needled to give the dressing a coherent structure.

Comfeel Seasorb, now discontinued in the UK, was somewhat different in that it was manufactured from a high M calcium/sodium alginate produced in a freeze-dried form carried on a high-density polyethylene net so that the dressing superficially resembles a fine soft foam sheet.

Fibracol Plus, which is not available in the UK, is a development of Fibracol which was marked for a while in the UK by Johnson and Johnson. The dressing consists of a mixture of 90% collagen with and calcium alginate presented as a freeze dried sheets. The rationale for the combined use of these two agents is that the alginate provides a moist wound-healing environment and the collagen a scaffold for the newly developing tissue.

The first modern alginate dressing was Sorbsan which was developed by Courtaulds Fibres Ltd, Coventry. Launched in 1983, it consisted of calcium alginate fibres with a high mannuronic acid content. These were formed into a loose fibrous fleece for dressing superficial wounds, but for cavity wounds the carded web was formed into a sliver that was subsequently cut to length to form pieces resembling a loose rope. A ribbon form of the dressing was also produced for narrow sinuses. The alginate fibre from which Sorbsan is produced rapidly gels and disintegrates in the presence of sodium ions in wound fluid or saline. As a result the dressing is easily removed from a wound by irrigation with Normal Saline.

Sorbsan alginate fibre was subsequently employed as a facing layer on a number of other products including the absorbent dressing pads Sorbsan Plus and Sorbsan Plus SA.. Originally marketed by N.I. Medical, the company was sold to Pharma-Plast which changed its name to Maersk Medical A/S, then Unomedical A/S. The product was then owned briefly by Convatec before being sold once again to the current owners, Aspen Surgical, in February 2009.

Kaltostat is a fibrous high-G calcium alginate, which like Sorbsan, is available in a variety of presentations. When it was first introduced to the market place in 1986 the dressing contained levels of a quaternary ammonium compound which were shown to impart pronounced cytotoxic properties to the dressing when tested by a cell culture method. This agent, arquad, was included to aid fibre handling during the manufacturing process. Following correspondence in the pharmaceutical press,[10-12] the manufacturing process was subsequently modified to ensure that the arquad was reduced to sub-toxic levels.

Kaltostat differs from Sorbsan in that the sheet dressing has a more stable structure and maintains its integrity when wet. In about 1988 Kaltostat was further modified so that the dressing contained a mixture of calcium and sodium alginate in the ratio of 80:20. This was done to improve the gel forming ability of the fibres.

Like Sorbsan, the dressing was made available in a number of different presentations including a sheet and rope form. A faster gelling form was subsequently introduced called Kaltogel which contained a higher content of mannuronic acid and was designed to approximate more closely to the performance of the original Sorbsan. This was discontinued in 2001, presumably because it was thought to compete with another newly introduced product from Convatec product called Aquacel.

Kaltostat fibre was also used to form an absorbent pad on a semipermeable film to form an island dressing called Kaltoclude, also discontinued, although smaller versions of film backed island dressings which bear a pad of alginate fibres are marketed by others as first aid dressings, e.g. Savlon Alginate Dressing.

Originally developed by Britcair, later a UK division of CV Laboratories, Kaltostat was purchased by E.R. Squibb in 1995 then ownership was transferred to Convatec in 2008.

Tegagel, launched in 1989 by 3M Healthcare, was subsequently renamed Tegagen. Two versions of the dressing were produced: Tegagen HG, later to be renamed Tegaderm High Gelling Alginate Dressing, which becomes an amorphous gel-like mass when saturated, and Tegagen HI, renamed Tegaderm High Integrity Alginate Dressing, which was designed to maintain its integrity so that it could be lifted in one piece from a wound even when saturated with blood or other fluids. This second product thus effectively aimed to combine the rapid gelling properties of Sorbsan with the stability of Kaltostat. This was originally achieved by exposing a nonwoven web of alginate fibre to a curtain of water streams at high velocity to hydroentangle the nonwoven alginate fibres but this process has since been has replaced by a needling technique.

It is also possible to prepare alginate dressings from mixtures of fibres produced from different types of alginates. Melgisorb, for example, consists of a blend of 60% high-M and 40% high-G alginate which is predominantly (96%) in the calcium form.

Other fibrous alginates, most of which are available in a number of forms include:

- Activheal Alginate
- Algisite M
- Algosteril
- Curasorb
- Curasorb Zn (contains zinc ions)
- Restore
- Sorbalgon
- Suprasorb A

In addition to the above some dressings are produced from a blend of calcium alginate and carboxymethylcellulose fibres. Examples of these mixed dressings include:

- Askina Sorb
- Seasorb Soft
- Nu-Derm (now discontinued)
- Urgosorb

The rapid proliferation of alginate dressings has made it necessary for the manufacturers of these products to seek a marketing advantage for their individual products. This is often related to an aspect of the fluid handling properties or absorbency of their particular brand.

When examining the fluid handling data presented by different companies, it is particularly important to take note of the fluid used during laboratory testing.

A study published in 1992[13] compared the absorbency of different alginate dressings using water, sodium chloride solution 0.9% and Solution A.

Under the conditions of test, the weight of each fluid absorbed by one gram of Sorbsan was 8, 21 and 14 grams for each of the three test solutions respectively. With Kaltostat the results were somewhat different, *viz.* 15, 14 and 13 grams respectively. These variations were due to differences in the gelling characteristics of the alginate fibres, largely a function of the previously described M:G ratio.

The absorbency and tensile properties of eight alginate dressings were compared in a laboratory study published by Johnson and Simpson,[14] and Ichioka *et al.*[15] who compared the gelling and fluid handling characteristics of alginates and hydrocolloid dressings using a method similar to that published previously by Thomas.[13]

In 1995, the British Pharmacopoeia (BP) published monographs for alginate fibre,[16] and alginate dressings, which included simple methods for assessing gelling, wet integrity (dispersible or non-dispersible), and fluid handling properties.[17-18]

The BP monograph classified dressings both in terms of their absorbency and their ability to maintain their structural integrity when wet. Flat dressings are described as high absorbency if they retain more than 12 grams of per 100 cm^2. For cavity wound dressings the limit is six grams/gram. The absorbency values quoted for flat dressings are expressed as grams/unit area rather than grams/gram because dressings are used as individual pieces of standard size as supplied by the manufacturer regardless of their weight. This is a more clinically relevant figure than the figure quoted previously.[13]

Previously unpublished values for the results of the BP absorbency and dispersion tests obtained with different alginate dressings and three products containing carboxymethylcellulose (CMC) or a CMC/alginate blend, are shown in Table 19 and summarised in Figure 51.

In normal use products that maintain their integrity are removed from a wound in one piece, those products that do not maintain their integrity can be irrigated away with saline. The results shown in this table are typical of those obtained with a dressing sample not subjected to any form of pressure. In the clinical situation, however, the use of compression bandages may substantially reduce the absorbent capacity of the individual products. High-G alginates generally form wet integral or non-dispersible dressings, and high-M alginates dispersible dressings. The situation has been made a little more complicated, however, by the production of high-M alginates, for example Tegagen, that are subjected to a fibre entanglement process that limits the ability of the fibres to swell and thus disperse during the integrity test.

Table 19: Absorbency and dispersibility of polysaccharide dressings.

Dressing	Absorbency grams/100cm^2	Dispersion characteristics
Algisite M	18.30 (0.71)	Non-dispersible
Aquacel*	18.46 (1.02)	Non-dispersible
Kaltostat	21.67 (1.89)	Non-dispersible
Kaltogel	17.86 (2.32)	Dispersible
Comfeel Seasorb [a]	21.24 (2.05)	Non-dispersible
Sorbsan	16.16 (0.75)	Dispersible
Sorbalgon	19.90 (1.40)	Dispersible
Tegagen HG	24.34 (3.19)	Dispersible
Tegagen HI	24.70 (1.89)	Non-dispersible
Urgosorb**	26.55 (2.96)	Non-dispersible

*Carboxymethylcellulose fibre ** Carboxymethylcellulose/alginate blend [a]Freeze dried alginate sheet*

Figure 51: Absorbency of polysaccharide dressings

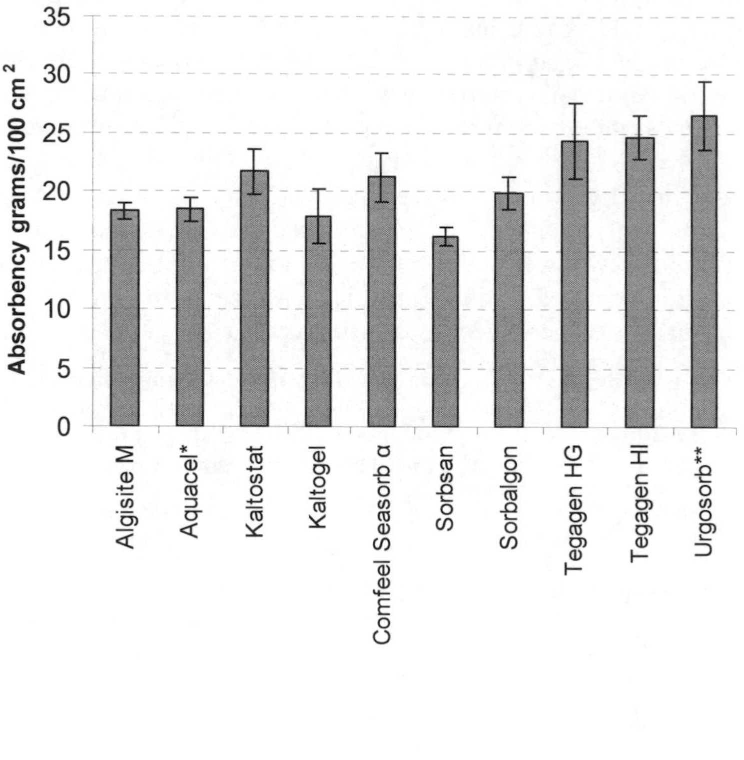

CLINICAL EXPERIENCE WITH ALGINATE DRESSINGS

Although the literature contains isolated historical allusions to the early use by sailors and others of seaweed as a dressing,[19-21] these reports are generally not well referenced and no authoritative medical texts have been found that confirm its application in this way. Given the range of materials that have been used historically for managing wounds, however, it would be surprising if seaweed had not been used for this purpose.

The first person in modern times to recognise the potential value of alginates extracted from seaweed in surgery and wound management was George Blaine, a major in the Royal Army Medical Corp. He showed them to be absorbable by tissue, Sterilizable by heat, and compatible with penicillin.[22] He also described how he had used alginate films clotted *in situ* for the treatment of wounds and burns in troopship hospitals in the Far East and described the use of alginate, sometimes in combination with plasma as an alginate-plasma film, as 'puncture patches' over scleral defects.

During a subsequent assessment of the use of alginates as haemostats and wound dressings, Blaine reported upon their apparent lack of toxicity following a series of animal studies in which fibres were implanted into animal tissues, and gels made from alginates were used to treat experimentally produced burns.[23] Clinical studies followed, and the successful use of alginate-derived materials in aural surgery and neurosurgery was reported by Passe and Blaine,[24] and Oliver and Blaine[25] respectively.

Other, more general applications were described in 1948, when Bray *et al.*[26] reported the results of a three-month trial into the use of alginate in the casualty department of Croydon Hospital. In this study, alginates - in the form of films, wool, gauzes, and clots (formed in situ by mixing sterile solutions of calcium chloride and sodium alginate), were applied to a wide range of wounds, including burns, lacerations, ulcers and amputations. In all cases, healing was found to be rapid and uneventful.

According to the results of a survey carried out by Stansfield and reported by Blaine,[27] in the late 1940s and early 1950s alginates were being used in some 70 hospitals over the range of surgical specialities. Overall, they were found to be highly satisfactory in use but where criticisms were recorded, they were directed mainly at the poor absorption properties of the material and its consequent tendency to induce fistula formation. It was noted that most of these criticisms related to cases in which the product had been used as packing for large cavities or dead spaces, a function for which it was never originally intended.

Following the early work of Blaine and others, a number of commercial medical alginate products were produced, including an absorbable swab called Calgitex but when the large-scale manufacture of alginate fibre ceased in the early 1970s, for reasons described previously, this product was discontinued owing to the high cost of production.

The first clinical reports describing the use of a 'modern' alginate dressing, Sorbsan, were published in 1983 by Fraser and Gilchrist[28] and Gilchrist and Martin,[20] who described their experiences with the dressing in the management of foot disorders and a variety of skin lesions, following a clinical evaluation in a group of hospitals in the Sunderland area.

The results of these studies were very positive and supported the findings of Blaine some 40 years earlier. Further papers followed which described the use of Sorbsan in the management of problem wounds including infected traumatic wounds and leg ulcers.[29-30] In 1988 alginate dressings finally gained widespread clinical acceptance when Sorbsan was included in the Drug Tariff. An introduction to the use of alginates and alginate fibres in all aspects of clinical practice was published by Sherr.[31]

Numerous reviews have been published on alginates[2] and alginate dressings,[32-37] and the literature also contains many references to their use.[21,29,38-45]

Imamura et al.[46] described how a calcium/sodium alginate dressing was successfully applied to extensive areas of skin loss caused by toxic epidermal necrolysis that spread from the scalp to the lower extremities and suggested that the dressing could be used to treat other disorders with widespread detached epidermis such as autoimmune blistering diseases.

Cannavo et al.[47] compared the performance of three different dressings in the management of 36 dehisced surgical abdominal wounds. These were a standard alginate; gauze moistened with 0.05% sodium hypochlorite solution, and a 'combine dressing pad', consisting of an absorbent pad to which is added a semipermeable film dressing. No statistically significant differences in healing rates between the three treatment groups were detected but there was a trend for the combine dressing protocol to produce a greater reduction in wound area. Maximum pain was significantly greater ($p = 0.011$), and satisfaction significantly lower, among patients who received the sodium hypochlorite treatment; associated treatment costs were also substantially higher for this group of patients. The authors suggested that, based upon these results, the use of sodium hypochlorite soaked dressings for surgical wounds should be abandoned.

Berry[48] compared Kaltostat with a polyurethane foam dressing, Allevyn, in the management of patients with non-infected cavity wounds. Both dressing regimes were found to be easy to use, effective and acceptable to patients and clinicians.

Patients with gaping abdominal wounds following Caesarian section[49] and radical vulvectomy,[50] were also managed successfully with alginate dressings.

When a patient with a ten-year history of heroin abuse and multiple ulcerations to his upper arm had his wounds dressed with a calcium alginate rope and covered with in a four-layer bandage, complete healing was achieved in 42 days.[51]

It has been suggested that alginates have a role in accident and emergency departments as an alternative to paraffin tulle dressings.[52] In the treatment of 'road rash' and other similar abrasions, following surgical toilet they have been applied moistened with 20 mL of a solution containing of bupivacaine 0.05% with adrenaline 1:200000, to provide initial pain relief and reduce bleeding.[53] When covered with paraffin gauze, Gamgee tissue and a bandage, it was suggested the dressing could be left undisturbed for up to ten days.

As previously identified, composite dressings containing alginate have been developed in a variety of forms that include simple adhesive island dressings, (Kaltoclude) to absorbent pads with an alginate wound contact layer (Sorbsan Plus). An alginate-faced dressing containing activated charcoal for used in the management of malodorous wounds has also been developed and the results of a laboratory-based evaluation to compare the performance of this dressing with other charcoal dressings have been described in the literature.[54]

The results of a small study to assess the performance of an alginate/film combination, were published by Moody,[55] who concluded that although the dressing is not suitable for wounds that produce copious amounts of exudate, it was satisfactory for moist chronic wounds that produce low to moderate levels of exudate.

Use of alginate dressings in specific wound types

Leg ulcers

The first controlled trial involving an alginate dressing was carried out as a Drug Tariff reimbursement study involving 64 community patients with leg ulcers. The patients were allocated to treatment with either Sorbsan or paraffin gauze dressings.[56] Only 4% of the ulcers treated with tulle healed during the course of the study whilst 31% of the ulcers treated with Sorbsan healed completely. The average healing rate achieved with Sorbsan (measured as a decrease in wound area per day) was over four times that recorded using tulle. Overall, 73% of patients on Sorbsan showed evidence of improvement during the trial, indicated by a reduction in wound area, compared with 43% of patients in the control group.

This study was later criticised on a number of grounds but principally because patients were not provided with sustained graduated compression.[57-58] At the time that the study was undertaken, however, no competent compression bandages were available on the Drug Tariff and for this reason they had been specifically excluded from the trial protocol.[59]

Moffat et al.[60] subsequently performed a randomized controlled trial in which they compared an alginate dressing, Tegagel with a simple knitted viscose primary dressing under a graduated compression bandaging system. Sixty patients were randomized to treatment the results of which were analyzed by life table. Twenty-six patients whose wounds were dressed with Tegagel healed compared with twenty-four patients on N-A Dressing. This difference was not statistically significant. All the ulcers included in this study were venous in origin and wounds greater than 10 cm^2 were excluded.

Scurr et al.[61] compared the effects of two different secondary dressings applied over an alginate dressing in the treatment of venous ulcers. A total of 20 patients were recruited to the study. Ten were dressed with Sorbsan and a polyurethane film dressing, Opsite, the remainder with an alginate and a thin sheet of adhesive polyurethane foam (Flexzan). This foam had a moisture vapour transmission rate in excess of 5000 g/m^2/24 hours, approximately six times that of Opsite.

Patients were assessed six times, at weekly intervals. The groups had similar results in terms of changes in ulcer size, wound condition scores and reduction of pain scores but patients treated with the foam secondary dressing required significantly fewer dressing changes than those in the film dressing group, 87 to 192, respectively (p = 0.0038). The group receiving the foam dressing also had fewer problems with edge roll and leakage, a lower incidence of sensitivity reactions, and higher patient acceptability. The authors concluded that while both the foam and film dressings are efficacious as secondary dressings when used with an alginate primary dressing in the management of venous ulcers, the foam dressings may offer some practical advantages.

In a second paper, Scurr et al.[62] compared Sorbsan with a hydrocolloid dressing (Granuflex) in the treatment of 40 patients with confirmed venous ulcers. Compression was provided by means of a Class III compression stocking. Wounds were evaluated weekly for six weeks or until healed. Of the wounds dressed with alginate, six healed and 70% improved (decreased in size by more than 40%). Of the wounds dressed with hydrocolloid, two healed and 45% improved, but these differences were not statistically different. Pain scores were significantly lower for patients dressed with alginates and all but two of the patients managed with hydrocolloid had a degree of maceration around the area of the wound.

Stacey et al.[63] compared Kaltostat with a zinc paste bandage, (Viscopaste) and a zinc oxide impregnated stockinette in a randomized controlled trial involving 113 patients with 133 ulcerated limbs. A minimal stretch bandage, Elastocrepe, was used to provide compression with an elasticated tubular stockinette (Tubigrip) applied over the top to hold the dressings in place.

Patients were followed for nine months or until the limbs had healed. Only ulcer size, ulceration on the right leg and the use of the paste bandage had any significant effect on the time to healing. At the 12-week stage 64% of ulcers dressed with the paste bandage had healed compared with 50% of those dressed with alginate and zinc oxide stockinette. The authors proposed that the difference in healing could be due to the extra layers of bandage that result from the use of the paste bandage, and suggested that these may well have produced sustained levels of compression, higher than those achieved with the other two dressing systems.

Limova[64] compared two calcium alginate dressings in a prospective, randomized, controlled clinical involving 19 patients. Ten patients (53%) were treated with Tegagen and nine patients (47%) with Sorbsan. Dressings were changed weekly and patients were followed for a maximum of six weeks or until the venous ulcer no longer required the use of an alginate dressing. Tegagen was rated significantly better than Sorbsan in all parameter assessed. Two patients treated with Sorbsan healed but no patients treated with Tegagen achieved closure during the study.

Burns and donor sites

An obvious potential use for alginate fibre is in the treatment of burns and donor sites, where the haemostatic and absorbent properties of the material should be at their most useful. Groves and Lawrence[65] described a study in which they compared Sorbsan with a standard gauze pad. They found that, in a simple laboratory test, the alginate absorbed nearly three times as much citrated blood as gauze when calculated on a weight for weight basis. When the dressings were applied to fresh, split-thickness donor sites for a period of five minutes after excision, the blood loss from sites treated with Sorbsan was almost half that recorded from comparable wounds treated with gauze.

The effect of longer-term application of alginates to donor sites was investigated by Attwood.[66] In an initial study 15 patients with split skin grafts had one half of their wound dressed with Kaltostat, the other half with paraffin gauze. Upon assessment every area dressed with alginate showed significantly better healing than the corresponding 'control' area.

The second phase of the study was designed to assess the time to complete healing of alginate-dressed areas and the patient acceptability of the dressing. A total of 155 donor sites were examined; 130 treated with alginate and 25 treated with traditional dressings. Sites treated with Kaltostat healed in 7.0 ± 0.71 days but paraffin gauze dressed wounds took 10.7 ± 51.6. Patient comfort and quality of healing with Kaltostat was significantly better than that achieved using the traditional material. Attwood also discussed the types of secondary dressing that could be used with Kaltostat, and suggested that it was not necessary to use the bulky dressings commonly used when dressing donor sites. For some wounds a film dressing applied over the alginate prevented desiccation and improved patient comfort providing that haemostasis and good adhesion to the surrounding skin could be achieved. Wounds on the torso dressed with alginate were sometimes left uncovered.

The importance of the choice of secondary dressings when using alginates in the management of donor sites was illustrated by the results of a blind randomized study involving 40 patients whose wounds were dressed with paraffin gauze, alginate plus gauze, alginate with a semipermeable film, or a film dressing.

The paraffin gauze dressing was found to be the most painful product used, and alginate covered with the film dressing was associated with the fastest healing rate. Alginate used alone tended to dry out, nevertheless, the healing times recorded were still superior to those achieved with paraffin gauze or the semipermeable film on its own.[67]

Rodier-Bruant et al.[68] published the results of an early evaluation of the use of Sorbsan which involved the treatment 52 patients who required a skin graft for various reasons. Healing times varied according the wound type but in 85% of cases, was achieved between one and 2.5 weeks. The authors commented that the speed of healing allowed multiple split skin grafts to be taken from the same donor site, facilitating the treatment of extensive skin burns. The dressing was said to be easy to remove causing only minimal discomfort to the patient. The incidence of side effects such as itching and scar hypertrophy or pigmentation was also low.

Basse et al.[69] compared Kaltostat with a paraffin gauze, Jelonet in 17 patients who had mirror-image donor sites on the thighs. Saline-soaked gauze was first applied to achieve haemostasis followed by the appropriate dressing. This in turn was covered by an elastic bandage. Because of the small numbers of patients involved no statistical test were performed on the resulting data but there was evidence to suggest that both blood loss and discomfort were reduced with the alginate product. The mean time to healing for Kaltostat was 8.3 days (range 7 - 11 days) and for Jelonet 10.2 days (range 7 - 17 days). The secondary dressings used in this study were not identified.

Further evidence for the superiority of alginate dressings over paraffin gauze on split skin graft donor sites was presented by Donoghue et al.,[70] following a prospective randomized control trial involving 51 patients, 30 of whom were randomized to treatment with calcium alginate and 21 to the paraffin gauze. In one group a single layer of paraffin gauze was applied covered with three layers of cotton gauze, cotton wool padding and secured with a bandage. In the other group Kaltostat, impregnated with

0.25% bupivacaine, was overlaid with paraffin gauze, then cotton gauze and padding as for the controls. Upon assessment, ten days post harvesting, it was found that 21 of the 30 patients dressed with calcium alginate were completely healed while only 7/21 in the paraffin gauze group were healed (p < 0.05). In their discussion the authors considered that the choice of day ten as the inspection period was probably inappropriate, following some further investigations in which they removed the alginate dressing on day seven as recommended by Attwood.[66] At this stage the dressing was still moist and separated painlessly from the wound but by day ten it had dried out and become more difficult to remove. They concluded that calcium alginate dressings provide a significant improvement over traditional treatments in healing split skin graft donor sites and recommended that the first dressing change should be carried out on day 7.

Cihantimur *et al.*[71] in a prospective, randomized, controlled study compared Kaltostat with Jelonet in the treatment of split-thickness skin graft donor sites in 40 patients. The healing time, quality of regenerated skin, ease of removal of dressing, the rates of infection and convenience of the dressing in clinical use were compared. Dressings were changed after eight days when healing of the donor site was assessed; the mean time from operation to observation of complete healing was 8.5 with Kaltostat and 11.5 days with Jelonet. Patient comfort and the quality of regenerated skin were better under Kaltostat dressings.

The use of alginate and paraffin gauze were compared in the treatment of scalp donor sites in 67 children in a controlled, randomized, clinical trial held in ten French plastic surgery departments.[72] Epithelialization occurred after ten and 11 days in the calcium alginate dressing group and the paraffin gauze group respectively (*ns*). Earlier reharvesting of the donor site was possible in the calcium alginate dressed group than in the control group (p = 0.003), and removal of the alginate dressing caused significantly less trauma and pain than the paraffin gauze. This same study was subsequently reported again some five years later by Pannier *et al.*[73]

Steenfos and Agren[74] compared a fibre-free alginate dressing, Comfeel SeaSorb, with a paraffin gauze, Jelonet, on donor sites in 17 patients. Both dressings were applied to parts of each wound and covered with gauze and a crepe bandage. The alginate dressing absorbed 40% more blood, measured as total iron content of used dressings, during the first ten minutes post-wounding than fine mesh gauze (p < 0.05). Light microscopic examination of punch biopsies obtained from ten wounds on post-operative day six showed that nine wounds treated with the alginate dressing had fully epithelialized compared with seven wounds treated with paraffin gauze. This difference did not reach statistical significance (p = 0.46). The authors concluded that although the fibre-free alginate dressing showed increased initial blood absorption and quicker haemostasis, it had no clear beneficial effect on epithelialization. They suggested that this might have been due to the small sample size and their failure to occlude the alginate dressing over the critical first two post-operative days.

Calcium alginate was compared with Scarlet Red Ointment Dressing by Bettinger *et al.*, in 12 paired wounds in seven patients undergoing skin grafting.[75] No significant differences in healing time were recorded, both groups taking 11.8 days. It is considered, however, that the dressing procedures used in this study may well have contributed to the extended healing time of the alginate dressings.

The same two dressings were compared in a second study, described by Lawrence and Blake, in which 46 patients had split thickness skin grafts harvested from the upper inner thigh. Kaltostat and scarlet red dressings were applied to each half of the wound and covered with gauze, cotton wool and a crepe bandage. The dressings changed after ten days when healing of the donor site was assessed. In this study, scarlet red was found to be significantly better than Kaltostat, for 84% of wounds dressed with scarlet red had healed compared with 72% dressed with alginate (p < 0.04).[76]

In a letter, commenting upon the paper by Lawrence and Blake, Lim and Walter[77] stated that when using Kaltostat on donor sites of 67 patients, they achieved an average healing rate of 6.2 days (range 5-14) and implied that the relatively poor results obtained by Lawrence might be due to desiccation of the primary dressing due to the use of an inappropriate secondary dressing.

The relative merits of Kaltostat and a porcine xenograft (E-Z Derm) were examined in a controlled, prospective study of split-thickness skin graft donor sites on 20 patients.[78] E-Z Derm is a meshed xenograft derived from pig skin in which the collagen has been cross linked chemically with an aldehyde. Time to complete healing, quality of regenerated skin and patient comfort were assessed. Time to healing was 8.1 days with alginate and 11.3 days with porcine xenograft (p < 0.001). The quality of the healed skin obtained with the alginate was superior to that under the xenograft in 95% of patients (p < 0.001). No hypertrophic scarring was noted in patients treated with alginates but was reported in 25% of xenograft-dressed sites (p < 0.01). The authors concluded that porcine xenograft is inferior to calcium sodium alginate as a dressing for split-thickness skin donor sites.

Deep burns of the hand represent a common serious surgical problem with major occupational and economic implications. The application of alginate dressings helped to control haemorrhage during excision and grafting and prevent desiccation of important deep structures such as extensor tendons or joints exposed during surgery.[79]

Kelly et al.[80] made use of the gel forming properties of alginate dressings to protect exposed tissue when they used them as a temporary recipient bed dressing prior to the delayed application of split skin grafts.

A novel use of an alginate dressing in the management of extensive burns on a seven year old boy was described by Varma et al.[81] In the absence of sufficient donor site material to cover the entire area with a conventional graft, small pieces of skin grafts (edges of meshed grafts and shredded skin) were cut into small pieces, formed it into a suspension and poured it evenly over a sheet of Kaltostat. This was then applied to the wound. Clear evidence of epithelial islands was visible after ten days and complete coverage was achieved by the 28th postoperative day.

The well recognised problem of donor site pain, was addressed by Butler et al.[82] in a study involving 45 patients undergoing split thickness skin grafting. After harvesting the graft each patient was randomized to one of three different treatment regimens, dry Kaltostat, Kaltostat moistened with 20 mL of saline and Kaltostat moistened with 20 mL of bupivacaine 0.5%. The dressing was then covered with an outer wound pad and secured with an adhesive dressing. A blinded medical observer unaware of the treatment provided then assessed post-operative wound pain at 24, 48 and 72 hours using a linear analogue pain scale. The dressing was removed on the 10th postoperative day and healing assessed. Ease of removal and the presence of infection were also recorded. There was a dramatic statistical difference in the pain scores between patients who received the bupivacaine soaked dressing and the other two treatment groups at 24 and 48 hours, but by 72 hours all patients reported only low levels of discomfort. No differences in ease of removal were recorded.

Porter compared alginate dressings with hydrocolloid dressings in the healing of split skin graft donor sites.[83] Sixty-five patients were randomized to treatment and the rate of epithelialization, discomfort experienced by the patients and the convenience of the two dressings in use were compared. The alginate dressings were applied to the raw donor areas and held in place by layers of dry gauze, plaster wool and a crepe bandage. In the second group the hydrocolloid dressing was applied after haemostasis was achieved and covered by plaster wool and a crepe bandage. At the time of the first dressing change 87% of the donor areas dressed with the hydrocolloid and 86% of the donor areas dressed with the alginate were found to be more than 90% healed. The mean time from operation to the observation of complete healing was 10.0 days for the donor areas dressed with the hydrocolloid and 15.5 days for wounds dressed with alginate; this difference was found to be statistically significant. Again it is considered that the poor performance of the alginate dressing was due the dressing technique and choice of secondary dressings.

Comfort and ease of use of Kaltostat, was compared with that of an adhesive retention tape Mefix, in two studies. In the first study,[84] 30 consecutive patients were randomized to treatment. Dressings were assessed by interview and questionnaire after 24 hours, 48 hours and two weeks. In the second study the dressings were applied to 50 patients and the performance similarly assessed. In both studies it was reported that Mefix required less nursing intervention and allowed patients easier mobility with a greater range of daily activities, especially washing, without compromising wound healing.[85]

Alginates have also been compared with more modern dressing in the treatment of donor sites. O'Donoghue et al.[86] in an open, randomized, prospectively controlled trial, compared healing, slippage rates and discomfort on removal of calcium alginate and a silicone-coated polyamide net dressing on split skin graft donor sites. Sixteen patients were randomized to the calcium alginate group and 14 to the silicone-coated group. The donor sites were assessed at days 7, 10, 14 and up to day 21. The mean time to healing in the calcium alginate group was 8.75 ± 0.78 days (range 7 - 14) compared to 12 ± 0.62 days (range 7 - 16) for the silicone-coated group ($p < 0.01$). More occurrences of slippage were encountered in wounds dressed with the silicone-coated dressings than the alginate (5 vs 1), but this difference was not statistically significant. Overlaid absorbent gauze adhered to the donor site through the fenestrations in the silicone coated dressing necessitating the placement of paraffin gauze between the experimental dressing and the overlying cotton gauze. Based on these results the authors recommend that calcium alginate remain the dressing of choice for split skin graft donor sites.

Vaingankar et al.[87] compared Kaltostat with Allevyn foam in 20 patients. The dressings were applied to equal halves of each donor site. Although sites dressed with Allevyn showed a tendency to earlier healing, this was not confirmed statistically, however, Allevyn was found to be more comfortable than Kaltostat and this difference was statistically significant.

More recently, Kaltostat has been compared with a new gel-based product, Tegaderm Absorbent, in a prospective randomized controlled trial in 40 patients with split thickness donor sites in 40 patients.[88] At the first assessment, 79% of the Tegaderm Absorbent donor sites had healed completely, compared with 16% of the Kaltostat ones (p < 0.001). Mean time to complete healing was also significantly less for Tegaderm Absorbent than Kaltostat, 14 vs 21 days, (p < 0.001) and postoperative pain was reduced. Tegaderm Absorbent was also judged significantly easier to apply and remove than Kaltostat. At one month post-surgery, Vancouver scar scores showed that Tegaderm Absorbent dressed wounds were less red, flatter, softer and less itchy. Once again the possibility that the choice of secondary dressings might have impacted upon treatment outcomes cannot be ignored.

In a review of clinical practice in the management of split skin graft donor sites in the British Isles conducted by means of a postal questionnaire,[89] it was found that for the 279 surgeons who responded, a response rate of 78%, alginates were the most popular dressings, especially in adult donor sites, being the treatment of choice for 167 respondents (60%). Adhesive fabrics were much less popular, first choice for small adult donor areas for 46 respondents (16%). Plastic film dressings and Biobrane were first choice for only approximately 5% of respondents for small and large donor areas. Ten percent of respondents said they avoided paraffin gauze and another 10% avoided plastic film dressings in all cases. Five percent avoid hydrocolloid and another 5% avoided adhesive fabric in all cases. Following their review the authors concluded that alginates should be the product of choice as the control treatment in any future study of donor-site dressings.

The use of alginate dressings is usually associated with minimal side effects but Davey et al.[90] reported that after 12 years uneventful use as the standard dressing for split skin donor sites, they had recently encountered five cases with the unusual and unexplained phenomenon of dermal calcification in the donor site following the use of two new, unidentified, varieties of calcium alginate dressing.

Pressure ulcers

An early account of the use of Kaltostat, in the management of a sacral pressure ulcer was provided by Mack.[91] Sayag et al.[92] subsequently compared the efficacy of Algosteril with that of dextranomer paste, an established local treatment, in a prospective, randomized, controlled trial of 92 patients with full-thickness pressure ulcers. They reported that a minimum 40% reduction in wound area was obtained in 74% of the patients in the alginate group compared with 42% of those in the dextranomer group. The median time taken to achieve this reduction with alginate dressings was four weeks compared with more than eight weeks with the dextranomer. Mean surface area reduction rates per week were 2.39 ± 3.54 cm2 and 0.27 ± 3.21 cm2 for the alginate and dextranomer treated wounds respectively. They concluded that 'This striking healing efficacy of an alginate dressing suggests it possesses pharmacological properties which require further investigation'.

The use of Sorbsan in the treatment of 19 patients with 30 pressure ulcers was described by Chapuis and Dollfus,[93] who concluded that the dressing appears to give good results in the treatment of patients with spinal cord lesions including the control of odour. Similar claims for the use of Kaltostat in the management of pressure ulcers was made by Young,[36] McMullen,[38] Motta,[39] and Fowler and Papen, who reported upon a small seven patient study involving 310 dressing changes.[94]

Belmin et al,[95] recognizing that some dressings are best suited for particular types of wounds, described an open, randomized, multicenter parallel-group trial involving 110 elderly patients with Grade III or IV ulcers in which they compared the efficacy of calcium alginate and hydrocolloid dressings applied sequentially, with hydrocolloids applied alone.

The control strategy consisted of applying a hydrocolloid dressing, Duoderm E, alone for eight weeks; the sequential strategy consisted of applying a calcium alginate dressing, Urgosorb, for the first four weeks, then a hydrocolloid dressing, Algoplaque, for the next four weeks.

During the study, ulcer areas were calculated weekly from tracing. The endpoints were the mean absolute surface area reduction during the 8-week study period and the number of patients achieving a 40% or more reduction in surface area. Fifty-seven and 53 patients were randomly allocated to sequential and control strategies respectively. Baseline patient characteristics and ulcer features at inclusion were similar in the two groups. Mean ± s.d. reduction in wound area was significantly larger in the sequential treatment group, 5.4 ± 5.7 cm^2 and 7.6 ± 7.1 cm^2 at four and eight weeks, than in the control group, 1.6 ± 4.9 cm^2 and 3.1 ± 7.2 cm^2 ($p < 0.001$). In the sequential treatment group, 68.4% of the patients achieved a 40% reduction by four weeks and 75.4% by eight weeks, significantly higher than in the control group, 22.6% vs 58.5% respectively ($p < 0.0001$). The authors concluded that in the treatment of Grade III or IV pressure ulcers, application of a calcium alginate dressings followed by a hydrocolloid dressing promotes faster healing than treatment with hydrocolloid dressings alone.

The results of this possibly unique study confirm the present author's strongly held opinion that dressing selection should be determined by the condition of the wound rather than its aetiology. In this instance the initial application of an alginate to an exuding wound followed by a hydrocolloid as healing progresses appears logical and is based upon a good understanding of the performance of the products concerned. It is perhaps a little unfortunate that the hydrocolloid dressing used was not the same in both treatment arms, for there remains the possibility, however unlikely, that some difference in the chemical composition or physical properties of the two hydrocolloids might have been responsible for the differences in the results obtained. It is to be regretted that this eminently sensible and rationale approach would be rejected by many who conduct clinical trials or undertake systematic reviews.

Foot care

Neuropathy and peripheral vascular disease are the two most common foot problems affecting 15% to 20% of all diabetic patients. Following the early success reported by Fraser and Gilchrist,[28] alginate dressings have been widely used for these and other wounds on the feet.[96] Their low-adherent properties also make them useful for dressing toes following surgery for in-growing toe nails.

Burrow and Lindsay[97] compared Kaltostat with Ultraplast, an adhesive island dressing with an integral alginate pad. No major differences were detected between the two products in terms of healing rates but Ultraplast was found to cause more maceration of the toe and surrounding tissue, due it was suggested to the presence of the adhesive carrier film.

Smith[98] described a study in which 67 patients undergoing partial or complete toenail avulsion had their wounds dressed with either Sorbsan or polynoxylin and a perforated film dressing, (Melolin). They found that the use of the alginate dressing reduced both healing time and the number of follow up visits.

Similar results were reported by Foley and Allen[99] who also compared Kaltostat with Melolin in 70 patients undergoing partial or complete toenail avulsion. They found that the use of the alginate dressing reduced both the number of dressing changes required and the time to healing (34 to 26 days). No difference in pain was detected between the two treatment groups.

Foster et al.[100] compared Kaltostat with a foam dressing, Allevyn, in 30 patients randomized to treatment with the different products. A total of seventeen patients (57%) were healed by the end of the eight week study, nine in the polyurethane foam treated group, and eight in the group dressed with alginate. Although no difference was detected in healing rates, the foam was found to be easier to use and more acceptable to patients.

When a collagen-alginate dressing (Fibracol) was compared with alginate alone in a small randomized control trial involving 24 patients with legs ulcers, a small but non-significant advantage was found to be associated with the use of the collagen-alginate, but the results of this study were severely limited by the small number of subjects and the fact that an unknown number of arterial ulcers were included.[101]

Fibracol was also shown to be superior to soaks and daily dressing changes in the postoperative management of chemical matricectomies reducing the average healing time from 36 days to 24 days.[102] Donaghue et al.[103] compared the efficacy and safety of the same collagen-alginate dressing with gauze moistened with normal saline for the treatment of diabetic foot ulcers. Seventy-five patients with foot ulcerations participated in the trial and assigned randomly in a 2:1 ratio to receive the collagen-alginate test dressing or the saline-moistened gauze control. At the initial examination, baseline characteristics of the wounds were assessed according to size, location, duration, and stage. Participants were seen weekly for a maximum of eight weeks or until the wounds healed. Although the mean percent reduction in the wound area and the incidence of complete healing were higher in the collagen-alginate-treated group, the differences did not reach statistical significance. At the end of the study, mean percentage reduction of the wound area was $80.6 \pm 6\%$ vs $61.1 \pm 26\%$ (p = 0.4692) for the collagen-alginate dressing group and the gauze dressing group respectively. Forty-eight percent (24/50) of patients in the collagen-alginate dressing group and 36% (9/25) in the gauze dressing group had complete ulcer healing, although the mean time to healing was longer for the collagen-alginate dressing group when compared with the control group, 6.2 ± 0.4 vs 5.8 ± 0.4 weeks respectively.

Bale *et al.*[104] undertook an initial assessment of Comfeel Seasorb dressing in 41 diabetic patients with an ankle brachial pressure index (ABPI) > 0.4 who had foot ulcers > 1 cm in diameter which were classified as Wagner Grade I or II. The patients were treated for a maximum of six weeks or until the ulcer healed. Evaluable data was obtained from 39 patients, eleven of whom healed within the six-week trial period. Overall, there was a significant reduction in mean ulcer area during this time from 2.8 cm^2 to 1.02 cm^2. Eleven patients experienced ulcer pain, the intensity of which decreased during the six week study. A total of 12 adverse events were reported: seven mild to moderate and five severe. None were directly attributed to the study dressing. Six patients required treatment for infection.

In an open-label randomized multicenter controlled study, alginate dressings were compared with Vaseline gauze in the treatment of 77 diabetic foot ulcers with a surface area of 1 - 50 cm^2.[105] Dressings were initially changed daily then every two to three days as the condition of the wound permitted. The selected primary outcome was the proportion of patients with granulation tissue over 75% of the wound area and having a 40% decrease in wound surface area. This was achieved in 42.8% of the alginate-treated wounds and of 28.5% of those dressed with Vaseline gauze (not statistically significant). Pain at dressing change was lower in the calcium alginate group (p = 0.047) and the total number of dressing changes tended also to be lower (p = 0.07). Adverse events, which occurred four times in the calcium alginate group and six times in the other, were judged independent of the treatments. The authors concluded that calcium alginate appeared to offer advantages over Vaseline gauze, in the treatment of diabetic foot ulcers both in terms of healing rate and patient acceptability.

Surgery

A number of studies have compared alginate dressings with traditional treatments in surgical wounds left to heal by secondary intention. Gupta *et al.*[106] showed that compared with proflavine soaked gauze, alginate dressings, Sorbsan, caused less pain and reduced the need for analgesia when used to pack post-surgical cavity wounds in 29 patients. The use of alginate also appeared to reduce bacterial counts within the wound. The authors felt that the advantages offered by the alginate outweighed the corresponding increase in cost.

In a second study,[107] 16 patients were randomized to receive calcium alginate and 18 patients received saline-soaked gauze dressings for packing abscess cavities following incision and drainage. At the first dressing change the patient marked on a linear analogue scale the pain experienced; the nurse noted similarly the ease of removal of the dressing. Calcium alginate was significantly less painful to remove after operation (p < 0.01), and also easier to remove (p < 0.01) than gauze dressings. The authors concluded that if abscess cavities are packed after incision and drainage, calcium alginate appears to be an improvement on conventional dressings.

Similar findings were recorded when alginate dressings were compared with gauze soaked in povidone iodine solution for the treatment of 70 pilonidal abscesses following incision and drainage.[108] Wounds treated with alginate reduced in size faster, (p < 0.05), and more became filled with granulation tissue during the trial period but this difference failed to achieve statistical significance. A major difference in wound pain and ease of use was reported in favour of the alginate dressings, (p = 0.0001 and p = 0.011 respectively).

Sorbsan and paraffin gauze/cotton were also compared in a prospective randomized study when used as packs following haemorrhoidectomy.[109] Fifty consecutive patients were prospectively randomized to treatment. Post-operative pain was assessed at six hours, on removal of rectal packing and at first bowel action. Haemorrhage was monitored at six hours and upon removal of pack. Patients who received the calcium alginate pack reported reduced pain at the time of removal/spontaneous discharge of rectal packing and first post-operative bowel action. No significant difference in post-operative haemorrhage between the two groups was reported. There was no difference in the hospital stay between the two groups. The authors concluded that compared to more bulky anal packs, the alginate effectively reduced post-operative pain with no adverse result upon blood loss.

Williams et al.[110] compared a high-M alginate dressing, Sorbsan, with a high-G dressing, Kaltostat, in the treatment of cavity wounds following surgical debridement left to heal by secondary intention. Four dressing changes were performed on each wound by four dedicated staff who removed Sorbsan by irrigation and Kaltostat using forceps. No differences were detected between treatments either in terms of pain or bacterial colonization.

Dental practice

A mixture of sodium alginate and calcium penicillin in powder form, was first used as a styptic in dental work by Blockley.[111] Rumble[112] later reported that when the minimum quantity of 'fast' alginate wool, required to stop post-extraction haemorrhage was lightly packed into a cavity, it was subsequently rapidly absorbed, often within 2-3 days. (Fast alginate wool contained a significant proportion of sodium alginate)

The haemostatic properties of Kaltostat, were compared with those of a gauze pad in standard wounds on the buccal mucosa in beagle dogs.[113] The authors concluded that although the alginate was more effective than cotton gauze at controlling bleeding, a piece of alginate sutured over the defect made no difference to the healing rate compared with uncovered control wounds.

The use of Kaltostat in modern dental practice was described in 1989 by Joy and Murray,[114] following its use in 100 cases. The dressing usually arrested haemorrhage within 45 seconds but always within 2.5 minutes. It was also reported that healing was accelerated and that post-operative pain was reduced. On this basis the authors suggested that it would seem appropriate to use Kaltostat routinely for this purpose.

Odell et al.[115] urged caution in the use of haemostatic agents, including alginates, following a florid foreign body giant cell reaction elicited by Kaltostat which had been used to obtain haemostasis in an apicectomy cavity on an upper lateral incisor approximately seven months earlier. The authors suggested that this case demonstrated that alginate fibres if left in situ may elicit a long-lasting and symptomatic adverse foreign body reaction. They proposed that the dressing should be reserved for problematic haemorrhage and be removed from the tooth socket soon after haemostasis.

This observation was consistent with that of others who had conducted animal studies in which they implanted an alternative alginate dressing, Astroplast, in bony cavities within rabbit mandibles - a situation analogous to an apicectomy.[116] In this situation it was found that the reaction lasted at least eight weeks and was associated with delayed bone healing.

A histopathological study to compare the response of tissue to Kaltostat and oxidised cellulose (Surgicel - Johnson and Johnson) in healing tooth sockets in beagles was carried out by Mathew *et al.*[117] Tooth sockets filled with blood clot acted as controls. The results showed that both dressings delayed wound healing in the early phase (1-4 weeks), giving rise to foreign body reactions. At 12 weeks there was little difference between the control sockets and the sockets containing the test materials, although remnants of retained dressing materials were identified. Healing of the tooth sockets was complete at 24 weeks.

In a further study, Mathew *et al.*[118] undertook a histological comparison of the tissue response to Kaltostat and Surgicel when implanted between bone and periosteum in the jaws of beagles at intervals up to 24 weeks. Both products caused a foreign body reaction, persisting up to 12 weeks after surgery. New bone formation was detected along the surface of the mandible in some specimens, but was not apparently related to the implants. It was concluded that the implantation of Kaltostat or Surgicel between bone and periosteum in the jaws caused a delay in wound healing, and had no effect on bone induction.

Surgical x-ray detectable swabs manufactured from alginate fibre were developed in the late 1980s. Following the success of an earlier implantation study on rabbits,[119] Blair *et al.*[120] compared these swabs, with traditional cotton gauze in 100 patients undergoing elective surgery. They reported that compared with cotton swabs, the median value for blood loss was reduced from 91 mL (range 3 - 329) to 72 mL (range 2 - 181). An unexpected finding was that operation times were also reduced by the use of the alginate swabs. The authors concluded that calcium alginate swabs were absorbent, strong enough to use in retraction of tissue and able to improve haemostasis.

Supporting evidence for the reduced blood loss associated with alginate swabs was presented by Davies *et al.*[121] following a study conducted in patients undergoing internal fixation of intertrochanteric fractures of the proximal femur. Patients in the gauze swab group lost 139.4 ± 9.6 mL per-operatively, whilst those in the alginate swab group lost 98.8 ± 9.9 mL ($p < 0.01$). The post-operative suction drainage loss was also reduced in the alginate group. The authors concluded that alginate swabs significantly decrease per-operative blood loss and post-operative suction drainage loss, and suggested that haemostatic swabs could have wider applications in orthopaedic surgery.

The conclusions of this paper were questioned by Jones,[122] who, whilst accepting that the measured values for blood loss were statistically different in the two treatment groups, argued that these differences were not clinically relevant. He also argued that the cost difference between the two swabs could not be justified for such a small clinical advantage.

Alginate swabs were compared with cotton gauze during tonsillectomy and inferior tonsillar pole ligation in the control of blood loss during tonsillectomy.[123] Ninety-nine tonsillectomy patients were randomized to gauze or alginate swab use. Mean total blood losses and operative times were similar for the two groups. Independent assessment showed no difference in the healing rate associated with the two swabs. The authors therefore concluded that alginate swabs offer no advantage over gauze in terms of blood loss, operative time or complications of tonsillectomy.

Despite the initial enthusiasm for the items that was expressed in the medical press,[124] surgical swabs made from alginate failed to make a major impact in the market place and production were discontinued in about 1997.

As haemostatic agents

In 1951 Blaine performed a comparative evaluation of absorbable haemostatic agents, including alginates.[27] He found that although calcium alginate fibres took up to 12 weeks to be fully absorbed, sodium calcium alginates were generally absorbed within ten days following implantation. In experiments involving minimal trauma with small implants, uneventful absorption took place within a few days. No evidence of adverse local histological changes was detected, although the rate of absorption varied with the location and vascularity of the surrounding tissue. In a further study it was shown that in the presence of antiseptic agents such as cetylpyridinium bromide, the absorption process was generally incomplete, and some histological changes were noted including encapsulation and giant cell production.[25]

The lack of adverse tissue reactions to alginates was described by Amies,[125] who evaluated sodium alginate as depot substance in active immunisation and showed in animal and volunteer studies that when the soluble sodium form is injected into living tissue it was converted into the calcium form. Although this gave rise to a foreign body-type reaction, in contrast to other agents in use at the time it did not lead to necrosis or abscess formation within in the tissue.

Jaros and Dewey,[126] formed similar conclusions following the long-term administration of sodium alginate as an adjuvant for repository hyposensitisation agents. They concluded that the material was 'well tolerated with less of a reaction rate than expected using regular allergenic extracts'.

Other, less favourable, observations upon the toxicity of alginates have also been reported in the literature. Frantz,[127] in a poorly designed and badly reported study, disregarded her own findings which showed that alginic acid fibres implanted into rats were absorbed completely within two days without any significant undesirable effects, and concluded that alginates were toxic on the basis of additional results obtained from studies involving a nitrated sodium alginate, a material that has no clinical application.

Chenoweth[128] tested the toxicity of alginic acid and sodium alginate in cats by both intravenous and intraperitoneal routes, and reported that dose levels of 250 and 500 mg/kg body-weight caused death or major damage to internal organs such as the heart and kidneys. Dose levels of 25 and 100 mg/kg were found to be much less toxic, although precise details were not given. As neither the method of test nor the dose of alginate used bears any relationship to the use of the material as a haemostat or wound dressing, the relevance of these observations is clearly open to question.

Gosset and Martin[129] in a presentation to the Academy of Surgery in Paris in 1949, considered that the two papers cited previously were primarily intended as a defence of oxycellulose and presented experimental data which showed that calcium alginate injected intramuscularly into both rabbits and rats, using volumes of 0.5 and 3 mL, failed to produce any of the effects described by the American authors; they concluded that calcium alginate was an excellent haemostatic agent that was well tolerated by living tissue.

Supporting evidence for the early findings of Blaine was provided by Blair et al.[119] who compared the haemostatic effect of four different materials in liver lacerations in the rabbit. The products examined were oxidised cellulose (Surgicel), porcine collagen, (Medistat), calcium alginate (Kaltostat) and surgical gauze. Calcium alginate stopped bleeding in less than three minutes compared with a mean ($\pm$ s.e.m.) of 5.7 ± 0.75, 12.5 ± 0.9, and > 15 minutes for porcine collagen, oxidised cellulose gauze respectively. Oxidised cellulose and calcium alginate reabsorbed within three months leaving a fibrous scar, but a vigorous foreign body reaction was observed with porcine collagen. In a further group of animals samples of all three haemostatic agents were left in situ on the liver and small bowel mesentery for three months. During this period the porcine collagen caused fatal intestinal obstruction in five animals within three months.

Sirmanna[130] investigated the use of calcium alginate fibre for packing the nasal cavity following surgical trimming of the inferior turbinates. In a pilot study 32 nostrils were packed with Kaltostat for 36-48 hours to achieve haemostasis. There was no bleeding while the packs were in place or after they were removed. These results were compared retrospectively with two other treatments, trousered paraffin gauze and glove finger packs both of which had been associated with bleeding in over 50% of cases either whilst the dressings were in situ or following their removal.

This pilot study was followed by a second in which the three treatments were compared prospectively.[131] All three types of packing material were found to be similarly effective in preventing bleeding whilst the packs were in situ, but the alginate caused significantly less bleeding on removal than the other two packing materials. Reduced bleeding was recorded with all three packs if they were left for 48 hours before removal. It was suggested that the observed reduction in bleeding might lead to a decrease in post operative infections.

In a third publication, which recorded the results of a follow up study on the same group of patients over a three-week period,[132] it was shown that packing for 48 hours resulted in significantly more complications for all types of packing materials than when packs were removed at 24 hours. It appeared that more infection, crusting and airway problems were associated with the use of the alginate than with the other two treatments if the packs were left in place for 48 hours but patient numbers were too small to test this statistically.

The original manufacturers of Kaltostat, BritCair, applied for a product licence for Kaltostat based upon its haemostatic activity in accordance with the requirements of the Medicines Act 1968. Manufacturers of other alginate dressings chose not to follow this route so these alternative products could never formally be marketed as haemostatic dressings.

The haemostatic activity of Kaltostat was investigated by Jarvis et al.,[133] who showed it to be associated with the exchange of calcium ions for sodium in the blood, stimulating both platelet activation and whole blood coagulation.

Segal and Gilding[134] compared the effects of different alginates containing calcium and zinc with non-alginate dressings on blood coagulation and platelet activation. They found that alginates activated coagulation more rapidly than non-alginate materials. Alginates rich in high-G had the greatest prothrombogenic effects, producing higher levels of thrombin generation and rapid platelet activation, an effect that was enhanced by the presence of zinc ions.

Evidence for the haemostatic activity of a high mannuronic alginate dressing, Sorbsan, was generated in a laboratory study in which the dressing was applied to experimental full and partial thickness wound models for periods up to 14 days to assess its effects on wound healing. Histological evaluation showed it to be an effective haemostat, generally well tolerated by body tissues. Good epidermal healing was seen on all wounds although cellular reactions could be provoked in full thickness wounds without occlusion, if there was an insufficient volume of wound exudate to completely wet the alginate fibres.[135]

The mechanisms by which alginate fibres are removed from tissue are not well understood. It has been suggested that the polysaccharide molecule is broken down to monomers or oligomers by lysozyme activity within the body but this is not supported by experimental evidence and is thought unlikely.[10,136]

Toxicity and biocompatibility issues

In a comparative study of the properties of three modern haemostatic agents used in current surgical practice, Blair[119] found Kaltostat to be more effective than either oxidized cellulose or porcine collagen in controlling bleeding from a surgically inflicted wound in rabbit liver. In addition, the material showed no tendency to cause intestinal obstruction when implanted into mesentery. In contrast, rabbits receiving porcine collagen had to be sacrificed. After six weeks, the oxidized cellulose had completely dissolved, but histological examination of the wound sites treated with alginate showed some evidence of calcium deposition and some fibrous reaction. It is possible that the fibrous reaction was due, in part, to the presence of Arquad in the material at that time.

Lansdowne et al., implanted samples of Kaltostat subcutaneously in rats to evaluate their biodegradability and ability to evoke local tissue reactions.[137] Implant sites were evaluated after 24 hours, 7, 28 and 84 days. Histological sections showed no noticeable degradation of the Kaltostat within is time: following subsidence of a modest foreign body reaction, implants became embedded in thin fibrous sheaths which were infiltrated with vascular channels and fibroblasts. The authors concluded that Kaltostat fibres in the rat model present no obvious toxic risk or contraindication to their use as wound dressings or as haemostatic agents in general surgery.

Suzuki et al.[138] reported that compared with a novel freeze-dried alginate gel dressing, extracts prepared from Kaltostat induced cytopathic effects when tested in vitro on L929 cells. In a second in vivo study, samples of the novel preparation, Kaltostat and cotton gauze were applied to circular full-thickness wounds on the backs of pigs. Wound tissue was harvested on day 18 for histological examination when the dressing treated with the freeze dried preparation showed more rapid wound closure compared to the Kaltostat and gauze dressed wounds in which a marked foreign-body reaction was noted. The authors concluded that based on these data, the new freeze dried alginate could reduce the cytotoxicity to fibroblasts and foreign body reaction that have been observed with currently available calcium alginate.

When four alginate dressings, Algosteril, Comfeel Alginate, Kaltostat and Sorbsan were compared in a partial thickness wound model in the pig, no difference was detected between the products in terms of healing rates or inflammatory changes but significant differences were noted in other aspects of their performance. Sorbsan tended to spread more exudate onto the surrounding skin, Algosteril tended to adhere more to the wound surface than Comfeel Alginate, and Kaltostat left significantly more dressing residues on the wound surface at dressing removal than the Comfeel Alginate dressing.[139]

The tissue compatibility of alginate dressings and their apparent lack of toxicity is illustrated by the work of Wu et al.[140] who showed that when alginate sponge was placed in a 5-mm gap created in the dorsal ramus of the facial nerve of each of five cats, movement of the upper eyelids and electrophysiological function were restored 12 weeks postoperatively. Histological examination confirmed that many new myelinated axons were observed in the original gap 16 weeks after operation, but no alginate residue was detected. In a control group of animals, no movement or electrophysiological restoration was recorded, and there were few regenerated axons accompanied by a large amount of scar tissue. The nerve repaired with alginate showed remarkable regeneration.

Cellular and biochemical effects

It has been observed that alginate-based microcapsules containing islets of Langerhans used as a bioartificial pancreas produce a foreign body reaction with fibrosis in an animal model. Pueyo et al.[141] demonstrated that macrophage cells involved in this process can be produced from monocytes activated by alginate-polylysine microcapsules in vitro.

Otterlei et al.[142] compared the ability of alginates to stimulate human monocytes to produce three important cytokines: tumour necrosis factor-α (TNF-α), interleukin-1 and interleukin-6. They reported that high-M alginates were approximately ten times more potent in inducing cytokine production than high G alginates and therefore proposed that mannuronic acid residues are the active cytokine inducers in alginates.

Others workers have also produced evidence to suggest that it is the β(1→ 4) glycosidic linkage (M Blocks) rather than the α(1→ 4) linkage (G Blocks) that is responsible for cytokine stimulation and anti-tumour activity. These β(1→ 4) bonds are found linking D-glucuronic acid in C-6-oxidised cellulose which also has demonstrable TNF-α stimulating activity although this is limited compared with that of alginate rich in mannuronic acid.[143]

Unpublished data from Shalby et al., cited in a review by Skjak-Braek and Espevik,[144] indicated that β(1→ 4) linked uronic-acid polymers such as poly M are potent cytokine inducers in vivo, able to protect mice against lethal infections with S. aureus or E. coli. It is also stated that they can provide a marked degree of protection against lethal irradiation by increasing the production of myeloid blood cells by stimulating haematopoietic cells in the bone marrow. Further evidence for the importance of high concentrations of M Blocks comes from the finding that treatment of alginate with a high mannuronic acid content with C-5 epimerase (which converts β-D-mannuronic acid into α-L-guluronic acid) results in a loss of TNF inducing ability.[144]

Zimmerman et al.[145] and Klock et al.[146] disputed the difference in activity of M and G alginates following studies in which they tested different types of alginates for mitogenic activity both in vivo and in vitro before and after purification by free flow electrophoresis and dialysis.[147] They found that material treated in this way lost all its mitogenic properties regardless of the M/G ratio of the raw material and suggested that this activity could be partly due to oligomers of mannuronic or guluronic acids. They also identified positively charged fractions with strong mitogenic activity that they proposed was LPS or LPS-related but this observation is not in accord with the earlier work conducted by Otterlei et al.[142] who demonstrated that mitogenic activity in alginates was not inhibited by the addition of Polymixin B which they showed, was able to inhibit LPS-induced cytokine production.

LPS consists of a lipid A, a core oligosaccharide and a polysaccharide part of varying size and complexity. In their review Skjak-Braek and Espevik[144] state that LPS and poly M alginate share a common binding site on the macrophage, reacting with the membrane protein CD-14 which is believed to have a broad specificity for compounds rich in various types of sugar residues. They also report that the binding of poly M and LPS to monocytes can be inhibited by addition of G-blocks. Unlike LPS which can stimulate cells that do not express membrane CD-14, poly M is unable to stimulate cell types that lack this membrane protein. Skjak-Braek and Espevik conclude their review by proposing that 'poly M may activate the non-specific immune system resulting in increased protection against various types of infections.'

Doyle et al.[148] investigated the effect of calcium alginate dressings upon other cell types and showed that low concentrations of an extract of one alginate dressing, Sorbsan, stimulated human fibroblasts upon extended contact but decreased the proliferation of human microvascular endothelial cells and keratinocytes. They proposed that this activity could be due to calcium ions released from the dressing during the gelling process.

The possibility that alginate might stimulate or accelerate healing by activating macrophages present within a wound was investigated by Thomas et al.[149] Alginate fibres taken from four commercially available dressings were co-cultured with the human histiocytic lymphoma cell line U937 following its differentiation with PMA. Activation was assessed by measurement of TNF alpha production.

Two of the dressings, Comfeel Seasorb and Tegagen, had a minimal effect, but Sorbsan, at one mg/mL, induced 302 ± 19 pg/mL TNF alpha. This effect was inhibited by polymyxin B indicating that activation was due to endotoxin contamination. Kaltostat induced production of 839 ± 36 pg/mL TNF alpha. This effect was induced both by polymyxin inhibitable endotoxin and a direct interaction with the alginate fibres. These data indicate that some alginate containing dressings have the potential to activate macrophages within the chronic wound bed and generate a pro-inflammatory signal which may initiate a resolving inflammation characteristic of healing wounds.

When later, Nakagawa et al.[150] produced aqueous extracts of alginates and subjected them to the Limulus amoebocyte lysate (LAL) test they detected high levels of activity in extracts from three products made from calcium alginate. These extracts also induced a pyrogenic response in rabbits and induced the release of a pro-inflammatory (pyrogenic) cytokine, interleukin-6 (IL-6), from human monocytic cells (MM6-CA8). These effects were eliminated when the extracts were treated with endotoxin-removing gel column chromatography or with an endotoxin antagonist, suggesting that the contaminating pyrogen was indeed due to the presence of endotoxins.

Summary of properties of alginate dressings

Calcium alginate dressings vary in structure and chemical composition. These differences influence the gelling and fluid handling properties of the products, which have important implications for their absorbency and method of use, particularly the removal of the dressing from the wound. The possibility that these differences may have implications for healing and infection rates in the wounds to which they are applied has not been seriously considered or investigated in the past

Despite the substantial number of alginate dressings used each year, relatively few publications have been produced to provide robust statistically convincing evidence to justify their use in any particular type of wound. Such randomized trials that have been performed often produce conflicting results, or are of limited value for other reasons. This may be because the comparator chosen is not widely used in clinical practice or the way in which the dressings have been applied has adversely affected their performance. Alginates require the application of an appropriate secondary dressing in order to function optimally. An absorbent pad is usually necessary for heavily exuding wounds, but for more lightly exuding wounds or wounds that are approaching the end of the healing process a semipermeable film or foam may be more appropriate to prevent desiccation of the primary dressing. The choice of secondary dressing is critical as it can have a major influence on treatment outcomes and should be considered when designing or undertaking studies with alginate dressings. This was elegantly demonstrated in an animal study conducted by Pirone et al.[151] who compared two types of alginate dressings covered with either a polyurethane film or gauze with a hydrocolloid dressing in partial thickness wounds in pigs. Twelve wounds were made on the backs of each of six pigs and the return of the epithelial barrier function was measured with an evaporimeter. They found that the resultant healing rate was related to the moisture retaining properties of the dressing system. The hydrocolloid dressing, the most occlusive of the systems evaluated produced the fastest rate of healing followed by the alginate and film combination. Healing was significantly slower beneath alginate and gauze, leading the authors to suggest that alginate dressings should not be used on dry wounds or under gauze dressings. Despite this excellent advice, several clinical studies have since been published using this dressing combination.

There is convincing evidence that when used appropriately, alginate dressings are superior to paraffin gauze in the management of donor sites, reducing healing times and pain and trauma associated with dressing changes. Moistening the alginate with a suitable local anaesthetic agent may provide further pain relief. The results of studies that suggest that scarlet red ointment dressing is superior to alginates should be regarded with caution in the light of the extended healing times recorded with both products. It is likely that these are due to the use of inappropriate secondary dressings.

There is also evidence to suggest that alginates may be superior to paraffin gauze in the treatment of leg ulcers but the influence of the primary dressing is minimal compared to that of external graduated compression in the treatment of ulcers that are venous in origin.

Alginate dressings also appear to a have role in the treatment of different types of wounds that are left to heal by secondary intention following some form of surgical procedure.

The literature on the use of alginates as haemostatic agents is confusing. Whilst there is little doubt that the material is an effective haemostatic agent, a number of publications suggest that if it is left *in situ*, it may cause a foreign body reaction and impede wound healing. Others workers have reported, however, that alginate is completely absorbed with no adverse effects.

From this review it seems likely that there are three factors which need to be considered. These are the chemical nature of the alginate, the amount of fibre implanted and the vascularity of the tissue at the site of implantation. The evidence would tend to suggest that small quantities of a fast-gelling alginate implanted into a very vascular area will be eliminated rapidly, but large amounts of fibres of a slow gelling material tightly packed into a relatively poorly vascularised area will remain in place for an extended period. Further work is probably required to answer this question.

There is evidence to suggest that alginate dressings may have an effect of wound healing at the cellular level. It is suggested that they are able to stimulate the production of cytokines and other biologically active molecules from key cells involved in the healing process. There is also some evidence to suggest that this effect is greatest in alginates that are rich in mannuronic acid, although some workers dispute this, claiming that the activity is related to the presence of a contaminant or breakdown product and is lost if the material is highly purified.

Any assessment of the value of alginates in wound care is made particularly difficult by the fact that there is no such thing as a 'standard' alginate dressing. Alginates, even those derived from a single species of seaweed, are subject to minor variations in composition and structure but this variation can be considerable when products from different species are compared.

Variations in the MG ratio will influence the nature of the gel that is formed when the dressing is applied to an exuding wound. A high-M product, particularly if it contains a proportion of sodium alginate will form a thick soft gel as the fibres take up liquid and swell. A high-G alginate, particularly one composed entirely of calcium alginate will change very little as it absorbs exudate for the degree of swelling of the individual fibres is very limited.

It is tempting to speculate that as the high-M alginate fibres swell they could absorb within their structure, agents present in wound fluid that have a deleterious effect on the healing process. These might include bacteria, proteolytic enzymes, toxins etc. This effect would occur to a much lesser extent with fibres that swell only slightly.

It is also not unreasonable to suppose that a fibre that gels readily and dissolves more easily in biological fluids would be eliminated from tissue more quickly than one which resisted the dissolution process. In 1949 Rumble[112] recognised the importance of selecting the right type of alginate for treating post-extraction haemorrhage to ensure rapid absorption of the fibre. Few if any of the authors of the modern clinical papers appear to be equally aware of the characteristics of the different types of alginates or recognise their importance. It is interesting to note that the majority of implantation studies involving alginates have been conducted using a high-G alginate.

The fluid-handling properties of alginate dressings have been discussed in some detail, particularly the importance that is given to the absorbency values determined experimentally. It is not uncommon to see publications that state that alginates are suitable for the management of heavily exuding wounds because they absorb up to 20 times their own weight of fluid. Whilst it is true that alginates are capable of taking up many times their own weight of solution, a standard 10×10 cm alginate dressing only weighs about 1-2 grams and therefore the total amount of fluid that it can absorbed will be limited.

To put this into context, leg ulcers have typically been found to produce up to 0.5 mL of exudate/cm^2/24 hours but in the presence of infection this may double. For a wound 20 cm^2 in area, that could be dressed with a single piece of alginate dressing measuring 10×10 cm, this would equate to the production of 10 - 20 mL of fluid per day.

The fluid handling capacity of alginate dressings ranges from about 15 - 25 grams/100 cm^2 (*not* grams per gram). Under a compression bandage this may be reduced to somewhere between five and 10 mL. A standard 10×10 cm dressing would therefore be unable to cope with the exudate produced from a 20 cm^2 wound for more than about 12 hours.

The application of a standard film dressing, which has a *maximum* moisture vapour transmission rate of approximately 1000 grams/m^2/24hours,[152] placed over an alginate sheet would in practice allow the loss of about a further five grams of fluid in 24 hours, making a total fluid handling capacity for an alginate/film dressing combination of 10 - 15 mL in the first day. This is still less than the volume of fluid produced by a heavily exuding leg ulcer or donor site. On the second day, however, the alginate dressing, being fully saturated, would be unable to absorb any further exudate and therefore fluid would rapidly accumulate beneath the dressing resulting in leakage and/or maceration of the surrounding skin. This effect was observed clinically by Moody.[55]

The application of a so-called 'intelligent' film dressing over a sheet of alginate might partially resolve the problems described above. In the presence of liquid, such films have an MVTR of 5,000-10,000 grams/m^2/24 hours, which would greatly enhance the ability of the dressing to cope with exudate production. As the wound begins to dry, the MVTR of the film would decrease and thus help to preserve moisture in the alginate fibre. Such a combination could prove particularly valuable in the treatment of donor sites.

The principal benefits to be gained from the use of alginate dressings lay in their ability to form a moist environment on the wound surface that facilitates optimal wound healing and permits pain and trauma-free removal. They should therefore be regarded as low-adherent, gel-forming interface layers rather than as absorbent dressings in their own right. This description emphasises the importance of an appropriate secondary dressing to control moisture vapour loss and provide a bacterial barrier function.

One of the principal criticisms often levelled at alginate dressings, in common with many other 'modern' wound management materials is one of price. Many modern materials are significantly more expensive than traditional dressings, when compared on a unit cost basis. However, such simple cost comparisons are artificial, as they take no account of the effectiveness of the materials concerned. The method of comparison is particularly important when calculating the total cost of managing chronic wounds. Leg ulcers that are claimed to be of 20 - 30 years' duration are commonly encountered, and it is obvious that any dressing or treatment that can facilitate healing in such wounds in a reasonable time, regardless of unit cost, must be worthy of serious consideration. Most financial arguments relating to the cost effectiveness of dressings, particularly in the community revolve around the nursing costs associated with dressing changes. Reducing the frequency of dressing changes can result in significant savings in nurse time and travelling costs.[153] A detailed costing system which took account of treatment failure as well as success has been described previously.[56]

The differences between the various types of alginates described within this review may not be limited to their physical properties. In 1992 a survey was conducted into the management of fungating wounds and radiation damaged skin by specialist centres throughout the UK.[154] The results revealed that although the 114 respondents considered that Sorbsan and Kaltostat were equivalent in terms of their fluid handling properties, Sorbsan was considered to be much superior to Kaltostat in the treatment of malodorous, necrotic or infected wounds, even scoring more highly than some products containing activated charcoal or recognised antimicrobial agents.

These subjective opinions may have some scientific basis, for the review has identified numerous references which suggest that the relatively small differences in the structure of the alginate dressings may have important implications for the way in which they perform at a cellular level within the wound.

Many of these references consider the interaction between the alginate molecule and macrophage cells that play a key role in many physiological and patho-physiological processes by synthesising various biologically active molecules called cytokines. A major cytokine secreted by macrophages is tumour necrosis factor-α (TNF-α) also known as cachectin, which is produced when the cells is exposed to endotoxins, lipopolysaccharide molecules (LPS) derived from bacterial cell walls. TNF-α was first described as a tumour cytotoxic agent when it was established it had cytotoxic properties against both tumour cells and normal cells infected with intracellular pathogens. It is also a very important inflammatory mediator which modulates many physiological and immunological functions and has been implicated in inflammatory conditions such as rheumatoid arthritis, Crohn's disease, multiple sclerosis and the cachexia associated with cancer or human immunodeficiency virus infections. Experimentally it has been shown that the production of endotoxin induced TNF-α inhibits the effect of growth factors in the area of a wound, which results in decreased collagen production and eventually to impairment of the healing process.[155] A reduction in collagen production has similarly been shown to result from the direct application of TNF-α to human and animal fibroblasts *in vitro*.[156] Paradoxically, however, it has been suggested that the ability of TNF-α to inhibit collagen formation may be beneficial in foetal wounds where it will limit fibroplasia and thus reduce scarring.[157]

The ability of a macrophage to function in this way depends upon the successful completion of the differentiation pathway of immature precursor cells to the mature macrophage. Circulating blood monocytes emigrate into extravascular tissue either to become resident organ-specific mature macrophages or to be recruited as immune effector cells at sites of inflammation, injury, and allograft or tumour rejection. Macrophages have been shown to be the main cell type that essentially regulates the wound-healing cascade. Their deactivation leads to termination of the wound healing process. Wound macrophages can be stimulated (activated) by both endogenous and exogenous factors including, it appears, alginates. It is interesting to speculate if this activity could be the reason for the preferred use of a high M alginate in the treatment of infected or malodorous wounds as highlighted in the survey described previously.

CARBOXYMETHYLCELLULOSE DRESSINGS

Development of carboxymethylcellulose dressings

Cellulose is a naturally occurring polymer which is the principal structural element of all plants. Native cellulose such as cotton fibre, is poorly degradable in living tissue but it is possible to chemically modify cellulose to form derivatives some of which are readily absorbed by animal tissue.[158]

A particularly useful cellulose derivative is carboxymethyl cellulose (CMC) which is widely employed in medical applications. Like salts of alginic acid, CMC it is used as a hydrophilic thickening agent in a variety of cosmetic and food products such as toothpaste and ice cream and has also been used as an absorbent in dressing pads and incontinence products and is the principal gel forming component of hydrocolloid dressings such as Granuflex (Duoderm). In the late 1990s, a process was developed which enabled sodium carboxymethylcellulose (CMC) to be produced in a fibrous form. This represented new opportunities in the wound care market, and in 1997 a new dressing, consisting of 100% CMC fibre, was launched by Convatec Ltd with the brand name of Aquacel.

Aquacel is available in sheet form for shallow or surface wounds, and in the form of a ribbon for packing deeper cavities. In both presentations the individual fibres have been entangled using an interlocking needling process, which imparts significant tensile strength to the final fabric.

The manufacturers of Aquacel have described the new fibre as a 'Hydrofibre', a trademarked term, which probably has more marketing value than scientific merit. In an attempt to differentiate Aquacel from the alginate products and capitalise upon the commercial success of the Granuflex (Duoderm) range, they have also described Aquacel as a 'hydrocolloid' fibre. Regrettably the Drug Tariff and British National Formulary (BNF) have unfortunately adopted this description. As a result in both these publications the dressing is listed with the hydrocolloid sheets dressings rather than with the alginate products, which it much more closely resembles in structure, function and usage. ActivHeal Aquafibre, Advanced Medical Solutions is also made from CMC.

Suprasorb X (previously Xcell) from Lohmann Rauscher (Activa Healthcare in UK) although similar in appearance to the other CMC dressings is manufactured from processed bacterial cellulose as described below.

As previously indicated, CMC fibre can also be blended with alginate fibre to improve the wet strength, fluid handling and cohesive properties of the final dressing. Products made from a blend of fibres include:

- Askina Sorb
- Carboflex
- Seasorb Soft
- Urgosorb
- Maxorb Extra

Effect of CMC fibre on the histology of experimental wounds

The effect of Aquacel on partial-thickness wounds in the rat was investigated by Hoekstra *et al.*,[159] who examined the acute inflammatory infiltrate of granulocytes and macrophages in the wound and the dressing using a partial-thickness wound model on the backs of 60 anaesthetized male Wistar rats. Half of the wounds were dressed with Aquacel and the remainder with paraffin gauze. The rats were sacrificed on postoperative days 1, 2, 3, 4, 7 and 10 (ten animals per day and five per dressing) and the excised wounds were examined for polymorphonuclear (PMN), fibronectin and macrophage activity; the degree of reepithelialization was also estimated.

Compared with wounds dressed with paraffin gauze, Aquacel-dressed wounds contained relatively few PMN leucocytes (granulocytes), but large numbers of active PMNs were detected in the dressing carried there by the flow of exudate and also possibly attracted by the presence of fibronectin, which was clearly detectable around the CMC fibres. It was postulated by the authors that the presence of these cells helped to create an appropriate antimicrobial environment within the dressing.

Somewhat later in the acute phase of the healing process, it was found that became adhered to the wound bed by a layer of fibrin, which also acted as a barrier, preventing the migration of macrophages from the wound into the dressing. It was suggested that this barrier might protect the wound from matrix metalloproteinases enzymes produced by the granulocytes trapped within the dressing. It was further proposed that the separation of the granulocytes from the PMNs meant that the macrophages received minimal direct stimulation from the granulocytes, which limited their inflammatory activity enabling them to function primarily in the repair mode. In comparison with Aquacel-dressed wounds where the dressing remained on top of the wound, those dressed with paraffin gauze showed a more disturbed pattern of epithelial outgrowth with evidence of incorporation of fibres into the wound bed.

The authors concluded that these histological findings correlated well with published clinical experiences in relation to the speed of reepithelialization and the level of scarring associated with the use of Aquacel.

Mechanisms of action

When brought into contact with liquid, the individual fibres of the Aquacel dressing absorb liquid directly into their structure causing them to swell and form a gel. The gelling properties of Aquacel are illustrated graphically in Figure 52 where they are compared with those of several different alginate dressings. (This figure has been constructed from the data in Table 18.) These results indicate that the diameter of the Aquacel fibre increases by a factor of ten as it absorbs fluid, twice as much as the nearest alginate product.

The swelling characteristics of the fibres and the volume of solution absorbed, is greatly influenced by its composition, for the presence of salts or proteins in the test solution significantly reduces the absorbent capacity of the dressing compared with values obtained with distilled water. The results of fluid handling studies, which compared the absorbent capacity of Aquacel with that of the alginate dressings, have been shown previously in Table 19 and Figure 51.

Figure 52: Swelling characteristics of polysaccharide fibres

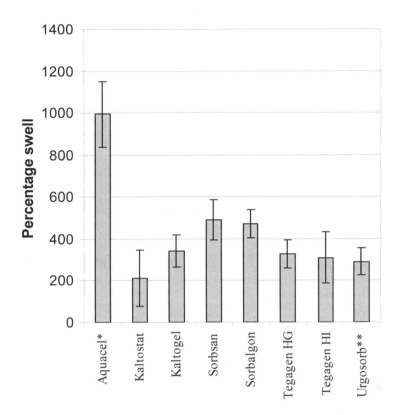

An intact dressing initially absorbs exudate by vertical wicking, which allows rapid uptake of wound fluid, preventing it from spreading over peripheral skin. As additional liquid is taken up it is gradually distributed laterally throughout the structure but remains within the body of the dressing and so is not released onto the surrounding skin where it might cause maceration.

The results of laboratory studies undertaken by Bowler *et al.*,[160] led the authors to suggest that this property of the dressing to absorb and retain fluid within the structure of the fibre might provide a passive mechanism for reducing the microbial load in wounds and the surrounding environment. They therefore used an *in vitro* model to investigate and compare such properties in a range of fibrous absorbent dressings (alginate, CMC and hydrophobic).

Dressings were challenged with a simulated wound fluid containing the common wound pathogens *S. aureus* and *P. aeruginosa*, and bacterial sequestering and binding levels were monitored over time. The CMC dressing and two calcium alginate dressings were shown to effectively sequester challenge organisms from a simulated wound fluid.

However, the hydrophobic and CMC dressings produced statistically significant different results in their ability to adsorb and retain the challenge organisms ($p < 0.05$). The authors showed that the ability of Aquacel to take up and retain bacteria was considerably greater than that of two alginate dressings tested in the same way, although they conceded that further studies were required to determine the clinical relevance of this observation.

The same team later used scanning electron microscopy to demonstrate that upon hydration of Aquacel, the resultant cohesive gel effectively encapsulated large populations of potentially pathogenic bacteria such as *P. aeruginosa* and *S. aureus* under the gelled surface and within the swollen fibres. In contrast, hydrated alginate wound dressings did not form a uniform, cohesive gel structure, with the result that fewer bacteria were immobilised within the gel matrix. It was intimated that this property of the dressing might have important clinical implications for combating or preventing the development of infection.[161]

This was later confirmed using an animal model in which pieces of alginate, Sorbsan and Kaltostat, and CMC dressings were applied to experimental wounds on the backs of rats which had been inoculated with either *S. aureus* or *P. aeruginosa* at a concentration of 1.5×10^6 colony-forming units per wound.[162] After 12 hours each dressing was divided into two pieces. Total viable bacterial count within the dressing was calculated using one piece, and bacterial count released from the dressing into physiological saline was determined using the other, enabling bacterial retention rate to be calculated. Bacterial counts in tissue were also determined. Each dressing was tested on each of ten wounds contaminated with each bacterium. Statistical analyses were performed using one-way analysis of variance (ANOVA). The CMC dressing was found to be the most effective in terms of its ability to retain both *S. aureus* and *P. aeruginosa* ($p < 0.05$). However, bacterial counts in tissue showed no significant change with respect to pathogen or the type of dressing used which calls into question the clinical relevance of these observations.

Unlike alginate dressings, Aquacel fibre is not thought to interact chemically with exudate and there is no suggestion that it has any effect upon angiogenesis or any of the cellular processes involved in wound healing.

Method of use

It is recommended that on shallow wounds a single sheet dressing should be cut or folded so that it overlaps the margin of the wound by at least 1 cm, but for larger wounds multiple dressings may be required. Deep cavity wounds may be dressed with the ribbon, which should be folded into the wound but not packed in too tightly to allow for swelling. A moisture-retentive secondary dressing is then added to complete the process. The interval between dressing changes will be determined by the condition of the wound. On clean lightly exuding wounds the dressing may remain undisturbed for up to seven days but on infected or heavily exuding wounds more frequent changes will be required. Under normal conditions of use the dressing may be regarded as non-adherent by virtue of its gel forming properties. If problems of adherence are encountered on lightly exuding wounds irrigation with sterile water or saline should facilitate removal.

Clinical indications

The marked similarities in the appearance and physical properties of Aquacel and alginate dressings such as Sorbsan, clearly suggest that the products will have a similar range of indications, specifically all types of exuding wounds including problem wounds which may or may not contain a limited amount of soft slough or necrotic tissue. Clinical experience to date supports this view and a number of papers have been published that describe the use of the dressing in the treatment of a many different wound types including necrotizing fasciitis,[163] a squamous cell carcinoma of the anal canal,[164] a recurrent pilonidal sinus,[165] a patient with complex multiple wounds,[166] a heavily exuding sinus in a breast,[167] Fournier's gangrene in an HIV-positive man,[168] and following surgery to correct Dupuytren pathology in 52 patients.[169]

More structured, prospective, studies involving Aquacel have also been reported that describe its use in the treatment of a variety of wound types.

Leg ulcers

Armstrong and Ruckley[153] reported upon a multicentre, prospective, randomized trial involving 44 patients with exuding leg ulcers in which they compared Aquacel with Kaltostat in terms of dressing performance, patient comfort, safety and cost-effectiveness. The groups were well matched with regard to sex and age. Although no statistically significant difference was detected in the healing rates achieved with the two dressings, a difference was recorded in mean wear time achieved with the two products, four days for Aquacel compared with three for Kaltostat.

This difference of 1.03 days was considered important as a full day is the minimum time difference that can realistically be expected to make any impact upon the work patterns of a community-based nurse. The authors suggested, however, that this difference could have been due to an imbalance in allocation to treatment in favour of the Aquacel, as five subjects in the alginate group had heavily exuding ulcers compared with one in the CMC-treated group. Nevertheless, they concluded from the results of this investigation that the CMC dressing might have clinical benefits that merit further investigation with larger patient numbers.

In this study, however, the primary dressing was covered by with a semipermeable film coated with a layer of a hydrocolloid adhesive, Duoderm Extra Thin, which has a relatively limited moisture vapour transmission rate. Dressing changes were performed if leakage of liquid had occurred from beneath the adhesive dressing. The end point of this study was therefore largely determined not just by the performance of the primary dressing but also by the strength of the adhesive bond between the adhesive film and the skin. This would be affected by the amount of liquid that accumulated at the lowest point of the dressing, which in turn would be determined by the size of the wound and the extent to which the film dressing overlaps onto the surrounding good skin.

Following a second larger multicentre leg ulcer study that compared Aquacel with Sorbsan involving 132 evaluable patients, lasting a maximum of 84 days, significant preference were reported for the Aquacel product in terms of ease of application and removal of the dressing. As in the previous study it was found that the use of the Aquacel was associated with increased intervals between dressing changes with beneficial effects upon treatment costs.[170]

Donor sites

Like alginate dressings, the gel forming ability of CMC fibrous dressings suggest that these materials could be of value in the treatment of painful exuding wounds such as split-thickness skin graft donor sites. This possibility was examined by Barnea et al.[171] who compared it with the standard paraffin gauze dressings in a study involving 23 adults. In each case one half of the donor sites were dressed with paraffin gauze, the remainder with Aquacel. CMC-dressed wounds produced significantly less pain and healed more rapidly than those dressed with paraffin gauze. One year later at follow up, the cosmetic appearance of Aquacel-treated wounds was superior to that achieved with paraffin gauze.

Burns

The value of Aquacel in the treatment of partial thickness burns was investigated by Vloemans et al.[172] in a study involving 84 patients with burns covering from 1% - 18% of the total body surface area (TBSA).

Of the 84 patients, 76 had previously received one or two days pre-treatment with a topical antimicrobial agent. Two patients developed signs of a clinical wound infection during treatment, but in general wound cultures were low or negative. The wounds of 42 patients healed completely within ten days but in six patients small defects remained that healed by further treatment with a topical antimicrobial cream. In 36 patients excision and grafting of the remaining deeper parts of the wounds was undertaken, the standard protocol in the centre for all burned areas that have not healed within 2-3 weeks post-injury. Even in these wounds however, the extent of the surgical procedures was limited since 66.1% of the wound area had healed during the initial phase of treatment.

After 2-3 months the wounds of 54 patients were examined using the Vancouver Scar Scale when generally favourable results were recorded particularly in those patients who did not require surgery. The authors concluded that the CMC dressing is a safe, suitable and easy to use material for treatment of partial thickness burns.

In a second study the same authors compared the fibrous CMC dressing with glycerol preserved allograft skin in a randomized trial involving 80 patients conducted over a two year period. As before burns that had not reepithelialized following 14 ± 3 days treatment were debrided and grafted or, if small enough, managed with a topical antimicrobial agent. No significant differences were detected between the groups in number of patients with superficial or deep burns. Of the wounds dressed with the CMC dressing, 24/40 healed completely compared with 27/40 in the group that received an allograft. It was recorded, however, that post-study more excision and grafting was required in the CMC group than in the allograft group, 45% vs 15%, (p = 0.004). At follow-up ten weeks later, no significant differences were seen in the appearance of the resultant scars but skin elasticity, was significantly greater in the allograft-treated group (p = 0.010). These differences were no longer detectable after six months and one year follow-up. The incidence of hypertrophy after six months was higher, but not significantly, in the CMC group compared to the allograft skin group, 52.5% *vs* 30%, (p = 0.09).

Based upon their experience with the CMC dressing, the authors concluded that allograft skin was to be preferred for larger burns of mixed depth, but for partial thickness and small burns the CMC dressing could be considered to be the treatment of choice.

Surgical wounds

Like alginate dressings, Aquacel also has potential value in surgical wounds. Moore and Foster[173] in a prospective randomized controlled trial compared the benefits of Aquacel and ribbon gauze soaked in proflavine in 40 patients with acute surgical wounds left to heal by secondary intention. The clinical results showed that although there was no significant difference in healing rates, patients treated with Aquacel experienced less pain and required less analgesia. An analysis of financial implications of the two treatments revealed that although the CMC dressing was more expensive than the gauze on a unit cost basis, the total cost of each patient episode was less, £295 *vs* £680 (p = 0.01) and early discharge was facilitated.[174] The authors concluded that in an average UK Health authority with a population of 300,000, one hundred bed days a year could be saved by the use of this treatment, equivalent to an overall potential saving of £55,000.

In a further study,[175] the same group then compared Aquacel with Sorbsan in a 100 patients with similar acute wounds healing by secondary intention. Although both dressings performed well, the authors reported that the CMC product outperformed the alginate in terms of ease of use and removal although this effect did not achieve statistical significance.

Vogt *et al.*[176] compared Aquacel with a simple absorbent island dressing in the management of primary closed wounds following vascular surgery to compare patient comfort, cost-effectiveness, infections, wound complications, and length of hospital stay. One hundred and sixty patients were randomized to receive either Mepore or Aquacel dressing. No significant difference was noted in patient comfort between the two groups, but treatment costs were higher in the Aquacel group despite significantly fewer changes of dressings in these patients. No difference was noted in the infection rate, 13% *vs* 11%, (p = 0.73), length of hospital stay, or wound complications between the two groups. However, the basic rational for undertaking this study is not clear as Aquacel would not normally be considered as a dressing for wounds that have been closed surgically.

. A more appropriate indication is for the treatment of open wounds healing by secondary intention. Cohn *et al.*[177] randomized 50 patients with open surgical wounds to treatment with Aquacel or wet-to-dry gauze. Wound healing was measured as a reduction in volume for deep wounds or the reduction in area for shallow wounds by an investigator blinded to treatment.

Seven patients were withdrawn from the study after the first evaluation. Of the remaining 43 patients, 21 were in the gauze group and 22 were treated with Aquacel. For deep wounds, a mean change in the wound healing rate of 1.9 ± 1.3 cm^3 per day was reported for the gauze group and 2.9 ± 2.3 cm^3 per day for the Aquacel group. These results approached, but did not achieve, statistical significance (p = 0.082). For superficial wounds, the mean change in the healing rate was 1.6 ± 1.5 cm^2 per day for the gauze group and 1.9 ± 2.2 cm^2 per day for the Aquacel group, suggesting that Aquacel appears to be at least as effective as wet-to-dry gauze in the healing of open surgical wounds.

The cost of treating wounds with Aquacel or gauze was compared using a theoretical model by Guest,[178] who, based upon published data, calculated that there were probably cost advantages associated with the use of the CMC dressing because of reduced nursing costs associated with a lower frequency of dressing changes compared to gauze.

Orthopaedic wounds

Aquacel, like the alginate dressings, has been successfully used together with a semipermeable film as a secondary dressing. Folestad[179] described the use of this combination in 27 patients undergoing total hip arthroplasty in the Molndal and Orebro hospitals and compared the results with those achieved in 14 patients whose wounds were dressed with traditional dressings consisting of an adhesive dressing and absorbent pad secured by tape and adhesive net. A further 17 patients undergoing total knee arthroplasty were also randomized to receive standard treatment (n = 8) or Aquacel and film (n = 9) dressing. The aims of the study were to determine whether the novel dressing would delay the first dressing change and reduce the frequency of changes thereafter. Following hip surgery, wounds dressed with the Aquacel/film combination required a mean 2.4 changes per patient compared with 6.2 for the comparator. The corresponding figures for knee surgery were 2.3 and 4.7 respectively. There was also a marked but non-significant difference in the number of blood soaked dressings that required changing. On the basis of these results, the authors reported that 60 of the 80 orthopaedic centres in Sweden have since adopted the Molndal dressing technique.

A common problem following hip or knee surgery is the development of a blister around the operation site. This problem is most commonly associated with the use of adhesive dressings, the limited extensibility of which can lead to the development of shear forces during movement of the affected limb. Harle *et al.*[180] compared the Molndal dressing with conventional management in a randomized trial involving 100 patients to determine if the two treatments varied in this regard. At the first dressing change, 59% of the patients dressed with Aquacel and film exhibited skin reactions such as blisters, erythema, oedema, skin injury and haematoma compared with 81% in the control group. (p = 0.02). The average cost of the materials used per patient by the third postoperative day was €14.70 for the Molndal dressing and €8.70 for the conventional treatment (p < 0.01) but this figure was considered insignificant given the fact that the cost of the dressings represented only about 0.02% of the total cost of hip replacement surgery.

In a similar study involving 200 patients undergoing an orthopaedic procedure, 183 of whom provided evaluable data, a self-adhesive island dressing, Cutiplast, was compared with Aquacel used with a semipermeable film. In this study it was reported that this combination was 5.8 times more likely to result in a wound with no complications compared to the application of a Cutiplast dressing (p < 0.00001). A significant difference in wound pain was also noted between the two treatments in favour of the alginate and film.[181]

Abuzakuk,[182] also compared Aquacel with and an adhesive island dressing, Mepore, in 61 patients receiving total hip or knee replacements. As in previous studies, compared with Mepore, the number of dressing changes in the Aquacel group was reduced before the fifth postoperative day (43% *vs* 77%). Fewer blister were detected in patients dressed with Aquacel (13% *vs* 26%)

Diabetic ulcers

Aquacel was evaluated in the treatment of diabetic ulcers by Piaggesi *et al.*[183] A group of consecutive out-patients with well perfused limbs and non-infected ulcers of > 3 weeks duration and deeper than one centimetre were recruited to the study. Twenty patients' lesions were surgically debrided and randomly assigned to treatment with saline-moistened gauze or Aquacel dressing. All patients in both groups received appropriate footwear and crutches until complete healing had been achieved.

After eight weeks the reduction in the volume of each wound was evaluated by an operator blinded to treatment. Ulcers dressed with Aquacel reduced in volume quicker (p < 0.01) and healed faster (p < 0.001) than those dressed with gauze, leading the authors to conclude that Aquacel was safe, effective and well tolerated in the management of non-ischaemic, non- infected deep diabetic foot ulcers.

HYALURONAN

Properties of hyaluronan

Hyaluronan, a glycosaminoglycan, also known as hyaluronic acid, hyaluronate or HA, is an extracellular matrix polysaccharide polymer that occurs widely in nature. Consisting of a linear polymer of alternating D-glucuronic acid N-acetylglucosamine disaccharide, it is found in all vertebrates and some lower marine organisms and bacteria.

Originally called hyaluronic acid, it was first isolated by Meyer and Palmer in 1934,[184] from the vitreous of the eye, although it has since been found in skin, synovial fluid, umbilical cord and rooster comb,[185] which is thought to be the principal commercial source. Significantly, the chemical structure of hyaluronan from all these different sources is identical, except for molecular weight differences. This means that material derived from one source or species will not be recognised as a 'foreign body' by another.

There exists a wealth of literature on hyaluronan, which has been comprehensively reviewed and summarised by Chen and Abatangelo.[186] The authors described its effects upon cytokine expression, cell proliferation, epithelial migration, reduction of scar formation, the production of granulation tissue and free radical scavenging, and concluded that hyaluronan has a 'multifaceted role in the mediation of the tissue repair process, from early in the inflammatory activation process through to granulation tissue formation and to the reepithelialization process'.

Hyaluronan is intensely hygroscopic, absorbing up to 3000 times its own weight of water to form a viscous hydrogel, which has a unique range of physical and chemical properties.[186]

Early studies with hyaluronic derivatives were reported by Davidson et al. in 1991[187] who used two animal models to compare the biological effects of hyaluronic acid and hyaluronic acid ethyl ester, a new hemisynthetic derivative in the form of a 0.2% (w/w) solution in a neutral sodium alginate vehicle. These preparations were examined in partial-thickness excisional wounds in pigs and full-thickness excisional wounds in the rabbit ear and applied daily under a polyurethane dressing. No evidence of toxicity or any other adverse effects were detected with either product but the rabbit ear model data suggested the possibility of a very slight inhibition of wound healing although clearly the effects of the alginate carrier could not be completely discounted. Hyaluronate-treated wounds tended to accumulate collagen more slowly, which the authors suggested, may reflect the ability of these materials to affect the scarring process.

The physical characteristics of hydrated hyaluronan combined with its limited stability meant that considerable practical difficulties had to be overcome in order to produce a product that was suitable for routine clinical use. This was eventually achieved by the controlled esterification of the carboxyl groups on the backbone of the molecule with benzyl alcohol to produce a family of biopolymers, the Hyaff series.[188]

By varying the degree of esterification it is possible to determine the solubility and biodegradation properties of the molecule which enables the material to be produced in a variety of physical forms such as microspheres, sponges, films or fibres from which various woven or nonwoven fabrics may be derived.

The physical characteristics of membranes made from benzyl hyaluronate esters, including their water vapour, oxygen and carbon dioxide transmission rates, were determined and compared with those of several commercial wound dressings by Ruiz-Cardona et al.[189] They concluded that the enhanced permeability of the benzyl hyaluronate membranes made them of potential value as wound dressings.

Several years later these membranes were used as a culture and transport medium for autologous keratinocytes obtained from three patients with chronic full-thickness ulcers of different aetiologies. The cells were isolated, cultured and then seeded on to the membrane and once sub-confluent, the sheets were then applied directly to the patients' ulcers. This technique was considered to improve graft handling, reduce total time required for tissue cultivation by facilitating grafting at a sub-confluent non-differentiated stage.[190]

The benzyl hyaluronate technology was later utilised to produce a three dimensional nonwoven scaffold designed to facilitate the culture of dermal fibroblasts, and a laser-drilled membrane that allowed migration of keratinocytes onto the wound bed.

These elements were utilised by Caravaggi, et al.,[191] to facilitate the production of autologous dermal and epidermal grafts for use in the management of diabetic foot ulcers. A total of 79 diabetics with dorsal (n = 37) or plantar (n = 42) ulcers were randomized to treatment with paraffin gauze (n = 36) or autologous tissue-engineered grafts (n = 43). A skin biopsy was taken from each patient randomized to the treatment group and sent to the TissueTech Autograft laboratory (Fidia Advanced Biopolymers, Abano Terme, Italy) for fibroblast and keratinocyte cell culturing. From the biopsy, fibroblasts and keratinocytes were isolated and propagated for subsequent passaging for 14 days. The cells were then seeded on the appropriate hyaluronate ester structure, and eight days after seeding, the resultant dermal grafts or epidermal sheets were ready for transplantation. Aggressive debridement, wound infection control procedures, and appropriate pressure relief were provided in both groups. Wounds were assessed weekly for up to 11 weeks. Complete ulcer healing was achieved in 65.3% of the treatment group and 49.6% of the control group (p = 0.191) and the mean time to closure was 57 vs 77 days for the treatment and control groups respectively. No adverse events attributable to either treatment were recorded. The authors suggested that the autologous tissue-engineered treatment exhibited improved healing in dorsal ulcers when compared with standard dressing treatment. For plantar ulcers, the use of the off-loading cast appeared to be of paramount importance and this masked or nullified the effects of the autologous wound treatment.

Given the expense and complexity of the treatment, however, it is argued that it would have been more appropriate to compare it with a more modern dressing, such as an alginates or CMC product, to ensure that it performed significantly better than these substantially cheaper treatment options for this indication.

An absorbent fibrous fleece manufactured from hyaluronan was marketed widely by Convatec under the brand name of Hyalofill. In this UK this arrangement has been discontinued but it is still believed to apply elsewhere, including the USA. Like the alginates and CMC dressings, Hyalofill is available in the form of a flat nonwoven matrix (Hyalofill-F) or a rope (Hyalofill-R) specifically designed for deeper irregular wounds or cavities. Both presentations are used in the same way as the other types of gel-forming fibrous absorbents. Upon contact with exudate the fibrous materials, forms a soft, cohesive gel on the wound surface. In this moist state, the esterification process is slowly reversed, resulting in the formation within the wound of hyaluronan and benzyl alcohol, a widely used pharmaceutical preservative with a well characterized, non toxic, metabolic route.[186] Hyalofill may last up to three days in the wound before completely degrading, depending upon amount of fluid present.

Davidson *et al.*[192] compared the effects of Hyalofill and an alginate dressing, Sorbsan, on the healing of experimental wounds in pigs. They found from morphometric and biochemical observations made upon the healing of deep excisional punch wounds in the Yutacan micro-pig that wounds dressed with Hyalofill healed much more quickly than those dressed with alginate (80% healed by day 9, compared with 40% at day 15).

Clinical experience with hyaluronan

Compared with many other types of modern dressings, the literature on the clinical use of hyaluronic acid and its derivates is relatively limited.

In an early publication Hollander *et al.*[193] described how it was used to treat a human bite and a haematoma, and in 2003 Vazquez *et al.*[194] described how 36 patients with foot ulcers associated with diabetes had their wounds surgically debrided and dressed with Hyalofill every other day for a maximum of 20 weeks. Hyalofill was applied until the wound bed was completely covered with granulation tissue at which point a moisture-retentive dressing was used until complete healing had occurred. In total, 75% of wounds healed in the 20-week evaluation period taking a mean 10 ± 4.8 weeks. The average duration of Hyalofill treatment in all patients was 8.6 ± 4.2 weeks. Deeper wounds were over 15 times less likely to heal than superficial wounds. The authors suggested that the hyaluronan-containing dressings may be a useful adjunct to appropriate diabetic foot ulcer care but suggested that the results of larger controlled trial were required to confirm this initial view.

An open, uncontrolled pilot study was performed by Colletta *et al.*,[195] to assess the value of Hyalofill-F in the treatment of venous leg ulcers when used in conjunction with compression bandaging. Twenty patients with venous insufficiency and a leg ulcer that had been refractory to treatment for one month were enrolled into the study and treated for up to eight weeks. Wounds were assessed weekly. During the study four ulcers healed completely and an average reduction in wound area of 53.5% was recorded in those wounds that did not achieved closure. The authors concluded that the dressing showed promised but once again concluded further studies were required to confirm its efficacy.

A year later the results of one such study were published when Hyalofill-F was compared with paraffin gauze dressings plus compression therapy in the treatment of 17 patients with 24 chronic venous leg ulcers.[196] Initially there were twelve ulcers in each group but six were withdrawn; one in the hyaluronan group because of a protocol violation and five in the paraffin gauze group because of a poor response to treatment and the development of a skin reaction. Hyalofill-F under compression performed significantly better than non-adherent gauze plus compression bandage in all of the parameters examined, which included levelling of wound margins and control of maceration. The mean reduction in ulcer area in the Hyalofill-F group was 8.1 cm^2 after eight weeks of treatment, compared with 0.4 cm^2 in the comparator group (p = 0.0019) leading the authors to concluded that that the dressing 'stimulates the healing response to compression therapy'.

Other preparations have also been developed that contain hyaluronan in various forms. In 2006 Voinchet[197] published the results of an open-label study designed to determine if hyaluronic acid could improve the healing of a range of acute wounds. Forty-three patients with traumatic wounds, surgical sutures, burns, and dermabrasions, were included in the study. Hyaluronic acid under the brand name Ialuset, Laboratoires Genévrier, was applied either in the form of a cream or as a dressing for a maximum of nine applications. During the course of the treatment, the mean surface area of the wounds decreased by an average 70%, from 556 mm^2 to 169 mm^2 by the sixth evaluation: complete healing occurred in 56%. Both presentation of hyaluronic acid were well tolerated and were rated highly by nurses and patients for ease of use and treatment satisfaction although the value of this study was limited by the relatively small number of patients, the variations in wound types and the lack of appropriate controls.

Meaume et al.[198] examined the effects of a preparation containing hyaluronic acid in the care of 125 patients with leg ulcers in a Phase III, prospective, randomized, multicentre, controlled study.

Ialuset Hydro - Laboratoires Genévrier, a hydrocolloid dressing containing hyaluronic acid, was compared with a standard hydrocolloid in the treatment of leg ulcers. Inclusion criteria included wounds of venous or mixed aetiology, active for at least two months with an area of 5 - 40 cm^2 and at least 50% of the wound area free of fibrinous deposits (slough). Sixty three patients were randomized to treatment with Ialuset Hydro and 62 to treatment with the reference hydrocolloid, Duoderm. Dressings were replaced when they reached saturation or after a maximum of seven days. Treatment was continued until closure or for a maximum of 42 days. Wounds were assessed after 1, 2, 7, 14, 28 and 42 days. The number of wounds that healed following treatment with Ialuset was over twice that in the control group, 15 vs 7 respectively. By day 42 the median reduction in the surface area of the ulcer was 42.6% in the Ialuset arm versus 31.0% in the reference hydrocolloid arm (p = 0.6). Improvements were also noted in other areas including the presence and severity of oedema, erythema, purpura and odours. The use of analgesics (paracetamol) was the same in the two groups.

The potential value of Ialuset cream as a treatment for pressure ulcers was investigated by Barrois et al.[199] in a multicentre, non-randomized, pilot study. Twenty one predominantly elderly patients with pressure ulcers of Grade II or above had their wounds treated with Ialuset cream over a 3-week period. Overall the treatment outcomes were described as 'good' or 'very good' by clinicians for 19/20 wounds reviewed, however, the authors acknowledged that further investigation in the form of large, randomized clinical trials were required to support these conclusions.

A cream containing 0.2% hyaluronic acid and 1% silver sulfadiazine (HA-SSD) (Connettivina Plus cream) was compared with a standard silver sulfadiazine cream in the treatment of 111 adult patients with recent superficial and deep dermal thermal burns. In a multicenter, randomized, double-blind, controlled, parallel-group study, patients were randomized to treatment with the appropriate cream which was applied daily for a maximum of four weeks or until the wounds healed. Both treatments were found to be effective and well tolerated. All burns healed, except one treated with SSD but on average wounds treated with HA-SSD healed in 4.5 days less than those in the control group. This difference was statistically significant (p = 0.0073).[200]

A high molecular weight complex prepared from sodium hyaluronate and an iodine salt, called Hyiodine, has been described by Sobotka,[201] and its properties evaluated both in the laboratory and in clinical studies. Frankova et al.[202] examined the effects of this material on several cell lines in culture. He found that it had no adverse effects upon viability and proliferation of the cells but it inhibited the PMA-activated oxidative burst and significantly increased the production of IL-6 and TNF-alpha by lymphocytes. Based upon these observations it was suggested that the hyaluronan content of Hyiodine reduces the toxic effect of KI3 complex on cells and speeds up the wound healing process by increasing the production of inflammatory cytokines.

The clinical benefits of Hyiodine were investigated by Sobotka et al.[201] in 22 patients suffering from complicated foot diabetic wounds. They reported that within 2-6 weeks following the initiation of treatment, all but two wounds were filled with granulation tissue and that complete healing was achieved in 18 patients within 6-20 weeks. They concluded that the preparation provided an effective treatment for difficult to heal diabetic defects without complete arterial occlusion.

CHITIN AND CHITOSAN

Chemistry of chitin

Chitin, poly-1,4-2-acetamido-2-deoxy-β-D-glucose is a naturally occurring polymer found in crustacean shells and the cell walls of fungi. It is produced commercially by deproteinisation and demineralization of shell waste of crabs, shrimps and krill, which typically contains about 15-25% of chitin.

Although chitin can be converted into a fibrous form, the process is complicated and not suited to large-scale production. Chitosan, a deacetylated derivative of chitin, which is freely soluble in acid, can easily be formed into fibres by extruding it into a coagulation bath of a dilute alkali. These fibres can then subsequently be converted back to chitin by re-acetylation with acetic anhydride.[203]

According to Muzzarelli[204] chitosan is unique among polysaccharides because of its susceptibility to enzymatic depolymerization within the body by lysozyme, N-acetylglucosaminidase and human chitinase, resulting in the formation of chito-oligomers and monomers that activate macrophages and stimulate fibroblasts respectively, resulting in production of smooth, vascularised and physiologically normal tissues.

Biochemical effects of chitin

Chung et al.[205] examined the effect of chitin/chitosan from a number of fungal sources on the rate of proliferation of human F1000 fibroblasts in culture. Extracts were prepared from *Aspergillus oryzae*, *Mucor mucedo*, and *Phycomyces blakesleeanus* cultures, which were estimated to contain 37, 52, and 91% chitin respectively. At 0.01% w/v, all three materials exhibited significant ($p < 0.05$) proproliferant activity over a period of 13 days. However, at 0.05% w/v, *P. blakesleeanus* further enhanced cell proliferation, whereas *A. oryzae* and *M. mucedo* produced a significant ($p < 0.05$) antiproliferant effect. Higher concentrations of *P. blakesleeanus* (0.1 and 0.5%) caused marked inhibition of F1000 cell proliferation when measured on days three and six. The authors concluded that only the proproliferant effect of these fungal materials appears to correlate to their chitin content. There was also evidence that the *P. blakesleeanus*, and to a lesser extent *M. mucedo*, possessed cell attractant properties which again correlated with chitin content. The authors proposed that the sporangiophores of *P. blakesleeanus* and the mycelium of *M. mucedo* could be used in wound management to promote fibroblast growth and provide a matrix for their anchorage.

Use of chitin as a dressing

Various derivatives of chitin and chitosan have been used as wound management materials with encouraging results. In laboratory studies reported by Muzzarelli[206] N-carboxybutyl chitosan was found to exhibit marked inhibitory activity against a large number of bacteria, producing morphological changes detectable by electron microscopy. Biagini et al.[207] in 1991, used this material in the form of soft freeze-dried pads to treat donor sites in a plastic surgery unit and reported that, compared with conventional treatment, the wounds showed better histoarchitectural order, improved vascularization and the absence of inflammatory cells at the dermal level. They concluded that N-carboxybutyl chitosan leads to formation of regularly organized cutaneous tissue and reduces anomalous healing. Similar benefits for the use of chitin in the treatment of donor sites were reported by Stone et al.[208]

Chitosan can be produced in a number of physical forms. Yusof et al.[209] prepared chitin beads with a carboxymethylated surface layer, capable of absorbing 95 times their dry weight of water, which the authors suggested had potential value as a component of wound dressings, and Hirano et al.[210] prepared chitin fibres containing 5 - 33% glycosaminoglycans some of which was released in the presence of tissue fluid.

Dai et al.[211] described a chitosan acetate bandage, HemCon, which when applied to full-thickness excisional wounds in mice that had been infected with pathogenic bioluminescent bacteria, P. aeruginosa, P. mirabilis, and S. aureus, rapidly killed the bacteria and prevented the mice from developing fatal infections. They also showed that it could act as a topical antimicrobial dressing for third-degree burns in mice contaminated with two of these bacterial species, P. aeruginosa and P. mirabilis. In the case of P. aeruginosa infections, the survival rate of mice treated with the chitosan acetate bandage was 73.3% compared with a survival rate of 27.3% for mice treated with a nanocrystalline silver dressing ($p = 0.0055$) and 13.3% for untreated animals ($p < 0.0002$). For P. mirabilis infections, the comparable survival rates were 66.7%, 62.5%, and 23.1% respectively.

Mi et al.[212] described the production of a novel asymmetric chitosan membrane which consists of a 'skin-like' top layer supported by a macroporous sponge-like sub-layer. This membrane showed controlled evaporative water loss, excellent oxygen permeability and promoted fluid drainage. It also provided an effective bacterial barrier. It was also claimed that the membrane had haemostatic properties and promoted rapid healing confirmed by histological examination. In a subsequent paper,[213] this membrane was used as a topical delivery system for silver sulfadiazine. It was found that although large amounts of sulfadiazine were released during the first day, these subsequently tailed off to give much slower release. However, the release of silver from the chitosan dressing displayed a slow release profile with a sustained increase of silver concentration.

Films with interesting properties made from chitin alone,[214-215] or from a chitosan-alginate polyelectrolyte complex have also been described.[216] The literature also contains numerous publications which suggest that some of these new developments may offer benefits in routine wound management the but despite these encouraging reports, no dressings prepared from chitin or chitosan have yet been launched commercially on the UK market.

BACTERIAL CELLULOSE

History of bacterial cellulose in medicine

The first attempts to produce bacterial cellulose (BC) on a commercial scale were made by Johnson and Johnson in the early 1980s,[217] but because of practical problems associated with the production process, no products were ever launched. Subsequently companies in Brazil, Japan Poland and the US began to invest in BC production and to date two of these have produced commercial products based upon BC for use in wound management although other organizations have developed alternative forms for use as thickening and stabilizing agents in the food industry.

Production of bacterial cellulose

The Gram-negative bacterium *Acetobacter xylinum* is an efficient producer of extracellular β-1,4-glucan chains forming a specific type of cellulose. The formation of bacterial cellulose has been described by Sanchavanakit *et al.*[218] and Czaja *et al.*,[217] who have stated that each single organism acts like a nano-spinneret, producing a bundle of sub-microscopic fibrils consisting of very pure cellulose with a high degree of crystallinity. The final material is free of any components of animal origin or any protein that is likely to induce sensitivity reactions in human.

Under the appropriate conditions, a liquid culture of the organism produces an entangled mesh of nanofibres 3 - 8 nm in diameter, which together form a gelatinous pellicle upon the surface of the culture medium. This can be removed, washed and purified to remove any residual microorganisms and used as a hydrated structure such as that used in Suprasorb X (previously Xcell). Alternatively the pellicle can be dried to form a thin membrane not dissimilar in appearance to tracing paper or baking paper as in the case of Veloderm. Suprasorb X PHMB is a medicated version of Suprasorb X that contains poly(hexamethylene biguanide hydrochloride), also known as polyhexanide, a potent broad spectrum antimicrobial agent.

Properties of bacterial cellulose

According to Czaja,[217] the unique nano-morphology of the fibrils results in a large surface area that can hold a large amount of water, about 200 times its dry mass. When the membrane used in Veloderm is moistened with a sterile solution of normal saline or some other physiological solution, it absorbs liquid and becomes soft and flexible, with a texture not unlike that of human skin. When fully hydrated, is absorbs five times its own weight of liquid, much more than normal plant cellulose.

In the dry state the diameter of the individual fibrils ranges from 0.01 - 1.0 μm, and the membrane has an effective pore diameter < 0.1 μm. In the hydrated form the fibrils swell and the effective pore diameter increases to around 0.2 -1.0 μm.

The hydrated product, Suprasorb, is said to be capable of absorbing or donating liquid according to the condition of the wound to which it is applied.

Clinical experience with bacterial cellulose

Bacterial cellulose is chemically inert but its physical properties have generated much interest in its potential value in a variety of biomedical applications. Not least of these is its possible role as a wound dressing. In 1990 Fontana *et al.*[219] described the production and use of a BC film as a temporary skin substitute, and according to Sanchavanakit, it was used with good effect for the treatment of wounds on horses.

Melandri *et al.*[220] published the results of a multi-centre, open study involving 23 adult patients with burns that required grafting. Each patient had three identical donor sites, formed by excision of 0.25 - 0.30 mm thickness of skin which were dressed with a bacterial cellulose dressing, Veloderm, an alginate dressing, Algisite, and Jaloskin, a film composed entirely of an ester of hyaluronic acid. In this way each patient acted as their own control. A single piece of dressing was applied in a single layer and covered with sterile dry gauze. Dressings were changed in accordance with clinical judgement. On days 10-13, when the dressings were removed for inspection, the areas completely healed were significantly higher with Veloderm than the other two dressings (47.6%, *vs* 26.3% and 10% for Veloderm, Algisite M and Jaloskin, respectively ($p < 0.03$).

Wounds dressed with Veloderm and Jaloskin required very few dressing changes during the first week of treatment, while Algisite M needed several multiple re-dressings. Veloderm was judged superior to the other treatments in terms of acceptability ($p < 0.001$), ease of use ($p < 0.001$) and efficacy ($p < 0.00001$).

Pain during application and removal and the formation of local infections were negligible with all dressings. The aesthetic outcome of the treated lesions after healing was judged to be significantly better with Veloderm ($p = 0.0016$) but no scars were formed in any skin donor site. The authors concluded that Veloderm is a safe and effective dressing for the reepithelialization of the skin graft donor sites and superior to the other products examined.

To date, however, most publications on Veloderm have consisted of individual case reports or uncontrolled studies involving a limited number of patients. The literature on the subject has been reviewed previously.[221]

Little has been published on Suprasorb X although Coerper *et al.*[222] reported the results of a single-centre, retrospective analysis of a database of 603 patients with 1,419 wounds treated at the outpatient clinic at the Department of Surgery, University Hospital Tübingen, Germany between 2003 and 2005. Eligible patients had to have had a wound with an initial wound > 0.1 cm^2 which had been treated for a minimum of two weeks using standard moist wound therapy followed by a minimum of four weeks using the bacterial cellulose dressing.

In total, 54 patients with 96 wounds were identified who met these inclusion criteria, 12 of whom (22%) had diabetic ulcers, 21 (39%) had venous ulcers, 14 (26%) had ischemic ulcers, and seven (13%) ulcers of other aetiologies.

According to the records, the 96 ulcers were treated with standard care for a median of 184.5 days (range 14 - 365), during which time the median area increased, but not significantly, from 6.7 to 7.39 cm^2, ($p = 0.22$). The median percentage of area reduction during this treatment period was 0.0%.

When the cellulose dressings were subsequently applied for a median of 172 (14 - 365) days, median ulcer size decreased significantly from 7.39 cm^2 to 2.9 cm^2 (p = 0.0001). The percentage reduction in wound area using standard care was +28.4% for venous ulcers, 0% for ischemic, and 0% for diabetic foot ulcers. Following the use of cellulose dressings, the average reduction in ulcer area was 40% for venous ulcers, 75% for ischemic ulcers and 14.7% for diabetic ulcers. No adverse events related to the dressing occurred, including allergy or skin irritation.

The authors advised that for a number of reasons their results be interpreted with caution, but concluded that the bacterial cellulose dressing appeared to be a viable option in chronic wound care, especially in the treatment of venous and ischemic ulcers.

OXIDISED CELLULOSE

Oxidized cellulose in various forms (gauze, lint, or knitted fabric) has been used as a surgical and dental haemostat for about half a century. When applied to a bleeding surface it forms a gelatinous mass, which is gradually absorbed by the tissues, usually within two to seven days. Traumacel, the calcium salt of oxidized cellulose, which is available as a woven gauze or powder, is used as a military haemostatic field dressing that is believed to facilitate haemostasis by donating calcium ions that have an important role in the clotting cascade.

Hofman *et al.*[223] carried out a small-scale, 12-week pilot study involving Traumacel, during which they examined the safety and efficacy of the dressing in the management of 11 patients with a total of 15 non-healing leg ulcers. Five ulcers healed within the study period and three patients reported significant pain relief. No patients experienced sensitization to the product or had to be withdrawn because of adverse effects. The authors concluded that the treatment was safe in the management of chronic wounds and appeared to promote healing in some recalcitrant ulcers.

The results of this clinical study were subsequently supported by those of a further study undertaken by the same group[224] in which they determined the effect of Traumacel P powder on human dermal fibroblasts *in vitro*. They found that concentrations of 0.5 mg/mL and 1.0 mg/mL stimulated the metabolic activity of the fibroblasts in a variety of different growth media and concluded that direct stimulation of fibroblast proliferation may be one mechanism by which Traumacel P facilitated the healing of ulcers as reported in the earlier study.

CURRENT STATUS OF POLYSACCHARIDE FIBRE DRESSINGS

Most of the polysaccharides perform similarly in terms of their fluid handling characteristics, but vary in terms of their biochemical effects within a healing wound. Dressings produced from CMC appear to be free from direct stimulatory activity, whilst hyaluronan and perhaps to a lesser extent chitin and its derivates, posses properties which, in theory, should accelerate wound healing and reduce scarring. Some alginates also appear to possess some biochemical activity but the clinical relevance of this remains the subject of some debate.

Despite the anticipated advantages associated with the use of dressings containing hyaluronan or chitin/chitosan, such dressings have so far failed to make much of a commercial impact and clinical publications supporting their use are scarce; fibrous dressings made from alginates and CMC that simply perform a more basic fluid control function continue to dominate this market sector.

The reason for this is unclear but it may be because the processes that are taking place within a healing wound are so complex and interdependent that the introduction of large amounts, in biochemical terms, of an active molecule such as hyaluronan simply does not induce the response predicted by laboratory-based studies and the dressings therefore fails to function as anticipated.

Alternatively, it may be that the dressing does accelerate wound healing but the improvement is insufficient to justify the significant costs involved, approximately £25 for a 10 × 10 cm sheet of Hyalofill. This issue could, perhaps, be resolved in the future, if the dressings become more widely used.

REFERENCES

1. Stanford ECC. On algin: a new substance obtained from some of the commoner species of marine algae. *Chemical News* 1883;47:254-257.
2. Gacesa P. Alginates. *Carbohydrate Polymers,* 1988;8:1-22.
3. Guiry MD. A brief history of the uses of seaweed. *http://seaweed.ucg.ie/* 1998.
4. Johnson FA, Craig DQ, Mercer AD. Characterization of the block structure and molecular weight of sodium alginates. *Journal of Pharmacy and Pharmacology* 1997;49(7):639-643.
5. Qin Y, Gilding DK. Alginate fibres and wound dressings. *Medical Device Technology* 1996(November):32--41.
6. Qin Y. The gel swelling properties of alginate fibres and their applications in wound management. *Polymers for Advanced Technologies* 2008;19:6-14.
7. Sherbrock-Cox V, Russell NJ, Gacesa P. The purification and chemical characterisation of the alginate present in extracellular material produced by mucoid strains of Pseudomonas aeruginosa. *Carbohydr Res* 1984;135(1):147-54.
8. Winter GD. Formation of the scab and the rate of epithelization of superficial wounds in the skin of the young domestic pig. *Nature* 1962;193:293-294.
9. Gilchrist T, Turner TD, Schmidt RJ, Harding KG. Sorbsan - the natural dressing, in Advances in Wound Management. *London,John Wiley* 1985:73-81.
10. Schmidt RJ, Turner TD, Spyratou O. Alginate dressings (letter). *Pharm. J.* 1986;236:36-37.
11. Fry JR. Alginate dressings (letter). *Pharm. J.* 1986;236:37.
12. Cair. Calcium alginate dressings. *Pharmaceutical Journal* 1986;236:578.
13. Thomas S. Observations on the fluid handling properties of alginate dressings. *Pharmaceutical Journal* 1992;248:850-851.
14. Johnson BJ, Simpson C. Laboratory comparison of alginate dressings. *Pharmaceutical Journal* 1993(November 6):R46.
15. Ichioka S, Harii K, Nakahara M, Sato Y. An experimental comparison of hydrocolloid and alginate dressings, and the effect of calcium ions on the behaviour of alginate gel. *Scand J Plast Reconstr Surg Hand Surg* 1998;32(3):311-6.
16. Alginate Fibre. *British Pharmacopoeia Addendum* 1995:1705-1706.
17. Alginate Dressing. *British Pharmacopoeia Addendum* 1995:1706.
18. Alginate Packing. *British Pharmacopeia Addendum* 1995:1706-1707.

19. Williams C. Sorbsan. *Br J Nurs* 1994;3(13):677-80.
20. Gilchrist T, Martin AM. Wound treatment with Sorbsan - an alginate fibre dressing. *Biomaterials* 1983;4:317-320.
21. Hinchley H, Murray J. Calcium alginate dressings in community nursing. *Practice Nurse* 1989;2(6):264-268.
22. Blaine G. The use of plastics in surgery. *Lancet* 1946;ccli(2):525-528.
23. Blaine G. Experimental observations on absorbable alginate products in surgery. *Annals of Surgery* 1947;125(1):102-114.
24. Passe ERG, Blaine G. Alginates in endaural wound dressing. *Lancet* 1948;2:651.
25. Oliver LC, Blaine G. Haemostasis with absorbable alginates in neurosurgical practice. *British Journal of Surgery* 1950;37:307-310.
26. Bray C, Blaine G, Hudson P. New treatment for burns, wounds and haemorrhage. *Nursing Mirror* 1948;86:239-242.
27. Blaine G. A comparative evaluation of absorbable haemostatics. *Postgraduate Medical Journal* 1951;27:613-620.
28. Fraser R, Gilchrist T. Sorbsan calcium alginate fibre dressings in footcare. *Biomaterials* 1983;4(3):222-4.
29. Thomas S. Use of a calcium alginate dressing. *Pharmaceutical Journal* 1985;235:188-190.
30. Odugbesan O, Barnett AH. Use of a seaweed-based dressing in management of leg ulcers in diabetics: a case report. *Pract. Diabet.* 1987;4:46-47.
31. Scherr GH. Alginates and alginate fibers in clinical practice. *Wounds* 1992;4(2):74-80.
32. Barnett AH, Odugbesan O. Seaweed-based dressings in the management of leg ulcers and other wounds. *Intensive Therapy and Clinical Monitoring* 1988;May/June:70-76.
33. Piacquadio D, Nelson DB. Alginates. A "new" dressing alternative. *J Dermatol Surg Oncol* 1992;18(11):992-5.
34. Morgan D. Alginate Dressings. *Journal of Tissue Viability* 1996;7(1):4-14.
35. Thomas S. Alginates. *Journal of Wound Care* 1992;1(1):29-32.
36. Young MJ. The use of alginates in the management of exudating, infected wounds: case studies. *Dermatol Nurs* 1993;5(5):359-63, 356.
37. Gensheimer D. A review of calcium alginates. *Ostomy Wound Manage* 1993;39(1):34-8, 42-3.
38. McMullen D. Clinical experience with a calcium alginate dressing. *Dermatol Nurs* 1991;3(4):216-9, 270.
39. Motta GJ. Calcium alginate topical wound dressings: a new dimension in the cost- effective treatment for exudating dermal wounds and pressure sores. *Ostomy Wound Manage* 1989;25:52-6.
40. Seymour J. Alginate dressings in wound care management. *Nurs Times* 1997;93(44):49-52.
41. Fanucci D, Seese J. Multi-faceted use of calcium alginates. *Ostomy and Wound Management* 1991;37:16-22.
42. Choate CS. Wound dressings. A comparison of classes and their principles of use. *J Am Podiatr Med Assoc* 1994;84(9):463-9.
43. Davis E. Care of a patient with rheumatoid arthritis and a vasculitic ulcer. *Journal of Wound Care* 1993;2(2):72-73.
44. Miller L, Jones V, Bale S. The use of alginate packing in the management of deep sinuses. *Journal of Wound Care* 1993;2(5):262-263.
45. Marghoob AA, Artman NN, Siegel DM. Calcium alginate dressings with second intention healing of surgical wounds: Our experience. *Wounds-a Compendium of Clinical Research and Practice* 1997;9(2):50-55.

46. Imamura Y, Fujiwara S, Sato T, Katagiri K, Takayasu S. Successful treatment of toxic epidermal necrolysis with calcium sodium alginate fiber letter. *Int J Dermatol* 1996;35(11):834-5.

47. Cannavo M, Fairbrother G, Owen D, Ingle J, Lumley T. A comparison of dressings in the management of surgical abdominal wounds. *Journal of Wound Care* 1998;7(2):57-62.

48. Berry DP, Bale S, Harding KG. Dressings for treating cavity wounds. *Journal of Wound Care* 1996;5(1):10-7.

49. Eagle M. The care of a patient after a Caesarean section. *Journal of Wound Care* 1993;2(6):330-336.

50. Roberts KJ, Rowland CM, Benbow ME. Managing a patient's infected wound site after a radical vulvectomy. *Journal of Wound Care* 1992;1(4):14-17.

51. Cortimiglia-Bisch L, Brazinsky B. Use of a four-layer bandage system in the treatment of an i.v. drug abuser with chronic upper extremity ulcerations: a case study. *Ostomy Wound Manage* 1998;44(3):48-52, 54-5.

52. Eyre G. Alternative wound dressings in A&E. *Nurs Stand* 1993;7(19):25-8.

53. La Hausse-Brown TP, Dujon DG. A dressing for 'road rash' letter. *Ann R Coll Surg Engl* 1997;79(2):154.

54. Thomas S, Fisher B, Fram PJ, Waring MJ. Odour-absorbing dressings. *Journal of Wound Care* 1998;7(5):246-50.

55. Moody M. Calcium alginate: a dressing trial. *Nurs Stand Spec Suppl* 1991(13):3-6.

56. Thomas S, Tucker CA. Sorbsan in the management of leg ulcers. *Pharmaceutical Journal* 1989;243:706-709.

57. Smith J, Lewis JD. Sorbsan and leg ulcers (letter). *Pharmaceutical Journal* 1990:468.

58. Franks PJ. Sorbsan and leg ulcers (letter). *Pharmaceutical Journal* 1990:468.

59. Thomas S. Sorbsan and leg ulcers (letter). *Pharmaceutical Journal* 1990:468-469.

60. Moffatt CJ. Assessing a calcium alginate dressing for venous ulcers of the leg. *Journal of Wound Care* 1992;1(4):22-24.

61. Scurr J, H. , Wilson LA, Coleridge -Smith PD. A Comparison of the Effects of Semipermeable Foam and Film Secondary Dressings
over Alginate Dressings on the Healing and Management of Venous Ulcers. *Wounds* 1993;5(6):259-265.

62. Scurr JH, Wilson LA, Coleridge-Smith PD. A comparison of calcium alginate and hydrocolloid dressings in the management of chronic venous ulcers. *Wounds* 1994;6(1):1-8.

63. Stacey MC, Jopp-Mckay AG, Rashid P, Hoskin SE, Thompson PJ. The influence of dressings on venous ulcer healing-a randomised trial. *Eur J Vasc Endovasc Surg* 1997;13(2):174-9.

64. Limova M. Evaluation of two calcium alginate dressings in the management of venous ulcers. *Ostomy Wound Manage* 2003;49(9):26-33.

65. Groves AR, Lawrence JC. Alginate dressing as a donor site haemostat. *Ann R Coll Surg Engl* 1986;68(1):27-8.

66. Attwood AI. Calcium alginate dressing accelerates split skin graft donor site healing. *British Journal of Plastic Surgery* 1989;42(4):373-9.

67. Beldon P. Comparison of four different dressings on donor site wounds. *Br J Nurs* 2004;13(6 Suppl):S38-45.

68. Rodier-Bruant C, Keller P, Herman D, Stricher R, Geiger D, Manunta A, et al. The use of Sorbsan in the treatment of the donor site of skin transplantations. *Minerva Chir* 1992;47(11):995-9.

69. Basse P, Siim E, Lohmann M. Treatment of Donor sites-calcium alginate versus paraffin gauze. *Acta Chir Plast* 1992;34(2):92-8.

70. O'Donoghue JM, O'Sullivan ST, Beausang ES, Panchal JI, O'Shaughnessy M, O'Connor TP. Calcium alginate dressings promote healing of split skin graft donor sites. *Acta Chir Plast* 1997;39(2):53-5.
71. Cihantimur B, Kahveci R, Ozcan M. Comparing Kaltostat with Jelonet in the treatment of split-thickness skin graft donor sites. *European Journal of Plastic Surgery* 1997;20(5):260-263.
72. Rives JM, Pannier M, Castede JC, Martinot V, LeTouze A, Romana MC, et al. Calcium alginate versus paraffin gauze in the treatment of scalp graft donor sites. *Wounds-a Compendium of Clinical Research and Practice* 1997;9(6):199-205.
73. Pannier M, Martinot V, Castede JC, Guitard J, Robert M, Le Touze A, et al. [Efficacy and tolerance of Algosteril (calcium alginate) versus Jelonet (paraffin gauze) in the treatment of scalp graft donor sites in children. Results of a randomized study]. *Ann Chir Plast Esthet* 2002;47(4):285-90.
74. Steenfos HH, Agren MS. A fibre-free alginate dressing in the treatment of split thickness skin graft Donor sites. *J Eur Acad Dermatol Venereol* 1998;11(3):252-6.
75. Bettinger D, Gore D, Humphries Y. Evaluation of calcium alginate for skin graft donor sites. *J Burn Care Rehabil* 1995;16(1):59-61.
76. Lawrence JE, Blake GB. A comparison of calcium alginate and scarlet red dressings in the healing of split thickness skin graft donor sites. *Br J Plast Surg* 1991;44(4):247-9.
77. Lim TC, Tan WT. Treatment of donor site defects letter; comment. *Br J Plast Surg* 1992;45(6):488.
78. Vanstraelen P. Comparison of calcium sodium alginate (KALTOSTAT) and porcine xenograft (E-Z DERM) in the healing of split-thickness skin graft Donor sites. *Burns* 1992;18(2):145-8.
79. Kneafsey B, O'Shaughnessy M, Condon KC. The use of calcium alginate dressings in deep hand burns. *Burns* 1996;22(1):40-3.
80. Kelly SA, Dickson MG, Sharpe DT. Calcium alginate as a temporary recipient bed dressing prior to the delayed application of split skin grafts. *Br J Plast Surg* 1988;41(4):445.
81. Varma SK, Henderson HP, Hankins CL. Calcium alginate as a dressing for mini skin grafts (skin soup). *Br J Plast Surg* 1991;44(1):55-6.
82. Butler PE, Eadie PA, Lawlor D, Edwards G, McHugh M. Bupivacaine and Kaltostat reduces post-operative donor site pain. *Br J Plast Surg* 1993;46(6):523-4.
83. Porter JM. A comparative investigation of re-epithelialisation of split skin graft donor areas after application of hydrocolloid and alginate dressings. *Br J Plast Surg* 1991;44(5):333-7.
84. Giele H, Tong A, Huddleston S. Adhesive retention dressings are more comfortable than alginate dressings on split skin graft donor sites--a randomised controlled trial. *Ann R Coll Surg Engl* 2001;83(6):431-4.
85. Hormbrey E, Pandya A, Giele H. Adhesive retention dressings are more comfortable than alginate dressings on split-skin-graft donor sites. *Br J Plast Surg* 2003;56(5):498-503.
86. O'Donoghue JM, O'Sullivan ST, O'Shaughnessy M, O'Connor TP. Effects of a silicone-coated polyamide net dressing and calcium alginate on the healing of split skin graft donor sites: a prospective randomised trial. *Acta Chir Plast* 2000;42(1):3-6.
87. Vaingankar NV, Sylaidis P, Eagling V, King C, Elender F. Comparison of hydrocellular foam and calcium alginate in the healing and comfort of split-thickness skin-graft donor sites. *J Wound Care* 2001;10(7):289-91.
88. Terrill PJ, Goh RC, Bailey MJ. Split-thickness skin graft donor sites: a comparative study of two absorbent dressings. *J Wound Care* 2007;16(10):433-8.
89. Geary PM, Tiernan E. Management of split skin graft donor sites--results of a national survey. *J Plast Reconstr Aesthet Surg* 2009;62(12):1677-83.

90. Davey RB, Sparnon AL, Byard RW. Unusual donor site reactions to calcium alginate dressings. *Burns* 2000;26(4):393-8.

91. Mack R. Treating a patient with a sacral pressure sore. *Journal of Wound Care* 1992;1(4):12-13.

92. Sayag J, Meaume S, Bohbot S. Healing properties of calcium alginate dressings. *Journal of Wound Care* 1996;5(8):357-62.

93. Chapuis A, Dollfus P. The use of a calcium alginate dressing in the management of decubitus ulcers in patients with spinal cord lesions. *Paraplegia* 1990;28(4):269-71.

94. Fowler E, Papen JC. Evaluation of an alginate dressing for pressure ulcers. *Decubitus* 1991;4(3):47-8, 50, 52 passim.

95. Belmin J, Meaume S, Rabus MT, Bohbot S. Sequential treatment with calcium alginate dressings and hydrocolloid dressings accelerates pressure ulcer healing in older subjects: a multicenter randomized trial of sequential versus nonsequential treatment with hydrocolloid dressings alone. *J Am Geriatr Soc* 2002;50(2):269-74.

96. Bradshaw T. The use of Kaltostat in the treatment of ulceration in the diabetic foot. *Chiropodist* 1989;September:204-207.

97. Burrow BA, Lindsay A. A limited evaluation of alginates and a small scale comparison between Kaltostat and a standard non-adherent dressing, Ultraplast Alginate, in the treatment of nail avulsion by matrix phenolisation. *Chiropodist* 1989(October):211-218.

98. Smith J. Comparing Sorbsan and polynoxylin/Melolin dressings after toenail removal. *Journal of Wound Care* 1992;1(3):17-19.

99. Foley GB, Allen J. Wound healing after toenail avulsion. *The Foot* 1994;4:88-91.

100. Foster AVM, Greenhill MT, Edmonds ME. Comparing two dressings in the treatment of diabetic foot ulcers. *Journal of Wound Care* 1994;3(5):224-228.

101. Chaloner D, Fletcher M, Milward P. Clinical trials: comparing dressings. *Nurs Stand Spec Suppl* 1992;7(7):9-12.

102. Van Gils CC, Roeder B, Chesler SM, Mason S. Improved healing with a collagen-alginate dressing in the chemical matricectomy. *J Am Podiatr Med Assoc* 1998;88(9):452-6.

103. Donaghue VM, Chrzan JS, Rosenblum BI, Giurini JM, Habershaw GM, Veves A. Evaluation of a collagen-alginate wound dressing in the management of diabetic foot ulcers. *Advances in Wound Care* 1998;11(3):114-9.

104. Bale S, Baker N, Crook H, Rayman A, Rayman G, Harding KG. Exploring the use of an alginate dressing for diabetic foot ulcers. *Journal of Wound Care* 2001;10(3):81-84.

105. Lalau JD, Bresson R, Charpentier P, Coliche V, Erlher S, Ha Van G, et al. Efficacy and tolerance of calcium alginate versus vaseline gauze dressings in the treatment of diabetic foot lesions. *Diabetes Metab* 2002;28(3):223-9.

106. Gupta R, Foster ME, Miller E. Calcium alginate in the management of acute surgical wounds and abscesses. *Journal of Tissue Viabilty* 1991;1(4):115-116.

107. Dawson C, Armstrong MW, Fulford SC, Faruqi RM, Galland RB. Use of calcium alginate to pack abscess cavities: a controlled clinical trial. *J R Coll Surg Edinb* 1992;37(3):177-9.

108. Guillotreau J, Andre J, Flandrin P, Moncade F, Duverger V, Rouffi J, et al. Calcium alginate and povidone iodine packs in the management of infected postoperative wounds: results of a randomized study [abstract]. *British Journal of Surgery* 1996;83:861.

109. Ingram M, Wright TA, Ingoldby CJ. A prospective randomized study of calcium alginate (Sorbsan) versus standard gauze packing following haemorrhoidectomy. *J R Coll Surg Edinb* 1998;43(5):308-9.

110. Williams P, Howells RE, Miller E, Foster ME. A comparison of two alginate dressings used in surgical wounds. *Journal of Wound Care* 1995;4(4):170-2.

111. Blockley CH. A penicillin-styptic for dental work. *British Dental Journal* 1947;82:213.

112. Rumble JFS. Twenty-five cases treated with absorbable alginate wool. *British Dental Journal* 1949;86:203-205.
113. Matthew IR, Browne RM, Frame JW, Millar BG. Alginate fiber dressing for oral mucosal wounds. *Oral Surg Oral Med Oral Pathol* 1994;77(5):456-60.
114. Joy RH, Murray JR. A new calcium alginate haemostatic dressing. *Dental Practice* 1989(Feb 16).
115. Odell EW, Oades P, Lombardi T. Symptomatic foreign body reaction to haemostatic alginate. *Br J Oral Maxillofac Surg* 1994;32(3):178-9.
116. Mattsson T, Anderssen K, Koendell P-A, Lindskog SA. A longitudinal comparative histometric study of the biocampatibility of three local hemostatic agents. *International Journal of Oral and Maxillofacial Surgery* 1990;19:47-50.
117. Matthew IR, Browne RM, Frame JW, Millar BG. Tissue response to a haemostatic alginate wound dressing in tooth extraction sockets. *Br J Oral Maxillofac Surg* 1993;31(3):165-9.
118. Matthew IR, Browne RM, Frame JW, Millar BG. Subperiosteal behaviour of alginate and cellulose wound dressing materials. *Biomaterials* 1995;16(4):275-8.
119. Blair SD, Backhouse CM, Harper R, Mathews J, McCollum CN. Comparison of absorbable materials for surgical haemostatis. *British Journal of Surgery* 1988;75(10):969-971.
120. Blair SD, Jarvis P, Salmon M, McCollum C. Clinical trial of calcium alginate haemostatic swabs. *British Journal of Surgery* 1990;77(May):568-570.
121. Davies MS, Flannery MC, McCollum CN. Calcium alginate as haemostatic swabs in hip fracture surgery. *J R Coll Surg Edinb* 1997;42(1):31-2.
122. Jones B. Calcium alginate as haemostatic swabs in hip fracture (comment). *J R Coll Surg Edinb* 1998;43(1):120-131.
123. Sharp JF, Rogers MJ, Riad M, Kerr AI. Combined study to assess the role of calcium alginate swabs and ligation of the inferior tonsillar pole in the control of intra- operative blood loss during tonsillectomy. *J Laryngol Otol* 1991;105(3):191-4.
124. Scalpel and seaweed, nurse. editorial. *Lancet* 1990;336(8720):914.
125. Amies CR. The use of topically formed calcium alginate as a depot substance in active immunization. *J.Path Bact.* 1959;77:435-442.
126. Jaros SH, Dewey JL. Use of an alginate in hyposensitization. *Annals of Allergy* 1964;22:173-179.
127. Frantz VK. Experimental studies of alginates as haemostatics. *Annals of Surgery* 1948;127:1165-1172.
128. Chenoweth MB. The toxicity of sodium alginate in cats. *Annals of Surgery* 1948;127:1173-1181.
129. Un nouvel hemostatique chirurgical: l'alginate de calcium,. Communication to the Academie de Chirurgie; 1949; Paris.
130. Sirimanna KS. Calcium alginate fibre (Kaltostat 2) for nasal packing after trimming of turbinates--a pilot study. *J Laryngol Otol* 1989;103(11):1067-8.
131. Sirimanna KS, Todd GB, Madden GJ. A randomized study to compare calcium sodium alginate fibre with two commonly used materials for packing after nasal surgery. *Clin Otolaryngol* 1992;17(3):237-9.
132. Sirimanna KS, Todd GB, Madden GJ. Early complications of packing after nasal surgery with three different materials. *Ceylon Med J* 1994;39(3):129-31.
133. How does calcium alginate achieve haemostasis is surgery. XI International Congress on Thrombosis and Haemostasis; 1987 July 6-10; Brussels.
134. Segal HC, Hunt BJ, Gilding K. The effects of alginate and non-alginate wound dressings on blood coagulation and platelet activation. *J Biomater Appl* 1998;12(3):249-57.

135. Barnett SE, Varley SJ. The effects of calcium alginate on wound healing. *Annals of the Royal College of Surgeons of England* 1987;69(4):153-5.

136. Schmidt RJ, Turner TD. Calcium alginate dressings (letter). *Pharmaceutical Journal* 1986;236:578.

137. Lansdown AB, Payne MJ. An evaluation of the local reaction and biodegradation of calcium sodium alginate (Kaltostat) following subcutaneous implantation in the rat. *J R Coll Surg Edinb* 1994;39(5):284-8.

138. Suzuki Y, Nishimura Y, Tanihara M, Suzuki K, Nakamura T, Shimizu Y, et al. Evaluation of a novel alginate gel dressing: cytotoxicity to fibroblasts in vitro and foreign-body reaction in pig skin in vivo. *J Biomed Mater Res* 1998;39(2):317-22.

139. Agren MS. Four alginate dressings in the treatment of partial thickness wounds: a comparative experimental study. *Br J Plast Surg* 1996;49(2):129-34.

140. Wu S, Suzuki Y, Tanihara M, Ohnishi K, Endo K, Nishimura Y. Repair of facial nerve with alginate sponge without suturing: an experimental study in cats. *Scand J Plast Reconstr Surg Hand Surg* 2002;36(3):135-40.

141. Pueyo ME, Darquy S, Capron F, Reach G. In vitro activation of human macrophages by alginate-polylysine microcapsules. *J Biomater Sci Polym Ed* 1993;5(3):197-203.

142. Otterlei M, Ostgaard K, Skjak-Braek G. Induction of cytokine production from human monocytes stimulated with alginate. *Journal of Immunotherapy* 1991;10:286-291.

143. Otterlei M, Sundan A, Skjak-Braek G, Ryan L, Smidsrod O, Espevik T. Similar mechanisms of action of defined polysaccharides and lipopolysaccharides: characterization of binding and tumor necrosis factor alpha induction. *Infection Immunology* 1993;61(5):1917-1925.

144. Skjak-Braek G, Espevik T. Application of alginate gels in biotechnology and biomedicine. *Carbohydrates in Europe* 1996;14:19-25.

145. Zimmermann U, Klock G, Federlin K, Hannig K, Kowalski M, Bretzel RG, et al. Production of mitogen-contamination free alginates with variable ratios of mannuronic acid to guluronic acid by free flow electrophoresis. *Elecrophoresis* 1992;13:269-274.

146. Klock G, Pfeffermann A, Ryser C, Grohn P, Kuttler B, Hahn HJ, et al. Biocompatibility of mannuronic acid-rich alginates. *Biomaterials* 1997;18(10):707-13.

147. Klock G, Frank H, Houben R, Zekorn T, Horcher A, Siebers U, et al. Production of purified alginates suitable for use in immunoisolated transplantation. *Appl Microbiol Biotechnol* 1994;40(5):638-43.

148. Doyle JW, Roth TP, Smith RM, Li YQ, Dunn RM. Effects of calcium alginate on cellular wound healing processes modeled in vitro. *Journal of Biomedical Materials Research* 1996;32(4):561-8.

149. Thomas A, Harding K, Moore K. Alginates from wound dressings activate human macrophages to secrete tumour necrosis factor-α. *Biomaterials* 2000;21:1797-1802.

150. Nakagawa Y, Murai T, Hasegawa C, Hirata M, Tsuchiya T, Yagami T, et al. Endotoxin contamination in wound dressings made of natural biomaterials. *J Biomed Mater Res B Appl Biomater* 2003;66(1):347-55.

151. Pirone LA, Bolton LL, Monte KA, Shannon RJ. Effect of calcium alginate dressings on partial-thickness wounds in swine. *J Invest Surg* 1992;5(2):149-53.

152. Thomas S, Loveless P, Hay NP. Comparative review of the properties of six semipermeable film dressings. *Pharm. J.* 1988;240:785-789.

153. Armstrong SH, Ruckley CV. Use of a fibrous dressing in exuding leg ulcers. *Journal of Wound Care* 1997;6(7):322-4.

154. Thomas S. *Current Practices in the Management of Fungating Lesions and Radiation Damaged Skin*. Bridgend: SMTL, 1992.

155. Kawaguchi H, Hizuta A, Tanaka N. Role of endotoxin in wound healing impairment. *Res Commun Mol Pathol Pharmacol* 1995;89(3):317-327.

156. Rapala KT, Vaha-Kreula MO, Heino JJ. Tumour necrosis factor-alpha inhibits collagen synthesis in human and rat granulation tissue fibroblasts. *Experimentia* 1996;51(1):70-74.

157. Boyce DE, Thomas A, Hart J. Hyaluronic acid induces tumour necrois factor-alpha production by human macrophages *in vitro*. *British Journal of Plastic Surgery* 1997;50(5):362-368.

158. Miyamoto T, Takahashi S, Ito H, Inagaki H, Noishiki Y. Tissue biocompatibility of cellulose and its derivatives. *J Biomed Mater Res* 1989;23(1):125-33.

159. Hoekstra MJ, Hermans MH, Richters CD, Dutrieux RP. A histological comparison of acute inflammatory responses with a hydrofibre or tulle gauze dressing. *Journal of Wound Care* 2002;11(3):113-7.

160. Bowler PG, Jones SA, Davies BJ, Coyle E. Infection control properties of some wound dressings. *Journal of Wound Care* 1999;8(10):499-502.

161. Walker M, Hobot JA, Newman GR, Bowler PG. Scanning electron microscopic examination of bacterial immobilisation in a carboxymethyl cellulose (AQUACEL((R))) and alginate dressings. *Biomaterials* 2003;24(5):883-90.

162. Tachi M, Hirabayashi S, Yonehara Y, Suzuki Y, Bowler P. Comparison of bacteria-retaining ability of absorbent wound dressings. *Int Wound J* 2004;1(3):177-81.

163. Foster L, Smith E, Moore P, Turton P. The use of a hydrofibre dressing in fulminating necrotizing fasciitis. *British Journal of Nursing* 2001;10 (suppl)(11):S36-S42.

164. Moore P, Foster L, Clark S, Parrott D. The role of a hydrofibre dressing in squamous cell carcinoma of the anal canal. *Journal of Wound Care* 1999;8(9):432-4.

165. Foster L, Moore P. The management of recurrent pilonidal sinus. *Nurs Times* 1997;93(32):64-8.

166. Russell L, Carr J. New hydrofibre and hydrocolloid dressings for chronic wounds. *Journal of Wound Care* 2000;9(4):169-172.

167. Bell ES. Managing a breast sinus wound in the community: a care study. *Br J Nurs* 2004;13(21):1276-9.

168. Licheri S, Erdas E, Pisano G, Garau A, Barbarossa M, Tusconi A, et al. [Fournier's gangrene in an HIV-positive patient. Therapeutic options]. *Chir Ital* 2008;60(4):607-15.

169. Cuesta Cuesta JJ. [Wet environmental cure for Dupuytren pathology. Evaluation and follow-up]. *Rev Enferm* 2008;31(5):16-20.

170. Robinson BJ. The use of a hydrofibre dressing in wound management. *Journal of Wound Care* 2000;9(1):32-4.

171. Barnea Y, Amir A, Leshem D, Zaretski A, Weiss J, Shafir R, et al. Clinical comparative study of aquacel and paraffin gauze dressing for split-skin donor site treatment. *Ann Plast Surg* 2004;53(2):132-6.

172. Vloemans AF, Soesman AM, Kreis RW, Middelkoop E. A newly developed hydrofibre dressing, in the treatment of partial- thickness burns. *Burns* 2001;27(2):167-73.

173. Foster L, Moore P. The application of a cellulose-based fibre dressing in surgical wounds. *Journal of Wound Care* 1997;6(10):469-73.

174. Moore P, Foster L. Cost benefit of two dressings in the management of surgical wounds. *British Journal of Nursing* 2000;9(17).

175. Foster L, Moore P, Clark S. A comparison of hydrofibre and alginate dressings on open acute surgical wounds. *Journal of Wound Care* 2000;9(9):442-445.

176. Vogt KC, Uhlyarik M, Schroeder TV. Moist wound healing compared with standard care of treatment of primary closed vascular surgical wounds: a prospective randomized controlled study. *Wound Repair Regen* 2007;15(5):624-7.

177. Cohn SM, Lopez PP, Brown M, Namias N, Jackowski J, Li P, et al. Open surgical wounds: how does Aquacel compare with wet-to-dry gauze? *Journal of Wound Care* 2004;13(1):10-2.
178. Guest JF, Ruiz FJ. Modelling the cost implications of using carboxymethylcellulose dressing compared with gauze in the management of surgical wounds healing by secondary intention in the US and UK. *Curr Med Res Opin* 2005;21(2):281-90.
179. Folestad A. The management of wounds following orthopaedic surgery: The Molndal dressing. *European Product News* 2002;March/April.
180. Harle S, Korhonen A, Kettunen JA, Seitsalo S. A randomised clinical trial of two different wound dressing materials for hip replacement patients. *Journal of Orthopaedic Nursing* 2005;9:205-210.
181. Ravenscroft MJ, Harker J, Buch KA. A prospective, randomised, controlled trial comparing wound dressings used in hip and knee surgery: Aquacel and Tegaderm versus Cutiplast. *Ann R Coll Surg Engl* 2006;88(1):18-22.
182. Abuzakuk TM, Coward P, Shenava Y, Kumar VS, Skinner JA. The management of wounds following primary lower limb arthroplasty: a prospective, randomised study comparing hydrofibre and central pad dressings. *Int Wound J* 2006;3(2):133-7.
183. Piaggesi A, Baccetti F, Rizzo L, Romanelli M, Navalesi R, Benzi L. Sodium carboxyl-methyl-cellulose dressings in the management of deep ulcerations of diabetic foot. *Diabet Med* 2001;18(4):320-4.
184. Meyer K, Palmer JW. The polysaccharides of the vitreous humor. *J Biol Chem* 1934;107:629-634.
185. Abatangelo G, Brun P, Cortivo R. Hyaluronan (Hyaluronic acid): an overview. In: Willams DF, editor. *Annual Meeting of the European Society for Biomaterials*. Pisa (Italy): University of Liverpool, 1994:8-18.
186. Chen JWY, Abatangelo G. Functions of hyaluronan in wound repair. *Wound Rep Reg* 1999;7:79-89.
187. Davidson JM, Nanney LB, Broadley KN, Whitsett JS, Aquino AM, Beccaro M, et al. Hyaluronate derivatives and their application to wound healing: preliminary observations. *Clin Mater* 1991;8(1-2):171-7.
188. Benedetti L, Bellini DR, Renier D, O'Regan M. Chemical modification of hyaluronan. In: Willams DF, editor. *Annual Meeting of the European Society for Biomaterials*. Pisa (Italy): University of Liverpool, 1994:20-29.
189. Ruiz-Cardona L, Sanzgiri YD, Benedetti LM, Stella VJ, Topp EM. Application of benzyl hyaluronate membranes as potential wound dressings: evaluation of water vapour and gas permeabilities. *Biomaterials* 1996;17(16):1639-43.
190. Hollander D, Stein M, Bernd A, Windolf J, Pannike A. Autologous keratinocytes cultured on benzylester hyaluronic acid membranes in the treatment of chronic full-thickness ulcers. *Journal of Wound Care* 1999;8(7):351-5.
191. Caravaggi C, De Giglio R, Pritelli C, Sommaria M, Dalla Noce S, Faglia E, et al. HYAFF 11-based autologous dermal and epidermal grafts in the treatment of noninfected diabetic plantar and dorsal foot ulcers: a prospective, multicenter, controlled, randomized clinical trial. *Diabetes Care* 2003;26(10):2853-9.
192. Davidson JM, Beccaro M, Pressato D, Dona M, Pavesio A. Biological reponse of experimental cutaneous wounds in the pig to hyaluronan ester biomaterials. In: Willams DF, editor. *Annual Meeting of the European Society for Biomaterials*. Pisa (Italy): University of Liverpool, 1994:44-51.
193. Hollander D, Schmandra T, Windolf J. Using an esterified hyaluronan fleece to promote healing in difficult-to-treat wounds. *Journal of Wound Care* 2000;9(10):463-466.

194. Vazquez JR, Short B, Findlow AH, Nixon BP, Boulton AJ, Armstrong DG. Outcomes of hyaluronan therapy in diabetic foot wounds. *Diabetes Res Clin Pract* 2003;59(2):123-7.

195. Colletta V, Dioguardi D, Di Lonardo A, Maggio G, Torasso F. A trial to assess the efficacy and tolerability of Hyalofill-F in non-healing venous leg ulcers. *Journal of Wound Care* 2003;12(9):357-60.

196. Taddeucci P, Pianigiani E, Colletta V, Torasso F, Andreassi L, Andreassi A. An evaluation of Hyalofill-F plus compression bandaging in the treatment of chronic venous ulcers. *Journal of Wound Care* 2004;13(5):202-4.

197. Voinchet V, Vasseur P, Kern J. Efficacy and safety of hyaluronic acid in the management of acute wounds. *Am J Clin Dermatol* 2006;7(6):353-7.

198. Meaume S, Ourabah Z, Romanelli M, Manopulo R, De Vathaire F, Salomon D, et al. Efficacy and tolerance of a hydrocolloid dressing containing hyaluronic acid for the treatment of leg ulcers of venous or mixed origin. *Curr Med Res Opin* 2008;24(10):2729-39.

199. Barrois B, Carles M, Rumeau M, Tell L, Toussaint JF, Bonnefoy M, et al. Efficacy and tolerability of hyaluronan (ialuset) in the treatment of pressure ulcers: a multicentre, non-randomised, pilot study. *Drugs R D* 2007;8(5):267-73.

200. Costagliola M, Agrosi M. Second-degree burns: a comparative, multicenter, randomized trial of hyaluronic acid plus silver sulfadiazine vs. silver sulfadiazine alone. *Curr Med Res Opin* 2005;21(8):1235-40.

201. Sobotka L, Velebny V, Smahelova A, Kusalova M. [Sodium hyaluronate and an iodine complex--Hyiodine--new method of diabetic defects treatment]. *Vnitr Lek* 2006;52(5):417-22.

202. Frankova J, Kubala L, Velebny V, Ciz M, Lojek A. The effect of hyaluronan combined with KI3 complex (Hyiodine wound dressing) on keratinocytes and immune cells. *J Mater Sci Mater Med* 2006;17(10):891-8.

203. Qin Y, Agboh C, Wang X, Gilding DK. Novel polysaccharide fibres for advanced wound dressings. In: Anand S, editor. *Medical Textiles 96*. Cambridge: Woodhead, 1996:15-20.

204. Muzzarelli RA. Human enzymatic activities related to the therapeutic administration of chitin derivatives. *Cell Mol Life Sci* 1997;53(2):131-40.

205. Chung LY, Schmidt RJ, Hamlyn PF, Sagar BF. Biocompatibilty of potential wound management products: Fungal mycelia as a source of chitin/chitosan and their effect on the proliferation of human F1000 fibroblasts in culture. *Journal of Biomedical Materials Research* 1994;28:463-469.

206. Muzzarelli R, Tarsi R, Filippini O, Giovanetti E, Biagini G, Varaldo PE. Antimicrobial properties of N-carboxybutyl chitosan. *Antimicrob Agents Chemother* 1990;34(10):2019-23.

207. Biagini G, Bertani A, Muzzarelli R, Damadei A, DiBenedetto G, Belligolli A, et al. Wound management with N-carboxybutyl chitosan. *Biomaterials* 1991;12(3):281-6.

208. Stone CA, Wright H, Clarke T, Powell R, Devaraj VS. Healing at skin graft donor sites dressed with chitosan. *Br J Plast Surg* 2000;53(7):601-6.

209. Yusof NL, Lim LY, Khor E. Preparation and characterization of chitin beads as a wound dressing precursor [In Process Citation]. *J Biomed Mater Res* 2001;54(1):59-68.

210. Hirano S, Zhang M, Nakagawa M. Release of glycosaminoglycans in physiological saline and water by wet- spun chitin--acid glycosaminoglycan fibers. *J Biomed Mater Res* 2001;56(4):556-61.

211. Dai T, Tegos GP, Burkatovskaya M, Castano AP, Hamblin MR. Chitosan acetate bandage as a topical antimicrobial dressing for infected burns. *Antimicrob Agents Chemother* 2009;53(2):393-400.

212. Mi FL, Shyu SS, Wu YB, Lee ST, Shyong JY, Huang RN. Fabrication and characterization of a sponge-like asymmetric chitosan membrane as a wound dressing. *Biomaterials* 2001;22(2):165-73.

213. Mi FL, Wu YB, Shyu SS, Schoung JY, Huang YB, Tsai YH, et al. Control of wound infections using a bilayer chitosan wound dressing with sustainable antibiotic delivery. *J Biomed Mater Res* 2002;59(3):438-49.

214. Yusof NL, Lim LY, Khor E. Flexible chitin films: structural studies. *Carbohydr Res* 2004;339(16):2701-11.

215. Yusof NL, Wee A, Lim LY, Khor E. Flexible chitin films as potential wound-dressing materials: wound model studies. *J Biomed Mater Res A* 2003;66(2):224-32.

216. Khor E, Lim LY. Implantable applications of chitin and chitosan. *Biomaterials* 2003;24(13):2339-49.

217. Czaja W, Krystynowicz A, Bielecki S, Brown RM, Jr. Microbial cellulose--the natural power to heal wounds. *Biomaterials* 2006;27(2):145-51.

218. Sanchavanakit N, Sangrungraungroj W, Kaomongkolgit R, Banaprasert T, Pavasant P, Phisalaphong M. Growth of human keratinocytes and fibroblasts on bacterial cellulose film. *Biotechnol Prog* 2006;22(4):1194-9.

219. Fontana JD, de Souza AM, Fontana CK, Torriani IL, Moreschi JC, Gallotti BJ, et al. Acetobacter cellulose pellicle as a temporary skin substitute. *Appl Biochem Biotechnol* 1990;24-25:253-64.

220. Melandri D, De Angelis A, Orioli R, Ponzielli G, Lualdi P, Giarratana N, et al. Use of a new hemicellulose dressing (Veloderm) for the treatment of split-thickness skin graft donor sites A within-patient controlled study. *Burns* 2006;32(8):964-72.

221. Thomas S. A review of the physical,biological and clinical properties of a bacterial cellulose wound dressing. *Journal of Wound Care* 2008;17(8):349-352.

222. Coerper S, Beckert S, Gängler M, Deutschle G, Küper M, Künigsrainer A. A retrospective evaluation of hydrocellulose dressings in the management of chronic wounds. *Ostomy and Wound Management* 2008;54(8).

223. Hofman D, Wilson J, Poore S, Cherry G, Ryan T. Can Traumacel be used in the treatment of chronic wounds? *Journal of Wound Care* 2000;9(8):393-6.

224. Hughes MA, Yang Y, Cherry GW. Effect of Traumacel P on the growth of human dermal fibroblasts in vitro. *Journal of Wound Care* 2002;11(4):149-54.

12. Hydrocolloid dressings

INTRODUCTION

The term 'hydrocolloid' was coined in the 1960s during the development of mucoadhesives, a class of gel-forming absorbent polymeric materials designed to adhere to the mucosal surfaces of the mouth, intestine or genitourinary tract. It was first used by Chen[1] in 1967 in a US patent, which described both a simple paste for treating mouth ulcers, and a preparation for topical use in which the paste was applied to a carrier such as a pliable water impermeable film.

In the 1980s the term was widely adopted by the international wound care community to describe a new family of dressings in which a gel-forming agent, typically carboxymethyl-cellulose (CMC), is dispersed in a mixture of adhesives and tackifiers applied to a foam or film carrier to form an absorbent, self-adhesive sheet.

Figure 53: The first hydrocolloid sheet dressing

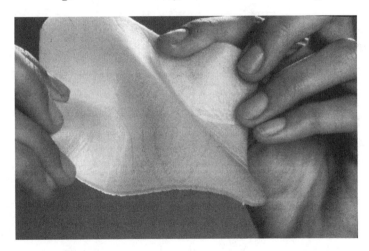

In scientific terms, a colloid is a defined as an intimate mixture of two substances one of which, called the dispersed phase (or colloid) is uniformly distributed in a finely divided state through the second substance, called the dispersion medium. The dispersion medium may be a gas, liquid or solid and the dispersed phase may be any of these, although it is not customary to refer to a system of one gas dispersed in another as a colloidal system.[2] A system consisting of a solid substance or water insoluble liquid colloidally dispersed in liquid water is called a 'hydrosol'.

Particles of the disperse phase are generally between 10^{-7} and 10^{-9} metre in diameter, imparting physical properties to colloidal mixtures that are intermediate between those of a true solution and a fine suspension. A hydrogel is a specific form of colloid in which the dispersed particles bind or react chemically together to form pores immobilizing the aqueous dispersion medium.

The use of the term 'hydrocolloid' to describe the dressings is actually somewhat misleading, for in their intact state they contain no water. In this context the term 'hydro' merely indicates that the colloidal particles are hydrophilic in nature and capable of absorbing water or other aqueous fluids into the matrix.

More recently, however, the term hydrocolloid has been used to describe two very different products, an amorphous hydrogel dressing and a fibrous dressing made from modified carboxymethylcellulose (CMC), both of which are totally dissimilar in structure and appearance to the adhesive sheets that were first described in this way. Whilst it is possible to argue that hydrogels are colloidal dispersions and that the CMC fibres form a colloidal dispersion or hydrogel in the presence of liquid, the same can also be said of other gel-forming fibres made from alginates, hyaluronidase, chitin or chitosan. Extending the use of the term in this way to materials with totally different physical characteristics and clinical indications from the original adhesive gel-forming sheets, causes confusion in the market place and cuts across existing, well-understood, dressing classification systems. Conversely there are also products available which, although they physically resemble hydrocolloid sheets, are actually more closely related to some of the foam products. Cutinova Hydro, for example, consists of a semipermeable film to which is applied a non-foamed hydrophilic polyurethane mass containing a dispersion of a sodium polyacrylate superabsorbent. For the purpose of this publication, however, this will be considered with the hydrocolloids, as it is widely perceived to be a member of this family of products.

DEVELOPMENT OF HYDROCOLLOID DRESSINGS

Early formulations

The hydrocolloid paste described by Chen in 1967 was subsequently marketed as Orabase. It has the ability to adhere firmly to moist surfaces, particularly those in the buccal cavity, where it absorbs water to form a protective gel over an ulcer or other lesion. It was this property that led to its experimental use in the treatment of skin excoriation caused by the effluent from surgical stomas and gastro-intestinal fistulae.[3] The treatment proved so successful that a more convenient presentation was developed, in which a semi-solid pliable wafer of material was backed with a thin polyethylene sheet. The new material, called Orahesive or Stomahesive, had two principal functions: it provided an effective protective barrier to the skin, and the polyethylene back also served as a good base for the attachment of an ostomy appliance.[4-5]

In 1973, the clinical benefits associated with the use of Stomahesive led to a preliminary study into the use of the adhesive base without the usual plastic backing in the treatment of 15 patients with venous ulcers.[6] This initial report was followed in 1975 by a further study in which Varihesive (as the new material was now called) was applied to a total of 22 leg ulcers of mixed aetiology.[7] The following year, two anecdotal reports were published that described the successful use of Stomahesive in the management of a small number of patients with pressure ulcers.[8-9]

Experience with both Stomahesive and Varihesive in the treatment of leg ulcers led eventually to the development of the first hydrocolloid dressing. After extensive pre-clinical and clinical trials, this was launched in the UK in 1982 as Granuflex, and introduced into the USA in the following year as Duoderm. The brand name 'Granuflex' is also used in South Africa, but in Canada and Australia the dressing is called 'Duoderm' and in Germany, Austria and Spain, 'Varihesive', all marketed by Convatec then part of Bristol-Myers Squibb.

In its original form, Granuflex/Duoderm consisted of gelatin, pectin, and sodium carboxymethylcellulose (NaCMC), dispersed as micro-granules in an adhesive mass of polyisobutylene which was applied to a thin layer of semi-open-cell polyurethane foam. The closed cells on the outer surface of the foam were initially thought to provide an effective bacterial barrier, but when the results of laboratory tests demonstrated that this was not the case, a semipermeable film dressing was soon added to the outer surface of the foam to provide this function. When applied to an exuding wound, the hydrocolloid components absorbed exudate and progressively decreased in viscosity until they eventually formed a soft mobile gel. During this process, the adhesive base underwent phase inversion, so that it ceased to consist of a dispersion of hydrophilic granules in an adhesive mass but become a dispersion of the adhesive in an aqueous hydrogel.

Figure 54: Removal of early hydrocolloid dressing

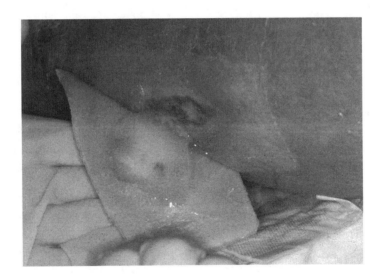

The resulting semi-solid material, which had a characteristic odour and a superficial resemblance to pus, had to be removed from the wound at each dressing change by irrigation or some other suitable means, and was considered by some to detract from the acceptability of the dressing. It was also suggested by some that these dispersed polyisobutylene residues might become trapped within the cellular structure of the wound during healing and lead to histological changes.

Second generation products

Recognizing the clinical and commercial potential of hydrocolloid dressings, other manufacturers developed products with a continuous phase which resisted disintegration, thereby eliminating some of the perceived disadvantages of the original Granuflex/Duoderm formulation. Some of these formulations used a styrene-isoprene-styrene (S-I-S) copolymer or some other thermoplastic elastomer such as an ethylene-propylene copolymer together with tackifiers and antioxidants. At room temperature these polymers effectively form cross-links resulting in a three dimensional lattice in which the absorbent gel-forming agent is contained. One example of a product based upon this technology is Comfeel Plus, which was launched in the United Kingdom in 1995 as an improved version of the original product Comfeel. The dressing contains calcium alginate and sodium carboxymethylcellulose as the absorbent gel forming agents, dispersed in an S-I-S copolymer with a plasticiser, (dioctyl adipate) and a hydrogenated hydrocarbon resin tackifier carried upon a permeable polyurethane film.

Other products have a continuous phase composed of a blend of polyisobutylene and ethylene-vinyl acetate (EVA) copolymer that forms cross-links when exposed to ionizing radiation.

The chemistry of different types of commercially available hydrocolloid dressings and the function of the various components used in their formulation has been comprehensively reviewed by Lipman.[10]

In order to overcome the problem of large quantities of liquefied hydrocolloid residues remaining in the wound when the dressing was removed, Granuflex/Duoderm was reformulated and relaunched in the UK in 1989 as 'Granuflex E' and in the US as Duoderm CGF (Controlled Gel Formulation). For a time the both formulations remained available but eventually the original formulation was discontinued, and in the UK the suffix 'E' was eventually dropped altogether.

The new presentation, which still contains gelatin, CMC and pectin, is based upon a formulation described in a second U.S. Patent of 1985.[11] This describes a medical-Grade pressure sensitive adhesive comprising a mixture of one or more polyisobutylenes or blends of polyisobutylenes and butyl rubber, one or more styrene radial or block copolymers, a pentaerythritol ester of hydrogenated rosin as a tackifying agent and mineral oil in addition to the water soluble gel forming agents. The mineral oil is said to improve the extensibility of the formulation and enhance the aggressiveness of the adhesive.

Effects of formulation changes

At the time of its introduction, it was claimed that the new formulation of Granuflex/Duoderm was more absorbent than the original presentation, however, the results of independent laboratory tests which showed that the fluid handling properties of the new formulation were considerably inferior to those of the original Granuflex, cast doubt on the validity of this claim.[12-13]

The hydration properties of the two formulations were similarly compared by Ferrari et al. over a four day period in two separate studies[14-15] using a passive uptake technique. They also found that, for the first two days at least, the weight of fluid taken up by the new formulation was considerably less than that absorbed by the original formulation, although by day four the total amount of fluid absorbed by both dressings was broadly equivalent. The differences in the rheological (viscoelastic) properties of the dressings were also highlighted in this study. The original formulation absorbed water rapidly and reached saturation after 12 hours during which time there was a marked reduction in both rheomechanical and adhesive properties. The modified formulation exhibited a linear water uptake profile over four days and its rheomechanical and adhesive properties remained unchanged after hydration under the conditions of test.

The possibility that such a fundamental change in formulation could have an effect upon the clinical performance of the dressing could not be discounted, for according to Rousseau,[16] these different physicochemical properties could affect the immune system, the healing rate and the appearance of the wound bed upon removal of the dressing. For this reason the results of laboratory and clinical studies performed upon the original formulation of Granuflex/Duoderm (i.e. those published prior to 1989/1990) are not actually applicable to product produced after that date. There was also some evidence to suggest that changes in formulation increased the potential for the dressing to cause adverse skin effects.

Presentation

Originally produced in small squares, hydrocolloid sheets are now available in a variety of shapes and sizes. In some the adhesive mass extends to the edge of the dressing but in others the mass is applied in the form of an island in the centre, forming a so-called bordered dressing.

Figure 55: Examples of shaped hydrocolloid island dressings

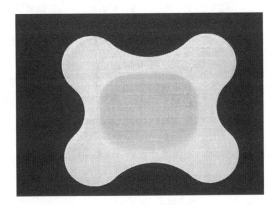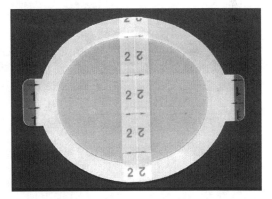

Dressings have also been developed that consist of a semipermeable film coated with a thin layer of a hydrocolloid adhesive. These are used as post-operative dressings or as secondary retention products over primary dressings such as alginates or hydrogels as alternatives to semipermeable polyurethane films with acrylic-based adhesive systems such as Opsite or Tegaderm.

When two such products, Duoderm Extra Thin and Tegaderm were compared as secondary dressings over an alginate dressing or a hydrogel dressing in a randomized controlled trial involving 100 patients,[17] they were considered to be broadly equivalent in performance as no significant differences were detected in their ability to prevent maceration or resist wrinkling (the primary outcome variables).

Powders, pastes and granules containing some of the components used in hydrocolloid sheets have also been developed.

Figure 56: Hydrocolloids pastes, powders and granules

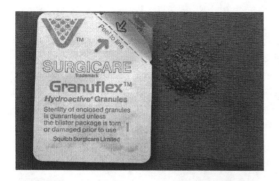 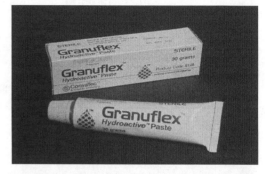
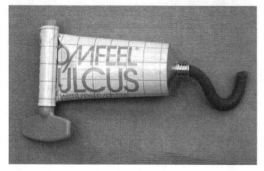 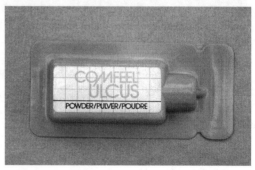

These are introduced into small cavities or sinuses, or used in conjunction with the dressing sheets to increase the absorbent capacity of the system when used on heavily exuding wounds. Hydrocolloid paste has also been evaluated as a vehicle for the administration of transforming growth factor–beta1 (TGF-beta 1).[18] The hydrocolloid granules have since been discontinued, but the powder and two formulations of paste are still available (Comfeel Powder and Paste and Granuflex Paste).

The use of these materials was judged to extend the range of indications for hydrocolloids in pressure sore therapy as they were thought to enable ulcers of any Grade to be treated, although even using the paste the dressings were better suited to ulcers on the limbs than on the sacrum.[19]

One hydrocolloid sheet has been developed with a foam layer six mm thick divided into three central concentric rings on the outer surface. One or more of these rings can be removed to match the size of the pressure ulcer beneath, the remaining foam rings cushion the region around the ulcer and may allow for a reduction of pressure around the wound tissue.

Figure 57: Comfeel Pressure Relieving Dressing

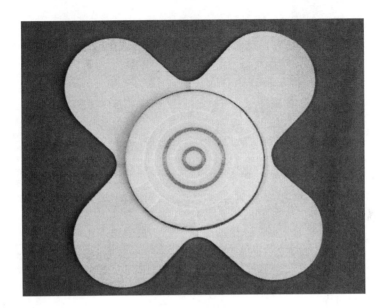

The use Comfeel Pressure Relieving Dressing (PRD) , was described by Stoker[20] and Clark,[21] who determined trochanteric and peritrochanteric interface pressures on 12 healthy volunteers and showed that the use of the PRD reduced the maximum pressure applied to the apex of the trochanter from a mean of 64.2 mm Hg to a mean of 52.2 mm Hg. It is unlikely, however, that the reduction in pressure is of sufficient magnitude to produce any significant clinical benefit unless it is used in conjunction with other pressure relieving measures. This product was subsequently reformulated to contain the same adhesive mass found in standard Comfeel Plus at which time it was renamed Comfeel Plus Pressure Relieving Dressing.

Another product, Dermasorb, consisted of a hydrocolloid/alginate mixture formed into a flat sheet cut into a spiral for use as a cavity dressing. The dressing was capable of absorbing large quantities of liquid, increasing dramatically in volume as it did so. Despite its novel design and some encouraging early clinical results when used as an alternative to paraffin gauze in the treatment of donor sites,[22] it proved not to be a commercial success and so was therefore discontinued.

Figure 58: Dermasorb before and after hydration

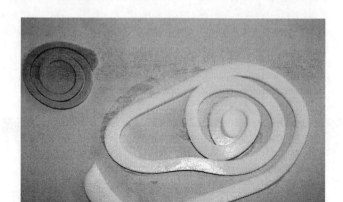

Examples of current hydrocolloid dressings include:

- Activheal Hydrocolloid (film backed)
- Activheal Hydrocolloid Foam Backed
- Comfeel Plus
- Comfeel Plus Pressure Relieving Dressing
- Comfeel Plus Transparent
- Cutinova Hydro
- Dermafilm
- Duoderm Extra Thin
- Duoderm Signal
- Flexigran Hydrocolloid
- Granuflex
- Hydrocoll
- Hydrocoll Basic
- Hydrocoll Thin
- Nu-Derm
- Nu-Derm - Thin
- Replicare
- Restore - Hollister
- Suprasorb H
- Suprasorb H Thin
- Tegaderm Hydrocolloid
- Tegaderm Hydrocolloid Thin
- Ultec Pro - Covidien

Anecdotal accounts of the use of some of these products have been published previously.[23-24] Some of these dressings are also available in multiple shapes and sizes, bordered and unbordered.

In addition to the above, a number of other products have been developed which consist of film or foam-backed absorbent pads, sometimes containing alginate or CMC fibre, which are coated with a thin layer of a hydrocolloid adhesive. These dressings are often classified incorrectly as 'hydrocolloids' for in reality have little in common with the products previously described. Examples include:

- Alione - Coloplast
- Combiderm - Convatec
- Combiderm N - Convatec
- Versiva - Convatec

PHYSICAL PROPERTIES

Fluid handling properties

Unlike simple adhesive polyurethane films dressings such as Opsite and Tegaderm, in their intact state the principal hydrocolloid dressings are virtually impermeable to moisture vapour. When applied to an exuding wound, however, the absorbent components of the adhesive mass gradually take up liquid to form a gel and as this process progresses throughout the thickness of the adhesive mass, the permeability of the dressing increases until it reaches a steady state determined principally by the permeability of the backing film. The ability of a dressing to dissipate a proportion of the aqueous component of wound fluid as water vapour in this way can, in some instances, significantly improve the product's fluid handling properties. The results of a laboratory study which compared the moisture vapour transmission rate (MVTR) of six hydrocolloid dressings was published in 1988 which showed that the permeability of those products backed with a polyurethane film varied from 79 to 956 g/m^2 over a 24 hour period.[25] A further dressing Biofilm which had a nonwoven fabric back transpired in excess of 4000 g/m^2 during this period. To put these results into context, when fully hydrated, the most permeable of the film-backed products, (Granuflex) was actually found to be more permeable than six polyurethane film dressings, investigated in an earlier study,[26] which included Opsite, the brand leader.

An early account of the ability of a dressing to change its physical properties in response to changes in the local environment was provided by Palamand.[27] Such products are sometimes referred to as 'smart' or 'intelligent' dressings. Polyurethane films, for example, are now available the permeability of which changes by several orders of magnitude in the presence of liquid. When used as backing layers for polyurethane foam dressings, these films greatly increase the fluid handling capacity of the product and thus greatly increase its wear time.[28]

Whilst the change in the permeability of hydrocolloid dressings is only a fraction of that of the new films, it is, nevertheless, an important property of the dressings which has significant clinical implications - particularly for the treatment of dry sloughy or necrotic wounds. In these situations the relatively impermeable nature of the intact dressing initially prevents loss of moisture vapour from the affected area, thereby increasing the moisture content of the underlying tissue and facilitating autolytic debridement - an effect that was noted in some of the earliest clinical studies with hydrocolloid dressings. As debridement progresses and the dead tissue separates from the healthy layers beneath, exudate produced by the wound will be taken up by the dressing causing an increase in its permeability as gel formation takes place.

In the practice of wound management, the fluid handling properties of a dressing (defined as the sum of its absorbency and MVTR) is of considerable clinical importance, as the effective management of the moisture content of a wound and the surrounding skin is, arguably, the most important requirement of any dressing system. For this reason, manufacturers of dressings of all types place considerable emphasis upon the results of comparative laboratory data to support their marketing or promotional activities.

In 1998 these and other techniques were used to compare the key properties of twelve hydrocolloid dressings. A full account of this study was published previously,[29] but the fluid handling results from this investigation are summarised in Figure 59 to illustrate the differences that existed between the various products available at that time.

These results clearly illustrate significant important differences between the various dressings. Not only do they differ in terms of the total volume of liquid absorbed, but considerable variation also exists in the rate of absorption. One product, (Number 3) absorbs well initially, but then the weight of liquid retained by the dressing appears to decrease over the next 48 hours due, it is assumed, to the gel forming component of the dressing passing into solution. Considerable differences also exist in the permeability of the various dressings which have important implications for the total fluid handling capacity of the products concerned.

Figure 59: Fluid handling properties of hydrocolloid dressings

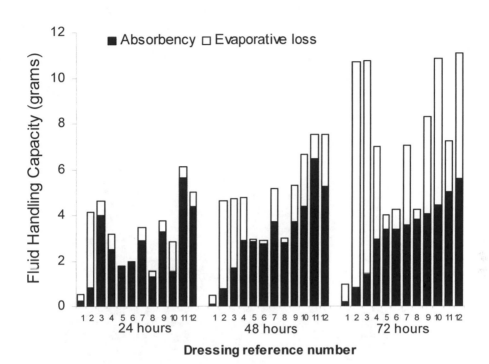

No.	Hydrocolloid	No.	Hydrocolloid
1	Askina Biofilm Transparent	7	Tegasorb Thin
2	Askina Transorbent	8	Algoplaque
3	Comfeel Plus Transparent	9	Comfeel Plus Flexible
4	Cutinova Hydro	10	Comfeel Plus Bevelled
5	Granuflex	11	Hydrocoll
6	Varihesive E	12	Tegasorb

Conformability

A further important physical property of hydrocolloid dressings is their ability to conform to hard-to-dress anatomical sites. This is determined, at least initially, by the thickness and rigidity of the adhesive mass, and also the extensibility of the material from which the backing layer is manufactured. The conformability results from the study cited previously, obtained using the method described in Chapter 7, are shown in Figure 60. In this test, conformability is considered to be inversely proportional to inflation pressure.

Figure 60: Conformability of hydrocolloid dressings

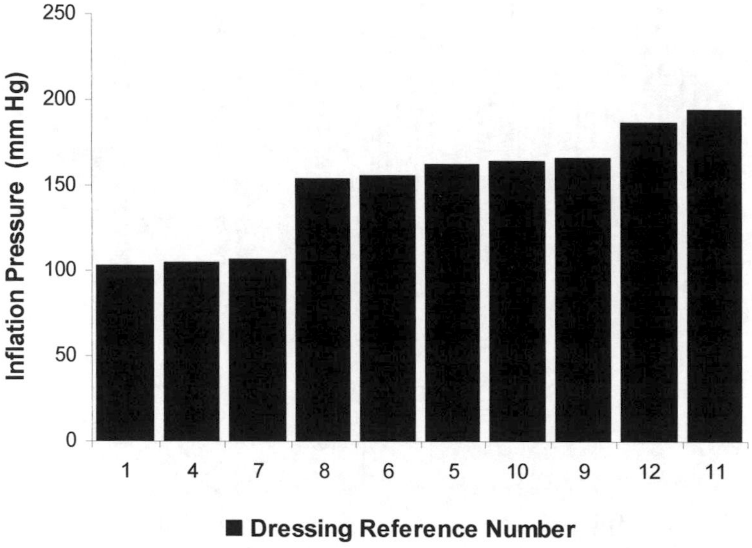

Dressing 2 was permeable to air and therefore could not be tested and the dimensions of Dressing 3 were too small for it to be tested using the standard test equipment.

EXPERIMENTAL STUDIES

Effect upon local wound environment

A detailed comparison of the local environment of chronic wounds under HCD and polyurethane film dressings (PUF) was carried out by Varghese *et al.*,[30] who examined fluid collected from nine patients with 14 chronic full thickness ulcers dressed with Duoderm or Opsite. They found that the oxygen tension (pO_2) was zero or very low beneath both dressings despite the relative permeability of the PUF to oxygen in laboratory studies. They therefore proposed that the low oxygen concentration required for the optimal growth of fibroblasts (5 - 10 mm Hg) and that the somewhat higher requirement of keratinocytes (40 - 140 mm Hg) can be met by the local blood supply.

The pH of the wound fluid beneath each dressing was also measured, and was found to be more acidic beneath the hydrocolloid material than under the polyurethane film, due, at least in part, to the chemical nature of the hydrocolloid base. The low pH under the hydrocolloid dressing was thought to have an inhibiting effect on the growth of some bacteria, particularly Pseudomonas species. An acidic environment also reduces the histotoxicity of ammonia, produced by enzymatic breakdown of urea by bacterial enzymes, and increases the dissociation of oxyhaemoglobin thereby raising the pO_2 of the wound. Viable neutrophils were found under both dressings, but in greater numbers beneath the polyurethane film.

In a pilot study,[31] seven patients with leg ulcers dressed with Duoderm had the pH of their wounds measured continuously over a 24-hour period. The mean pH value was 6.7 at the beginning of the trial period falling to a minimum of 5.6 after 24 hours although this trend failed to reach statistical significance. This is perhaps not surprising, given the fact that an extract of Duoderm has a pH of around 4.5 - 5.0,[29] and that it takes many hours to complete the gelling process of Duoderm.

The low pO_2 beneath Granuflex/Duoderm was thought by Cherry and Ryan[32] to be responsible for the increase in the rate of formation of vascular tissue that they observed in the chorio-allantoic membrane (CAM) of the chick embryo, and also in experimental wounds in pigs. This increase in vascularity was elegantly confirmed by Pickworth and De Sousa[33] who used an immunohistological technique to compare the degree of angiogenesis in full thickness wounds in pigs dressed with a dry dressing, Opsite or Duoderm. After three, six and nine days, the degree of angiogenesis was greater under the HCD than the PUF or dry dressing but on days three and six angiogenesis under the PUF was not significantly different from that seen under the dry dressing although this reached significance on day nine.

Samuelsen and Nielsen[34] also used the CAM model to examine the angiogenic effects of hydrocolloid dressings using an angiogenic growth factor as a positive control. In contrast to Cherry and Ryan,[32] they found no significant stimulatory effect associated with the use of the dressings and concluded that the increased levels of angiogenesis reported clinically were probably due to an indirect effect caused by the low oxygen tension and the general influence of the products upon the local wound environment rather than any substances released from the hydrocolloids themselves.

Because of their relatively impermeable nature, hydrocolloid dressings applied to wounds filled with slough or covered with a dry necrotic layer, prevent the loss of moisture vapour from the underlying skin to the external environment and thus increase the moisture content of the devitalised tissue. This in turn facilitates natural wound cleansing by the action of proteolytic enzymes and macrophage activity, a process termed 'autolytic debridement'. Early reports of the ability of hydrocolloids to promote wound debridement were made in 1977 by Tracy,[35] and in 1984 by Johnson.[36]

Lydon et al.[37-38] suggested that Granuflex/Duoderm also has fibrinolytic activity, breaking down human fibrin clots by both tissue-plasminogen-activator-dependent and independent mechanisms. This activity was thought to be due to the presence of pectin, and it was proposed that this property makes Granuflex/Duoderm contribute in an active or positive way to the wound cleansing process. Some support for this suggestion came from in vivo studies, which revealed that Granuflex/Duoderm accelerated the clearance of labelled fibrin clots in porcine full thickness wounds. It was therefore proposed that the dressing might help to restore normal capillary function in humans by causing dissolution of the fibrin cuffs often found around blood vessels in patients with lipodermatosclerosis or venous ulceration which are believed to prevent the diffusion of oxygen from affected vessels, leading to tissue necrosis and cell death.

This possibility was investigated by Mulder et al.,[39] who took tissue biopsies from the rims of 19 venous ulcers before and after treatment with Duoderm covered by an Unna's boot and compression bandage, and compared them with those from wounds dressed similarly but without the hydrocolloid dressing. Frozen sections of all biopsies were stained with an immunofluorescent antibody to fibrin to determine thickness of shallow and deep dermal pericapillary fibrin cuffs (PFCs). Separate sections were stained with haematoxylin and eosin to assess capillary frequency, histopathology, and inflammation. All ratings and pathology assessments were performed blinded to treatment conditions. Both deep and shallow PFCs were reduced in 89% of ulcers treated with Duoderm plus Unna's boot compared with 40% of ulcers treated with Unna's boot alone (p < 0.04). No other significant differences in inflammation, histopathology, or capillary frequency were observed. The authors concluded that the presence of the hydrocolloid had a marked effect upon PFCs but cautioned that, as not all hydrocolloid dressing are fibrinolytic, these results may not apply to other dressings.

Samuelsen and Nielsen[40] questioned the clinical relevance of the reported fibrinolytic effects of hydrocolloid dressings. Using a chromogenic assay they showed that the activation, by extracts of hydrocolloid dressings, of tissue-plasminogen activator (t-PA), which is responsible for the conversion of proteolytically inactive plasminogen into the fibrinolytic enzyme plasmin, was very weak compared with the activation of t-PA by purified fibrin. They argued that as fibrin is a natural constituent of the tissue repair process, the contribution made by the constituents of hydrocolloid dressings has no clinical relevance.

The benefits of a moist wound-healing environment with particular reference to the use of hydrocolloid dressings were discussed in a review published by Field and Kerstein in 1994.[41]

Healing rates

When hydrocolloid dressings were first developed it was perhaps inevitable that they would be compared with film dressings in both animal and clinical studies. In 1983 Alvarez et al.,[42] compared Duoderm, with Opsite, 'wet to dry' gauze dressings, and air exposure, on superficial experimental wounds in the domestic pig. Compared with the other two groups, collagen synthesis was enhanced under both HCD and PUF. The differences were detectable from the first day after wounding and remained evident throughout the course of the study. Although the rate of epithelialization beneath both these 'occlusive' dressings was greater than that in wounds dressed with gauze or exposed to air, the hydrocolloid produced a significantly greater number of resurfaced wounds in the early days of treatment, and had a lower HT_{50} (time to heal 50% of wounds) than the polyurethane film. The relative rate of healing for HCD, PUF and gauze relative to air exposure was +36%, +21% and -5% respectively. Alvarez and his co-workers also confirmed that, as might be predicted, the hydrocolloid was less likely than the film dressing to cause occasional re-wounding as exudate production decreased on or after day three of the study.

Numerous animal studies have been reported in which the wound healing properties of hydrocolloids have been compared with other types of dressings. Leipziger[43] compared the effects of a film dressing and a hydrocolloid dressing with a collagen sponge produced from purified bovine tendon type I collagen on the healing and scarring of full-thickness excision wounds in pigs. Granulation tissue production within the wounds was estimated by measuring ^{14}C proline incorporation into collagenase-sensitive protein; epidermal resurfacing and wound contractions were measured by computerised morphometric image analysis of wounds made on a tattooed grid. The authors found that, compared with air-exposed wounds, collagen synthesis in occluded wounds was significantly enhanced and that epidermal resurfacing of wounds dressed with the film or hydrocolloid dressing was accelerated by 40%. Wound contraction was significantly reduced by the collagen matrix but remained unaffected by the occlusive dressings.

Chvapil *et al.*[44] compared a similar range of dressings, Duoderm, Opsite and collagen sponge, on sixteen shallow wounds on pigs caused by a fast-rotating abrasive disc an injury which is similar to a second-degree burn. The collagen sponge dressings were moistened with saline before use and covered with either an occlusive or semi-occlusive polyurethane film. They reported that the rate of epithelization, determined by planimetry, was the same in all groups after three to five days but that the epithelial layer was thicker in wounds treated with Duoderm. Wounds dressed by either of the collagen sponge materials showed a better appearance when visually scored. They also suggested that wounds dressed with Duoderm or Opsite were often macerated and stated that the residue from Duoderm was difficult to remove from the wound without inflicting discomfort to the subject.

When Reuterving[45] compared the effects of three dressings Mezinc, (an occlusive plaster containing zinc), Duoderm, or saline soaked gauze on full thickness wounds on 86 rats. The wounds were examined clinically, histologically and biochemically four, eight or twelve days after wounding. Four days postoperatively, the Duoderm-treated wounds differed significantly from the other two groups. An adherent discoloured gelatinous mass remained after removal of the Duoderm which, upon histological examination, corresponded to a superficial exudate containing polymorphonuclear leukocytes (PMNs), macrophages and condensed foreign material. They also showed evidence of a more extensive inflammatory reaction in the underlying tissues compared with saline gauze or Mezinc, and debris was seen in extracellular vesicles and in foamy macrophages. These macrophages were mainly confined to the granulation tissue, which was about twice as thick as in the other two treatment groups twelve days after excision.

When In a second study, Chvapil[46] compared the effects of eight dressing regimens on the rate of reepithelialization of 92 split-thickness wounds on pigs. Changes in wound dimensions were recorded using a morphometric technique and the inflammatory reaction produced within the wound by each dressing was scored from histological slides. Moderate to severe inflammatory changes were induced by dressings such as collagen sponge, polyethylene glycol, Duoderm, and a lanolin ointment; these wounds also reepithelialized significantly faster than gauze-covered wounds acting as controls. Dressings such as a hydrated hydrogel membrane, Carbopol 934P, or Silvadene cream, which did not elicit a significant inflammatory response, also did not affect the rate of reepithelialization compared with control wounds. Only when the inflammatory reaction to a wound dressing (methylcellulose) became excessive was the rate of reepithelialization significantly inhibited in comparison with the controls. The authors hypothesised that wound dressings that induce an inflammatory reaction, enhance healing by activating cells such as macrophages or fibroblasts that produce growth factors and other mediators of the repair process.

When Gokoo and Burhop,[47] compared the healing rates obtained with Duoderm, with those of a hydrogel sheet dressing, Clearsite, on eight full-thickness circular surgical wounds 20 mm in diameter produced on the backs of each of four micropigs. Wounds dressed with the hydrogel dressing exhibited a more rapid rate of closure and reepithelialization than those dressed with the hydrocolloid. Histological examination of the wounds confirmed the presence of much larger numbers of vacuoles granulomas and foam cells in the hydrocolloid-treated wounds compared with those dressed with the hydrogel.

Wound histology

The effects of various dressings, including hydrocolloids, upon the inflammatory status of wounds, sometimes recorded over an extended period, have been examined by a number of researchers.

Young et al.[48] in 1991, using a variety of histological techniques, compared Opsite and Granuflex/Duoderm on full-thickness excised wounds on pigs for up to six months after injury. Film-dressed wounds showed a decrease in the number of inflammatory cells (polymorphonuclear leukocytes and macrophages) from five to 60 days after wounding; whereas the numbers of proliferative phase cells (fibroblasts and endothelial cells) increased from days five to seven. The total cellularity per unit area showed an increase between days five and seven, during the proliferative phase of repair, and then progressively decreased as the proliferative phase was succeeded by the remodelling phase. Wound repair in the hydrocolloid-dressed wounds was more complex. The number of inflammatory cells remained relatively high throughout and there were consistently fewer endothelial cells present. Fibroblast numbers showed an initial fall from day five to 14 but then started to increase in number from day 21 to 60. The authors suggested that the chronic inflammatory reaction appeared to be caused by the presence of particulate matter that had been incorporated into cavities or vacuoles in the wound bed and hypodermis, which was similar to that previously reported by Reuterving[45] and Gokoo.[47] These artifacts were still apparent six months after injury.

The findings and conclusions of this paper were vigorously challenged by Witkowski,[49] and Phillips et al.,[50] who questioned the design of the study and the assumption that the material in the vacuoles was a hydrocolloid residue. They also expressed concerns over the clinical relevance of the observations to human patients given that in blinded examination of 13 biopsies from chronic wounds in human patients, no significant difference in histology or particle-containing cavities were detectable with either product. These criticisms were addressed in further communication from the original authors who argued that given the depths at which the cavities were detected in the porcine model, these would not have been found in standard shallow punch biopsies and reported that intradermal injection of hydrocolloid produces a similar response to that induced when the dressing is used topically. They acknowledged, however, that as the rate of granulation production in the porcine model is significantly greater than in a chronic wound, this could increase the likelihood of the effect previously reported.

Additional evidence that appeared to support of the findings of Young et al.,[48] was published in a number of further papers. In 1992, using the same pig model, Leek et al.[51] compared the histological changes produced by four different hydrocolloids, Duoderm, Intrasite HCD (now discontinued), Tegasorb and Replicare. Animals were sacrificed at 4, 10, 21 and 90 days post-wounding and the excision sites were examined histologically. Granulomatous lesions were observed following treatment with each of the dressings. These lesions developed between four and ten days after wounding and showed little evidence of resolution after 90 days. Duoderm and Intrasite HCD induced the most marked reactions resulting in granulomata with a distinct and different morphology. The authors concluded that the results of this experimental study may, if reflected in the clinical environment, 'question the efficacy and indication of HCD dressings in the treatment of wounds having a number of different aetiologies'.

Chakravarthy et al.[52] also used full-thickness wounds on pigs to compare three new hydrocolloid dressing formulations with two commercial preparations, Restore and Duoderm. Two of the new formulations consisted of conventional absorbents dispersed in a maceration-resistant adhesive matrix; the third contained the same matrix, mixed with potentially biodegradable dextran microspheres. Wound tissue was harvested 18 days after wounding and compared histomorphometrically. Gross disintegration of the dressings within the wound ranged from minimal, for the product with the biodegradable microspheres, to severe for Restore. Disintegration of other dressings was described as 'moderate'. The percentage of tissue sections containing giant cells reflected the degree of dressing disintegration; 38% of wounds dressed with the dextran product contained giant cells compared with 74% of wounds dressed with Duoderm and 100% of wounds dressed with Restore. The wounds dressed with the dextran microsphere product had relatively fewer chronic inflammatory cells than other dressings and were also characterized by a well-organised collagen matrix and complete reepithelialization. Wound closure was similar with all dressings examined except Restore, which was delayed compared with wounds dressed with alternative products. Two of the prototype materials elicited an inflammatory tissue response that was comparable to Duoderm but the material containing the dextran microspheres caused minimal tissue reactions.

Vogt[53] examined the effect of moisture upon wound healing in a porcine partial-thickness wound model when he compared the effects of 'wet' wounds, produced by saline contained in a vinyl chamber, and 'moist' wounds produced by the application of hydrocolloid dressing, with 'dry' wound dressed with sterile gauze. The saline-filled chambers were replaced daily with normal saline containing penicillin and streptomycin to prevent infection, but the hydrocolloid and gauze dressings were left undisturbed. The time to achieve complete closure was six, seven, and eight days in wet, moist, and dry environments respectively. Thickness of the epidermis in wet, moist, and dry wounds was 204 ± 23, 141 ± 12, and 129 ± 18 (mean $\pm$ SEM), respectively. The authors also found that moist wounds had more sub-epidermal inflammatory cells than wet wounds, and that compared to dry wounds, the moist or the wet healing environment resulted in less necrosis and faster and better quality of healing in the formation of the newly regenerated epidermis.

Agren[54] compared the effects of Comfeel and Duoderm on key aspects of the wound healing process in full-thickness skin wounds in rats, and in a further study the same hydrocolloids were compared with Opsite on 20 mm full thickness punch biopsy in pigs.[55] In both studies they showed that hydrocolloid residues were phagocytosed as indicated by the presence of foam cells in the granulation tissue. Granulomatous tissue reactions around extracellular vacuoles were present in ten of twelve pig wounds dressed with Duoderm but only one dressed with Comfeel. None of the ten wounds dressed with the film dressing showed any evidence of this reaction. In the rat model, extra cellular vacuoles (100-400 microns in size) occupied about 25% of the granulation tissue volume in the Duoderm group but less than 5% in the Comfeel group, a statistically significant difference ($p < 0.001$). In both species the vacuoles contained hydrophobic polymers derived from the respective hydrocolloid dressing, as analyzed by Fourier Transform Infrared (FT-IR) microscopy. Although there was a tendency for Duoderm to delay entry into the contraction phase in pigs, there was no significant difference in epithelialization between the three dressings. In the rat, wounds treated with Comfeel were significantly more reepithelialized (mean: 78%) than those treated with Duoderm (mean: 41%). The authors concluded that extensive incorporation of hydrophobic dressing material from hydrocolloid dressings may render the wound bed less suitable for epithelial migration during acute secondary wound healing.

Biochemical effects

When In 1993 Schmidt[56] and Chung[57] had suggested that the clinical inflammatory reaction associated with the use of Granuflex/Duoderm might be mediated by the *in-situ* generation of hydrogen peroxide, following a laboratory study in which they were able to demonstrate that the auto-oxidative production of very low concentrations of this material from Granuflex/Duoderm granules had a significant effect on the rate of proliferation of murine (L929) fibroblasts *in vitro*. This activity was shown to be associated with the gelatin and pectin components of the dressing but not the sodium carboxymethylcellulose. The dressing also displayed some evidence of superoxide savaging activity which they postulated could also benefit wound healing.

Wollina *et al.*[58] later questioned these conclusions and proposed an alternative mechanism for the possible wound healing stimulatory properties of hydrocolloids, following a study in which they compared the effects of seven wound dressings on human keratinocytes and mouse 3T3 fibroblast cells in culture. Morphological changes were noted within the first day of exposure to some of the dressings and after 72 hours, inhibition of cell growth was observed in the presence of three products, Algoplaque, Cutinova Plus and Varihesive (Granuflex). Interestingly the same three dressings were also shown to be responsible for inducing the production by both cell types of interleukin-6 (IL-6), a cytokine involved in the initiation of wound healing. As production of IL-6 did not correlate to cell injury or proliferative activity, it was proposed that it came from 'activated' cells rather than from passive release from damaged cells. This effect was most pronounced with Varihesive.

The *in vitro* effects of the hydrophilic components isolated from six commercial hydrocolloid dressings on fibroblast proliferation were examined by Agren.[59] The dressings were extracted using an organic solvent (xylene) to remove the hydrophobic adhesive matrix and the hydrophilic residues were dissolved in complete cell growth medium to provide a final concentration of 0.1% and 0.01% w/v. These extracts were added to confluent human dermal fibroblasts grown in a monolayer culture and incubated for 24 hours. Cell proliferation was estimated by the incorporation into the cells of the thymidine analogue 5-bromo-2'-deoxyuridine (BrdU) determined using an ELISA technique. Apart from Comfeel Plus, the hydrophilic components of hydrocolloid dressings significantly inhibited fibroblast proliferation by varying amounts at 0.1% compared to control-treated fibroblasts ($p < 0.05$) although no obvious morphological changes could be detected in the treated cells when these were examined by phase-contrast microscopy. The authors concluded that the results of this study 'may provide an objective basis for prescribing the appropriate hydrocolloid dressing for wound management.'

When Achterberg[60] in an '*in vitro*' study compared the way in which different absorbent/gel-forming dressings interacted with artificial wound fluid (human plasma). The test fluid was incubated with Cutinova Hydro, Varihesive E, Comfeel Ulcer Dressing and Allevyn, and the concentrations of total protein, albumin, immunoglobulin and growth factors determined. Considerable differences were recorded in the total weight of fluid taken up by Cutinova hydro and Allevyn which absorbed 4-5 times as much as the hydrocolloids. Rather more interesting, was the finding that the products also differed significantly in the way in which this fluid was handled. Cutinova hydro selectively took up water, effectively increasing the concentrating of the dissolved proteins in the remaining free fluid - presumably by preventing high molecular weight material from entering into the superabsorbent gel contained within the dressing. In contrast, Allevyn and the hydrocolloids had no significant effect upon the concentration of the proteins in the unabsorbed solution, indicating that the gelling process was not selective.

The significance of this observation is not clear. Whilst it is possible that in some instances selective absorption is desirable, because it leaves potentially important molecules within the wound, it could equally be argued that if a chronic wound contains high levels of proteolytic enzymes, which have a deleterious effect upon healing, concentrating these further would only make a bad situation worse. This is clearly an area that requires further investigation.

When Quirinia and Viidik[61] used a rat model to examine the effect of Duoderm on the healing of ischaemic incisional wounds and on flap survival in rats. They found that after ten days, ischaemic wounds dressed Duoderm decreased in strength by 41% - 44%. Following removal of Duoderm on day ten, the biomechanical properties had improved but not returned to normal by day 20. In the dressed animals the shrinkage of ischaemic wounds and the extension of necrosis on the ischaemic flaps were reduced.

Matsumura[62] used hairless descendants of Mexican hairless dogs to compare the rate of healing of deep dermal burns dressed with Vaseline gauze or a hydrocolloid dressing. They reported that wounds treated with hydrocolloid dressings were reepithelialized on day 24, whereas wounds treated with VG were not reepithelialized until day 30.

In a unique study Agren et al.[63] compared Comfeel Plus, Duoderm CGF and Opsite with air exposure in four full thickness 4 mm biopsy wounds on each of ten human volunteers. Each wound was subsequently rebiopsied with a 6 mm punch on seven and fourteen days post wounding, and epithelialization was assessed histologically. Epithelial coverage increased significantly ($p = 0.007$) with all of the dressings tested ($62 \pm 6\%$, mean $\pm$ SEM) compared with air exposure ($39 \pm 7\%$) on day seven, but by day 14 no difference could be detected between the treatments. The thickness of the epithelium was significantly increased in the occluded wounds by day 7. This enhanced epithelial cover was shown by immunohistochemical techniques to be due principally to increased migration rather than enhanced proliferation. Although it appeared that there might be differences in the healing rates and epithelial proliferation rates between the various occlusive dressings, the number of volunteers who took part was not large enough for these to reach statistical significance.

Effect of dressing additives on healing

The hydrocolloid adhesive mass can be medicated with a variety of agents. Agren et al.,[64] investigated the possible benefits of adding zinc oxide in a study involving surgical wounds in pigs, following an earlier study in which they demonstrated that zinc oxide accelerated wound closure when applied with gauze or a collagen sponge.[65]

Forty partial-thickness wounds were treated with different zinc oxide concentrations, and epithelialization was evaluated morphometrically in 320 histological sections. Wound closure, bacterial growth, and inflammation were studied in eight full-thickness wounds. The level of serum zinc was determined before and after treatment. In partial-thickness wounds, concentrations of zinc oxide at or below 1.0% w/w inhibited epithelialization, whereas no effect was observed at zinc oxide concentrations from 2% to 6%. In full-thickness wounds, 6% zinc oxide reduced bacterial growth by about two log units and increased the inflammatory response in the granulation tissue, but had no effect on healing when compared with control (hydrocolloid alone). Serum zinc levels remained unchanged throughout the treatment period. The authors concluded that apart from a mild antibacterial effect, the addition of zinc oxide to hydrocolloid dressings produced no beneficial effects on wound healing in pigs receiving a normal diet. Other hydrocolloids contain silver salts to impart antimicrobial activity, and hydrocolloid paste has been used as a carrier for pharmaceuticals and growth factors.[18]

Hydration of intact skin

When Wu et al.[66] investigated the effects of occlusion on evaporative water vapour loss from exposed skin wounds. They found that the degree of water loss depends mainly on the wound depth and is similar in chronic leg ulcers and full thickness burns. They also showed that compared with exposed wounds, hydrocolloid dressings reduce evaporative water loss by 70 - 80%.

Berardesca et al.[67] reviewed the effects of occlusion on skin function and concluded that, under certain conditions, it represents a powerful treatment, 'capable of inducing several changes on epidermal metabolism, skin flora, sweat glands and epidermal morphology'. In a subsequent paper,[68] they compared the effects of hydrocolloid and polyurethane film dressings with a polyethylene film and a plastic chamber on the skin barrier and the stratum corneum water holding capacity using the Plastic Occlusion Stress Test (POST). Each device was applied on the forearm for 24 hours in ten healthy volunteers and after which the water holding capacity, measured as skin surface water loss (SSWL), was recorded continuously for 25 minutes using an evaporimeter. The results showed significant differences between the occlusive materials. Higher SSWL values were recorded in sites occluded with the plastic chamber, but the polyurethane film had limited occlusive capacity. The hydrocolloid dressing and polyethylene film produced similar results that were significantly higher than those produced with the polyurethane film. These results are entirely consistent with the findings of the laboratory studies described previously and could easily have been predicted.

Skin reactions

Skin reactions thought to be associated with the change to the original formulation of Granuflex/Duoderm were identified by Sasseville et al.[69] who proposed that the inclusion of the hydrogenated rosin ester increased the sensitization potential of the dressing. They described three patients who developed eczematous lesions beneath the dressing and subsequently displayed positive patch tests to both colophony and to the dressing itself. They argued that the addition of the rosin derivative could adversely affect the good safety record of this family of dressings. A further 27 cases of skin reactions to the new formulation of Granuflex/Duoderm were reported by Hausen et al.,[70] who showed, by means of patch tests, that these were also all due to the presence of the hydrogenated rosin ester. Other isolated reports of reactions to this agent in Granuflex/Duoderm were reported in Korea,[71] and Germany,[72] and following the application of Combiderm, a product which also has a hydrocolloid-type adhesive. A similar skin reaction has also been reported in a patient treated with Comfeel Plus transparent hydrocolloid dressing but the constituent responsible in this case could not be identified.

Despite these adverse reports, overall the incidence of skin reactions to all types of hydrocolloids, including Granuflex/Duoderm, remains extremely low given the millions of dressings that are used annually. In two studies designed to determine the prevalence of contact sensitivity in a total of 69 patients with venous disease of the leg (often assumed to be a group at particular risk) to materials commonly used in wound care, none of the patients tested showed any reaction to hydrocolloid dressings.[73-74]

MICROBIOLOGICAL CONSIDERATIONS

Infection rates

When hydrocolloid dressings were originally introduced, many clinicians were initially concerned that the relatively occlusive environment produced beneath the dressing would tend to promote wound infections, particularly those caused by anaerobic bacteria but in clinical practice, this has not proved to be the case.

Annoni[75] studied thirty patients with leg ulcers of different aetiologies, who were treated with a hydrocolloid dressing changed about twice a week for a maximum period of 12 weeks. The average interval between dressing changes was 4.1 days and the average duration of treatment was 67 ± 11 days by the end of which time 26 patients had healed. The bacterial flora of each wound was examined prior to treatment, then weekly or twice weekly thereafter. The results of the initial microbiological investigation revealed mixed flora with prevalence of S. aureus. Subsequent bacterial cultures showed a persistence of the original flora, but there was no correlation between the type of flora present and clinical evidence of infection or between the type of flora present and the rate of healing of the ulcer.

Gilchrist[76] also monitored the bacterial flora of chronic ulcers treated with a hydrocolloid over an eight week period, using a novel sampling method in an attempt to isolate anaerobic bacteria which, at the time, were considered at the time to represent a potential threat, given the low oxygen tension beneath the dressing. The flora was found to be generally stable, although P. aeruginosa appeared to be inhibited by the dressing. Anaerobic organisms were isolated from 12 of the 20 wounds examined but these did not appear to have a significant influence on healing.

Mulder et al.[77] examined the effects of different types of dressings on bacterial growth in 48 ulcers of different aetiology and found that bacterial proliferation was significantly lower in wounds dressed with Duoderm, compared with wounds dressed with gauze or a polyurethane film. They concluded that although there was evidence to suggest that increased bacterial growth delays wounds closure, the mere presence of bacteria in wound does not indicate the potential for infection as the pathogenicity of the organism must also be considered.

Although heavy colonization by skin and wound flora is often seen under certain types of occlusive products, clinical infection is not a frequent occurrence and is most often found in wounds compromised by devitalised tissue or the presence of drains or sutures which can facilitate bacterial proliferation. Hutchinson et al. addressed this issue in detail.[78-81] In a retrospective review they examined 69 papers in which 'occlusive' dressings, defined as polyurethane films, hydrocolloids, hydrogel sheets etc., were compared with other more traditional materials such as gauze, or low-adherent dressings including paraffin gauze in both controlled and uncontrolled studies. They found that, overall, the infection rate for wounds dressed with conventional dressings was 7.1% compared with 2.6% for those dressed with 'occlusive' dressings. In several controlled studies, both groups of dressings were used and in these cases non-occlusive and occlusive treatment resulted in infection rates of 7.6% and 3.2% respectively. Both differences were highly significant (p < 0.001). When the data were analyzed according to wound type, the difference between conventional and occlusive products was significant for ulcers (p < 0.001), donor sites (p = 0.01) and for 'miscellaneous' wounds (p = 0.001). For burns no significant difference could be detected between treatment groups, but the authors noted that for this indication some film dressings were associated with high infection rates which may have contributed to the overall lack of significance. When the study data were analysed according to treatment type, the infection rates were 1.3% for hydrocolloids, 4.5% for films, and 2.2% for foams and hydrogels combined.

Wound infection may be caused by proliferation of organisms already present within the wound or on the periwound skin, or by the uncontrolled growth of pathogenic organisms from the external environment. The ability of hydrocolloid dressings to act as a bacterial barrier in order to prevent the ingress of pathogenic organisms into experimental wounds in an animal model was investigated in 1985 by Mertz et al.[82] Two common skin pathogens, the non-motile, S. aureus, and the motile, P. aeruginosa, were used to challenge three different types of dressings placed on 48 partial-thickness rectangular wounds each measuring 7 × 5 cm and 0.3 mm deep in three pigs. The wounds were dressed with pieces of dressing measuring 4 × 4 cm. A 0.1 mL sample of bacterial culture containing $> 10^8$ cfu of the test organisms was applied to a 5 × 5 cm area on and around each dressing on one, two or three occasions twenty four hours apart.

The dressings were removed and the wounds sampled and cultured at 24, 48 and 72 hours. S. aureus was recovered in large numbers from 100% of air-exposed wounds, from 50% of wounds covered with either a polyurethane film dressing, (Opsite) or a hydrogel dressing, Vigilon. The organism was not isolated from wounds dressed with Duoderm. Similarly, P. aeruginosa was recovered from 100% of all air-exposed wounds and from all those dressed with the film or hydrogel but was not recovered from Duoderm-covered wounds. The total numbers of organisms isolated from the Duoderm-treated wounds (principally Gram-positive skin flora) were broadly similar to those found in air-exposed wounds but at 24 and 48 hours the number of organisms isolated from beneath Opsite (S. aureus and skin flora) was reduced compared with untreated controls. Wounds dressed with the hydrogel showed a marked propensity to the increased growth of primarily Gram-negative organisms in addition to the challenge organisms.

As semipermeable films can be shown to form an effective barrier to bacteria in laboratory studies, the wound contamination must have resulted from migration of the organisms through channels formed between the skin and the adhesive film. It is be postulated that the thicker, more malleable, adhesive mass present on the hydrocolloid effectively prevents the formation of these channels and therefore the migration of bacteria.

Some five years later, the same group investigated the effects of different dressings upon wounds which had been inoculated with pathogenic organisms.[83] A total of 24 partial-thickness wounds each measuring 11 × 7 mm and 0.6 mm deep on eight domestic pigs were inoculated with 0.05 mL of cultures each containing approximately

10^8 cfu of *S. aureus*, *Clostridium perfringens*, *Bacteroides fragilis*, or *P. aeruginosa*. Each wound was covered with 4 × 4 cm pieces of one of three dressings, Duoderm, Opsite, Vigilon, or left exposed to air. Groups of wounds were sampled at 24, 48, and 72 hours. Although no wounds became infected, high levels of *S. aureus* were detected beneath all of the dressings and also in the air-exposed wounds. The numbers of *C. perfringens* and *B. fragilis* decreased in the air-exposed wounds and slightly reduced in the Opsite covered wounds, but remained high in wounds dressed with Vigilon or the hydrocolloid. The numbers of *P. aeruginosa* were greatest in the Opsite and Vigilon covered wounds. On the basis of these results the authors suggested that occlusive dressings are not indicated in wounds that appear to be grossly contaminated or that may contain anaerobic organisms. It is interesting to note that the first study was undertaken on the original formulation of Granuflex/Duoderm whilst the second might have been performed on the modified formulation.

Soderberg *et al.*[84] compared the effects of three different dressings, two occlusive and one non-occlusive, on the bacterial flora of 120 excised wounds in 60 rats. They reported that although no clinical signs of infection were observed in any of the wounds, the number of organisms per gram of granulation tissue was significantly lower four, eight and 12 days postoperatively in wounds treated with Mezinc, a zinc-medicated occlusive dressing compared with wounds treated with Duoderm or a wet-to-dry non-occlusive gauze dressing. When the minimum inhibitory concentration (MIC) of zinc sulphate was determined on different strains of bacteria isolated from the wounds of rats and on strains isolated from humans, the most susceptible species isolated from both rat wounds and humans were Streptococcus sp., *S. aureus* and *E. coli*; Proteus and Enterococcus sp. were less sensitive and *P. aeruginosa* showed no evidence of inhibition under the conditions of test. Based upon the results of these investigations, the authors suggested that the use of an occlusive dressing containing of zinc might reduce the risk of wound infection in man.

Bioburden of intact skin

Lawrence and Lilly[85] compared the effect of Granuflex, Opsite, paraffin gauze and an impermeable plastic tape (Sleek) on the bacteriology of normal human skin.

They found that although skin covered with the impermeable tape showed a significant increase in the number of bacteria present, the application of Granuflex/Duoderm did not produce a similar increase, despite the equally occlusive nature of the dressing. Neither of the other products examined caused a significant increase in the number of organisms present.

Bacterial barrier properties 'in vivo'

In a further paper, Lawrence[86] reviewed the physical properties of Granuflex/Duoderm and concluded that it formed an effective dressing for minor wounds, acting as a bacterial barrier and enhancing patient comfort. Patients were able to shower or wash, and volunteers who wore the dressing for up to ten days showed no evidence of sensitivity reactions or any other adverse response.

The barrier properties of hydrocolloid dressings were used to good effect by Wilson *et al.*,[87] who used them in seven patients to control the spread of methicillin-resistant *S. aureus* from leg ulcers colonised by the organism to other carriage sites such as axillae and nares. The authors suggested that the use of these products represented an important method for helping to prevent the spread of infection.

Lawrence[88] in both laboratory and clinical studies, compared the effect of dressings upon the spread of airborne microorganisms. He found that the removal from wounds colonised with bacteria of conventional fibrous dressings such as gauze, liberated large numbers of microorganisms into the air but interestingly, removal of wet dressings resulted in fewer numbers of airborne bacteria than the removal of dry dressings, presumably because the production of airborne particles to which the bacteria were attached was reduced when the dressing was wet. Hydrocolloid dressings reduced contamination levels still further, to approximately 20% of the number observed for gauze.

Lawrence's work was taken a stage further by Suzuki *et al.*[89] who examined the spread of the varicella zoster virus (VZV) in from hospitalised patients with herpes zoster infections localised to the thoracic region. Patients had their skin lesions covered with either a hydrocolloid dressing or conventional gauze bandages. Using a sensitive polymerase chain reaction assay, the presence of VZV DNA was sought in swab samples from dressings, the subject's throat, and filters of air purifiers. The viral DNA was not detected in any samples taken from dressings or air purifier filters for patients dressed with the hydrocolloid, but VZV DNA was detected in samples from dressings and air purifier filters for all six patients in the gauze group. VZV DNA was detected less frequently in throat samples from patients in the hydrocolloid group than in those from patients in the gauze group. The authors concluded that hydrocolloid dressings effectively prevent dissemination of aerosolised VZV DNA from skin lesions of patients with localised herpes zoster.

The work of Lawrence and Suzuki could have important implications for the management of patients who are carrying, or believed to be carrying, pathogenic blood borne bacterial or viral infections which could be spread via airborne particulates within the local environment.

In one unique study,[90] the ability of hydrocolloid dressings to control the release of pathogenic organisms from pressure ulcers on para and tetraplegic patients undergoing hydrotherapy was examined. Twelve patients with spinal cord lesions participated, six of whom had healed ulcers and constituted a control group. The evaluation was performed both with and without the wounds covered with a hydrocolloid dressing, Duoderm. Bacterial samples were taken from the bath-water before and after a 30 minute period of exercise. Additionally, specimens were obtained from the ulcer, the patients' skin and urine, and from the skin of the physiotherapist who exercised the patient. The microbiological study revealed no significant difference in the contamination of the bath-water after exercising with or without a hydrocolloid dressing in place. Post exercise, the water was found to be contaminated with facultative aerobic intestinal flora. In nearly one-third of the sessions, the bath water was contaminated with *P. aeruginosa* before starting and after exercise 25% of the ulcers were colonised with these pathogens. The authors concluded that intestinal flora were more important that bacteria coming from the ulcers and suggested that the pressure ulcers contributed little contamination to the bath-water and therefore the presence of the wounds ought not to prohibit patients from receiving the potential benefits of water exercise, although they commented that adequate chlorination of the water in the pool was important.

Bacterial barrier properties 'in vitro'

A simple 'in vitro' method for assessing the ability of a hydrocolloid to provide an effective bacterial barrier was described in 1985 by Lawrence.[86] He applied a small piece of Granuflex to the neck of small glass containers (Bijou bottles) containing a culture of test organism. Swabs taken from the outer surface of the dressing over a seven day period showed no evidence of bacterial growth, suggesting that the dressing was indeed able to prevent the passage of microorganisms. In 1987 he used a similar technique to examine the bacterial barrier properties of four hydrocolloid dressings, Granuflex, Comfeel, and the now discontinued Dermiflex and Biofilm.[91] A bacterial culture applied to a filter paper, was used to challenge a piece of each dressing which formed a closure to an open ended tube containing sterile growth medium. Three dressing resisted the passage of the test microorganisms in all instances but Biofilm, which unlike the others had a thick hydroentangled nonwoven fabric backing made from hydrophobic polyester fibre, failed both tests. The clinical significance of the test method, and therefore these results, subsequently formed the subject of a spirited exchange of letters in the Pharmaceutical Journal.[92-99]

Lawrence subsequently published a brief review in which he compared the likely barrier properties of a variety of dressings.[100]

The ability of five different hydrocolloid dressings to resist penetration by multi-resistant strains of MRSA were compared in a laboratory study reported by Dunn and Wilson.[101] The products included in this study were Granuflex, Comfeel, Dermiflex and Intrasite. The test involved the use of two sterile glass hemispheres between which the dressing was held. One hemisphere (to which the inner or wound contact surface of the dressing was attached) contained a bacterial culture; the other had a number of access ports through which a microbiological swab could be introduced to sample the outer surface of the dressing over a fourteen day period.

They found that whilst none of the brands of dressings tested formed an absolute barrier to bacteria, with the exception of Granuflex, the degree of penetration was very limited, a maximum of one or two failures out of fifteen tests performed on each product. With Granuflex, however, there were major failures in the three manufacturing batches tested. This was said to be due to a manufacturing problem which, when corrected, resulted in product that had a comparable performance to the other products examined. The authors argued that this test method offered advantages over previous methods because it examined a much larger surface area, virtually an entire dressing. Evidence was also presented to suggest that the ability of the organism to penetrate all the dressing was inversely proportional to its antibiotic resistance although no explanation for this observed effect was offered.

A possible disadvantage of the method as described is that the weight of fluid in the one chamber can cause the dressing to become distorted and stretched, potentially contributing to its failure. This problem can be overcome by placing sterile growth medium in the second chamber to equalise the pressure. The development of turbidity in this sterile solution indicates that bacteria have penetrated through the dressing. Although this change increases the sensitivity of the test and overcomes at least one of the potential problems, it impossible to estimate the number of points at which penetration has occurred. This modified technique, described elsewhere, has been adopted as a standard method by a leading medical device testing laboratory and is currently being proposed for consideration as the basis of a European standard.

Wilson and Dunn[102] subsequently published a second paper in which they described the testing of different batches of Biofilm which had been manufactured using different components and sterilised by different methods (ethylene oxide and beta-irradiation). They showed that, as predicted previously by Thomas,[95] the ability of Biofilm to resist penetration by bacteria was greatly influenced by its ability to transpire moisture away from its outer surface, but concluded that even when this occurred, the dressing was unlikely to provide the same degree of impermeability as dressings that incorporate a semipermeable membrane.

The apparatus described by Wilson and Dunn was used in a later study[103] to compare the barrier properties of a number of foam and film dressings. The results, which suggested that one dressing, Tielle, failed to provide an effective barrier, stimulated a very strongly worded response from the manufacturer who questioned the validity and clinical relevance of the method.[104]

CLINICAL EXPERIENCE WITH HYDROCOLLOID DRESSINGS

In catheter care

Hydrocolloid dressings have been trialled as alternatives to polyurethane films for dressing catheter sites in order to prevent catheter related sepsis, a not uncommon and potentially life threatening complication of total parenteral nutrition. A new hydrocolloid dressing Visiband was compared with a standard polyurethane film in eight patients with central venous catheters.[105] Dressings and lines were changed every changed every 3rd day for the first month then every 5th day for the second month. Skin swabs were collected from the exit sites for microbiological analysis. No growth was detected during 17 of 64 dressing changes in the first month, 11 of which were in the Visiband group and six in the PUF group (p = 0.12) During the second month, seven of 40 dressing changes showed no growth, six of which were in the Visiband group (p = 0.04). At both time intervals the growth of *S. aureus* and *S. epidermidis* was higher in the PUF group, although these differences did not always reach statistical significance. *Candida* species were detected five times under the PUF but were not isolated from beneath the hydrocolloid. The authors concluded that PUF dressings should be changed after three days but that the hydrocolloid could be left *in situ* for up to five days.

In a second study,[106] adult patients requiring the insertion of a multilumen central venous catheter in an intensive care unit were randomized to receive either a standard polyurethane dressing or a transparent hydrocolloid dressing. Cultures were obtained from 125 skin insertion sites, 141 catheter hubs, 128 catheter tips, and blood samples from 132 patients. Extensive data on patient and catheter characteristics were collected. Skin and hub cultures revealed no significant difference in degree of colonization. However, the hydrocolloid group had a significantly higher level of catheter colonization than the polyurethane group (p = 0.048). Conversely, there was a significantly higher frequency of positive blood cultures in the polyurethane group (p = 0.03) although the majority were considered to be potential contaminants. There were only six cases in which the same species was simultaneously isolated from a positive blood culture and a colonised catheter, five from the hydrocolloid group and one from the polyurethane group. The results of this study suggest that an increased risk of catheter colonization is associated with the use of hydrocolloid dressings, despite previous research suggesting that they significantly reduce microbial growth compared with standard polyurethane.

In wound management

Leg ulcers

The first reported use of a hydrocolloid for the treatment of leg ulcers was published in 1973 by Allen[6] who used an ostomy product, Stomahesive, held in place with elastic bandages to treat the wounds of 15 patients. Normally produced with a polyethylene backing, Allen obtained samples without this film which he cut into pieces the size and shape of the wound, and applied them in a series of layers until the upper surface was level with the surrounding skin. He reported that the dressing used in this way appeared to promote both granulation and epithelialization and also facilitated wound debridement, a process which, it was suggested, might be due either to the activity of microorganisms on the ulcer floor or some element in the discharge which acted as the dissolving agent.

This initial report was followed in 1975 by a further study in which Varihesive, as the new material was now called, was applied to a total of 22 ulcers of mixed aetiology, with and without occlusion provided by means of a zinc paste bandage.[7] As before the dressing was cut to the size and shape of the wound and changed after either one, two or four days. In most instances the periwound skin was protected by the use of zinc paste and ichthammol but in two of three cases where the trial dressing was applied directly to the surrounding skin it dried out or caused an adverse skin reaction. As before it was observed that the hydrocolloid appeared to stimulate the formation of granulation tissue, but it was recorded that in a number of instances this became so exuberant that it had to be destroyed by the application of silver nitrate. Overall, however, the material was well tolerated and produced no general adverse reactions, although a change of treatment was sometimes required to bring about epithelialization.

In 1977, Tracy et al.[35] in an open non-comparative study applied Varihesive to 43 patients with indolent ulcers of varying aetiology that had proved resistant to local therapy for more than ten weeks and found that 84% of the ulcers healed in an average of 10.2 weeks. The authors noted that the dressing appeared to reduce pain and promote liquefaction of slough but found no evidence that occlusion lead to problems of infection. They concluded that Varihesive formed an excellent covering for wounds in which there was minimal suppurative infection, and suggested that it might also be of value in the treatment of abrasions, donor sites and pressure ulcers.

The first attempt at a randomized controlled trial to compare Varihesive with a conventional treatment, paraffin gauze, was reported by Baxter in 1980[107] but randomization procedures were not correctly followed and allocation to treatment was seriously biased which made the results of the study of questionable value.

The early success with Varihesive led directly to the development of Granuflex/Duoderm which was subjected to an early open, non-comparative multicentre study reported by Cherry et al. in 1984.[108] Data from 54 patients were analysed, 11 of whom had bilateral ulcers. In one centre 19/37 (51%) of wounds healed following treatment with the hydrocolloid in an average of 56 days (range 12 - 133). In the second centre 10/19 (53%) ulcers in 17 patients healed in an average of 62 days (range 39 - 140). The authors also commented that, in general, the use of the hydrocolloid resulted in decreased wound pain, although one patient was removed from the study because of pain issues.

In the same year, Friedman et al.[109] described an uncontrolled comparative study involving 22 patients with 31 leg ulcers. Patients were divided into two groups. The first comprised 15 patients (11 outpatients) with 19 ulcers 12 of which (63%) healed in an average of 57 days when treated solely with the hydrocolloid. The second group comprised seven hospitalised patients with at least two leg ulcers of similar size and distribution. The 20 ulcers in the seven patients were treated with either mild topical antimicrobial wet dressings, hydrocolloid dressings, or both treatments applied sequentially. All 20 ulcers eventually healed but the design of the study made prevented meaningful comparisons of the outcomes of the various forms of therapy.

In 1985, Mulder et al.[110] successfully used Duoderm to treat 18 patients with 24 ulcers that had failed to respond to conventional treatments. All wounds eventually healed although it was reported that in the early stages of treatment the wounds often appeared to increase in size due to the debriding action of the dressing.

Also in 1985 Ryan et al.[111] reported the results of a multicentre uncontrolled study involving 28 patients with venous stasis ulcers. During a three-month period 43% of ulcers healed, and there was a mean decrease in ulcer size of 75%. An unspecified small number of patients failed to respond favourably, and showed an increase in ulcer size during the third month of treatment. It was considered that, in these patients, the improved local conditions produced under the dressing remained inadequate to overcome the underlying problems caused by the venous stasis. The major problems associated with the use of the hydrocolloid were odour, and leakage of liquefied gel from beneath the dressing. In addition, two ulcers produced excessive amounts of granulation tissue, which was dealt with by the application of a foam pad and a pressure bandage.

Around this time a number of anecdotal reports and case studies were published describing the successful use of Comfeel,[112-114] and Granuflex,[115] in leg-ulcer management. In the last of these publications, the author compared the treatment costs associated with the hydrocolloid with those of conventional treatments, and suggested that considerable savings could be made by switching to this form of therapy and as a result urged that the dressings should be made available on prescription in the community.

In a non-comparative multicentre study,[116] involving 152 ulcers drawn from seven centres in six countries all dressed with Duoderm, 62% of ulcers healed in an average of 51 ± 5 days. Of 69 ulcers that had deteriorated during previous therapy, 42 (61%) healed with hydrocolloid treatment. A reduction in pain was reported by 79% of patients and no cases of wound infection were recorded despite the fact that a wide variety of organisms were cultured from the ulcers. The authors noted that diabetic patients and those in poor health appeared to have a lower chance of complete healing and they also reported a statistically significant difference in healing rates between ulcers present less than or longer than one year prior to inclusion in the study ($p < 0.05$).

Most published clinical studies involving hydrocolloid dressings have been undertaken in temperate climates and little information is available concerning their performance under tropical conditions. Furthermore, it is known from laboratory studies that temperature can affect both the fluid handling properties and gelling rate of these materials which could impact upon their fluid handling ability.

This issue was addressed by Zeegelaar et al.[117] who undertook a study to assess the performance of a hydrocolloid (Comfeel Plus) used in combination with short stretch compression bandages under more extreme environmental conditions in Surinam, which has a tropical climate with annual temperatures between 22.8° and 32.2°C. The study was conducted during the rainy season when the humidity was fluctuating around 95%. Seventeen patients with venous leg ulcers attending an outpatient clinic were enrolled in the study, three of whom dropped out. The study lasted for six weeks and dressings were changed twice weekly. All ulcers made good progress towards healing as indicated by an increase in the percentage of the wound base covered with granulation tissue from 27% to 92% during the course of treatment. The mean circumference of the wounds fell from 9.9 cm to 4.9 cm during this time. In general, the dressing was very well accepted, pain was never reported. Exudate production diminished, although leakage was noted 39 times in the 164 dressing changes. Swabs for bacterial cultures were taken at the beginning and end of the study revealed no differences in the rate of bacterial infections or colonization of wounds compared with studies performed in temperate regions. The authors concluded that these results confirm that hydrocolloid dressings can be used under tropical conditions.

These early studies were largely uncontrolled and often paid little or no attention to the choice of control therapy and the importance of treating underlying venous disease by the application of some form of graduated external compression. Gradually a number of studies which addressed these and other issues began to be published. To facilitate comparisons these are grouped together below according to the nature of the comparator

Hydrocolloids vs povidone iodine

In 1985 a randomized controlled trial was undertaken in South Africa[118] in which hydrocolloid dressings were compared with conventional materials in 36 patients with long-standing ulcers. Over an eight-week period, ulcers treated with the hydrocolloid reduced in size by 67.6%, but those treated by with povidone-iodine, covered with a foam rubber pad and compression bandaging showed a mean reduction in size of only 23%. Although no serious problems were reported with the use of the hydrocolloid, some leakage of fluid from beneath the dressing did occur, and some patients developed a degree of skin maceration and minor fungal infections. Based upon the results of this study, the author considered that hydrocolloid dressings were best suited to application to non-infected wounds that do not produce excessive quantities of exudate.

Hydrocolloids vs knitted fabric dressing

The value of occlusive dressings, and Granuflex/Duoderm in particular, was questioned by Backhouse et al.,[119] who carried out a clinical trial in which they compared a simple knitted textile primary dressing (N-A Dressing) with Granuflex, in the treatment of 56 patients with chronic venous ulcers. All dressing were covered with a multi-layer bandage system and by 12 weeks complete healing occurred in 21 out of 28 (75 percent) of patients with occlusive dressings and 22 of 28 patients (78 percent) dressed with N-A Dressings. The authors concluded that careful graduated compression bandaging achieves healing in the majority of venous ulcers, and there is little to be gained by applying occlusive dressings. It is interesting to note, however, that the ulcers were very small, with an average area of less than 3.5 cm^2 as wounds larger than 10 cm^2

were specifically excluded from this study even though it is these larger wounds that are most difficult to heal in normal clinical practice.

The effect of hydrocolloid dressings on the healing rates of more extensive wounds was investigated by Moffat et al.[120] in a subsequent study in which they compared Comfeel ulcer dressing with N-A Dressing in sixty patients with ulcers that had previously failed to respond to high compression therapy. This study, which included wounds up to 66.3 cm^2, was conducted over a 12-week period with time to healing as the primary outcome variable. Despite a relatively short follow-up period, seven ulcers (23%) in the non-adherent group and 13 (43%) in the hydrocolloid group had healed completely. This just failed to achieve statistical significance (p = 0.077). The authors concluded that hydrocolloids might prove of great benefit to this small, difficult group of patients who fail to respond satisfactorily to other treatments.

Nelson et al.[121] similarly compared the effectiveness of knitted viscose or hydrocolloid dressings, pentoxifylline (1200 mg), and single-layer or four-layer bandaging for venous ulceration in a factorial randomized controlled trial with 24-week follow-up involving 245 adults with venous ulcers. The main outcome measure was time to complete healing. Secondary outcomes included proportions healed, withdrawals, and adverse events. The authors reported no difference in healing between wound treated with knitted viscose and hydrocolloid dressings, 58% vs 57% (p = 0.88). Pentoxifylline was associated with nonsignificant increased ulcer healing, 62% vs 53%, (p = 0.21) and four-layer bandages were associated with significantly higher healing rates than single-layer bandaging, 67% vs 49%, (p = 0.009).

Hydrocolloids vs paraffin gauze, saline and betadine soaks

In the latter part of the 20th Century, granulating wounds were commonly dressed with gauze impregnated with paraffin (Vaseline) or soaked in saline or Betadine solution. Several studies were therefore undertaken which compared these simple products with a hydrocolloid dressing to determine if differences existed in healing rates and treatment costs.

In the first study,[122] Granuflex/Duoderm was compared with paraffin gauze (Jelonet) in a randomized sequential crossover trial involving eight patients with ten ulcers. Following an initial preparatory period of one week for cleaning and debridement, the ulcers were randomized to receive either Granuflex/Duoderm or the control dressing for three weeks, followed by crossover to the alternative therapy for a further three weeks. All patients were hospitalised and provided with compression throughout the course of the study. Wounds dressed with Jelonet were dressed daily, but the hydrocolloid dressings were changed as dictated by leakage of exudate. All ulcers decreased in area by the end of each 3-week period. Those dressed with Granuflex/Duoderm decreased by 22% compared with a 17% reduction recorded with paraffin gauze. This difference was not significant, a not unexpected finding given the study design and the small number of patients involved. In five of seven wounds subjected to bacteriological analysis, counts of aerobic organisms were significantly higher in Granuflex/Duoderm treated wounds (p < 0.02). Anaerobes were also present in higher numbers in six of seven wounds (p < 0.01). P. aeruginosa was isolated from three of the wounds dressed with hydrocolloids. Despite the higher bacterial counts in ulcers dressed with hydrocolloid, no adverse effects (infections) were recorded.

A second study,[123] also compared a hydrocolloid (Comfeel) with paraffin gauze (Jelonet) in a 12 week study involving patients with leg ulcers and pressure ulcers. Initially 38 patients with leg ulcers were recruited into each treatment group. A total of 35 patients completed the study, 19 in the hydrocolloid group and 16 in the control group. Twelve of the wounds treated with hydrocolloid healed in three months compared with only three dressed with paraffin gauze.

The effect of wound size on the healing rate of leg ulcers dressed with a hydrocolloid dressing or a conventional treatment was examined in more detail in a randomized controlled trial involving 200 patients.[124] Wounds were dressed either with a combination of a hydrocolloid powder and self-adhesive hydrocolloid sheet dressing (Biofilm) or paraffin gauze dressing used with Betadine. Compression was provided to both groups by means of a Venosan stocking or two layers of shaped Tubigrip. Using the proportional hazards model, four variables were found to be associated with the time to ulcer healing ($p < 0.01$). These were: initial ulcer area, ulcer duration, age and deep vein involvement. No difference was detected between healing rates in small ulcers 2 - 4 cm in diameter, but for larger ulcers, > 4 cm diameter, a marked difference in healing rate for the first month of the study was recorded, 34% with Biofilm, and 10% with Betadine, although this did not achieve statistical significance ($p = 0.09$). These observations may explain the earlier findings of Backhouse et al.[119]

An unexpected finding was that episodes of acute infection were more common in wounds dressed with Betadine than Biofilm, (12 to 1 respectively). In contrast to the observations of Eriksson,[125] who reported that the bacterial population of wounds remained relatively constant, the authors of this study found that the bacterial population changed from month to month.

The results of this investigation and that of Moffat, together provide support for the theory that although the choice of primary dressing may be of little importance in the treatment of small ulcers; for larger wounds a hydrocolloid may offer real clinical benefits.

A Swedish study published in 1994,[126] compared Duoderm with saline soaked gauze in 30 community patients with venous or mixed venous/arterial ulcers using a short-stretch bandage, Comprilan, to provide compression. Seven patients in the hydrocolloid group and two in the gauze-group healed during the study. Ulcers dressed with gauze reduced in area by 19% compared with 51% in the hydrocolloid group ($p < 0.16$). Despite the apparent advantages associated with the use of hydrocolloid dressings, this did not achieve statistical significance because of the small sample size. Patients dressed with hydrocolloid reported significantly less pain at dressing changes than patients in the gauze-group ($p < 0.003$), and there were considerable financial benefits associated with the use of the hydrocolloid.

In a multicentre study[127] involving two treatment centres in the United States and the United Kingdom, 70 patients with 90 venous ulcers were randomly assigned to hydrocolloid or conventional dressing and compression therapy at four study centres. In all treatment centres the hydrocolloid dressing (Duoderm CGF) was covered with a zinc oxide paste bandage and a graduated compression bandage (reapplied daily by the patient) whilst patients in the control arm were treated with a paraffin gauze dressing in the U.S. and a saline/Betadine-impregnated gauze in the U.K. Although overall wounds were comparable in terms of their initial area, large differences were recorded in the duration of the ulcers prior to admission to the study between the two countries. Ulcers in patients in the United Kingdom were also larger and less likely to heal (p = 0.001). A total of sixteen patients failed to complete the study, seven in the control and nine in the hydrocolloid group. Ulcers treated with the hydrocolloid reduced in area by 71%, and control-treated wounds by 43%. Mean time to healing was seven weeks for the hydrocolloid dressing group and eight weeks for the control group, but the total number of wounds which actually achieved closure was 25 (34%) of which 11 were treated with hydrocolloid and 14 treated with the standard therapy. size of the ulcer at baseline was associated with treatment response and time to healing (p = 0.002). Percent reduction in ulcer area after two weeks was also correlated with treatment outcome (p=0.004) and time to healing (p = 0.002). When all treatment outcome predictors were analyzed together, only percent reduction in area after two weeks remained statistically significant (p = 0.002), with percent reduction during the first two weeks of treatment > 30% predicting healing. Most ulcers were less painful at final evaluation, but reduction in pain was more pronounced in hydrocolloid-dressed ulcers (p = 0.03).

The relative costs of treating wounds with hydrocolloids and paraffin gauze were compared by Augustin et al.[128] who also compared the effect of treatment upon the patients' quality of life (QoL). Twenty five patients aged 61.4 ± 12.3 years with venous ulcers were followed for six months. Eleven patients treated with paraffin gauze had daily dressing changes, whilst the 14 patients treated with hydrocolloid dressings had their wounds dressed every two to four days. The median healing times were 15.6 weeks for paraffin gauze and 14.3 weeks for the hydrocolloid. Treatment costs in Deutch Marks (DM) calculated per cm reduction in ulcer diameter were DM 482 and 300 for the paraffin gauze and hydrocolloid treated patients respectively. Costs for a 10% reduction in pain were DM 538 and DM 359 and costs for 10% improvement in QoL: DM 1046 and DM 672. In each case staff costs formed the major part of the expenditure.

Hydrocolloids vs zinc oxide impregnated bandages (Unna's Boot)

Bandages impregnated with zinc oxide paste have long been regarded as a standard treatment for leg ulcers. A particularly widely regarded treatment based upon this material is the formation of an 'Unna Boot' developed by a German physician and dermatologist, Paul Gerson Unna, (1850 - 1929). This was originally produced by the application to the lower leg of a paste made of zinc oxide, gelatin, glycerin, and water which was then covered with a bandage; an additional layer of paste completed the dressing. When this preparation dried it formed a relatively inextensible structure - a forerunner of the modern short stretch bandaging technique. Now commercially-available bandages already impregnated with paste tend to be used for this application.

In a Swedish study,[125] the healing rates of leg ulcers dressed with Duoderm and an elastic bandage were compared with those obtained with a double layer bandage system consisting of a stocking impregnated with zinc oxide paste (ACO-salvastrump) and an elastic outer bandage, Tensoplast. A total of 34 outpatients with chronic venous ulcers were randomized to treatment and their wounds measured using a stereophotogrammetric technique. Over a period of eight weeks, both groups of ulcers decreased in volume by an average of 40% and reduced in area by about 55%. There was no statistically significant difference between the two treatment groups at any point in the study. Microbiological studies undertaken at the same time indicated that *S. aureus* was the most common isolate. It was also found that the patients who healed kept their initial flora until healing. Gram-negative bacteria were found in ulcers that healed as well as in ulcers that did not. Three diabetic patients were included in the study all of which happened to be randomized to the hydrocolloid group and the wounds of two of these patients deteriorated, which probably introduced an element of bias into the study results.

Brandrup[129] also compared a hydrocolloid dressing, Duoderm, with a zinc oxide medicated bandage, Mezinc, in a prospective, randomized trial over a period of eight weeks. All patients were patch-tested before the study and colophony allergy (a component of Mezinc) was an exclusion criterion. Of the 43 patients enrolled, 31 completed the trial and six patients randomized to each treatment group were withdrawn. Ulcers decreased in area by 64% after eight weeks of treatment with Mezinc, and by 48% following treatment with Duoderm. This difference did not achieve significance. Both dressings were said to reduce wound pain by a similar amount but Mezinc treatment had to be discontinued in two cases due to sensitization to colophony.

The Unna Boot has been used as a comparator in a number of published studies with variable results. In one early randomized controlled trial published in 1988 by Kikta *et al.*[130] which involved a total of 69 ulcers, 21/30 wounds (70%) dressed with the traditional treatment healed compared with 15/39 (38%) treated with the hydrocolloid ($p < 0.01$) although the mean time required to heal just failed to reach significance ($p = 0.51$). Life-table healing rates at 15 weeks were 64% for Unna's Boot compared with 35% for hydrocolloid ($p = 0.01$, log rank test). Of the 39 patients dressed with hydrocolloids ten (26%) developed complications. No complications were observed in patients dressed with Unna's Boot ($p = 0.004$), but overall patients treated with hydrocolloids reported a significantly greater level of convenience than those treated with Unna's Boot ($p = 0.004$).

A second study involving the same two treatments produced different results.[131] A total of 30 patients were enrolled in a clinical trial to compare Unna's boot to Duoderm CGF over which was applied a cohesive bandage, Coban, a product that if applied with significant stretch provides comparable support to the Unna boot. The two patient groups were well matched with respect to age, sex, initial ulcer area, ulcer duration. Eight of 16 ulcers (50%) in the Duoderm group healed completely compared with 6/14 ulcers (43%) in the Unna's boot group (p=0.18). Healing rates (cm^2/week) correlated significantly with initial ulcer area and initial ulcer perimeter for both groups. After adjusting for differences in initial ulcer perimeter, healing rates were significantly faster for Duoderm treated patients during the first four weeks of therapy, 0.384 ± 0.059 cm^2/wk/cm perimeter for Duoderm *vs* 0.135 ± 0.043 cm^2/wk/cm perimeter for Unna's boot, ($p = 0.002$). At 12 weeks patients on Duoderm again appeared to heal faster than those on Unna's boot, although the result did not reach statistical significance,

0.049 ± 0.007 cm^2/wk/cm perimeter for Duoderm versus 0.020 ± 0.017 for Unna's boot, (p = 0.11).

Similarly positive results for the hydrocolloid therapy were obtained in 2000 when Unna's Boot, a hydrocolloid dressing and saline gauze were compared in a longitudinal study involving 81 patients with venous ulcers.[132] In this study there was marked variation in recurrence rates and treatment costs. Of the wounds treated with saline, 88% either did not heal or recurred, compared to 21% of ulcers treated with Unna's boot and 13% of ulcers dressed with the hydrocolloid dressing. The authors suggested that hydrocolloid dressings appeared more cost-effective than Unna's boot or saline-gauze dressings but cautioned that controlled clinical studies were required to ascertain the cost-effectiveness of different forms of venous ulcer care in different settings.

In a further study,[133] sixty patients with venous ulcers well matched for size and duration were randomly assigned to receive Comfeel plus elastic compression or to treatment with the Unna boot. Healing rates of patients who completed the study were comparable in the two groups, 20/27 (74%) for the Unna Boot and 21/26 (81%) for the hydrocolloid (p > 0.05). The weekly reduction in wound area for both treatment groups was also comparable but the hydrocolloid dressing was found to be easier to use (p < 0.0001) and required less time to apply (p > 0.05). Patients treated with the Unna boot, also experienced significantly more pain both during application and subsequently.

Hydrocolloids vs calcium alginate

Most of the studies described thus far have compared a hydrocolloid with a traditional treatment such as zinc paste or paraffin gauze. Of rather more interest are studies in which the hydrocolloid is tested against an alternative 'modern' dressing.

An early example of such a study was published in 1993 when Comfeel was compared with an alginate dressing, Kaltostat, in the treatment of heavily exuding ulcers.[134] In total 19 patients were randomized to compare the ease of use and acceptability of the two treatments. No healing data was presented. The authors reported that for the hydrocolloid the average treatment time was 8.3 minutes compared with 12.9 minutes for the alginate, and the average cost of materials used was £10.96 for the hydrocolloid and £17.02 for the alginate. The results of this study suggested that the use of hydrocolloids appeared to enhance healing rates, reduce pain and offer other advantages over conventional dressings but these observations were either not tested or found to be significant statistically.

Hydrocolloids vs foam/hydropolymer

Granuflex was compared with Tielle in a randomized controlled clinical study involving 100 community patients with leg ulcers and 99 patients with pressure ulcers.[135] Although statistically significant differences in favour of the foam dressing were detected for dressing leakage and odour production, no statistically significant differences were recorded in the number of patients with either leg ulcers or pressure ulcers who healed in each treatment group. In order to permit comparisons for wounds that did not achieve complete healing during the treatment period, an analysis was undertaken to compare the mean percentage change in wound area at the time of each weekly assessment. More leg ulcers treated with Tielle, (44/49, 90%) reduced in area compared to those treated with the hydrocolloid (34/47, 72%). This result was statistically significant (p = 0.028) and considered noteworthy especially in view of the fact that the initial ulcer size was greatest in the Tielle group.

Hydrocolloids vs cadexomer iodine

Granuflex/Duoderm was compared with a cadexomer iodine paste, Iodosorb/Iodoflex or paraffin gauze dressing in a 12-week, randomized, open, controlled, multicenter, multinational trial in patients with venous leg ulcers.[136] All patients used short-stretch compression bandages, Comprilan, throughout the study. The primary efficacy variable was the percentage reduction in ulcer size, and the secondary end-point was the time taken to stop exudation, when the patient had completed the study according to the protocol.

A total of 153 patients entered the study and were treated for 12 weeks or until cessation of exudation. The mean reduction in ulcer size in all patients was 62% with cadexomer iodine vs 41% and 24% for hydrocolloid and paraffin gauze respectively. These results failed to achieve significance. Of those treated for 12 weeks (n = 51), ulcer area reduction was 66% for cadexomer iodine and 18% for hydrocolloid (p = 0.0127). Overall the rate of healing expressed as a reduction in area per week, was significantly higher for cadexomer iodine than for paraffin gauze, 0.64 cm^2/week vs 0.19 cm^2/week, (p = 0.0353). The treatment costs were similar in all groups but when the costs were correlated with healing over a 12-week period, cadexomer iodine paste was found to be more cost effective than hydrocolloid dressing or paraffin gauze dressing. The authors concluded that cadexomer iodine paste appears to be an efficient, cost-effective and safe alternative to hydrocolloid dressing and paraffin gauze for the treatment of venous leg ulcers.

Comparisons between hydrocolloid dressings

Studies discussed thus far describe the results of comparisons between a particular brand of hydrocolloid and a product from a different family of dressing. Information on the relative performance of different hydrocolloid dressings is harder to find. In one such study,[137] the original formulation of Granuflex/Duoderm was compared with the newer Granuflex (Duoderm) Improved Formulation (Granuflex E or Duoderm CGF) and Comfeel Ulcer Dressing.

A total of 120 patients were randomly assigned to one of the three treatment groups and compression provided by means of Class 2 compression stockings to eliminate operator variability in the application of compression bandages. Before the study, the principal benefit was defined as healing, and the final figures demonstrated that a minimum of 88% of all patients recruited received benefit from the dressing regimen to which they were assigned. At best, 96% of a group of patients in a treatment group improved during the 13-week study period. Regular measurements using an accurate tracing technique were made of all leg ulcers in the trial. Analysis of the results revealed that patients dressed with the new formulation of Granuflex/Duoderm healed 16% faster than those given standard Granuflex/Duoderm and 35% faster than those treated with Comfeel. Both Comfeel and the new formulation of Granuflex/Duoderm produced less leakage than the original formulation. None of these findings were tested statistically.

Two unidentified hydrocolloid dressings, 'A' and 'B', were compared in the treatment of venous ulcers in 31 patients at two clinical sites.[138] Complete wound closure was observed in 59% of the patients treated with Hydrocolloid 'A', compared with 15% of the patients in the Hydrocolloid 'B' group (p = 0.03). Investigators also rated Hydrocolloid 'A' significantly better in ease of application, adhesion, conformability, exudate absorption, barrier properties, transparency, and patient comfort (p = 0.02). Significantly fewer patients in the Hydrocolloid 'A' group required unscheduled, product-related dressing changes (P < 0.02). In this clinical study, Hydrocolloid 'A' demonstrated excellent performance characteristics and was highly effective in treating venous insufficiency ulcers

Duoderm E was used as the comparator in a trial of Urgotul in the treatment of leg ulcers. After eight weeks of treatment wound area had reduced by a mean of 61.3% in the Urgotul group and 52.1% in the Duoderm group. This difference was not significant. Dressings were changed more frequently with the hydrocolloid, 2.54 ± 0.57 times per week, vs 2.31 ± 0.45 in the Urgotul group, (p = 0.047). Thirty-three local adverse events were recorded in 27 patients: ten in the Urgotul group and 23 in the control (p = 0.039). Pain on removal, maceration and odour were significantly better in the Urgotul group (p < 0.0001).

Hydrocolloids and ultrasound

Exposure to low-dose ultrasound has been suggested to assist the healing of venous leg ulcers. Twenty-four leg ulcer patients were randomized in a placebo-controlled parallel groups in a single-blind clinical study to receive conventional therapy consisting of the topical application of hydrocolloid dressings and compression, or conventional therapy with additional ultrasound treatment for 12 weeks.[139]

The ultrasound treatment consisted of ten minutes of foot bathing, and the application of 30 kHz continuous ultrasound 100 mW/cm^2 three times a week. All ulcers were measured by planimetry at intervals throughout the study and from these values changes in ulcer radius were calculated. After 12 weeks treatment ulcers in the control group had decreased in area by 16.5%. In contrast the area of wounds treated with ultrasound decreased by 55.4% (p < 0.007). When calculated on a daily basis the reduction in the ultrasound-treated patients was $0.08 \text{ mm} \pm 0.04 \text{ mm}$, and in the placebo patients $0.03 \text{ mm} \pm 0.03 \text{ mm}$. Patients recorded only minor side-effects such as a tingling feeling and occasionally pinhead-sized bleeding in the ulcer area. The authors concluded that the application of low-frequency and low-dose ultrasound is a potentially valuable adjunct to leg ulcer care for wounds that do not respond to conventional treatment.

Hydrocolloids vs epidermal allografts

Cultured epidermal allografts have been used to treat a variety of wounds. It is suggested that they function by releasing cytokines that stimulate epithelialization. Cryopreserved cultured allografts (CCAs) with compared with a hydrocolloid dressing in 43 patients with 47 ulcers in a randomized controlled trial.[140] Ulcers not healed by six weeks were changed to the alternative treatment. No difference in the number of healed ulcers between the two groups was observed at six weeks but healing rate, percent reduction of initial ulcer size, and radial progression toward wound closure were significantly greater for CCAs than for the hydrocolloid. Pain relief was not significantly different.

Predicting ulcer healing with hydrocolloid dressings

A principal problem in the management of leg ulcers is predicting which are likely to respond to treatment at an early stage in order to maximize treatment effectiveness or contain costs by curtailing an expensive form of therapy if this is likely to prove ineffective. Duoderm, was used in the treatment of 61 patients with 72 full-thickness ulcers,[141] in order to identify those patient and wound characteristics which might be used to predict healing. During a mean treatment time of 56 days, 54% of the full-thickness ulcers healed. Ulcers in males were less likely to heal than in females (p =.02). Healing was also impaired in patients with diabetes mellitus (p < .003). A reduction in ulcer area > 30% after two weeks of treatment was a predictor of both treatment outcome (p= 0.016) and time required for healing (p = 0.004). Odour at baseline and advanced age also were associated with increased time required for healing, (p = 0.005 and p = 0.017, respectively). It was also recorded that patients with full-thickness ulcers were more likely to be overweight (p < 0.001) and not fully mobile (p = 0.016).

As accurate measurement of wound area is key to assessing progress towards healing, it is important that a measurement technique is adopted which provides an objective record of wound size. Computerised planimetry can be useful but it is important that key parameters are standardised. This issue was addressed in a study designed to revisit the methods of morphometric analysis with emphasis on the suitability of the data to predict healing.[142] Leg ulcers from 53 outpatients were measured before and after a four week treatment with hydrocolloid dressing and compression bandages. From 43 of the same patients, measurements were also taken after a one and two week treatment period. Nine morphometric variables were used for comparison: six dealt exclusively with variations in ulcer size and three focused upon adjusted healing rates for the shape of ulcers. As in the previous study, analysis revealed that most parameters related to healing correlated significantly with the initial ulcer size. These relationships were not found in non-healing ulcers. The authors concluded that chronic leg ulcers of similar sizes heal at fairly uniform rates, though not in a linear fashion since they follow a proportional change process. Non-healing ulcers have an unpredictable course.

The value of initial healing rate as a prognostic indicator for eventual healing was further investigated by Margolis et al.[143] Twenty-seven venous ulcers treated with a hydrocolloid dressing and compression bandaging were monitored to obtain information on healing rates during the initial four week treatment period and the overall healing rates using the Gilman method (delta A/p where A is area in cm^2 and p is perimeter length in cm). They found that the average *initial* healing rate for all ulcers combined, the healed group, and the non-healing group was 0.069, 0.087, and 0.005 cm/wk, respectively. Similarly, the average *overall* healing rate for all ulcers combined, the healed group, and the non-healing group was 0.062, 0.089, and 0.043 cm/wk, respectively. These results suggest that the initial healing rate may represent an appropriate end point for clinical investigations when comparing therapies for the treatment of chronic venous leg ulcers.

Pressure ulcers

The wide variation in the nature of wounds caused by pressure damage means that dressings may be required to fulfil different functions according to the size, depth and state of hydration of the affected area.

The ability of some hydrocolloids to change in permeability according to the state of hydration of the underlying tissue makes them particularly useful for the treatment of superficial ulcers or those in the early stages of development whilst they are still covered with a dry necrotic layer. The impermeable nature of the intact dressing prevents evaporative loss and thus facilitates autolytic debridement. If the wounds are relatively superficial, hydrocolloids may continue to be of value as this process continues and leads to the formation of an exuding wound, but exudate production becomes significant, a change to an alternative form of treatment is probably indicated. If, however, exudate formation declines as healing progresses, it may be appropriate to reapply a hydrocolloid dressing at this stage.

The use of hydrocolloids in specific stages of pressure ulcer treatment has been described in a number of publications. In 1994 the results of a survey of 15 extended care facilities with access to ET nurse consulting services in the United States was published by Ballard-Krishnan et al.[144] They reported that although gauze-type dressings were used most frequently on all stages and types of pressure ulcers, a significant correlation between ulcer type and dressings used was found for stage II pressure ulcers only. Hydrocolloid (and polyurethane film) dressings were more likely to be used on stage II ulcers without exudate than on any other type of ulcer ($p < 0.001$).

Early experiences

In 1984 Johnson[36] first described the successful use of hydrocolloids in the treatment of a small number of patients with pressure ulcers. In the same year Yarkony et al.[145] reported the results of an uncontrolled trial involving 21 patients with a total of 25 pressure ulcers that had previously been treated with alternative therapies. In this study, the average length of treatment with hydrocolloids was 27 ± 3 days. During this time 14/25 ulcers, (56%) demonstrated marked improvement or complete healing with the hydrocolloid, although only 2/25 ulcers, (8%) had improved with previous treatments. Of the 16 ulcers that had failed to improve previously, seven (44%) had either healed or showed marked improvement with the use of the occlusive dressing.

Tudhope[146] reported results of a similar study involving 25 patients with 38 ulcers. All wounds were dressed with Duoderm after cleansing with 3% hydrogen peroxide. During the course of the study 14 (47%) of the wounds healed and 10 (33%) showed marked improvement. A further two (7%) showed a moderate improvement and one (3%) deteriorated. The average treatment time was 52 days.

In 1993, van Rijswijk[147] treated 48 patients with 56 full thickness pressure ulcers with Duoderm. During the study 21 (37.5%) of the ulcers healed and 16 (28%) showed marked or moderate improvement. The mean time to healing was 70.3 days and the mean treatment time was 56 days (range 13 - 243). Ulcers that subsequently progressed to healing initially showed a reduction in wound area of 47% in two weeks. The author proposed that in clinical practice ulcers that do not decrease in size within two weeks should be re-evaluated for additional or alternate treatment.

A hydrocolloid sheet dressing was used in conjunction with Dermasorb, a hydrocolloid/alginate spiral dressing, in the management of 30 exuding Grade III and IV pressure ulcers.[148] After a mean treatment time of 12.9 days, all wounds had a significant increase in the amount of granulation tissue/epithelium and a decrease in the amount of devitalised tissue. It was reported that the absorbent spiral helped to manage exudate, was easy to use and comfortable for the patients although the use of an air-fluidised bed or mattress was found to significantly reduce wear time of the dressing ($p < 0.01$).

These uncontrolled preliminary investigations were later supported by more structured randomized trials. Gorse[149] prospectively followed twenty-seven patients with 76 pressure ulcers treated with hydrocolloid dressings and 25 patients with 52 pressure ulcers who received treatment with Dakin's solution (chloramine-T)-soaked wet-to-dry dressings. In the hydrocolloid group, 66 (86.8%) pressure ulcers improved compared with 36 (69.2%) in the wet-to-dry dressings group, ($p = 0.026$).

An alternative approach was adopted by J. Belmin et al,[150] who, in an open, randomized, multicenter parallel-group trial involving 110 elderly patients with Grade III or IV ulcers, compared the efficacy of calcium alginate and hydrocolloid dressings applied sequentially, with hydrocolloids applied alone. The control strategy consisted of applying Duoderm E alone for eight weeks; the sequential strategy consisted of applying a calcium alginate dressing, Urgosorb for the first four weeks followed by a hydrocolloid dressing, Algoplaque, for the next four weeks. During the study ulcer areas were measured weekly by tracing. The endpoints were the mean absolute surface area reduction during the 8-week study period and the number of patients achieving a 40% or more reduction in surface area. Fifty-seven and 53 patients were randomly allocated to sequential and control strategies respectively. Baseline patient characteristics and ulcer features at inclusion were similar in the two groups. Mean ± s.d. reduction in wound area was significantly larger in the sequential treatment group, 5.4 ± 5.7 and 7.6 ± 7.1 cm^2 at four and eight weeks, than in the control group, 1.6 ± 4.9 and 3.1 ± 7.2 cm^2 ($p < 0.001$). In the sequential treatment group, 68.4% of the patients achieved a 40% reduction by four weeks and 75.4% by eight weeks, significantly higher than in the control group, 22.6% vs 58.5% respectively, ($p < 0.0001$). The authors concluded that in the treatment of Grade III or IV pressure ulcers, application of a calcium alginate dressings followed by a hydrocolloid dressing promotes faster healing than treatment with hydrocolloid dressings alone.

The results of this possibly unique study appear to confirm the author's opinion that dressing selection should be determined by the condition of the wound. The initial application of an alginate to an exuding wound followed by a hydrocolloid as healing progresses seems logical and based upon a good understanding of the products concerned. It is perhaps a pity that the hydrocolloid dressing used was not the same in both treatment arms for there remains the possibility that some difference in the chemical composition or physical properties of the two hydrocolloids might have been responsible for the results obtain. It is to be regretted that this eminently sensible and rationale approach would be rejected by many who conduct clinical trials or undertake systematic reviews.

Hydrocolloids *vs* saline gauze

Several workers have compared hydrocolloid dressings with saline-soaked gauze, once a standard treatment for pressure ulcers. Alm *et al.*[151] compared Comfeel with saline gauze in a controlled, randomized and partially single-blind study with parallel groups of 50 patients with 56 pressure ulcers. After six weeks treatment, compared with the original wound area, the median remaining ulcer area was 0% in the hydrocolloid dressing group and 31% in the group treated with saline gauze (p = 0.016). Although there appeared a marked difference in the number of wounds healed in the two treatment groups, this failed to achieve statistical significance.

When hydrocolloid dressing were compared with conventional wet-to-dry gauze dressing technique in 44 patients with Grade I and II ulcers by Kim,[152] 80.8% of the hydrocolloid dressed wounds and 77.8% of the conventional wet-to-dry gauze dressing group healed completely with no statistically significant difference between the two groups. However, the time required for complete healing was shorter with hydrocolloids 18.9 *vs* 24.3 days and ulcer healing speed was also slightly faster in group 9.1 *vs* 7.9 mm^2/day. Average time spent by staff in wound management was significantly shorter with the hydrocolloid and the costs were lower, even without taking into consideration the labour cost, leading the authors to conclude that the use of hydrocolloids for this indication provides a less time consuming and less expensive option than conventional techniques.

Further evidence for the financial benefits associated with hydrocolloids was offered by Colwell who also compared a hydrocolloid dressing, Duoderm with moist gauze in the treatment of patients with Grade II and/or Grade III pressure ulcers.[153] A total of 94 patients were initially recruited to the study 24 of whom failed to complete eight days of treatment leaving 70 evaluable patients with a total of 97 ulcers. These were randomized to treatment, which consisted of moist gauze, scheduled to be changed every six hours, or hydrocolloid wafer scheduled to be changed every four days. The daily cost of treating patients with moist gauze dressing was $12.26; compared with $3.55 for the hydrocolloid dressing. During the period of the study one ulcer healed in the moist gauze-dressing group, and 11 healed in the Duoderm group but problems with the distribution of Grade II and Grade III ulcers between the groups and the experimental design cast some doubts upon the statistical significance of these results.

Xakellis[154] also compared the cost of hydrocolloid dressings with saline-gauze wet-to-moist dressings in the treatment of 39 patients with pressure ulcers. Over a 21-month period 89% of wounds dressed with hydrocolloid healed compared with 86% of those dressed with non-sterile saline-soaked gauze. The median healing time for the hydrocolloid group was nine days, with 75% of wounds healed within 14 days. In the saline-gauze group, the median healing time was 11 days with 75% of wounds healed within 26 days, although this difference did not reach statistical significance. For the hydrocolloid treatment, the median nursing time was one eighth that of the saline-gauze treatment, but the material costs were 3.3 times higher. When nursing costs were included the authors concluded that there was a real although relatively modest financial saving associated with the use of hydrocolloid dressings.

In an open comparative randomized study Chang[155], compared Duoderm with saline gauze dressings in the treatment of 34 patients, 21 with Grade II and 13 with Grade III ulcers. Over an eight week period, subjects assigned to the hydrocolloid dressing experienced a mean reduction from their baseline surface area measurement of 34% compared with a 9% increase in subjects assigned to gauze dressings although this difference did not achieved statistical significance. In other performance areas, adherence to wound bed, exudate handling ability, overall comfort and pain during dressing removal the hydrocolloid was found to be statistically superior to the gauze.

Not all trial results have proved so favourable for hydrocolloids, however, for in 1996 Mulder[156] found no difference in wound healing rates when 67 patients with pressure ulcers were randomized to of three treatment modalities: hydrogel sheet, hydrocolloid, or wet-to-moist gauze.

It is perhaps not surprising that hydrocolloid dressings have been found to be superior to simple gauze packs in most studies as gauze is now widely regarded as outmoded form of treatment by many leading wound management centres. More relevant information on the performance of specific hydrocolloid dressings is obtained from comparisons with similar products or other modern dressings.

Hydrocolloids vs foam dressings

Banks and her co-workers published the results of two studies in which they compared Granuflex/Duoderm with a thin foam dressing, Spyrosorb. In the first study,[157] 29 patients with Grade II or 3 pressure ulcers were randomized to treatment, which lasted a maximum of six weeks. During the course of the investigation the wounds of ten of 13 patients dressed with the foam dressing healed compared with 11 of 16 wounds dressed with the hydrocolloid. No significant difference was detected in the healing rates or the number of wounds that healed, but significant differences were detected in favour of Spyrosorb in terms of ease of removal and lack of pain during dressing changes. In a second community-based study,[158] the same dressings were compared on 40 patients, 20 in each group. Of the patients treated with foam, 12 healed and a further six were judged to have improved. In the hydrocolloid group ten patients healed but the remainder were withdrawn from the study. No significant difference in healing rates was detected for the wounds that actually healed in the two groups although a trend was detected in favour of the polyurethane foam.

Bale *et al.*[159] compared Granuflex/Duoderm with Allevyn Adhesive in a randomized multicentre study involving 61 patients with Grade II or III pressure ulcers to evaluate ease of application and removal, adhesion, conformability, absorbency and wear time. Forty patients were withdrawn prior to completion of the study but in the patients that remained, each dressing was applied for up to 30 days and assessments were carried out at each dressing change. The results indicated that both dressings are easy and convenient to apply but absorbency and ease of removal were judged to be significantly better with the polyurethane foam dressing than the hydrocolloid dressing. Wear times were similar in both groups but the small number of patients who completed this investigated greatly diminished its value.

In a further study Bale et al.[160] compared Granuflex/Duoderm with Allevyn in single-centre randomized parallel group trial involving 100 community-based patients with a variety of wound types. Similar healing rates were observed in the leg ulcer and 'other wound' groups, the nature of which was not reported. Secondary objectives included a comparison of dressing durability; time to complete healing, ease of wound cleansing and dressing removal. In the pressure sore group 10/17 (59%) of patients treated with foam healed during the study compared with 4/15 (27%) treated with the hydrocolloid. For all aetiologies except pressure ulcers, the costs of the hydrocolloid dressing were less than the costs of the foam, but patient comfort and lack of leakage favoured the foam dressing.

Seeley et al.[161] also compared a hydrocolloid dressing with Allevyn, in the management of pressure ulcers. Forty adult patients of both sexes who had Grade II or Grade III pressure damage were enrolled in the study and randomized to treatment with one of the primary dressings under investigation. Dressings were replaced as required, and each ulcer was assessed on a weekly basis for a maximum of eight weeks or until ulcer closure was achieved. Although no differences were detected between the two dressing in terms of wound pain, odour, and changes in ulcer appearance and ulcer area, the foam dressing was found to be significantly easier to remove and quicker to change than the hydrocolloid dressing.

Comparisons of hydrocolloid dressings

One hundred and three patients with Grade II and III sacral pressure ulcers were enrolled into a prospective, controlled, multi-centre clinical study to compare dressing performance, safety and efficacy.[162]

Fifty-two patients were randomized to treatment with a triangle-shaped bordered version of Granuflex and 51 patients were randomized to an oval shaped Tegasorb dressing. The majority of patients in both groups (> 80%) had Grade II ulcers, which had existed for less than one month, and most wounds were relatively small. The duration of the study was limited to six dressing changes for each subject. By the end of the study 17 (36%) patients in the group dressed with Granuflex/Duoderm had healed compared with 11 (22%) of patients dressed with Tegasorb (p = 0.017). A total of six (13%) patients failed to respond favourably to treatment with Granuflex/Duoderm compared with 18 (37%) of patients dressed with Tegasorb. The remaining patients in each group were reported to have shown varying signs of improvement but not achieved complete healing during the period of the study. Patients in the oval dressing group were found more likely to exhibit a product related adverse reaction resulting in discontinuation of treatment as compared to patients treated with Granuflex/Duoderm (p = 0.057). These reactions were principally deterioration in the appearance of the wound and erythema/inflammation of the surrounding skin. Wear time was longest for wounds dressed with the triangle dressing applied point down. Incontinence reduced the interval between dressing changes in both groups. During this study it was recorded, somewhat paradoxically, those ulcers which healed were treated for a longer period of time than those that did not heal. This difference was 5.5 days (13.5 - 8) in the case of wounds dressed with Granuflex/Duoderm and 1.3 days (11 - 9.7) for wounds dressed with Tegasorb. Although the reasons for this were not discussed in the publication, it is possible that the increased frequency of change could be due to the production, by some of the more extensive wounds, of larger volumes of exudate, which would reduce the useful life of the dressing.

Banks et al.[163] compared Granuflex/Duoderm with a bordered version of Tegasorb in a small three week study involving 32 subjects with a variety of wound types and reported that the dressings performed similarly in terms of their conformability and fluid-handling properties, although the fact that the Tegasorb became transparent in use was considered to be an advantage. No effort was made to compare healing rates or cost of treatment.

Two thin hydrocolloids Tegasorb thin and Duoderm Extra Thin - were compared in clinical practice for their ease of application and removal, conformability, wear time and patient comfort. Both dressings were found to be highly acceptable in clinical practice, with advantages and disadvantages to each type of dressing. There was a high level of patient acceptability and no adverse reactions were noted during this evaluation.[164]

Hydrocolloids vs hydrogels

A hydrocolloid dressing and a synthetic hydrogel were compared in ten patients with Grade II or III pressure ulcers. Dressings were changed as required and the wounds were assessed weekly. The overall healing rate for the two groups was similar, but the hydrogel was judged to offer advantages in terms of debridement and cost in use.[165]

Duoderm was compared with a transparent dressing, Tegaderm Absorbent Clear acrylic dressing, in the management of Grade II and shallow Grade III pressure ulcers in a prospective, open-label, randomized, comparative, multisite clinical evaluation.[166] A total of 72 patients, 35 dressed with the acrylic dressing and 37 with the hydrocolloid, were followed up for a maximum of 56 days or until their ulcers healed. Wound assessments and dressing performance evaluations were conducted weekly. The acrylic product was judged to have outperformed the hydrocolloid in nearly all parameters examined, including ease of use, patient comfort, dressing wear time, and wound healing rates. A high value was also placed upon its transparent nature. Mean wear time for the acrylic dressing was 5.7 (s.d. 2.55) days compared with 4.7 (s.d. 2.29) days for the hydrocolloid, a difference that was judged to be clinically relevant by the investigators.

In an open, randomized, multicentre study, 168 patients suffering from Grade II to Grade IV pressure ulcers were treated with a Comfeel, or Inerpan a wound dressing consisting of a polymer of L-leucine and methyl-L-glutamate impregnated with a mixture of physiological serum and propylene glycol. Treatment was continued for eight weeks or until the ulcer healed.[167] Thirty-one Inerpan-treated patients and 23 Comfeel- treated patients achieved healing (P = 0.089), with median healing times of 32 and 38 days respectively. When healing times were compared using survival curves for the whole population adjusted for ulcer depth effect, they showed a significant difference in favour of Inerpan.

Hydrocolloids vs collagenase preparations

When hydrocolloid dressings were compared with collagenase gel, a wound cleansing agent, in two separate studies, conflicting results and conclusions were produced.

In the first,[168] Burgos *et al.* compared Varihesive, with a collagenase gel, Iruxol, (Smith and Nephew) in the treatment of 37 patients with pressure ulcers. The gel was applied daily to the wound in a layer 1-2 mm thick. The hydrocolloid was left in place for three days. After 12 weeks treatment six patients had healed, three in each treatment group. Wounds treated with the collagenase showed a mean reduction in ulcer area of 9.1 ± 12.7 cm^2 compared with 6.2 ± 9.8 cm^2 for those dressed with hydrocolloid – a difference that was not statistically significant. The material costs for the two treatments were broadly comparable, but staff costs were considerably greater for the collagenase group because of the need for more frequent dressing changes.

In the second study Duoderm and a collagenase-containing ointment were compared in the treatment of pressure sores on the heel in a randomized clinical trial conducted in the Netherlands.[169] A total of 24 females with Grade IV pressure sores on the heel following orthopaedic surgery were recruited to treatment. Wound healing was achieved, on average, within a shorter time period with the collagenase treatment (10 weeks) compared with the hydrocolloid treatment (14 weeks). Although treatment costs were similarly distributed within both groups, (34% for materials and 66% for personnel), the average cost per patient for treatment with the hydrocolloid dressing was about 5% higher than with the collagenase-containing ointment. The robustness of the results was tested using a sensitivity analyses which confirmed that collagenase offered a better cost-effectiveness ratio than hydrocolloid treatment.

Hydrocolloid dressings vs miscellaneous applications

The effectiveness of hydrocolloid dressings was compared with alternative materials on pressure ulcer healing in patients with spinal cord injuries.[170] Ninety-one Grade I and Grade II pressure ulcers of 83 young paraplegic males, some with multiple ulcers, victims of the Iran-Iraq war were randomly allocated to three treatment groups, a hydrocolloid dressing, phenytoin cream and simple dressing. All were managed in long term care units or in their homes for eight weeks by a team of general practitioners and nurses. At the end of this period and the ulcer status was assessed and simply recorded as 'completely healed', 'partially healed', 'without improvement' and 'worsening'. Complete healing of ulcers, regardless of location and stage, was better in the hydrocolloid group, 23/31 (74%) than either the phenytoin cream group 12/30 (40%) ($p < 0.01$), or the simple dressing group 8/30 (27%). This difference was statistically significant ($p < 0.005$). The authors concluded that the application of a hydrocolloid represents the most effective method investigated for treating Grade I and II pressure ulcers in young paraplegic men.

In 2003 a hydrocolloid was compared with topical collagen in a well designed randomized, single-blind controlled trial involving 65 nursing home residents with Grade II or III pressure ulcers over an 8-week period.[171] Thirty-five patients were allocated to topical collagen daily and 30 to topical hydrocolloid twice weekly. The primary outcome was complete healing within eight weeks. Secondary outcomes were time to heal, ulcer area healed per day, linear healing of wound edge, and cost of therapy. Analysis by intention to treat revealed similar complete ulcer healing within eight weeks in collagen (51%) and hydrocolloid (50%) recipients. Mean healing time was also similar. Cost analysis favoured the hydrocolloid leading the authors to conclude that as here were no significant differences in healing outcome between the two dressings collagen and offered no major benefits to patients otherwise eligible for hydrocolloid treatment.

Prevention of tissue damage

In one small study, Granuflex/Duoderm was shown to be more effective than Spenco Dermal in the prevention of nasal bridge ulcers caused by face masks in patients receiving intermittent positive pressure ventilation.[172]

Comfeel Pressure Relieving Dressing (PRD) was tested on 12 healthy volunteers to determine trochanteric and peritrochanteric interface pressures.[21] Use of the PRD reduced the maximum pressure applied to the apex of the trochanter from a mean of 64.2 mm Hg to a mean of 52.2 mm Hg. The author speculates that this statistically significant difference may have clinical relevance for 79% of pressure ulcers but not for the 21% of pressure ulcers with cavities.

Whilst it is possible to believe that the addition of the removal foam rings to the back of the Comfeel dressing may impart some small benefit in terms of pressure reduction, it is difficult to imagine how a standard hydrocolloid dressing might function in this way. Nevertheless, the ability of such a dressing to prevent ulcer formation on the heels of elderly orthopaedic patients, a group known to be at particular risk of developing this condition was examined in two clinical studies.

In the first study,[173] four commonly used devices were employed to determine their ability to decrease or remove pressure on the heels of patients with damaged femurs. In total 41 patients were randomly allocated to treatment with one of the selected devices, and their efficacy evaluated by continuously assessing the skin integrity of both heels on a daily basis over a period of 12 days. The devices employed were Duoderm, foam splints, eggshell foam, and heel protector boots. In this study foam splints and eggshell foam proved to be the most effective devices in relieving pressure exerted on the heel.

In a second study[174] published in 1997 using a similar group of patients, 15 patients received routine nursing care, and treatment groups of 15 and 20 patients received routine nursing care combined with the use of hydrocolloid dressing and egg crate foam respectively. The combination of routine nursing care and the use of egg crate foam was found to be a more effective method of maintaining skin integrity than either nursing care alone or nursing care combined with the use of hydrocolloid dressing, leading the author to recommend the routine use of this treatment in hospital. The results of these two investigations could have been largely predicted as hydrocolloid dressings have little or no elastic or cushioning properties, and it is difficult to see how they might have been expected to reduce interfacial pressure.

Diabetic ulcers

The treatment of ulcers and other lesions on the feet of patients with diabetes is perhaps the most controversial application for the use of hydrocolloid dressings.[175] The relatively limited bulk and good adherence characteristics of hydrocolloid dressings and their ability to form an effective bacterial barrier would tend to suggest that these materials should be of particular value for this indication, but some workers have expressed reservations, concerned about the risk that serious infections may be overlooked in wounds that are not regularly monitored.

Lithner[176] reported two cases of deterioration of infected diabetic ulcers following the application of a hydrocolloid dressings which in one case at least was left undisturbed for seven days. Foster *et al.*,[177] described eight wounds that had deteriorated following the extended use of hydrocolloid dressings in wounds with a pre-existing infection and argued that the resulting problems outweigh the practical and financial arguments for their use, concluding that hydrocolloid dressings should never be used on deep, infected or discharging wounds on the diabetic foot or in circumstances that preclude frequent dressing changes and wound inspection. Vowden[178] also suggested that diabetic ulcers judged to be at risk of serious infection should be monitored on a daily basis.

Under these conditions, the application of a hydrocolloid is inappropriate, for apart from the risk of infection, in order to function optimally, these dressings normally should be left *in situ* for at least 48 hours. Too frequent replacement can lead to traumatic stripping of the surrounding skin whilst preventing the dressing from gelling correctly.

Others workers have expressed a contrary view on the value of hydrocolloids for this indication. Laing[179] argued that accurate diagnosis is the first step towards successful treatment of these wounds and suggested that provided adequate pressure relief is provided and any necrotic material is removed, the wounds may safely be dressed with a hydrocolloid. If, however, signs of a clinical infection are present and/or bone is exposed, osteomyelitis should be suspected in which case aggressive surgical debridement and systemic antibiotics may be required to prevent amputation, the most serious complication of these wounds.

Knowles *et al.*[180] carried out a retrospective study to evaluate the use of Granuflex/Duoderm for this indication. Information was collected on 250 diabetic ulcers involving 2316 dressing changes. Dry dressings were used most frequently, followed by Granuflex. Healing and infection rates were comparable in Granuflex/Duoderm and non-Granuflex treated wounds.

Lazareth[181] emphasised the need to distinguish between limb or life threatening infections and non limb-threatening infections in diabetic wounds and recommended that for severe infections appropriate antibiotic therapy be initiated the duration of which depends on the nature of the infection and the need for surgical debridement. He also suggested that non-infected, free of necrotic material can be covered by modern dressing including hydrocolloids but that necrotic wounds should be dried until they can be treated surgically.

Few controlled studies have been published describing the use of hydrocolloid dressings in the treatment of diabetic ulcers. In one published report,[182] 44 diabetic patients with necrotic foot ulcers were treated with adhesive zinc oxide tape (Mezinc) or Duoderm in a randomized control trial. During the course of the 5-week study, the ulcers of 14 of 21 patients treated with Mezinc improved by at least 50% compared to six out of 21 with the hydrocolloid dressing ($p < 0.025$). During the same period 15 patients showed an increase in the area of necrosis ten of whom had been treated with the hydrocolloid.

A major factor in determining the suitability or otherwise of a hydrocolloid, or any other dressings, for a wound on the foot of a diabetic is the nature and underlying cause of the lesion itself. The neuropathic changes commonly associated with diabetes can lead to partial or complete loss of sensation in the toes or feet and this in turn may result in skin damage caused by unrelieved pressure or friction which remains unnoticed by the patient. There appears to be no reason why hydrocolloid dressings should *not* be used to treat these wounds as the results of microbiological studies contained in the literature and discussed previously actually suggest that wounds dressed in this way are no more likely to develop an infection when managed in this way than with any other form of topical treatment.

In marked contrast, necrotic areas which are caused by vascular damage, or toes that have become discoloured and 'dusky' looking, are probably not candidates for hydrocolloid therapy. In the absence of an adequate blood supply to a digit or part of a limb, the tissue will become devitalised and have to be removed, either by surgical means or sometimes by a process of mummification and autoamputation. The application of any dressing that retains moisture in this dead tissue will prevent this process and may lead to wet necrosis which will seriously increase the risk of infection. Ischaemic changes (with or without neuropathy) caused by microvascular damage can occur or deteriorate quite rapidly and it is for this reason that existing wounds or other areas of tissue at risk should be regularly monitored. The management of the diabetic foot has been comprehensively reviewed previously.[183]

Burns

An early account of the use of hydrocolloids in the treatment of thermal injuries was provided by Hermans and Hermans.[184] They described the use of Granuflex/Duoderm in the management of 24 patients, seven of whom had multiple burns which enabled comparisons to be made with other treatments. In 1986 and 1987, these data formed the basis of two further publications[185-186] involving 66 and 75 patients respectively. They concluded that healing rates with hydrocolloids compared very favourably with silver sulphadiazine cream (SSD) and allografts in both superficial and deep partial-thickness burns.

Hydrocolloids vs paraffin gauze with chlorhexidine

Phipps and Lawrence,[187] in a prospective randomized controlled trial, compared Granuflex/Duoderm with a chlorhexidine-impregnated paraffin gauze dressing (Bactigras), in 196 patients with burns involving less than 5% body area. Dressings were changed at weekly intervals or earlier if they became displaced or leaked. A total of 119 patients were followed to complete healing, which took 14.2 days for wounds dressed with hydrocolloid compared with 11.8 days for the alternative therapy, but the authors acknowledged that these times were imprecise because of the extended intervals between dressing changes. Although the hydrocolloid had a tendency to leak, patients reported that it was comfortable to wear and provided relief from pain.

Wright et al.[188] similarly treated 98 patients with partial-thickness burns suitable for outpatient management with Granuflex/Duoderm or Bactigras to compare the safety, efficacy and performance characteristics of the two products. A total of 31 patients were withdrawn for various reasons leaving 67 evaluable patients. Although time to healing was comparable in this study, median 12 days in each case, the quality of healing was rated as 'excellent' in 56% of patients treated with Granuflex/Duoderm compared with only 11% in the group treated with the chlorhexidine-impregnated paraffin gauze ($p < 0.0001$). Both investigators and patients showed a significant preference for the hydrocolloid despite greater problems of leakage with the hydrocolloid, leading the authors to suggest that Granuflex/Duoderm 'should be used as the first-choice dressing in the management of partial skin thickness burns'. Following a brief review of the literature, this view was supported by Smith et al.,[189] who concluded that superficial burns without necrosis or infection might benefit from the moist wound environment produced by the application of a hydrocolloid.

Hydrocolloids vs silver sulphadiazine

Wyatt et al.[190] compared Granuflex/Duoderm with a standard burn treatment, silver sulfadiazine cream, Silvadene, in the outpatient management of 50 patients with second-degree burns. Healing times were 10.23 ± 0.68 vs 15.59 ± 1.86 days ($p < 0.01$) for Granuflex/Duoderm and Silvadene respectively. Granuflex/Duoderm-treated burns required fewer dressing changes, caused less pain and produced fewer restrictions upon mobility, leading the authors to conclude that Granuflex/Duoderm was superior to Silvadene cream for this indication.

In a similar prospective, open, randomized and parallel group trial, Afilalo et al.[191] compared Granuflex/Duoderm with Bactigras and silver sulphadiazine (Flamazine), used together in the outpatient management of small partial skin thickness burns. Forty-eight patients with burns less than 48 hours old and below 15% TBSA were randomly allocated into the two treatment groups. Eighteen subjects dropped out leaving 15 in each group. The wounds were followed until complete reepithelialization occurred. Time to healing for the Granuflex/Duoderm group was 10.7 ± 4.8 days vs 11.2 ± 4.2 days for SSD/Bactigras. This difference was not statistically significant although statistically significant differences were reported in other areas. The hydrocolloid was found to be easier to apply but harder to remove than the control. Fewer dressing changes were also required, with a mean of three changes per subject in the hydrocolloid group compared with eight in the SSD/Bactigras group ($p = 0.117$). Two burn wounds became infected in the hydrocolloid group, and one in the SSD/Bactigras group. The authors concluded that the design of the protocol, which required wounds to be assessed at set intervals of increasing length, meant that a difference in healing rates may not have been detected. Despite this limitation, the two treatments appeared equally suitable and effective for small partial skin thickness burns.

The potential advantages of combining a hydrocolloid dressing with SSD in the management of scalds and other thermal injuries were investigated by Thomas and Lawrence.[192] A total of 54 burns on 50 patients were randomly allocated to treatment with Granuflex/Duoderm E alone, hydrocolloid plus silver sulphadiazine, or a medicated paraffin gauze dressing, Bactigras. All wounds were swabbed frequently during the treatment period. Wounds dressed with Bactigras required an average of 4.1 dressing changes and had a mean healing period of 11.1 days. Those dressed with hydrocolloid alone required an average of 2.3 dressing changes per patient and healed in an average of 10.6 days; the hydrocolloid and cream-dressed wounds required an average of 3.9 dressings per patient and took an average of 14.2 days to heal. The difference in healing rates between the hydrocolloid and the hydrocolloid/cream dressed wounds was statistically significant ($p < 0.05$) but no significant difference was detected between the hydrocolloid and the medicated paraffin gauze. The bacterial burden of the wounds in all three groups increased during the course of treatment with the smallest increase in the medicated paraffin gauze group. The increase in the number of pathogenic organisms was similar in all three groups.

Hydrocolloids vs Biobrane

Cassidy et al[193] compared Granuflex/Duoderm with Biobrane which is widely used for the treatment of superficial or partial-thickness burns. Biobrane is a composite dressing consisting of a silicone film and nylon fabric laminate to which collagen has been chemically bound. Seventy-two children aged 3-18 with burns, which covered less than 10% of the total body area, were included in the study. Although the authors found no significant difference either in pain scores or in the time to heal, 11.21 ± 6.5 vs 12.24 ± 5.1 days for Granuflex/Duoderm and Biobrane respectively ($p = 0.47$), they reported that the hydrocolloid is statistically less expensive than Biobrane and should be considered a first-line treatment option for intermediate-thickness burn wounds in children.

Donor sites

In patients with extensive burns, delayed healing of skin donor sites may be both costly and life threatening. A donor site dressing should facilitate healing without increasing the risk of a local infection which may either slow the healing process or ultimately convert the donor site to a full-thickness wound.[194] Donor sites have traditionally been dressed with simple materials such as gauze, sometimes impregnated with white soft paraffin or soaked in saline solution, all of which tend to adhere to the wound surface causing pain and trauma upon removal.

Hydrocolloids vs saline gauze

In 1985, Biltz et al.[195] compared Granuflex/Duoderm with saline gauze in the treatment of 24 patients with donor sites and reported a significant reduction in average healing rates, 7.2 ± 1.1 vs 13.3 ± 1.6 days, ($p < 0.01$). In addition, patients treated with

Granuflex/Duoderm reported a statistically significant reduction in pain scores, 2.1 ± 1.9 *vs* 6.5 ± 2.0 (p < 0.01). Madden *et al.*[196] also compared Granuflex/Duoderm with fine mesh gauze in the treatment of 20 donor sites and reported comparable benefits in terms of healing rates, 7.4 *vs* 12.6 days, p < 0.001), accompanied by greatly reduced infection rates.

Champsaur *et al.*[197] compared Granuflex/Duoderm with paraffin gauze in 20 patients with virtually symmetrical donor sites. The hydrocolloid dressed wounds healed in 6.8 ± 1.1 days *vs* 10.4 ± 1.7 days with paraffin gauze, (p < 0.01). Sites could also be reharvested five days earlier with hydrocolloid treatment in 10 *vs* 15 days.

Doherty *et al.*[198] reported similar benefits from the use of Granuflex, following a small study involving 14 patients with donor sites, 13 of which healed in seven days compared with the 10-14 days normally required for paraffin gauze. They also reported that the hydrocolloid produced better cosmetic results, as the healed donor sites were soft and supple in marked contrast to the dry sensitive areas that had formed beneath the conventional dressing. They concluded that the accelerated healing rates, and the reduced time spent in hospital, more than offset the high initial cost of the hydrocolloid. The advantages of hydrocolloid dressings over standard paraffin gauze in the treatment of donor sites were highlighted in further small scale studies by Donati *et al.*[199] and Demetriades and his co-workers.[200]

Tan *et al.*[201] in a prospective, randomized controlled study involving 60 patients with split skin graft donor sites compared Granuflex/Duoderm E with fine mesh paraffin gauze impregnated with 5% scarlet red. When the wounds were inspected on the tenth postoperative day, 27 (90%) of Granuflex/Duoderm wounds had healed, compared with 17 (57%) in the scarlet red group (p < 0.01). All wounds were completely healed by day 15. Donor site comfort was also significantly better in patients treated with the hydrocolloid. No clinical infections occurred in either group although wounds dressed with the hydrocolloid dressing required more frequent dressing changes than those dressed with scarlet red.

Smith *et al.*[202] compared Granuflex/Duoderm with a bismuth tribromophenate-impregnated gauze dressing, Xeroform, and found that healing rates in 25 evaluable patients were significantly different, 4/12 (33%) of hydrocolloid dressed wounds were healed in 5-8 days compared with 1/13 (8%) of the Xeroform treated wounds. Infection rates were also less in wounds dressed with hydrocolloid (0% *vs* 25%).

Leicht *et al.*[203] investigated the use of Granuflex/Duoderm as a dressing for donor sites on the scalp in a study involving 18 children with minor burns. Wounds dressed in this way healed normally, with a median healing time of 7.1 days enabling the patient to be mobilised very quickly after the operation. Good cosmetic effects were also achieved as the scar is hidden and invisible one month after the operation.

Comparison of hydrocolloids

Hydrocolloids have also been compared with other more 'modern' dressings. In one study Granuflex/Duoderm was compared with a second hydrocolloid, SureSkin, and paraffin gauze.[204] Ten patients with donor sites with a minimum size of 12 × 4 cm had their wound dressed with portions of all three dressings placed side by side. Punch biopsies taken on day eight from the central part of each wound were examined histologically. Healing times for Granuflex/Duoderm and SureSkin were identical (8.5 ± 0.8 days), but wounds dressed with paraffin gauze took 12 ± 1.6 days to heal. This difference was highly significant ($p < 0.0035$). The authors concluded that compared with the conventional treatment, hydrocolloids reduce healing times by 33%, but suggested that the frequent dressing changes associated with hydrocolloids limited their acceptability.

Hydrocolloids vs Omiderm and Biobrane

Leicht *et al.*[205] compared Granuflex/Duoderm with Omiderm, a highly permeable, hydrophilic, polyurethane membrane in patients with mirror image donor sites on both thighs. The trial was terminated when eight patients had been treated as the Granuflex/Duoderm dressing resulted in solid reepithelialization almost three days earlier than Omiderm, 7.8 (range 7 - 10) *vs* 10.6 (range 9 - 13). Granuflex/Duoderm was also more comfortable for the patients as crusts formed under the Omiderm which made it uncomfortable and difficult to remove. No such crusting occurred with the hydrocolloid, but leakage was a major problem from Granuflex/Duoderm during the first two days, which resulted in additional dressing changes. No signs of clinical infection were noted with either dressing.

In 1991, Feldman *et al.*[206] compared Granuflex/Duoderm with Biobrane and Xeroform in a prospective randomized study of 30 donor sites. Wounds dressed with Xeroform healed in an average of 10.5 days, which was significantly less than Granuflex/Duoderm, 15.3 days, or Biobrane, 19.0 days. Granuflex/Duoderm was reported to be the most comfortable dressing in use. No infections occurred in wounds dressed with Xeroform, but two wounds dressed with Biobrane became infected. One patient with Granuflex/Duoderm developed a donor site infection during a drug-related neutropenic reaction. Xeroform was the least expensive dressing to use ($1.16 per patient), followed by Granuflex/Duoderm ($54.88 per patient) and Biobrane ($102.57 per patient). The authors concluded that their study confirmed the usefulness of Xeroform as a donor site dressing as it promoted relatively rapid healing and was inexpensive and easy to use. Granuflex/Duoderm was considered to be ideal for smaller wounds when pain could be significantly reduced with minimal increase in cost. Biobrane was not considered suitable for routine use as a skin graft donor site dressing. Unfortunately the results of this study were of limited value because the wounds dressed with the hydrocolloid were only examined at seven day intervals, which artificially extended the recorded healing times in this group and thus the validity of this part of the study.

Hydrocolloids vs alginate

Porter[207] compared hydrocolloid dressings with alginate dressings in 65 patients to investigate the differences in the rate of epithelialization, discomfort experienced by the patients and the convenience of the dressings in normal clinical use. The alginate dressings were applied to the raw donor areas and held in place by layers of dry gauze, plaster wool and a crepe bandage.

At the time of the first dressing change 87% of the donor areas dressed with the hydrocolloid and 86% of the donor areas dressed with the alginate were found to be more than 90% healed. The mean time from operation to the observation of complete healing was 10.0 days for the donor areas dressed with the hydrocolloid and 15.5 days for wounds dressed with alginate; this difference was found to be statistically significant. The relatively poor performance of alginates in this study was almost certainly due to the use of an inappropriate secondary dressing system that caused the alginate to dry out during the later stages of the treatment. The healing times quoted in this investigation were greater than in most other studies because dressings were left undisturbed for longer periods. The investigators acknowledged that many wounds might have been healed long before they were inspected. They concluded that alginates are to be preferred as they are easier to apply and the need to achieve haemostasis prior to application is not as critical as with hydrocolloids.

Hydrocolloids vs hydrogel sheet

In a prospective randomized controlled study Tan et al.[208] compared Zenoderm, an acrylamide gel sheet containing a polysaccharide and a phospholipid, with Granuflex/Duoderm E in the treatment of split skin graft donor areas in 64 patients. Patient comfort was similar in the two groups but by the tenth postoperative day, 97% of wounds dressed with the hydrocolloid had healed compared with 75% of those dressed with Zenoderm ($p = 0.02$). Two patients in the Zenoderm group developed infection in their donor sites.

General surgery

Hydrocolloid dressings also have a role in the management of surgical wounds, both as primary and secondary dressings for sutured wounds and for those healing by secondary intention. One early report described the successful use of Granuflex/Duoderm to promote granulation in five patients following extensive excision of skin and subcutaneous tissue for large perianal lesions of *hidradenitis suppurativa*.[209] and a second described the use of Granuflex/Duoderm Extra Thin as a dressing following partial and total nail avulsions.[210]

Hydrocolloids vs traditional dressings

Healings rates of superficial wounds formed by surgical removal of seborrheic keratoses were compared in 16 patients who had their wounds dressed with a hydrocolloid, Avery H2460, or Fucidin cream used with an absorbent dressing, Cutiplast.[211] Wound healing was evaluated after seven and ten days and then daily until complete closure of the wound area. In seven of 16 patients, biopsies were taken after 14 days of reepithelization. Wounds dressed with the hydrocolloid healed significantly faster than the controls, median 8.5 *vs* 10 days ($p < 0.05$). No differences were detected in the histology of biopsies wounds taken from both groups.

Hydrocolloids have similarly been used following excision of pilonidal sinuses. Viciano et al.[212] compared Comfeel with Varihesive/Duoderm and conventional gauze in a prospective randomized trial involving 38 patients. The median healing time was 68 days (range 33 - 168) in the control group, compared with 65 days (range 40 - 137) in the two hydrocolloid groups combined. There were no differences between the hydrocolloid groups. A third of the postoperative cultures in the control group grew pathogens compared with 1/23 of the patients treated with hydrocolloid dressings (p = 0.03). This was considered to be of no clinical relevance. A significant number, 14/23 of wounds dressed with hydrocolloids developed leaks. Pain was significantly less in the first four postoperative weeks among the patients in the hydrocolloid groups compared with those in the control group (p < 0.05).

More positive results for hydrocolloids in this indication were reported by Estienne[213] who compared Granuflex/Duoderm with traditional dressings (hypochlorite irrigation and packing with paraffin gauze), for the treatment of 40 patients with pilonidal fistulae. The Granuflex/Duoderm was first applied on the third postoperative day after removal of an iodoform gauze pack applied in theatre. Granuflex/Duoderm granules (gel-forming particles, similar in composition to the adhesive mass on the hydrocolloid sheet) were introduced into the wound for the initial dressings, although subsequently the sheet was used in isolation. Initially, dressings were changed on alternate days, but this interval was later extended to 3-5 days. Wounds dressed with Granuflex/Duoderm achieved complete healing in an average of six weeks compared with the ten weeks required for traditionally treated wounds.

Hydrocolloids and sutured wounds

Standard hydrocolloids have also been used successfully as postoperative dressings following primary closure. Hulten[214] described the successful use of Granuflex/Duoderm in a series of 100 patients following colorectal surgery, and Young[187] reported the results of a small randomized study involving 49 patients with 54 wounds in which the performance of Granuflex/Duoderm was subjectively compared with that of unspecified standard treatments following clean elective surgery. Following both investigations it was concluded that hydrocolloid dressing offers an acceptable alternative to conventional products following primary closure.

Hermans[215] reported upon the clinical benefits of Granuflex/Duoderm Extra Thin in an open non-comparative multicentre trial involving a total of 95 patients with 102 sutured wounds of varying aetiologies. The study focused on patient quality of life issues, safety (incidence of infection), effectiveness (healing time) and ease of use. A total of 160 dressings were applied with an average wear time of 6.84 days (range 1 - 18). The overall incidence of wound infection was 2% but the dressing was not thought to be a causal factor. In five wounds, treatment had to be stopped before the scheduled time. Overall patients rated the comfort of the dressing as 'good' or 'very good' in 95% of cases, and they were able to shower with the dressing in place. In all of these studies the hydrocolloid was reported to be easy to use whilst increasing patient mobility and reducing pain.

Granuflex/Duoderm Extra Thin, was compared with Xeroform in 28 patients with 40 wounds who had undergone elective surgery.[216] One-half of every incision was covered with each of the dressings under investigation so that each patient served as their own control. Wounds were evaluated after 2-3 days, 7–10 days, four weeks, and seven months postoperatively. None of the incisions showed any evidence of infection. At the time of suture removal, the hydrocolloid dressings' ability to contain exudate, protect the wound, and facilitate mobility and personal hygiene were more highly rated compared with the gauze-type dressings (p<0.001, for all variables). At the four-week review, both the patient and the surgeon rated the scar segments covered with the hydrocolloid dressing better with respect to colour, evenness and suppleness, but these differences were no longer apparent seven months after surgery.

Comfeel, was compared with a conventional postoperative island dressing, Mepore, in a prospective randomized study involving 73 patients with clean incisions longer than 5cm.[217] The hydrocolloid was left in place until the sutures were removed but the Mepore was removed two days postoperatively. A total of 29 patients were withdrawn from the study, 20 dressed with Mepore and nine with Comfeel. Wound infections developed in one patient in the Comfeel group and five in the Mepore group (p = 0.2). The authors concluded that 'occlusive dressings stay in place and stay transparent, and do not increase the risk of wound infection', but the somewhat unusual design of the study and the large number of withdrawals made the result of this investigation of limited value.

Hulten[218] found that the waterproof backing of Granuflex/Duoderm Extra Thin offered particular benefits to 340 patients who had undergone surgery to form a stoma. Problems of soiling and maceration that commonly occur when such wounds are dressed with traditional gauze were not encountered in 89% of hydrocolloid-dressed wounds and wound infections were limited to 8% of patients studied.

Cardiac surgery

Several authors have described the use of hydrocolloid dressings following cardiac surgery with varying results. Alsbjorn[219] compared healing rates achieved with Granuflex/Duoderm and paraffin gauze on drainage wounds in 21 patients each of whom had two drains introduced through incisional wounds in the infrasternal area. The drains were removed 1-2 days postoperatively resulting in two identical wounds about 30 × 15 mm that were dressed with the products under examination. An operator, unaware of the nature of the treatment provided, examined the wounds on postoperative day 10. At this point, 13 hydrocolloid dressed wounds had healed compared with six wounds dressed with paraffin gauze. No differences in wound infection rates were detected.

Two hundred and fifty patients undergoing heart surgery were randomized to treatment with Granuflex/Duoderm, Cutinova Hydro or gauze and tape in a randomized controlled study described by Wikblad.[220] The conventional absorbent dressing was found to be more effective in achieving wound healing than Cutinova Hydro and fewer skin changes and less redness in the wounds was detected. The differences were not significant with the hydrocolloid dressing. The conventional dressing was less painful to remove than Cutinova Hydro and Granuflex/Duoderm. More frequent dressing changes, however, were needed when using the conventional dressing. Despite this, it was the least expensive alternative.

A further group of 737 patients were randomized to treatment with a Granuflex/Duoderm Thin, a simple island dressing (Primapore), or Opsite following a median sternotomy for cardiac surgery.[221] The dressings were assessed in terms of their ability to protect against infection and promote healing and patient comfort. There was no difference in the rate of wound infection or wound healing between treatment groups but the Primapore dressing was judged to be the most comfortable and least painful to remove. Granuflex/Duoderm Thin required the most frequent dressing changes (p < 0.001) and tended to be associated with the most discomfort upon removal. It was also the most expensive treatment of the three (p < 0.001).

According to Wilson,[222] thin hydrocolloid dressings can be used effectively as an alternative to sutures for graft fixation where the more traditional techniques are difficult or inappropriate. They have the additional advantage that they decrease slough and are less conspicuous than most other dressings.

Traumatic wounds

In addition to their role in the treatment of major acute wounds, hydrocolloid dressings have also been used with success in the management of superficial sports injuries and other traumatic wounds.

One report described how pieces of Granuflex/Duoderm were used to treat 39 soldiers who developed a total of 70 abrasions to their feet during a 160 km, 4-day road hike.[223] Estimation of pain levels before treatment showed that 28% had severe pain, 4% moderate pain and 8% no pain. Of those with initial severe or moderate pain, 92% reported 'good' and 8% 'moderate' pain relief after application of the dressings. The pain relief provided by the dressing enabled 35 of the 39 soldiers to complete the exercise.

A review of the pathophysiology, prevention and treatment of blisters that appeared in the journal *Sports Medicine,*[224] recommended the use of hydrocolloids for treating deroofed blisters, stating that this treatment 'provides pain relief and may allow patients to continue physical activity if necessary.'

Racing cyclists who had suffered partial thickness abrasions also gained benefit from the use of hydrocolloid dressings. Twenty-three individuals with 38 abrasions were treated with a hydrocolloid dressing and 24 individuals with 41 abrasions were treated with paraffin gauze.[225] The results showed that the occlusive dressing produced a shorter healing time, 5.6 *vs* 8.9 days, reduced pain, 91% *vs* 30% pain free, and had a lower incidence of infection (0% *vs* 10%). Athletes could also shower with the hydrocolloid in place, and comfort was judged to be good in 94% of instances. Showering comfort for wounds dressed with paraffin gauze was judged to be bad in 100% of cases.

The application of a hydrocolloid dressing can also offer other advantages to the sportsman for even relatively minor wounds such as lacerations that commonly occur during competitive contact sports such as competitive wrestling may limit the ability of the athlete to continue competition. When Granuflex/Duoderm Thin was trialled for this application it was found to support the skin, protect the laceration from further injury, shield the wound from exposure to infectious agents, and prevent transmission of blood or serum to other wrestlers, enabling two contestants to continue competition and/or practice without adverse effects.[226]

Knapman and Bache[227] described the use of Comfeel in an accident and emergency setting in the treatment of three patients with severe friction burns and gravel rash. They concluded that compared with conventional dressings the hydrocolloid appeared to promote healing and reduce discomfort experienced by the patient.

Similar benefits resulting from the use of a hydrocolloid dressing in the treatment of excoriations was reported by Andersson et al.[228] who showed that seven patients dressed with a hydrocolloid experienced less pain or discomfort than nine dressed with paraffin gauze.

Granuflex/Duoderm Extra Thin was compared with a non-adherent perforated film absorbent dressing in the management of 96 patients with lacerations, abrasions and minor operation incisions. Although time to heal was similar for both groups, patients using Granuflex/Duoderm Extra Thin experienced less pain ($p < 0.001$), required less analgesia ($p = 0.0154$) and were able to carry out their normal daily activities including bathing or showering without affecting the dressing or the wound.[229]

This important practical benefit associated with the use of hydrocolloid dressings was also noted by Hermans and van Wingerden,[230] following the use of Granuflex/Duoderm bordered dressing in a prospective study involving 30 patients with minor industrial wounds. Of these, 28 were partial thickness burns, one a combined cut/abrasion and one a combined cut, burn and abrasion. In 28 of the 30 wounds treatment with the hydrocolloid commenced immediately; in the remaining instances the wounds received two days of pretreatment with an antiseptic due to heavy contamination. Two patients had their treatment discontinued because of suspected infection and one because of a suspected allergic reaction to the dressing (not confirmed). Over 80% of patients rated the dressing as comfortable or very comfortable, enabling them to continue their daily activities.

Paediatric wounds

Hydrocolloid dressings offer important practical advantages in paediatric wound management, promoting healing and reducing pain.[231]

Three children who suffered from recessive dystrophic epidermolysis bullosa (RDEB) were treated with an impermeable hydrocolloid, paraffin gauze, or a perforated plastic film dressing, Telfa. The HT_{50} values obtained with hydrocolloids and Telfa were 3.0 days vs 4.2 days. For paraffin gauze it was 12.6 days.[232] In addition to the enhanced rate of healing, the use of the hydrocolloid also resulted in pain-free movement of the injured part, fewer dressing changes and a reduction in scar tissue formation. It is unlikely, however, that an adhesive hydrocolloid dressing would now find widespread use for this indication, as products made from silicone tend to be used for the treatment of very fragile skin.

A hydrocolloid dressing was compared with adhesive skin tapes on a variety of postoperative wounds in 170 children. Although effective skin closure was comparable in both groups, the hydrocolloids were more secure, remaining in place in 69 children, (81.2%), compared with 38 children (44.7%), in the control group ($p < 0.001$). No product-related maceration, infection or adverse events were reported during the study. The cosmetic results achieved in both groups was said to be very satisfactory.[233]

Similar benefits associated with the use of a hydrocolloid were reported by Rasmussen et al.[234] when they compared Granuflex/Duoderm with their standard treatment, which consisted of adhesive wound closures (Steristrips), covered with an island dressing with a non-woven fabric back (Cutiplast), in a randomized trial which focused on the psychological aspects of the treatment of 88 children who had undergone minor outpatient surgery. They found that the hydrocolloid dressing required fewer dressing changes, and readily permitted bathing or washing, whilst minimising the physical and psychological trauma to the infant or child and reducing the disruption to the child's and the parents' daily routines.

Hydrocolloids also have a very useful role to play in the treatment of skin lesions resulting from meningococcal septicaemia. The traditional approach of allowing such areas to dry out and demarcate prior to surgery or autoamputation may be appropriate where vascular studies have shown that a significant portion of a limb has become totally ischaemic and will definitely require amputation. For isolated areas or digits where the full extent of the damage cannot be accurately determined, intervention at an early stage with the application of a simple dressing such as a hydrocolloid that prevents further desiccation and the formation of dry eschar is worthy of serious consideration.[231,235]

Nagai et al.[236] described the successful use of a hydrocolloid (Duoderm) as an alternative to elastic bandages following urethroplasty for repairing hypospadias in 12 infants and suggested that the use of the dressing offers significant clinical advantages and a reduction in complications.

Hypertrophic scars

A small percentage wounds, fail to heal normally leading to the formation of hypertrophic or keloid scars. Hypertrophic scars take the form of a red raised lump on the skin, but do not grow beyond the boundaries of the original wound, but keloid scar scars are more serious as they can continue to develop forming benign tumours or growths. Keloid scars are most common in dark-skinned races and can be caused by surgery, or a traumatic injury. The causes of such scarring are not clearly understood, but when problems do arise, management can be difficult and usually involves the long term application of compression or even further surgical intervention.

Numerous papers describing the use of hydrocolloid dressings have commented that the incidence of hypertrophic scar formation appears to be low but little work has been done to confirm this in formal studies. Andersen et al.,[237] monitored the development of hypertrophic scarring in 38 children undergoing thoracic surgery over an average of 14 months. They found that wounds dressed with a hydrocolloid dressing appeared to be less likely to develop hypertrophic scars than those dressed conventionally although the difference between the groups did not reach statistical significance.

Phillips et al.[238] compared a hydrocolloid with silicone gel sheeting, an agent that is widely used to treat or prevent keloids and hypertrophic scars. Patients were allocated to receive hydrocolloid dressing or moisturiser to keloids or hypertrophic scars in a randomized controlled prospective study which monitored scar size and volume, colour, patient symptoms, and transcutaneous oxygen measurements. Hydration of the scars for two months resulted in symptomatic improvement, indicated by reduced itching, reduced pain and increased pliability, but produced no change in the principal physical appearance.

The available evidence therefore suggests that although the application of a hydrocolloid increases the hydration of the affected area and may relieve symptoms; such dressings are unlikely to offer major long-term benefits in the treatment of these sometimes distressing conditions.

Dermatology

Because of the occlusive nature of hydrocolloid dressings, it was recognized at an early stage that these materials could find application in the treatment of psoriatic plaques in the treatment of *psoriasis vulgaris*. In one very early study,[239] it was reported that in 26 patients with symmetric lesions, 16/34 (47%) resolved and 14/34 (41%) improved following prolonged application of a hydrocolloid dressing alone. Furthermore the hydrocolloid was therapeutically superior to twice-daily applications of fluocinolone acetonide cream a potent corticosteroid.

It was subsequently determined that the benefits of hydrocolloid treatment could be further enhanced by the combined use of the dressing and an appropriate corticosteroid in a variety of skin disorders,[240-243] and that this effect could also be demonstrated using objective techniques including measurement of O_2 consumption and blood flow,[244-245] and the biochemical markers keratin 10 and keratin 6.[246]

When Gonzalez,[247] compared two different hydrocolloid dressings, Duoderm and Actiderm, to occlude psoriasis plaques treated with triamcinolone acetonide cream in a prospective randomized controlled trial, they were unable to detect any difference between them. In a second comparative study,[248] Duoderm was compared with a highly permeable semipermeable film, Opsite IV 3000 over a topically applied steroid. As might be anticipated, it was found that the occlusive hydrocolloid was far superior to the permeable film for this indication.

The rapid improvement in clearance rates achieved with hydrocolloid occlusion does not, however, appear to impact greatly on time to relapse.[249]

Summary of clinical experience

Compared with more basic dressings such as paraffin gauze (both plain and medicated), the use of hydrocolloid dressings appears to result in improved healing rates in partial thickness wounds such as burns, donor sites, superficial traumatic injuries and some types of surgical wounds). There is also a body of evidence to suggest that their use is associated with a reduction in wound pain,[190,195,197-198,201,203,208,212,223-225,227-229,232,234] enhanced quality of life, (including the ability to wash or shower),[216,218,222-230] and also an improvement in the quality of the healed wound.[188,199,213-214,216-217,232]

With the exception of Biobrane, the hydrocolloids tended to be more expensive than products with which they were compared, although a number of authors proposed that the reduction in treatment time resulting from their use more than compensated for this increased initial cost.[193,198,206,208,216]

The principal advantage offered by this unique group of products is that in their intact state they are virtually impermeable to water vapour and therefore provide an effective barrier to transepidermal moisture loss when applied to intact skin or devitalised tissue. In the presence of exudate, the dressings absorb liquid and form a gel. As they do so they become permeable to moisture vapour which further increases their ability to cope with wound exudate. In most instances, however, they still require frequent replacement if applied to heavily exuding wound such as donor sites in the early stages of treatment as illustrated in this review. In contrast, alginates combined with appropriate secondary absorbent layers are well able to cope with such wounds initially, but as exudate production diminishes after the first couple of days of treatment, the fibrous dressing has a tendency to dry out leading to adherence and the possibility of secondary trauma. A logical approach to the management of these wounds would therefore seem to be the initial application of alginate, followed by a change to a hydrocolloid as exudate production is decreased in order to continue the provision of a moist wound healing environment.

Many of the references cited were published before the change in the formulation of Granuflex/Duoderm which may have some relevance to their findings and conclusions. Furthermore they also precede the introduction of foam dressings which in many centres have largely replaced hydrocolloids for the treatment of moderate to heavily exuding wounds. Nevertheless, the more occlusive nature of the hydrocolloids and their proven ability to conserve moisture, prevent infection and promote healing means that they remain worthy of very serious consideration for the treatment of all types of superficial wounds in which the production of excess exudate is unlikely to be a significant problem. The 'thin' versions of the hydrocolloid dressings are essentially similar to the standard semipermeable film dressings and are probably best reserved for use as secondary dressings.[17]

REFERENCES

1. Chen JL. 1967 1967. USA patent 3,339546.
2. Lide DR. *Handbook of Chemistry and Physics 88th Edn*. London: CRC, 2007.
3. Sircus W. Orabase in the management of abdominal-wall digestion by ileostomy and fistulas. *Lancet* 1964;2:762.
4. Kyte EM, Hughes ESR. Peristomal skin protection with "Orahesive". *Medical Journal of Australia* 1970;2:186.
5. Todd IP, Saunders B. Care of fistulous stomata. *British Medical Journal* 1971;4:747.
6. Allen S. Varicose ulcers: preliminary report on a new material to assist regranulation. *Curr Med Res Opin* 1973;1(10):603-4.
7. Ashurst PJ. Granulation in chronic leg ulcers: a trial with a new material. *Practitioner* 1975;215:353-358.
8. Leeson M. Stomahesive: the astounding new cure for decubitus ulcers. *Nursing* 1976;6:13-15.
9. Ryan DM. Pressure sores: treatment using Stomahesive. *Nurs. Times* 1976;72:299-300.
10. Lipman R. Hydrocolloid PSAs: New formulation stratergies. *Medical Device and Diagnostic Industry* 1999(June 1999):132-148.

11. Doyle A, Freeman FM. November 5th 1985 1985. USA patent 4,551,490.
12. Thomas S, Loveless P. A comparative study of the properties of six hydrocolloid dressings. *Pharmaceutical Journal* 1991;247:672-675.
13. Lee MG, Haines-Nutt F, Thomas S. Granuflex E (letter). *Pharmaceutical Journal* 1991;246(March 23):350.
14. Ferrari F, Bertoni M, Carmella C, Maring MJ, Aulton ME. The hydration and transmission properties of hydrocolloid dressings over extended periods. *Pharmaceutical Technology Europe* 1993;November:28-32.
15. Ferrari F, Bertoni M, Rossi S, Bonferoni MC, Caramella C, Waring MJ, et al. Comparative rheomechanical and adhesive properties of two hydrocolloid dressings: Dependence on the degree of hydration. *Drug Development and Industrial Pharmacy* 1996;22(12):1223-1230.
16. Rousseau P, Niecestro RM. Comparison of the physicochemical properties of various hydrocolloid dressings. *Wounds: A compendium of clinical research and practice* 991;3(1):43-48.
17. Thomas S, Banks V, Fear M, Hagelstein S, Bale S, Harding K. A study to compare two film dressings used as secondary dressings. *Journal of Wound Care* 1997;6(7):333-336.
18. Puolakkainen PA, Twardzik DR, Ranchalis JE, Pankey SC, Reed MJ, Gombotz WR. The enhancement in wound healing by transforming growth factor-beta 1 (TGF-beta 1) depends on the topical delivery system. *J Surg Res* 1995;58(3):321-9.
19. Dobrzanski S, Kelly CM, Gray JI, Gregg AJ, Cosgrove CA. Granuflex dressings in treatment of full thickness pressure sores. *Prof Nurse* 1990;5(11):594-9.
20. Stoker FM. A major contributor. Evaluation of Comfeel Pressure Relieving Dressing. *Prof Nurse* 1990;5(12):644-53.
21. Clark M. The effect of a pressure-relieving wound dressing on the interface pressures applied to the trochanter published erratum appears in Decubitus 1990 Nov;3(4);24. *Decubitus* 1990;3(3):43-6.
22. Cadier MA, Clarke JA. Dermasorb versus Jelonet in patients with burns skin graft donor sites. *J Burn Care Rehabil* 1996;17(3):246-51.
23. Thomas S. Making sense of hydrocolloid dressings. *Nursing Times* 1990;86:36-38.
24. Thomas S. Hydrocolloids. *Journal of Wound Care* 1992;1(2):27-30.
25. Thomas S, Loveless P. Moisture vapour permeability of hydrocolloid dressings. *Pharmaceutical Journal* 1988;241:806.
26. Thomas S, Loveless P, Hay NP. Comparative review of the properties of six semipermeable film dressings. *Pharm. J.* 1988;240:785-789.
27. Palamand S, Brenden RA, Reed AM. Intelligent wound dressings and their physical characteristics. *Wounds: A Compendium of Clinical Research and Practice* 1992;3(4):149-156.
28. Thomas S. Fluid handling properties of Allevyn foam dressing. *http://www.medetec.co.uk/Documents/Fluid%20handling%20properties%20of%20Allevyn%20foam%20dressing24-4-07.pdf* 2007.
29. Thomas S, Loveless P. A comparative study of the properties of twelve hydrocolloid dressings. *World Wide Wounds* 1998;247(17-Mar-1998).
30. Varghese MC, Balin AK, Carter DM, Caldwell D. Local environment of chronic wounds under synthetic dressings. *Arch Dermatol* 1986;122(1):52-7.
31. Henry M, Byrne PJ, Dinn.E. Pilot study to investigate the pH of exudate on varicose ulcers under Duoderm. In: Ryan TJ, editor. *Beyond Occlusion: Wound Care Proceedings*. London: Royal Society of Medicine, 1988:67-70.

32. Cherry GW, Ryan TJ. Enhanced wound angiogenesis with a new hydrocolloid dressing. In: Ryan TJ, editor. *An Environment for Healing: The Role of Occlusion,.* London: Royal Society of Medicine, 1985:61-68.
33. Pickworth JJ, De Sousa N. Differential wound angiogenesis: quantitation by immunohistological staining for Factor VII-related antigen. In: Ryan TJ, editor. *Beyond Occlusion: Wound Care Proceedings.* London: Royal Society of Medicine, 1988:19-23.
34. Angiogenetic effect of hydrocolloid dressings(Poster Presentation). Clinical Dermatology in the year 2000; 1990 May 22-25; London.
35. Tracy GD, Lord RS, Kibel C, Martin M, Binnie M. Varihesive sealed dressing for indolent leg ulcers. *Med J Aust* 1977;1(21):777, 780.
36. Johnson A. Towards rapid tissue healing. *Nurs. Times* 1984;80:39-43.
37. Lydon MJ, Cherry GW, Cederholm-Williams SA, Pickworth JJ, Cherry C, Scudder C, et al. Fibrinolytic activity of hydrocolloid dressings. In: Ryan TJ, editor. *Beyond Occlusion: Wound Care Proceedings.* London: Royal Society of Medicine, 1988:9-17.
38. Lydon MJ, Hutchinson JJ, Rippon M, Johnson E, de Sousa N, Scudder C, et al. Dissolution of wound coagulum and promotion of granulation tissue under Duoderm. *Wounds* 1989;1(2):95--106.
39. Mulder G, Jones R, Cederholm-Williams S, Cherry G, Ryan T. Fibrin cuff lysis in chronic venous ulcers treated with a hydrocolloid dressing. *Int J Dermatol* 1993;32(4):304-6.
40. Fibrinolysis and hydrocolloid dressings (Poster Presentation). Clinical Dermatology in the year 2000; 1990 May 22-25; London.
41. Field FK, Kerstein MD. Overview of wound healing in a moist environment. *Am J Surg* 1994;167(1A):2S-6S.
42. Alvarez OM, Mertz PM, Eaglstein WH. The effect of occlusive dressings on collagen synthesis and re-epithelialization in superficial wounds. *J Surg Res* 1983;35(2):142-148.
43. Leipziger LS, Glushko V, DiBernardo B, Shafaie F, Noble J, Nichols J, et al. Dermal wound repair: role of collagen matrix implants and synthetic polymer dressings. *J Am Acad Dermatol* 1985;12(2 Pt 2):409-19.
44. Chvapil M, Chvapil TA, Owen JA. Comparative study of four wound dressings on epithelization of partial- thickness wounds in pigs. *J Trauma* 1987;27(3):278-82.
45. Reuterving CO, Agren MS, Soderberg TA, Tengrup I, Hallmans G. The effects of occlusive dressings on inflammation and granulation tissue formation in excised wounds in rats. *Scand J Plast Reconstr Surg Hand Surg* 1989;23(2):89-96.
46. Chvapil M, Holubec H, Chvapil T. Inert wound dressing is not desirable. *J Surg Res* 1991;51(3):245-52.
47. Gokoo C, Burhop K. A comparative study of wound dressings on full-thickness wounds in micropigs. *Decubitus* 1993;6(5):42-3, 46, 48 passim.
48. Young SR, Dyson M, Hickman R, Lang S, Osborn C. Comparison of the effects of semi-occlusive polyurethane dressings and hydrocolloid dressings on dermal repair: 1. Cellular changes. *Journal of Investigative Dermatology* 1991;97(3):586-92.
49. Witkowski JA. Comparison of the effects of semi-occlusive polyurethane dressings and hydrocolloid dressings on dermal repair: 1. Cellular changes letter; comment. *Journal of Investigative Dermatology* 1992;98(5):816; discussion 816-7.
50. Phillips T, Colbert D, Palko MJ, Bhawan J. Comparison of the effects of semi-occlusive polyurethane dressings and hydrocolloid dressing on dermal repair: 1. Cellular changes letter; comment. *Journal of Investigative Dermatology* 1992;98(5):816; discussion 816-7.
51. Leek MD, Barlow YM. Tissue reactions induced by hydrocolloid wound dressings. *J Anat* 1992;180(Pt 3):545-51.

52. Chakravarthy D, Rodway N, Schmidt S, Smith D, Evancho M, Sims R. Evaluation of three new hydrocolloid dressings: retention of dressing integrity and biodegradability of absorbent components attenuate inflammation. *J Biomed Mater Res* 1994;28(10):1165-73.

53. Vogt PM, Andree C, Breuing K, Liu PY, Slama J, Helo G, et al. Dry, moist, and wet skin wound repair. *Ann Plast Surg* 1995;34(5):493-9; discussion 499-500.

54. Agren MS, Everland H. Two hydrocolloid dressings evaluated in experimental full-thickness wounds in the skin. *Acta Derm Venereol* 1997;77(2):127-31.

55. Agren MS, Mertz PM, Franzen L. A comparative study of three occlusive dressings in the treatment of full-thickness wounds in pigs. *J Am Acad Dermatol* 1997;36(1):53-8.

56. Schmidt RJ, Chung LY, Turner TD. Quantification of hydrogen peroxide generation by Granuflex (DuoDERM) Hydrocolloid Granules and its constituents (gelatin, sodium carboxymethylcellulose, and pectin). *Br J Dermatol* 1993;129(2):154-7.

57. Chung LY, Schmidt RJ, Andrews AM, Turner TD. A study of hydrogen peroxide generation by, and antioxidant activity of, Granuflex (DuoDERM) Hydrocolloid Granules and some other hydrogel/hydrocolloid wound management materials. *Br J Dermatol* 1993;129(2):145-53.

58. Wollina U, Knoll B, Prufer K, Barth A, Muller D, Huschenbeck J. Synthetic wound dressings--evaluation of interactions with epithelial and dermal cells in vitro. *Skin Pharmacol* 1996;9(1):35-42.

59. Agren M. The cytocompatibility of hydrocolloid dressings. *Journal of Wound Care* 1997;6(6):272-4.

60. Achterberg V, Meyer-Ingold W. Hydroactive dressings and serum proteins: an in vitro study. *Journal of Wound Care* 1996;5(2):79-82.

61. Quirinia A, Viidik A. The influence of occlusive dressing and hyperbaric oxygen on flap survival and the healing of ischaemic wounds. *Scand J Plast Reconstr Surg Hand Surg* 1998;32(1):1-8.

62. Matsumura H, Yoshizawa N, Kimura T, Watanabe K, Gibran NS, Engrav LH. A burn wound healing model in the hairless descendant of the Mexican hairless dog. *Journal of Burn Care and Rehabilitation* 1997;18(4):306-312.

63. Agren MS, Karlsmark T, Hansen JB, Rygaard J. Occlusion versus air exposure on full-thickness biopsy wounds. *Journal of Wound Care* 2001;10(8):301-304.

64. Agren MS, Franzen L, Chvapil M. Effects on wound healing of zinc oxide in a hydrocolloid dressing. *J Am Acad Dermatol* 1993;29(2 Pt 1):221-7.

65. Agren MS, Chvapil M, Franzen L. Enhancement of re-epithelialization with topical zinc oxide in porcine partial-thickness wounds. *J Surg Res* 1991;50(2):101-5.

66. Wu P, Nelson EA, Reid WH, Ruckley CV, Gaylor JD. Water vapour transmission rates in burns and chronic leg ulcers: influence of wound dressings and comparison with in vitro evaluation. *Biomaterials* 1996;17(14):1373-7.

67. Berardesca E, Maibach HI. Skin occlusion: treatment or drug-like device? *Skin Pharmacol* 1988;1(3):207-15.

68. Berardesca E, Vignoli GP, Fideli D, Maibach H. Effect of occlusive dressings on the stratum corneum water holding capacity. *Am J Med Sci* 1992;304(1):25-8.

69. Sasseville D, Tennstedt D, Lachapelle JM. Allergic contact dermatitis from hydrocolloid dressings. *Am J Contact Dermat* 1997;8(4):236-8.

70. Hausen BM, Kulenkamp D. Allergic contact dermatitis from hydrocolloid dressing in colophony- sensitive patients. *Aktuelle Dermatologie* 1998;24(6):174-177.

71. Jeong Ho L, Kim S-C. A case of allergic contact dermatitis from Duoderm hydrocolloid dressing. *Korean Journal of Dermatology* 2000;38(9):1256-1258.

72. Korber A, Kohaus S, Geisheimer M, Grabbe S, Dissemond J. [Allergic contact dermatitis from a hydrocolloid dressing due to colophony sensitization]. *Hautarzt* 2006;57(3):242-5.
73. Gallenkemper G, Rabe E, Bauer R. Contact sensitization in chronic venous insufficiency: modern wound dressings. *Contact Dermatitis* 1998;38(5):274-8.
74. Tomljanovic-Veselski M, Lipozencic J, Lugovic L. Contact allergy to special and standard allergens in patients with venous ulcers. *Collegium Antropologicum* 2007;31(3):751-756.
75. Annoni F, Rosina M, Chiurazzi D, Ceva M. The effects of a hydrocolloid dressing on bacterial growth and the healing process of leg ulcers. *Int Angiol* 1989;8(4):224-8.
76. Gilchrist B, Reed C. The bacteriology of chronic venous ulcers treated with occlusive hydrocolloid dressings. *Br J Dermatol* 1989;121(3):337-44.
77. Mulder G, Kissil M, Mahr JJ. Bacterial growth under occlusive and non-occlusive wound dressings. *Wounds* 1989;1(1):63-69.
78. Hutchinson JJ. Prevelance of wound infection under occlusive dressings: a collective survey of reported research. *Wounds* 1989;1(2):123-133.
79. Hutchinson JJ, McGuckin M. Occlusive dressings: a microbiologic and clinical review. *Am J Infect Control* 1990;18(4):257-68.
80. Hutchinson JJ, Lawrence JC. Wound infection under occlusive dressings. *J Hosp Infect* 1991;17(2):83-94.
81. Hutchinson JJ. Infection under occlusion. *Ostomy Wound Manage* 1994;40(3):28-30, 32-3.
82. Mertz PM, Marshall DA, Eaglstein WH. Occlusive wound dressings to prevent bacterial invasion and wound infection. *J Am Acad Dermatol* 1985;12(4):662-8.
83. Marshall DA, Mertz PM, Eaglstein WH. Occlusive dressings. Does dressing type influence the growth of common bacterial pathogens? *Arch Surg* 1990;125(9):1136-9.
84. Soderberg T, Agren M, Tengrup I, Hallmans G, Banck G. The effects of an occlusive zinc medicated dressing on the bacterial flora in excised wounds in the rat. *Infection* 1989;17(2):81-5.
85. Lawrence JC, Lilly HA. Bacteriological properties of a new hydrocolloid dressing on intact skin of normal volunteers. In: Ryan TJ, editor. *An Environment for Healing: The Role of Occlusion,*. London: Royal Society of Medicine, 1985:51-57.
86. Lawrence JC. The physical properties of a new hydrocolloid dressing. In: Ryan TJ, editor. *An Environment for Healing: The Role of Occlusion,*. London: Royal Society of Medicine, 1985:71-76.
87. Wilson P, Burroughs D, Dunn LJ. Methicillin-resistant Staphylococcus aureus and hydrocolloid dressings. *Pharm. J.* 1988;241:787-788.
88. Lawrence JC. Dressings and wound infection. *Am J Surg* 1994;167(1A):21S-24S.
89. Suzuki K, Yoshikawa T, Tomitaka A, Matsunaga K, Asano Y. Detection of aerosolized varicella-zoster virus DNA in patients with localized herpes zoster. *J Infect Dis* 2004;189(6):1009-12.
90. Biering-Sorensen F, Schroder AK, Wilhelmsen M, Lomberg B, Nielsen H, Hoiby N. Bacterial contamination of bath-water from spinal cord lesioned patients with pressure ulcers exercising in the water. *Spinal Cord* 2000;38(2):100-5.
91. Lawrence JC, Lilly A. Are hydrocolloid dressings bacteria proof? *Pharm. J.* 1987;239:184.
92. Piercey DA. Are hydrocolloid dressings bacteria proof? *Pharm. J.* 1987;239:223.
93. Cherry GW. Are hydrocolloid dressings bacteria proof? *Pharm. J.* 1987;239:281.
94. Lawrence JC. Are hydrocolloid dressings bacteria proof? *Pharm. J.* 1987;239:310.
95. Thomas S, Hay NP. Are hydrocolloid dressings bacteria proof? *Pharm. J.* 1987;239:388-389.
96. Cherry G. Are hydrocolloid dressings bacteria-proof. *Pharmaceutical Journal* 1987;239:456.
97. Lawrence JC, Lilly HA. Are hydrocolloid dressings bacteria proof? *Pharm. J.* 1987;239:486.

98. Moores J. Are hydrocolloid dressings bacteria proof? *Pharm. J.* 1987;239:486.

99. Johnson A. Are hydrocolloid dressings bacteria proof? *Pharm. J.* 1987;239:486.

100. Lawrence JC. Bacterial barrier properties of dressings. *Pharm. J.* 1990(November 1990):695-697.

101. Dunn LJ, Wilson P. Evaluating the permeability of hydrocolloid dressings to multi-resitant *Staphylococcus aureus*. *Pharmaeutical Journal* 1990;245(August 25):248-250.

102. Wilson P, Dunn L. The development of Biofilm hydrocolloid dressing-permeability to bacteria. *Pharmaceutical Journal* 1995;254(Feb 18):232-234.

103. Ameen H, Moore K, Lawrence JC, Harding KG. Investigating the bacterial barrier properties of four contemporary wound dressings. *Journal of Wound Care* 2000;9(8):385-388.

104. Harvey RE. Clinical trials versus laboratory studies. *Journal of Wound Care* 2000;9(9):414.

105. Haffejee AA, Moodley J, Pillay K, Singh B, Thomson S, Bhamjee A. Evaluation of a new hydrocolloid occlusive dressing for central catheters used in total parenteral nutrition. *S Afr J Surg* 1991;29(4):142-6.

106. Nikoletti S, Leslie G, Gandossi S, Coombs G, Wilson R. A prospective, randomized, controlled trial comparing transparent polyurethane and hydrocolloid dressings for central venous catheters. *Am J Infect Control* 1999;27(6):488-96.

107. Baxter R. Varihesive and the treatment of chronic leg ulcers. *Aust Fam Physician* 1980;9(9):599-601.

108. Cherry GW, Ryan T, McGibbon D. Trial of a new dressing in venous leg ulcers. *Practitioner* 1984;288:1175-1178.

109. Friedman SJ, Su WP. Management of leg ulcers with hydrocolloid occlusive dressing. *Arch Dermatol* 1984;120(10):1329-36.

110. Mulder GD, Albert SF, Grimwood RE. Clinical evaluation of a new occlusive hydrocolloid dressing. *Cutis* 1985;35(4):396-7, 400.

111. Ryan TJ, Given HF, Murphy JJ, Hope-Ross M, Byrnes G, editors. *The use of a new occlusive dressing in the management of venous stasis ulceration*. London: Royal Society of Medicine, 1985.

112. Milward P. Doing the legwork. *Nurs. Times* 1986;82:35-36.

113. Milward P. The use of hydrocolloid dressings for the treatment of leg ulcers in the community: Drug Tariff considerations. *Care Sci. Pract.* 1987;5:31-34.

114. Patrizi P, Silvagni M, Fiori SD, Morganti I. The treatment of superficial trophic ulcerations with Comfeel Ulcus. *Clin. Eur.* 1984;23:19-26.

115. Pottle B. Trial of a dressing for non-healing ulcers. *Nurs. Times* 1987;83:54-58.

116. van Rijswijk L, Brown D, Friedman S, Degreef H, Roed-Petersen J, Borglund E, et al. Multicenter clinical evaluation of a hydrocolloid dressing for leg ulcers. *Cutis* 1985;35(2):173-6.

117. Zeegelaar IE, Langenberg W, Hu R, Lai AFRF, Fabert WR. Tolerability and efficacy of hydrocolloid dressings in the treatment of venous leg ulcers under tropical conditions: an open prospective study. *J Eur Acad Dermatol Venereol* 2001;15(3):234-7.

118. Groenewald JH. Comparative effects of HCD and conventional treatment on the healing of venous ulcers. In: Ryan TJ, editor. *An Environment for Healing: The Role of Occlusion,.* London: Royal Society of Medicine, 1985:105-109.

119. Backhouse CM, Blair SD, Savage AP, Walton J, McCollum CN. Controlled trial of occlusive dressings in healing chronic venous ulcers. *Br J Surg* 1987;74(7):626-7.

120. Moffatt CJ. A trial of a hydrocolloid dressing in the management of indolent ulceration. *Journal of Wound Care* 1992;1(3):20-22.

121. Nelson EA, Prescott RJ, Harper DR, Gibson B, Brown D, Ruckley CV. A factorial, randomized trial of pentoxifylline or placebo, four-layer or single-layer compression, and knitted viscose or hydrocolloid dressings for venous ulcers. *J Vasc Surg* 2007;45(1):134-41.

122. Handfield-Jones SE, Grattan CE, Simpson RA, Kennedy CT. Comparison of a hydrocolloid dressing and paraffin gauze in the treatment of venous ulcers. *Br J Dermatol* 1988;118(3):425-7.

123. Winter A, Hewitt H. Testing a hydrocolloid. *Nursing Times* 1990;86(50):59-61.

124. Smith JM, Dore CJ, Charlett A, Lewis JD. A randomized trial of Biofilm dressing for venous leg ulcers. *Phlebology* 1992;7:108-113.

125. Eriksson G. Comparison of two occlusive bandages in the treatment of venous leg ulcers. *Br J Dermatol* 1986;114(2):227-30.

126. Ohlsson P, Larsson K, Lindholm C, Moller M. A cost-effectiveness study of leg ulcer treatment in primary care. Comparison of saline-gauze and hydrocolloid treatment in a prospective, randomized study. *Scand J Prim Health Care* 1994;12(4):295-9.

127. Arnold TE, Stanley JC, Fellows EP, Moncada GA, Allen R, Hutchinson JJ, et al. Prospective, multicenter study of managing lower extremity venous ulcers. *Ann Vasc Surg* 1994;8(4):356-62.

128. Augustin M, Siegel A, Heuser A, Vanscheidt W. Chronic leg ulcers: Cost evaluation of two treatment strategies. *Journal of Dermatological Treatment* 1999;10 Supplement 1:S21-S25.

129. Brandrup F, Menne T, Agren MS, Stromberg HE, Holst R, Frisen M. A randomized trial of two occlusive dressings in the treatment of leg ulcers. *Acta Derm Venereol* 1990;70(3):231-5.

130. Kikta MJ, Schuler JJ, Meyer JP, Durham JR, Eldrup-Jorgensen J, Schwarcz TH, et al. A prospective, randomized trial of Unna's boots versus hydroactive dressing in the treatment of venous stasis ulcers. *J Vasc Surg* 1988;7(3):478-83.

131. Cordts PR, Hanrahan LM, Rodriguez AA, Woodson J, LaMorte WW, Menzoian JO. A prospective, randomized trial of Unna's boot versus Duoderm CGF hydroactive dressing plus compression in the management of venous leg ulcers see comments. *J Vasc Surg* 1992;15(3):480-6.

132. Kerstein MD, Gahtan V. Outcomes of venous ulcer care: results of a longitudinal study. *Ostomy Wound Manage* 2000;46(6):22-6, 28-9.

133. Koksal C, Bozkurt AK. Combination of hydrocolloid dressing and medical compression stockings versus Unna's boot for the treatment of venous leg ulcers. *Swiss Med Wkly* 2003;133(25-26):364-8.

134. Rainey J. A comparison of two dressings in the treatment of heavily exuding leg ulcers. *Journal of Wound Care* 1993;2(4):199-200.

135. Thomas S, Banks V, Bale S, Fear-Price M, Hagelstein S, Harding KG, et al. A comparison of two dressings in the management of chronic wounds. *Journal of Wound Care* 1997;6(8):383-386.

136. Hansson C. The effects of cadexomer iodine paste in the treatment of venous leg ulcers compared with hydrocolloid dressing and paraffin gauze dressing. Cadexomer Iodine Study Group. *Int J Dermatol* 1998;37(5):390-6.

137. Burgess B. An investigation of hydrocolloids A comparative prospective randomised trial of the performance of three hydrocolloid dressings. *Professional Nurse* 1993;8(7):suppl 3-6.

138. Limova M, Troyer-Caudle J. Controlled, randomized clinical trial of 2 hydrocolloid dressings in the management of venous insufficiency ulcers. *J Vasc Nurs* 2002;20(1):22-34.

139. Peschen M, Weichenthal M, Schopf E, Vanscheidt W. Low-frequency ultrasound treatment of chronic venous leg ulcers in an outpatient therapy. *Acta Dermato-Venereologica* 1997;77(4):311-314.

140. Teepe RG, Roseeuw DI, Hermans J, Koebrugge EJ, Altena T, de Coninck A, et al. Randomized trial comparing cryopreserved cultured epidermal allografts with hydrocolloid dressings in healing chronic venous ulcers. *J Am Acad Dermatol* 1993;29(6):982-8.

141. van Rijswijk L. Full-thickness leg ulcers: patient demographics and predictors of healing. Multi-Center Leg Ulcer Study Group. *J Fam Pract* 1993;36(6):625-32.

142. Pierard GE, Pierard-Franchimont C. Planimetry of the healing rate of leg ulcers. *Journal of the European Academy of Dermatology and Venereology* 1995;5:S177.

143. Margolis DJ, Gross EA, Wood CR, Lazarus GS. Planimetric rate of healing in venous ulcers of the leg treated with pressure bandage and hydrocolloid dressing. *J Am Acad Dermatol* 1993;28(3):418-21.

144. Ballard-Krishnan S, van Rijswijk L, Polansky M. Pressure ulcers in extended care facilities: report of a survey. *J Wound Ostomy Continence Nurs* 1994;21(1):4-11.

145. Yarkony GM, Kramer E, King R, Lukanc C, Carle TV. Pressure sore management: efficacy of a moisture reactive occlusive dressing. *Arch Phys Med Rehabil* 1984;65(10):597-600.

146. Tudhope M. Management of pressure ulcers with a hydrocolloid occlusive dressing: results in twenty-three patients. *J. enterostom. Ther.* 1984;11:102-105.

147. van Rijswijk L. Full-thickness pressure ulcers: patient and wound healing characteristics. *Decubitus* 1993;6(1):16-21.

148. Barr JE, Day AL, Weaver VA, Taler GM. Assessing clinical efficacy of a hydrocolloid/alginate dressing on full-thickness pressure ulcers. *Ostomy Wound Manage* 1995;41(3):28-30, 32, 34-6 passim.

149. Gorse GJ, Messner RL. Improved pressure sore healing with hydrocolloid dressings. *Arch Dermatol* 1987;123(6):766-71.

150. Belmin J, Meaume S, Rabus MT, Bohbot S. Sequential treatment with calcium alginate dressings and hydrocolloid dressings accelerates pressure ulcer healing in older subjects: a multicenter randomized trial of sequential versus nonsequential treatment with hydrocolloid dressings alone. *J Am Geriatr Soc* 2002;50(2):269-74.

151. Alm A, Hornmark AM, Fall PA, Linder L, Bergstrand B, Ehrnebo M, et al. Care of pressure sores: a controlled study of the use of a hydrocolloid dressing compared with wet saline gauze compresses. *Acta Derm Venereol Suppl (Stockh)* 1989;149:1-10.

152. Kim YC, Shin JC, Park CI, Oh SH, Choi SM, Kim YS. Efficacy of hydrocolloid occlusive dressing technique in decubitus ulcer treatment: a comparative study. *Yonsei Med J* 1996;37(3):181-5.

153. Colwell JC, Foreman MD, Trotter JP. A comparison of the efficacy and cost-effectiveness of two methods of managing pressure ulcers. *Decubitus* 1993;6(4):28-36.

154. Xakellis GC, Chrischilles EA. Hydrocolloid versus saline-gauze dressings in treating pressure ulcers: a cost-effectiveness analysis. *Arch Phys Med Rehabil* 1992;73(5):463-9.

155. Chang KW, Alsagoff S, Ong KT, Sim PH. Pressure ulcers--randomised controlled trial comparing hydrocolloid and saline gauze dressings. *Med J Malaysia* 1998;53(4):428-31.

156. Mulder GD, Altman M, Seeley JE, Tintle T. Prospective randomized study of the efficacy of hydrogel, hydrocolloid, and saline solution-moistened dressings on the management of pressure ulcers. *Wound Repair Regen* 1993;1(4):213-8.

157. Banks V, Bale S, Harding KG. The use of two dressings for moderately exuding pressure sores. *Journal of Wound Care* 1994;3(3):132-134.

158. Banks V, Bale SE, Harding KG. Comparing two dressings for exuding pressure sores in community patients. *Journal of Wound Care* 1994;3(4):175-178.

159. Bale S, Squires D, Varnon T, Walker A, Benbow M, Harding KG. A comparison of two dressings in pressure sore management. *Journal of Wound Care* 1997;6(10):463-6.

160. Bale S, Hagelstein S, Banks V, Harding KG. Costs of dressings in the community. *Journal of Wound Care* 1998;7(7):327-30.

161. Seeley J, Jensen JL, Hutcherson J. A randomized clinical study comparing a hydrocellular dressing to a hydrocolloid dressing in the management of pressure ulcers. *Ostomy Wound Manage* 1999;45(6):39-44, 46-7.

162. Day A, Dombranski S, Farkas C, Foster C, Godin J, Moody M, et al. Managing sacral pressure ulcers with hydrocolloid dressings: results of a controlled, clinical study. *Ostomy Wound Manage* 1995;41(2):52-4, 56, 58 passim.

163. Banks V, Hagelstein S, Thomas N, Bale S, Harding KG. Comparing hydrocolloid dressings in management of exuding wounds. *Br J Nurs* 1999;8(10):640-6.

164. Baxter H. A comparison of two hydrocolloid sheet dressings. *Br J Community Nurs* 2000;5(11):572, 574, 576-7.

165. Motta G, Dunham L, Dye T, Mentz J, O'Connell-Gifford E, Smith E. Clinical efficacy and cost-effectiveness of a new synthetic polymer sheet wound dressing. *Ostomy Wound Manage* 1999;45(10):41, 44-6, 48-49.

166. Brown-Etris M, Milne C, Orsted H, Gates JL, Netsch D, Punchello M, et al. A prospective, randomized, multisite clinical evaluation of a transparent absorbent acrylic dressing and a hydrocolloid dressing in the management of Stage II and shallow Stage III pressure ulcers. *Adv Skin Wound Care* 2008;21(4):169-74.

167. Honde C, Derks C, Tudor D. Local treatment of pressure sores in the elderly: amino acid copolymer membrane versus hydrocolloid dressing. *J Am Geriatr Soc* 1994;42(11):1180-3.

168. Burgos A, Gimenez J, Moreno E, Lamberto E, Utrera M, Urraca EM, et al. Cost, efficacy, efficiency and tolerability of collagenase ointment versus hydrocolloid occlusive dressing in the treatment of pressure ulcers. A comparative, randomised, multicentre study. *Clinical Drug Investigation* 2000;19(5):357-365.

169. Muller E, van Leen MW, Bergemann R. Economic evaluation of collagenase-containing ointment and hydrocolloid dressing in the treatment of pressure ulcers. *Pharmacoeconomics* 2001;19(12):1209-16.

170. Hollisaz MT, Khedmat H, Yari F. A randomized clinical trial comparing hydrocolloid, phenytoin and simple dressings for the treatment of pressure ulcers [ISRCTN33429693]. *BMC Dermatol* 2004;4(1):18.

171. Graumlich JF, Blough LS, McLaughlin RG, Milbrandt JC, Calderon CL, Agha SA, et al. Healing pressure ulcers with collagen or hydrocolloid: a randomized, controlled trial. *J Am Geriatr Soc* 2003;51(2):147-54.

172. Callaghan S, Trapp M. Evaluating two dressings for the prevention of nasal bridge pressure sores. *Prof Nurse* 1998;13(6):361-4.

173. Zernike W. Preventing heel pressure sores: a comparison of heel pressure relieving devices. *J Clin Nurs* 1994;3(6):375-80.

174. Zernike W. Heel pressure relieving devices how effective are they? *Aust J Adv Nurs* 1997;14(4):12-9.

175. Gill D. The use of hydrocolloids in the treatment of diabetic foot. *Journal of Wound Care* 1999;8(4):204-6.

176. Lithner F. Adverse effects on diabetic foot ulcers of highly adhesive hydrocolloid occlusive dressings. *Diabetes Care* 1990;13:814 -815.

177. Foster AVM, Spencer S, Edmonds ME. Deterioration of diabetic foot lesions under hydrocolloid dressings. *Practical Diabetes International* 1997;14(2):62-64.

178. Vowden K. Diabetic foot complications. *Journal of Wound Care* 1997;6(1):4-8.

179. Laing P. Diabetic foot ulcers. *Am J Surg* 1994;167(1A):31S-36S.

180. Knowles EA, Westwood B, Young MJ, Boulton AJM. A retrospective study of the use of Granuflex and other dressings in the treatment of diabetic foot ulcers. In: Harding KG, Cherry G, Dealey C, Gottrup F, editors. *Proceedings of the 3rd European Conference on Advances in Wound Management* European Wound Management Association meeting, London: Macmillan Magazines, 1993.

181. Lazareth I. [Local care and medical treatment for ischemic diabetic ulcers]. *J Mal Vasc* 2002;27(3):157-63.

182. Apelqvist J, Larsson J, Stenstrom A. Topical treatment of necrotic foot ulcers in diabetic patients: a comparative trial of DuoDerm and MeZinc. *Br J Dermatol* 1990;123(6):787-92.

183. Boulton AJM, Cavanagh PR, Rayman G, editors. *The Foot in Diabetes (Fourth Edition)*. Chichester: John Wiley and Sons Ltd, 2006.

184. Hermans MH, Hermans RP. Preliminary report on the use of a new hydrocolloid dressing in the treatment of burns. *Burns Incl Therm Inj* 1984;11(2):125-9.

185. Hermans MH, Hermans RP. Duoderm, an alternative dressing for smaller burns. *Burns Incl Therm Inj* 1986;12(3):214-9.

186. Hermans MH. Hydrocolloid dressing (Duoderm) for the treatment of superficial and deep partial thickness burns. *Scand J Plast Reconstr Surg Hand Surg* 1987;21(3):283-5.

187. Phipps AR, Lawrence JC. Comparison of hydrocolloid dressings and medicated tulle-gras in the treatment of outpatient burns. In: T.J. R, editor. *Beyond Occlusion:wound Care Proceedings*. London: Royal Society of Medicine, 1988:121-126.

188. Wright A, MacKechnie DW, Paskins JR. Management of partial thickness burns with Granuflex 'E' dressings. *Burns* 1993;19(2):128-30.

189. Smith DJ, Jr., Thomson PD, Garner WL. Burn wounds: infection and healing. *American Journal of Surgery* 1994;167(1a(suppl.)):46s-48s.

190. Wyatt D, McGowan DN, Najarian MP. Comparison of a hydrocolloid dressing and silver sulfadiazine cream in the outpatient management of second-degree burns. *J Trauma* 1990;30(7):857-65.

191. Afilalo M, Dankoff J, Guttman A, Lloyd J. DuoDERM hydroactive dressing versus silver sulphadiazine/Bactigras in the emergency treatment of partial skin thickness burns. *Burns* 1992;18(4):313-6.

192. Thomas SS, Lawrence JC, Thomas A. Evaluation of hydrocolloids and topical medication in minor burns. *Journal of Wound Care* 1995;4(5):218-20.

193. Cassidy C, St Peter SD, Lacey S, Beery M, Ward-Smith P, Sharp RJ, et al. Biobrane versus duoderm for the treatment of intermediate thickness burns in children: a prospective, randomized trial. *Burns* 2005;31(7):890-3.

194. Smith DJ, Jr., Thomson PD, Garner WL, Rodriguez JL. Donor site repair. *Am J Surg* 1994;167(1A):49S-51S.

195. Biltz H. Comparison of hydrocolloid dressing and saline gauze in the treatment of skin graft donor sites. In: Ryan TJ, editor. *An Environment for Healing: The Role of Occlusion,*. London: Royal Society of Medicine, 1985:125-128.

196. Madden MR, Finkelstein JL, Hefton J.M., Yurt R. Optimal healing of donor site wounds with hydrocolloid dressings. In: Ryan TJ, editor. *An Environment for Healing: The Role of Occlusion,*. London: Royal Society of Medicine, 1985:133-136.

197. Champsaur A, Amamou R, Nefzi A, Marichy J. Use of Duoderm in the treatment of skin graft donor sites. Comparative study of Duoderm and tulle gras. *Ann Chir Plast Esthet* 1986;31(3):273-8.

198. Doherty C, Lynch G, Noble S. Granuflex hydrocolloid as a donor site dressing. *Care Crit. Ill* 1986;2:193-194.

199. Donati L, Vigano M. Use of the hydrocolloidal dressing Duoderm for skin donor sites for burns. *Int J Tissue React* 1988;10(4):267-72.
200. Demetriades D, Psaras G. Occlusive versus semi-open dressings in the management of skin graft donor sites. *S Afr J Surg* 1992;30(2):40-1.
201. Tan ST, Roberts RH, Blake GB. Comparing Duoderm E with scarlet red in the treatment of split skin graft donor sites. *Br J Plast Surg* 1993;46(1):79-81.
202. Smith DJ, Jr., Thomson PD, Bolton LL, Hutchinson JJ. Microbiology and healing of the occluded skin-graft donor site. *Plast Reconstr Surg* 1993;91(6):1094-7.
203. Leicht P, Siim E, Dreyer M, Larsen TK. Duoderm application on scalp donor sites in children. *Burns* 1991;17(3):230-2.
204. Steenfos H, Partoft S, Timshel S, Balslev E. Comparison of SureSkin, DuoDerm E and Jelonet Gauze in split skin donor sites - a clinical and histologial evaluation. *Journal of the European Academy of Dermatology and Venereology* 1997;8(1):18-22.
205. Leicht P, Siim E, Sorensen B. Treatment of donor sites-Duoderm or Omiderm? *Burns Incl Therm Inj* 1989;15(1):7-10.
206. Feldman DL, Rogers A, Karpinski RH. A prospective trial comparing Biobrane, Duoderm and xeroform for skin graft donor sites. *Surg Gynecol Obstet* 1991;173(1):1-5.
207. Porter JM. A comparative investigation of re-epithelialisation of split skin graft donor areas after application of hydrocolloid and alginate dressings. *Br J Plast Surg* 1991;44(5):333-7.
208. Tan ST, Roberts RH, Sinclair SW. A comparison of Zenoderm with DuoDERM E in the treatment of split skin graft donor sites. *Br J Plast Surg* 1993;46(1):82-4.
209. Michel L. Use of hydrocolloid dressing following wide excision of perianal hidradenitis suppurativa. In: Ryan TJ, editor. *An Environment for Healing: The Role of Occlusion,*. London: Royal Society of Medicine, 1985:143-148.
210. Ashford RL, Fullerton C. The use of Granuflex Extra Thin (hydrocolloid) dressing on partial and total nail avulsions - clinical observations. *JBPM* 1991;October:190-192.
211. Goetze S, Ziemer M, Kaatz M, Lipman RD, Elsner P. Treatment of superficial surgical wounds after removal of seborrheic keratoses: a single-blinded randomized-controlled clinical study. *Dermatol Surg* 2006;32(5):661-8.
212. Viciano V, Castera JE, Medrano J, Aguilo J, Torro J, Botella MG, et al. Effect of hydrocolloid dressings on healing by second intention after excision of pilonidal sinus. *Eur J Surg* 2000;166(3):229-32.
213. Estienne G, Di Bella F. The use of DuoDerm in the surgical wound after surgical treatment of pilonidal fistulae using the open method. *Minerva Chir* 1989;44(19):2089-92.
214. Hulten L. Wound dressing after colorectal surgery. In: Ryan TJ, editor. *An Environment for Healing: The Role of Occlusion,*. London: Royal Society of Medicine, 1985:149-151.
215. Hermans MH. Clinical benefit of a hydrocolloid dressing in closed surgical wounds. *J ET Nurs* 1993;20(2):68-72.
216. Michie DD, Hugill JV. Influence of occlusive and impregnated gauze dressings on incisional healing: a prospective, randomized, controlled study. *Ann Plast Surg* 1994;32(1):57-64.
217. Holm C, Petersen JS, Gronboek F, Gottrup F. Effects of occlusive and conventional gauze dressings on incisional healing after abdominal operations. *Eur J Surg* 1998;164(3):179-83.
218. Hulten L. Dressings for surgical wounds. *Am J Surg* 1994;167(1A):42S-44S; discussion 44S-45S.
219. Alsbjörn BF, Ovesen H, Walther-Larsen S. Occlusive dressing versus petroleum gauze on drainage wounds. *Acta Chir Scand* 1990;156(3):211-3.
220. Wikblad K, Anderson B. A comparison of three wound dressings in patients undergoing heart surgery. *Nurs Res* 1995;44(5):312-6.

221. Wynne R, Botti M, Stedman H, Holsworth L, Harinos M, Flavell O, et al. Effect of three wound dressings on infection, healing comfort, and cost in patients with sternotomy wounds: a randomized trial. *Chest* 2004;125(1):43-9.

222. Wilson PR. Dressed to heal: new options for graft site dressing. *Australas J Dermatol* 1996;37(3):157-8.

223. Hedman LA. Effect of a hydrocolloid dressing on the pain level from abrasions on the feet during intensive marching. *Mil Med* 1988;153(4):188-90.

224. Knapik JJ, Reynolds KL, Duplantis KL, Jones BH. Friction blisters. Pathophysiology, prevention and treatment. *Sports Med* 1995;20(3):136-47.

225. Hermans MH. Hydrocolloid dressing versus tulle gauze in the treatment of abrasions in cyclists. *Int J Sports Med* 1991;12(6):581-4.

226. Hazen PG, Grey R, Antonyzyn M. Management of lacerations in sports: use of a biosynthetic dressing during competitive wrestling. *Cutis* 1995;56(5):301-3.

227. Knapman L, Bache J. Hydrocolloid dressings in accident and emergency. *Nurs Stand Spec Suppl* 1989(6):8-11.

228. Andersson AP, Puntervold T, Warburg FE. Treatment of excoriations with a transparent hydrocolloid dressing: a prospective study. *Injury* 1991;22(5):429-30.

229. Heffernan A, Martin AJ. A comparison of a modified form of Granuflex (Granuflex Extra Thin) and a conventional dressing in the management of lacerations, abrasions and minor operation wounds in an accident and emergency department. *J Accid Emerg Med* 1994;11(4):227-30.

230. Hermans MH, van Wingerden S. Treatment of industrial wounds with DuoDERM Bordered: a report on medical and patient comfort aspects. *J Soc Occup Med* 1990;40(3):101-2.

231. Forshaw A. Hydrocolloid dressings in paediatric wound care. *Journal of Wound Care* 1993;2(4):209-212.

232. Eisenberg M. The effect of occlusive dressings on re-epithelializations of wounds in children with epidermolysis bullosa. *J Pediatr Surg* 1986;21(10):892-4.

233. Schmitt M, Vergnes P, Canarelli JP, Gaillard S, Daoud S, Dodat H, et al. Evaluation of a hydrocolloid dressing. *Journal of Wound Care* 1996;5(9):396-9.

234. Rasmussen H, Larsen MJ, Skeie E. Surgical wound dressing in outpatient paediatric surgery. A randomised study. *Dan Med Bull* 1993;40(2):252-4.

235. Thomas S, Humphreys J, Fear-Price M. The role of moist wound healing in the management of meningococcal skin lesions. *Journal of Wound Care* 1998;7(10):503-507.

236. Nagai A, Nasu Y, Watanabe M, Kusumi N, Tsuboi H, Kumon H. Clinical results of one-stage urethroplasty with parameatal foreskin flap for hypospadias. *Acta Med Okayama* 2005;59(2):45-8.

237. Andersen AS, Hjellestad M, Drevdal J, Segadal L, Rottingen JT, Skolleborg KC. [Prevention of scars. A controlled long-term study of the effect of hydrocolloid occlusive bandages after thoracic surgery in children]. *Tidsskr Nor Laegeforen* 1991;111(6):701-3.

238. Phillips TJ, Gerstein AD, Lordan V. A randomized controlled trial of hydrocolloid dressing in the treatment of hypertrophic scars and keloids. *Dermatol Surg* 1996;22(9):775-8.

239. Friedman SJ. Management of psoriasis vulgaris with a hydrocolloid occlusive dressing. *Arch Dermatol* 1987;123(8):1046-52.

240. Juhlin L. Treatment of psoriasis and other dermatoses with a single application of a corticosteroid left under a hydrocolloid occlusive dressing for one week. *Acta Derm Venereol* 1989;69(4):355-7.

241. David M, Lowe NJ. Psoriasis therapy: comparative studies with a hydrocolloid dressing, plastic film occlusion, and triamcinolone acetonide cream. *J Am Acad Dermatol* 1989;21(3 Pt 1):511-4.
242. Wilkinson RD, Ohayon M. Therapeutic response to a dermatologic patch and betamethasone valerate 0.1 percent cream in the management of chronic plaques in psoriasis. *Cutis* 1990;45(6):468-70.
243. Volden G. [Effective treatment of chronic inflammatory skin diseases. Once a week occlusion therapy with clobetasol propionate and Duoderm]. *Tidsskr Nor Laegeforen* 1992;112(10):1272-4.
244. Broby-Johansen U, Kristensen JK. Antipsoriatic effect of local corticosteroids--O2-consumption and blood flow measurements compared to clinical parameters. *Clin Exp Dermatol* 1989;14(2):137-40.
245. Broby-Johansen U, Karlsmark T, Petersen LJ, Serup J. Ranking of the antipsoriatic effect of various topical corticosteroids applied under a hydrocolloid dressing--skin-thickness, blood-flow and colour measurements compared to clinical assessments. *Clin Exp Dermatol* 1990;15(5):343-8.
246. Mommers JM, van Erp PE, van De Kerkhof PC. Clobetasol under hydrocolloid occlusion in psoriasis results in a complete block of proliferation and in a rebound of lesions following discontinuation. *Dermatology* 1999;199(4):323-7.
247. Gonzalez JR, Caban F. Treatment of psoriasis with triamcinolone acetonide 0.1% under occlusion: a comparison of two hydrocolloid dressings. *Bol Asoc Med P R* 1990;82(7):288-91.
248. Van de Kerkhof PCM, Chang A, Van der Walle HB, Van Vlijmen-Willems I, Boezeman JBM, Huigen-Tijdink R. Weekly treatment of psoriasis with a hydrocolloid dressing in combination with triamcinolone acetonide. A controlled comparative study. *Acta Dermato-Venereologica* 1994;74(2):143-146.
249. Volden G, Kragballe K, Van De Kerkhof PC, Aberg K, White RJ. Remission and relapse of chronic plaque psoriasis treated once a week with clobetasol propionate occluded with a hydrocolloid dressing versus twice daily treatment with clobetasol propionate alone. *J Dermatolog Treat* 2001;12(3):141-4.

13. Polysaccharide beads

INTRODUCTION

In the early 1970s a new type of absorbent dressing was introduced, totally different from anything that had been seen before. Unlike simple dressings made from cellulose fibre, which were in general use at that time to cover wounds and absorb exudate, this new material, Debrisan, took the form of free-flowing microbeads which had a more complex mode of action, functioning as a molecular sieve by selectively absorbing solutes according to their molecular weight.

In hindsight it is perhaps surprising that the product was ever considered for use as a dressing for the idea of introducing very small, insoluble, non-biodegradable beads into a deep wound or sinus appears to conflict with normal wound care practice which generally dictates the complete removal of particulate contamination which could become incorporated into new tissue or act as a focus for infection. Furthermore the practical problems associated with the application and removal of the beads also reduced their clinical acceptability. Nevertheless, the dressing was claimed to possess unique wound cleansing properties which provided some rationale for its use.

Although the handling problems associated with the beads were later largely overcome by the development of a paste, and subsequently a tea-bag presentation, this change in formulation almost certainly had an effect upon the performance of the beads themselves. Furthermore, the introduction of hydrogel dressings, which were shown to possess equivalent if not superior wound cleansing properties at much lower cost, combined with the widespread use of alginates and other dressings which were better suited for treating cavity wounds, seriously impacted upon the commercial success of Debrisan and in 2006 the manufacturer announced that when stocks were exhausted in March 2007 the product would be discontinued.

The Iodosorb/Iodoflex range, although superficially similar to Debrisan in that it is available as microspheres, a paste and a dressing, has the advantage that the beads from which the dressing is formed are biodegradable. They also contain iodine which imparts antimicrobial activity (including the ability to kill resistant strains of bacteria such as MRSA) and may also deliver other benefits to the healing process as described below.

STRUCTURE AND MODE OF ACTION

Dextranomer beads

Debrisan, (Debrisorb in Germany) was manufactured from a derivative of dextran, a linear polymer of glucose produced by a microorganism *Leuconostoc mesenteroides*. In its unmodified form, dextran is soluble in water but when treated with epichlorhydrin under controlled conditions, cross-links are formed between the chains which impart a three-dimensional structure to the molecule, rendering it insoluble. The resulting polymer was given the approved name 'dextranomer'.

The dressing was initially marketed by Pharmacia and Upjohn (later Pfizer) and supplied in the form of spherical beads, 0.1 - 0.3 mm in diameter, composed of dextranomer, poloxamer 187, polyethylene glycol 300, and a small quantity of water.[1]

Figure 61: Debrisan Beads

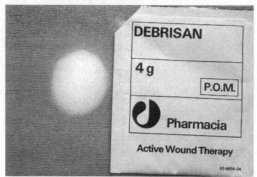

The beads, which were supplied in four gram sachets and 60 gram castors, were highly hydrophilic; one gram taking up about four grams of liquid. Fluid was initially rapidly drawn up by capillary action into the small spaces between the beads which gradually absorbed some of the liquid together with low molecular weight solutes, increasing in diameter as they did so. About 60% of the fluid taken up was held within the internal structure of the beads and the remainder retained in the spaces between them. Water, and solutes with a molecular weight of less than 1000, passed freely into the structure of the beads; materials with molecular weights in the range 1000 - 5000 penetrated only to a limited extent; and molecules larger than this were excluded. This ability of the beads to separate dissolved materials by their molecular weight forms the basis of their use in column chromatography where they are used under the name of Sephadex.

As the beads in contact with the wound became saturated, excess liquid was drawn up by the next dry layer, taking with it the high molecular weight material that could not penetrate their structure. In this way, exudate was drawn progressively away from the surface of the wound, carrying with it bacteria and cellular debris.[2]

The transport of bacteria away from the wound surface was neatly demonstrated in a laboratory model by Jacobsson et al,[2] following earlier work by Juhlin.[3] They allowed a column of Debrisan in a glass cylinder to take up a suspension of microorganisms in a mixture of plasma and normal saline until the beads became fully saturated. The column was then pressed out of the cylinder and divided into four segments which were examined by standard microbiological techniques. It was found that - regardless of the type of organism studied - at the end of the experiment, approximately 80% of the bacteria taken up by the dressing were present in the upper segment of the column.

The affinity of Debrisan for aqueous solutions was such that it initially created a suction pressure of up to 200 mmHg, but as the beads become saturated the suction pressure returned to zero. At this point, bacteria that had been transported to the outer layer of the dressing could start to spread back through the dressing. For this reason, it was recommended that Debrisan beads applied to moist wounds were changed regularly, preferably before they become totally saturated: for heavily exuding wounds, twice daily changes were sometimes required.

Because it was chemically inert, Debrisan was thought unlikely to cause any allergic reactions. In a study of 192 patients with dermatitis and leg ulcers, 69% were found to be sensitive to one or more components of commonly used topical preparations such as the antibiotics neomycin and framycetin. When the ulcers of 86 of these patients were treated with Debrisan, no irritant or allergic reactions were encountered. About 90% of all the patients treated reported a reduction in pain once treatment was initiated.[4]

The possible consequences of small numbers of beads becoming trapped in living tissue were investigated by Falk and Tollerz,[5] who implanted approximately 500 mg of the beads intramuscularly, and 100 mg subcutaneously, into rabbits and guinea pigs. Upon subsequent examination, each bead was found to be loosely encapsulated by connective tissue. Apparently unchanged beads were present up to three years after implantation. No granuloma formation was detected, and the lack of inflammatory signs and the limited proliferation of fibroblasts led the authors to conclude that Debrisan was well tolerated with an insignificant locally irritating effect.

Cadexomer beads

Iodosorb, originally introduced by Perstorp Pharma, but subsequently marketed by Smith and Nephew, is broadly similar in appearance and mode of action to Debrisan, consisting of microspheres 0.1-0.3 mm in diameter, formed from a three-dimensional network of cadexomer-starch chains cross-linked by ether bridges. The hydrophilic beads contain 0.9% w/w of elemental iodine, which is firmly held within the structure of the microspheres and is not liberated from them in the dry state, despite its high vapour pressure.

Figure 62: Iodosorb Beads

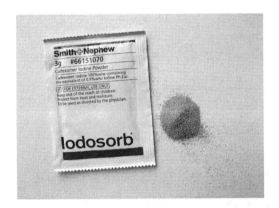 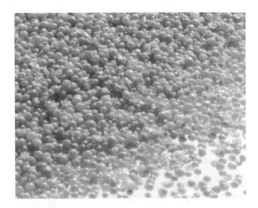

The beads are presented in individual sachets each containing three grams. Laboratory studies have shown that the release of iodine from the beads is governed both by the physico-chemical characteristics of the carrier and by the solubility of iodine in the solvent medium.[6] Solvents such as polyethylene glycol and propylene glycol are not taken up by the beads and no detectable levels of iodine can be found in them, despite the fact that iodine is soluble in both solvents.

In contrast water or an aqueous solution is rapidly taken up by the beads which are capable of absorbing about seven times their own weight of liquid. During this process the beads swell and iodine is slowly liberated. Within a wound the iodine is carried away from the damaged tissue by the capillary movement of fluid, resulting in a concentration gradient with the lowest levels of iodine at the surface of the wound.

Lawrence showed in laboratory studies that, although the mechanisms of fluid transport and the removal of debris and bacteria from the surface of a wound were generally similar in both Iodosorb and Debrisan, cadexomer iodine has the advantage of considerably reducing the number of viable organisms present.[7]

As with Debrisan, there were initially significant practical problems associated with the use of the original presentation of the dressing. These were alluded to by Shuttleworth and Mayho,[8] who commented that 'much of the dressing finds its way onto the floor'. They addressed this problem by the development of a paste containing three grams of Iodosorb and 0.5 mL of polyethylene glycol 400 which they found easier to apply and remove: glycerol was not suitable for this purpose because it would be taken up by the beads and lead to the premature release of the iodine. They reported that this formulation was much easier to use and appeared to reduce the stinging sensation which sometimes followed the application of the Iodosorb beads themselves.

Eventually a commercial preparation based on this formula was introduced. Called Iodosorb Ointment, it consisted of a poloxomer and polyethylene glycol base incorporating the sterile microspheres supplied in collapsible tubes containing 20 or 30 grams of the ointment. The iodine content of the beads used to produce the ointment is higher than that of standard Iodosorb in order to produce a final concentration of iodine in the paste of 0.9% w/w. In the presence of aqueous solutions or wound fluid, the beads in the ointment take up liquid and swell, slowly releasing the iodine, which imparts antibacterial properties to the dressing.

A third preparation, Iodoflex, consists of individual applications of cadexomer iodine ointment presented between two layers of gauze fabric which act as carriers and facilitate application. The dressing is supplied in three sizes, 5, 10 and 17 grams and like Iodosorb is intended primarily for the treatment of chronic leg ulcers.

Figure 63: Iodoflex Dressing

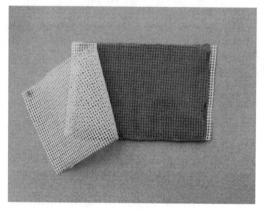

Unlike Debrisan, Iodosorb is biodegradable - being sensitive to enzymatic hydrolysis by an alpha-amylase that is present in most body fluids. The breakdown products are low molecular weight fractions consisting mainly of maltose and glucose.[9]

Because of the iodine content, there exists a theoretical possibility that excessive use of the dressing could affect thyroid function and a warning to this effect is provided on the instructions. Although this is considered very rare, the literature contains reports of two elderly patients who developed hyperthyroidism after cadexomer iodine treatment of small leg ulcers and who required symptomatic treatment and anti-thyroid medication.[10]

EFFECT UPON WOUND HEALING

Dextranomer beads

Published studies suggest that Debrisan beads had a positive effect upon developing granulation tissue, causing increased cellularity and vascularization, and enhanced accumulation of connective tissue ground substance.[11] Examination of Debrisan beads removed from the surface of wounds revealed high levels of fibrinogen degradation products, indicating marked fibrinolytic activity. No clottable fibrinogen was detected, suggesting that stable clots would not be formed on the surface of a wound dressed with Debrisan which would remain soft and free-draining.[12]

Frank *et al.*[13] examined the effect of Debrisan on experimental wounds in 20 rats which had been inoculated with 10^7 *S. aureus* or *P. aeruginosa*. Twenty four hours after inoculation the wounds were irrigated and dressed either with a moist saline dressing or Debrisan beads covered with a dry dressing. All dressings were changed daily, and on alternate days each was biopsied for quantitative bacteriological analysis. Under the conditions of the study, no difference could be detected between the two treatments in terms of the numbers of viable organisms present at each time point. It was noted, however, that the Debrisan treated wounds formed heavier scabs, and that the beads tended to become incorporated into the granulation tissue, requiring vigorous irrigation and scrubbing to effect removal. Furthermore the saline treated wounds appeared to close more quickly than those dressed with Debrisan beads.

Jacobsson *et al.*[2] utilised the ability of Debrisan beads to take up relatively low molecular weight material to estimate the concentration of prostaglandins in the fluid produced by leg ulcers. They found that the highest values were observed in beads removed from highly inflamed wounds, and noted that these levels often decreased as the wounds became cleaner and less oedematous. The constant removal of mediators like prostaglandins from within a wound has been claimed to limit the inflammatory reaction, and hence reduce wound pain. Comparative studies of human donor sites and experimental burns in pigs showed that, histologically, the inflammatory reaction to trauma was less pronounced in wounds dressed with the beads than in comparable wounds dressed with Vaseline gauze, although no difference in the rate of epithelialization was detected.[14]

Lundberg *et al.*[15] compared the effects of Debrisan and gauze in experimental wounds in the rat and reported that the results suggested that Debrisan is more effective than gauze for absorbing wound exudate when applied on an openly secreting wound. The inflammatory processes taking place in Debrisan-treated wounds also appeared to be less severe than in wounds treated with gauze.

Oredsson *et al.*[16] demonstrated that Debrisan caused activation of chemotactic factors in human serum and wound fluid via the alternate complement pathway which attracted both polymorphonuclear leukocytes (PMNs) and mononuclear leukocytes (MNs) in an agarose migration assay. They suggested that the formation of these factors at the wound surface could conceivably augment wound healing and influence the inflammatory response to infection.

Debrisan was also used as a diagnostic aid in clinical microbiology. Heggers *et al.*[17] developed a rapid slide technique to provide quantitative bacteriologic assessment of wounds to determine their suitability for grafting. The method involved the microbiological examination of Debrisan beads taken from a wound to detect the presence of bacteria. In 27 patients an 81% correlation was demonstrated between the bacterial count as determined by the new method and that determined by the more complicated tissue biopsy.

Cooper *et al.*[18] used Debrisan as a convenient technique for facilitating measurement of endogenous levels of cytokines in chronic wounds, as they were able to confirm in experimental studies that > 90% of cytokines applied to the beads could be recovered. Using this technique they found that although protein concentrations were remarkably similar, endogenous levels of cytokine growth factors in 20 pressure ulcers varied greatly.

Cadexomer beads

The iodine content of the Iodosorb range is generally assumed to help to prevent or combat wound infection. Mertz *et al.*[19] examined the effect of a cadexomer iodine wound dressing on methicillin resistant *S. aureus* (MRSA) in experimental partial thickness wounds on the backs of three pigs, inoculated with a known quantity of the organism. Wounds were dressed with either the cadexomer iodine dressing, a cadexomer which contained no iodine, or left untreated. Three wounds from each treatment group per animal were cultured using quantitative scrub techniques after 24, 48, or 72 hours of treatment. Compared to both the control and vehicle, the cadexomer iodine dressing significantly reduced both MRSA and total bacterial numbers within the wounds. No significant differences were observed in the number of bacteria recovered between the no treatment control and cadexomer (vehicle) treated wounds

In a second study using confocal laser scanning microscope, it was shown in experimental wounds in the rat that cadexomer iodine appears to inhibit the formation of the glycocalyx biofilm produced by *S. aureus*. Furthermore, if the dressing is brought into contact with microbial cells surrounded by glycocalyx, the dressing destroys the biofilm structure and kills the microorganism within.[20]

Iodine released by Iodosorb also appears to have other important effects in that it modulates the secretion of cytokines by human macrophages responding to bacterial lipopolysaccharide. In an experimental study a human macrophage cell line (U937), was co-cultured with Iodosorb, Iodosorb conditioned medium, or elemental iodine in the presence of optimal and sub-optimal stimulatory concentrations of bacterial lipopolysaccharide (LPS). The concentrations of tumour necrosis factor-alpha (TNF alpha) and interleukin-6 (IL-6) were assayed in the culture medium after 24 hours incubation. Co-culture with 0.25% Iodosorb, Iodosorb conditioned medium, or 20 µg/mL iodine, enhanced TNF alpha secretion by U937 cells stimulated with sub-optimal concentrations of LPS (0.25 ng/ml) from $48 \pm 3\%$ to $78 \pm 2\%$ cytotoxicity in L929 bioassay. The test substrates also inhibited secretion of IL-6 from cells stimulated with 10 ng/mL LPS (> 750 pg/mL to 267 ± 52 pg/ml). The authors further demonstrated, by immunohistological staining of sections prepared from biopsies of chronic leg ulcers, that the majority of macrophages present were negative for TNF alpha. They therefore proposed that Iodosorb provides a pro-inflammatory stimulus within wound tissue by activation of the resident macrophage population which would result in a localised production of pro-inflammatory cytokines and generate an influx of monocytes and T-lymphocytes into the wound which could trigger a chronic wound into a healing phase.[21]

Lamme et al.[22] showed that the dressing appeared to have a positive effect on epidermal regeneration during the healing of full-thickness, non-infected experimental wounds in the pig compared with a cadexomer iodine-free ointment, and saline treatment. The dressings were applied for 30 days followed by 30 days of wound assessment. The rate of epithelialization, wound contraction, systemic iodine absorption and several immunohistochemical markers were evaluated. All 36 wounds healed without macroscopic signs of wound infection and reepithelialized within 21 days. During the first nine days of treatment, wounds treated with cadexomer-iodine ointment showed significantly more epithelialization than the wounds treated with either cadexomer or saline, and the epidermis of wounds treated with cadexomer-iodine had significantly more epithelial cell layers from day 12 to day 30. No negative effects were observed that were associated with the use of cadexomer-iodine ointment.

Ohtani et al.[23] demonstrated that cadexomer with and without iodine induced the production of some pro-inflammatory cytokines and vascular endothelial growth factor by human macrophages, suggesting that the dressing has beneficial effects on wound healing unrelated to the presence of iodine and its recognised antibacterial activity.

CLINICAL EXPERIENCE

Dextranomer beads

Debrisan was recommended for the treatment of infected wounds, and for cleansing wounds containing pus, debris and soft yellow sloughy tissue. Once the dressing had achieved this objective, and healthy granulation tissue was obtained, a change of treatment was generally indicated.

It was recommended that Debrisan beads were poured into a wound to a depth of about 3 mm, and covered with a simple dressing pad or a semipermeable plastic film. The mobile nature of the beads often made this procedure difficult in shallow wounds and hard to dress areas. In the treatment of wounds to the hand including burns[24-25] and infected wounds following surgery or trauma,[26] the beads were sprinkled onto the hand, which was then inserted into a plastic bag. In the early stages, the dressings had to be changed three times a day, but the interval between changes was increased as healing progressed. The treatment was relatively painless and the hand and fingers could be moved freely within the bag. No crusts were formed and the areas remained soft and pliable throughout.

Gang et al.[27] also investigated the use of Debrisan in the treatment of discharging burns in a controlled study involving 48 patients. They found that, in this indication, Debrisan was able to reduce inflammation and bring about healing faster than saline dressings.

Frank et al.[13] as part of their assessment of Debrisan also undertook a study in which they compared saline gauze with Debrisan in 20 patients with a variety of different wounds during which the moist saline gauze was replaced every four hours, and the Debrisan beads changed every eight hours. Quantitative bacteriological studies were performed on tissue biopsies three times per week until the counts reached $\leq 10^5$. Debrisan appeared more effective than saline gauze in reducing the bioburden of ulcers caused by venous disease, and wounds treated in this way also improved more quickly than those dressed with saline gauze. However, patients with ischaemic ulcers did poorly with both treatments as expected. Several patients treated with Debrisan complained of a burning sensation and Debrisan dressings took twice as long to change as saline gauze because of problems associated with the removal of the dried crust of beads.

The results of a prospective trial comparing Debrisan beads with a silicone foam dressing in the treatment of 50 open surgical wounds were reported by Young and Wheeler.[28] Healing times for 25 wounds treated with Debrisan and an equivalent number dressed with elastomer were similar, 40.92 ± 98 and 36.90 ± 3.18 days respectively. The time taken for wounds to become pain-free was also comparable in both treatment groups, as was the persistence of signs in the wounds of erythema, oedema and slough; a comparison of costs reveals the elastomer dressing to be considerably cheaper than Debrisan.

Similar beneficial effects were recorded in a trial in which the beads were compared with Eusol and paraffin in the treatment of infected bowel wounds. Time to wound closure was eight days for Debrisan, compared with 12 days for the control group, and patients treated with Debrisan had a shorter hospital stay by a median of 2.2 days. The authors considered that this reduction in the time spent in hospital compensated for the high cost of the Debrisan treatment.[29]

In a small clinical study involving 20 patients following haemorrhoidectomy and fistulectomy[30] Debrisan was applied to ten patients and the other ten served as controls. Healing times were said to be considerably reduced in the Debrisan-treated wounds and the patients resumed a normal lifestyle earlier than expected.

The principal benefits of Debrisan appeared to be in the management of infected wounds and or sloughy wounds.[31-32] In a comparative study reported by Goode et al.[33] Debrisan pads were compared with ribbon gauze soaked in saline in the treatment of 67 patients with infected surgical wounds. It was found that the dextranomer-treated wounds were cleaned 32% quicker than the saline control group, and the authors concluded that the use of the pads provided a simple and efficient method of managing moist infected wounds.

When Hulkko et al.[34] compared Debrisan with streptokinase-streptodornase (Varidase) in a controlled study involving 87 infected wounds, although both treatments proved to be effective overall the dextranomer acted more quickly and appeared to stimulate more effective growth of granulation tissue.

The use of Debrisan was also described in a variety of case studies and trials involving other wound types. In one study involving 82 patients with infected sockets following tooth extraction,[35] cavities dressed with Debrisan, held in place with Orabase, became pain-free in five days, compared with the 12 days required for the control group whose wounds were treated with a paste made from zinc oxide and clove oil. In this particular study, however, it is not certain whether it was the beads or the Orabase paste that was mainly responsible for the rapid healing reported by the authors. Other slightly unusual applications included the treatment of an extensive laceration to the to the upper eye lid, which was successfully treated with a Debrisan pad changed twice daily,[36] and wounds produced following destruction of the nail bed by the application of phenol,[37] for which indication the beads were said to be more costly but broadly equivalent in performance terms to other products used for this purpose.

A major indication for Debrisan was claimed to be the treatment of leg ulcers, particularly moist wounds associated with venous disease,[38-41] for in drier ulcers associated with ischemia, the dressing was considered less useful.[13] It was suggested that once the slough was removed the dressing offered no advantage over more traditional methods in promoting ulcer healing.[42]

Numerous authors similarly described the use of Debrisan in the treatment of pressure ulcers.[43-45] When Shrosbree and Engel[46] treated 25 patients with 35 pressure ulcers of varying severity, most of the severe ulcers healed rapidly or were cleansed and ready for surgery at an average of 14.6 days and the superficial ulcers were completely healed within three weeks. Treatment of the sinuses with dextranomer using a catheter/syringe technique resulted in wound closure within 28 days.

The free-flowing nature of the Debrisan beads undoubtedly presented practical problems during application and removal. In an attempt to overcome these difficulties, the beads were sometimes formed into a paste with a suitable carrier to make them easier to handle. Mummery and Richardson[47] used Debrisan mixed with glycerin (4:1 by volume) in the treatment of 30 patients with a variety of wound types following surgical debridement. This preparation was said to be effective in cleansing the wound, reducing bacterial colonization, and decreasing local inflammation and oedema. The authors emphasised however, that the treatment was probably most appropriate for exuding wounds and should be discontinued as they became progressively drier. Johnson[48] described an alternative formulation using Debrisan beads and Macrogol, (polyethylene glycol 400) which proved very successful in the treatment of a number of infected wounds.

A commercial preparation of Debrisan paste was launched in 1985, in the form of sachets which consisted of dextranomer 6.4 g with polyethylene glycol 600 and water to 10 g. This was followed, in 1986, by the introduction of a Debrisan pad, in which a dextranomer paste was enclosed in a non-woven textile bag measuring 6×4 cm weighing about three grams.

As with the beads it was recommended that Debrisan paste or pad dressings should be changed before they became saturated with exudate. Depending upon the condition of the wound, this could vary from twice daily to every other day.

The pads were compared with the simple paste in 80 patients with leg ulcers randomized to one or other of the treatment groups.[49] Using a spatula, the paste was applied over a sterile mesh laid into the wound to a minimum depth of 3 mm; the pads were simply laid in the wound and held in place with a compression dressing. Wounds were monitored for the presence of pus and debris, pain and the formation of granulation tissue. During the course of the investigation patients in both groups reported a reduction in wound-related pain over time, and the two treatments produced a comparable reduction in wound size. Both were assessed as good or excellent by 70% of patients and 60% of assessors. Although the two formulations were equivalent therapeutically, the pads were found easier to use. The disadvantage of this presentation was that it was less suited to wounds of irregular shapes and sizes than the paste.

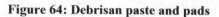

Figure 64: Debrisan paste and pads

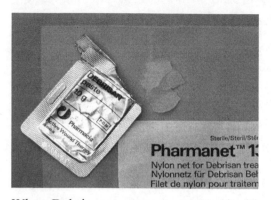 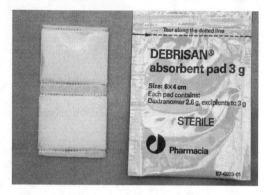

When Debrisan paste was compared with standard treatment in post-operative wounds in 20 patients in a randomized study the paste performed well, particularly in wounds with large amounts of pus and debris.[50] Debrisan 'teabags' were found to be useful following cryosurgery of cutaneous malignancies,[51] which can result in wounds that produce significant volumes of exudate.

Debrisan paste was compared with a hydrogel dressing, Intrasite Gel, in a randomized controlled trial involving 39 patients with Grade III or Grade IV pressure ulcers containing a significant amount of slough or necrotic tissue.[52] In accordance with the trial protocol wounds were assessed at 14 days at which point those which showed no evidence of improvement were withdrawn from the study for ethical reasons and treated as treatment failures. Wounds which showed clear evidence of debridement but which required further time to complete this process were treated for a further 14 days. At the mid point eight wounds dressed with gel were fully cleansed compared with one dressed with Debrisan (p = 0.008). During the subsequent 14-day treatment period a further four wounds in the Debrisan group became slough-free but there was no change in the number of fully-cleansed wounds in the Intrasite group. The eight wounds that were completely cleansed by Intrasite took an average of 11 days but the five wounds that were cleansed by Debrisan took an average of 18.2 days. Overall 12 of 20 wounds (60%) dressed with Debrisan improved compared with 16 of 19 wounds (85%) dressed with Intrasite Gel. Treatment costs were also substantially less (*circa* 50%), with the hydrogel treatment.

Debrisan paste was compared with a hydrogel in the management of sloughy pressure sores in a second study conducted by Colin *et al.*[53] who monitored efficacy, safety, ease of handling and patient comfort. The clinical investigation was restricted to the debridement of sloughy non-viable tissue only. The two treatments were similar in terms of debridement times for non-viable tissue; at day 21, however, the median reduction in wound area was 35% in the amorphous hydrogel group compared with 7% in the dextranomer paste group.

Sayag et al.[54] in a prospective, randomized, controlled trial involving 92 patients with full-thickness pressure ulcers compared dextranomer paste with an alginate dressing. During treatment, a minimal 40% reduction in wound area was obtained in 42% of those in the dextranomer group compared with 74% of the patients in the alginate group. The median time taken to achieve this was four weeks with alginate and more than eight weeks in the control group. The mean reduction in wound area per week was 2.39 ± 3.54 cm^2 and 0.27 ± 3.21 cm^2 in the alginate and dextranomer groups respectively (p = 0.0001).

Debrisan paste was compared with conventional saline dressings in an open-label, parallel-group study, involving 23 male spinal cord injury patients with a total of 30 pressure ulcers. Treatment was applied at least once every 12 hours and continued for a maximum of 15 day until the ulcer was clean and covered with new granulation tissue and suitable for skin grafting. Treatment with dextranomer paste resulted in significantly greater improvement in ulcer drainage compared with saline; 73% versus 13% of the ulcers, respectively, showed $\geq 25\%$ improvement in drainage from baseline to the end of the study. Both treatments were well tolerated, with no evidence of any local irritation.[55]

Cadexomer beads

Although cadexomer dressings have been used to treat wounds throughout the entire healing process, there is little doubt that their major value lies in the early part of the healing cycle - for promoting the cleansing and removal of infected material. Once this objective has been achieved, a change to an alternative treatment may be considered desirable.

In an early randomized trial of the treatment of 38 pressure ulcers,[56] it was found that cadexomer iodine was superior to standard treatments in removing pus and debris from the surface of the ulcer; wound healing rates, as measured by a decrease in wound area, were also significantly improved. No serious side effects were reported but during the course of the study, a small number of patients complained of transient smarting during the first hour following the application of the dressing.

Iodosorb is promoted particularly for the management of leg ulcers. In a multicentre trial involving 93 patients with this condition carried out in Sweden over a six-week period,[57] it was found that cadexomer iodine was more effective than the standard treatment in terms of reduction of pain, removal of exudate and debris, stimulation of granulation and reduction of erythema. Overall, the mean area of the ulcers treated with the beads decreased by over 30%, while those in the control group showed a small increase in area. A significant correlation was also observed between the use of the beads and a reduction in infection with S. aureus and other pathogenic species.

In a second optional crossover trial,[58] involving 61 selected patients with venous ulcers, Iodosorb was compared with a standard treatment regimen, which included the use of gentian violet and an ointment containing polymyxin and bacitracin. In this study, patients were encouraged to manage their ulcers by themselves, and although both treatments were found to be effective, ulcers dressed with the beads healed nearly twice as quickly as those in the control group. The authors concluded that daily bandaging and renewal of a non-adherent dressing may have distinct advantages over less demanding regimens.

In a further multicentre randomized crossover trial,[59] 72 patients had their ulcers managed entirely in the community by general practitioners. In the first four weeks of the study, ulcers treated with standard dressings and changed daily decreased in area by 10%, whereas those dressed with Iodosorb decreased by 36%. This trend toward increased healing continued after the crossover point. It was also recorded that ulcers dressed with cadexomer iodine produced less odour and pain than those in the control group.

A similar study to that described above was carried out by Lindsay *et al.*[60] In this investigation dressings were changed on alternate days and once again Iodosorb proved to be superior to the alternative treatments, in terms of wound debridement, odour control, pain relief and reduction of erythema and oedema. Ulcers dressed with traditional materials reduced in size by about 4% in four weeks, but those dressed with Iodosorb reduced in size by over 33%, a figure that is in close agreement with the results of earlier studies.

Iodosorb was compared with Debrisan in an eight-week study, involving 27 patients with venous leg ulcers.[61] Of the patients treated with Iodosorb, 65% healed completely, compared with 50% of those in the Debrisan group. Relative wound reduction also appeared to be greater in the cadexomer iodine group, but this did not reach statistical significance. The authors concluded that, although both products effectively reduced the symptoms caused by venous leg ulcers, the overall clinical response was significantly better in the cadexomer iodine group. It was suggested that this might be due to the enhanced absorbency of the beads and the antibacterial properties of the iodine, although the results of the bacteriological studies did not correlate well with ulcer healing.

Laudanska and Gustavson[62] compared cadexomer iodine beads with conventional treatments in a randomized trial involving 67 patients, 60 of whom provided data that was appropriate for statistical analysis. In both treatment groups mean ulcer area was reduced significantly compared with baseline, but after six weeks the reduction was significantly greater in the cadexomer treated group 71% *vs* 54% (p < 0.01). At this point 16 ulcers in the cadexomer group had healed compared with six in the control group, a difference that failed to achieve statistical significance. The iodine preparation was also more effective in improving the general condition and appearance of the wound. Five patients on cadexomer reported a stinging sensation in their wound associated with dressing usage.

Holloway[63] described a crossover study designed to assess the effect of cadexomer iodine on healing rates of venous stasis ulcers in which 75 patients were prospectively randomly assigned to receive either cadexomer iodine or standard treatment consisting of saline wet-to-dry compressive dressing. Thirty eight wounds dressed with cadexomer iodine healed more than twice as quickly as 37 wounds treated with the control, (p = 0.0025). There was also evidence of a trend toward reduced pain, exudate, pus, and debris, and a more rapid development of granulation tissue. Twelve patients crossed over from control treatment to the use of cadexomer iodine because of a failure to heal, but no patients switched to control therapy from the use of cadexomer iodine (p = 0.01). The only side effect reported with the iodine preparation was an occasional mild local burning sensation.

The effect of cadexomer iodine in ulcers colonised by *P. aeruginosa* was investigated by Danielsen *et al.*[64] in an open, uncontrolled, multicentre pilot study. Nineteen patients with venous leg ulcers were treated with cadexomer iodine paste and short-stretch bandaging for a maximum of 12 weeks or until the ulcer was healed. Ulcer area measurements and bacteriological cultures for growth of *P. aeruginosa* were regularly performed during the study period. In total seven patients were withdrawn for various reasons.

By the end of one week swabs taken from 11/17 patients (65%) proved negative for *P. aeruginosa*. After 12 weeks, 6/8 patients (75%) had a negative culture and complete healing was achieved in three patients (16%). The median ulcer area reduction obtained at 12 weeks was 32.9%. The authors concluded that their findings suggested that cadexomer iodine paste could be considered the treatment of choice for venous leg ulcers colonised with Pseudomonas sp but suggested that a larger controlled clinical study was required to confirm their observations.

One of the largest published studies involving cadexomer iodine was described by Hansson *et al.*[65] The dressing, in the form of a paste (Iodosorb/Iodoflex), was compared with Granuflex E, and paraffin gauze dressing (Jelonet) in a 12-week, randomized, open, controlled, multicenter, multinational trial in patients with exuding venous leg ulcers with compression provided by means of a short-stretch compression bandage, Comprilan. A total of 153 patients entered the study and were treated for 12 weeks or until exudate production ceased. The mean reduction in ulcer size was 62% with cadexomer iodine *vs* 41% and 24% for the hydrocolloid and paraffin gauze respectively. This difference failed to achieve significance. Of those wounds treated for 12 weeks (n = 51), ulcer area reduction was 66% for cadexomer iodine and 18% for hydrocolloid (p = 0.0127). Overall, the rate of healing, reduction in ulcer area per week, was significantly higher for cadexomer iodine than for paraffin gauze (0.64 cm^2/week *vs* 0.19 cm^2/week, (p = 0.0353). Although material costs were similar in all groups, when the costs were correlated with healing over a 12-week period, cadexomer iodine paste was found to be more cost effective than either the hydrocolloid dressing or paraffin gauze.

Similar financial benefits resulting from the use of cadexomer iodine ointment had been reported earlier by Apelqvist[66] following a study in which it was used to treat diabetic foot ulcers with exposed tendon, muscle, or bone. Patients were included in a 12-week open, randomized, comparative study in which the cadexomer iodine paste was compared with treatment consisting of gentamicin solution, streptodornase-streptokinase, or dry saline gauze. Treatment was continued until the ulcers stopped exuding at which point Vaseline gauze was used in both groups until the end of the study and the costs of dressing materials; staff and transportation were collected for comparison purposes.

Clinically relevant improvement was seen in 12 patients treated with cadexomer iodine and in 13 patients treated with standard treatment. The average weekly cost was

SEK 903 and SEK 1,421, respectively, of which the major part was the cost of staff and transportation determined by the frequency of dressing changes. No clinical difference was detected between the treatment groups but cadexomer iodine resulted in considerably lower weekly treatment costs.

Published evidence supporting the use of cadexomer iodine was critically reviewed by Bianchi in 2001[67] who concluded although the various publications provide some evidence to suggest that it can influence wound healing many of the paper were over 10 years old at that time and suggested that further more formal studies were required to strengthen the evidence base in support of the use of cadexomer on leg ulcers.

REFERENCES

1. Turner TD, Schmidt RJ, Harding KG, editors. Xerogel dressings - an overview. Advances in Wound Care; 1985; Cardiff. John Wiley.
2. Jacobsson S, Rothman U, Arturson G, Ganrot K, Haeger K, Juhlin I. A new principle for the cleansing of infected wounds. *Scand J Plast Reconstr Surg* 1976;10(1):65-72.
3. Juhlin I. Distribution of micro-organisms in a Debrisan column, . *Sv. Kir.* 1974;31:69-71. .
4. Fräki JE, Peltonen L, Hopsu-Havu VK. Allergy to various components of topical preparations in stasis dermatitis and leg ulcers. *Contact dermatitis* 1979;5:97-100.
5. Falk J, Tollerz G. Chronic tissue response to implantation of Debrisan: an experimental study. *Clinical Therapeutics* 1977;1(3).
6. Gustavson B. Cadexomer iodine: introduction,. In: Fox JA, Fischer H, editors. *Cadexomer Iodine,*. Munich,: Stuttgart, Schattauer Verlag, 1983:35-41.
7. Lawrence C. Bacteriology and wound healing. In: Fox JA, Fischer H, editors. *Cadexomer Iodine,*. Munich,: Stuttgart, Schattauer Verlag, 1983: 19-31.
8. Shuttleworth GJ, G.V. M. Controlled trial of Iodosorb in chronic venous ulcers, (letter). *Br. med J.* 1985;291:605-606.
9. Perstorp A. Personal communication from Perstorp AB, on the in-vitro enzymatic hydrolysis of Iodophore gel and other modified starch gels by endogenous alpha amylase. .
10. Michanek A, Hansson C, Berg G, Maneskold-Claes A. [Iodine-induced hyperthyroidism after cadexomer iodine treatment of leg ulcers]. *Lakartidningen* 1998;95(50):5755-6.
11. Niinikoski J, Renvall S. Effect of dextranomer on developing granulation tissue in standard skin defects of rats. *Clinical Therapeutics* 1980;3(4):273-278.
12. Åberg M, Hedner U, Jacobsson S, Rothman U. Fibrinolytic activity in wound secretions. *Scandinavian Journal of Plastic and Reconstructive Surgery* 1976;10.
13. Frank DH, Robson MC, Heggers JP. Evaluation of Debrisan as a treatment for leg ulcers. *Ann Plast Surg* 1979;3(5):395-400.
14. Jacobsson S, Jonsson L, Rank F, Rothman U. Studies on healing of Debrisan-treated wounds. *Scand J Plast Reconstr Surg* 1976;10:97-101.
15. Lundberg C. Inflammatory reaction and collagen accumulation in an experimental model of open wounds in the rat. A comparison between gauze and Debrisan treatment. *Scand J Plast Reconstr Surg* 1985;19(1):11-6.
16. Oredsson SU, Gottrup F, Beckmann A, Hohn DC. Activation of chemotactic factors in serum and wound fluid by dextranomer. *Surgery* 1983;94(3):453-7.

17. Heggers JP, Robson MC, Frank DH, Ko F. Rapid slide technique with dextranomer beads for bacteriologic assessment of wounds in the elderly: comparison with quantitative biopsy method. *J Am Geriatr Soc* 1979;27(11):511-3.
18. Cooper DM, Yu EZ, Hennessey P, Ko F, Robson MC. Determination of endogenous cytokines in chronic wounds. *Ann Surg* 1994;219(6):688-91; discussion 691-2.
19. Mertz PM, Oliveira-Gandia MF, Davis SC. The evaluation of a cadexomer iodine wound dressing on methicillin resistant Staphylococcus aureus (MRSA) in acute wounds. *Dermatol Surg* 1999;25(2):89-93.
20. Akiyama H, Oono T, Saito M, Iwatsuki K. Assessment of cadexomer iodine against Staphylococcus aureus biofilm in vivo and in vitro using confocal laser scanning microscopy. *J Dermatol* 2004;31(7):529-34.
21. Moore K, Thomas A, Harding KG. Iodine released from the wound dressing Iodosorb modulates the secretion of cytokines by human macrophages responding to bacterial lipopolysaccharide. *Int J Biochem Cell Biol* 1997;29(1):163-71.
22. Lamme EN, Gustafsson TO, Middelkoop E. Cadexomer-iodine ointment shows stimulation of epidermal regeneration in experimental full-thickness wounds. *Arch Dermatol Res* 1998;290(1-2):18-24.
23. Ohtani T, Mizuashi M, Ito Y, Aiba S. Cadexomer as well as cadexomer iodine induces the production of proinflammatory cytokines and vascular endothelial growth factor by human macrophages. *Exp Dermatol* 2007;16(4):318-23.
24. Paavolainen P, Sundell B. The effect of dextranomer (Debrisan) on hand burns. *Annales Chirurgiae et Gynaecologiae* 1976;65:313-317.
25. Arturson G, Hakelius L, Jacobsson S, Rothman U. A new topical agent (Debrisan) for the early treatment of the burned hand. *Burns* 1978;4:225-232.
26. Lohmann H, Buck-Gramcko D. [Debrisorb therapy of severe hand infections]. *Handchirurgie* 1980;12(1-2):89-92.
27. Gang R, K. Debrisan and saline dressing. *Chir Plast* 1981;6:65-68.
28. Young HL, Wheeler MH. Report of a prospective trial of dextranomer beads (Debrisan) and silicone foam elastomer (Silastic) dressings in surgical wounds. *Br J Surg* 1982;69(1):33-4.
29. Goode AW, Glazer G, Ellis BW. The cost effectiveness of dextranomer and eusol in the treatment of infected surgical wounds. *Br J Clin Pract* 1979;33(11-12):325, 8.
30. Gallegos Gonzalez L, Verdin Lopez Arce F, Hernandez Chavez MR. [Dextranomer in the postoperative of anorectal surgery]. *Rev Gastroenterol Mex* 1980;45(1):35-42.
31. Bewick B, Anderson J. A new method for treating infected wounds: studies on dextranomer (Debrisan): case reports. *Clinical Trials Journal* 1978;15(4):120-126.
32. Soul J. A trial of Debrisan in the cleansing of infected surgical wounds. *Br. J. clin. Pract.* 1978;32:172-173.
33. Goode AW, Welch NT, Boland G. A study of dextranomer absorbent pads in the management of infected wounds,. *Clin. Trials J.* 1985;22(5):431-434.
34. Hulkko A, Holopainen YV, Orava S, Kangas J, Kuusisto P, Hyvarinen E, et al. Comparison of dextranomer and streptokinase-streptodornase in the treatment of venous leg ulcers and other infected wounds. *Ann Chir Gynaecol* 1981;70(2):65-70.
35. Mathews RW. An evaluation of dextranomer granules as a new method of treatment of alveolar osteitis. *Br. dent. J.* 1982;152:157-159.
36. Jaross N. Treatment of extended lid lacerations with dextranomer beads. *Eur J Ophthalmol* 1993;3(4):223-5.
37. Drago JJ, Jacobs AM, Oloff L. A comparative study of postoperative care with phenol nail procedures. *J Foot Surg* 1983;22(4):332-4.

38. Floden C, Wikström K. Controlled clinical trial with dextranomer (Debrisan) on venous leg ulcers. *Current Therapeutic Research* 1978;24(7):753-760.
39. Sawyer PN, Dowbak G, Sophie Z, Feller J, Cohen L. A preliminary report of the efficacy of Debrisan (dextranomer) in the debridement of cutaneous ulcers. *Surgery* 1979;85(2):201-4.
40. Groenewald JH. An evaluation of dextranomer as a cleansing agent in the treatment of the post-phlebitic stasis ulcer. *S Afr Med J* 1980;57(20):809-15.
41. Groenewald JH, Booysen JN. Practical aspects of the use of Dextranomer (Debrisan) as a cleansing agent for venous stasis ulcers. *S Afr J Surg* 1981;19(1):65-70.
42. Morrison JD. Debrisan: an effective new wound cleanser. *Scott Med J* 1978;23(4):277-8.
43. McClemont EJW, Shand IG, Ramsay B. Pressure sores: a new method of treatment. *Br. J. clin. Pract.* 1979;33:21-25.
44. Parish LC, Collins E. Decubitus ulcers: a comparative study. *Cutis* 1979;23:106-110.
45. Nasar MA, Morley R. Cost effectiveness in treating deep pressure sores and ulcers. *Practitioner* 1982;226(307-310).
46. Shrosbree RD, Engel P. The treatment of decubitus ulcers with dextranomer. *S Afr Med J* 1981;59(25):902-4.
47. Mummery RV, Richardson WW. Clinical trial of Debrisan in superficial ulceration. *J Int Med Res* 1979;7(4):263-71.
48. Johnson A. Cleansing infected wounds. *Nursing Times* 1986;82:30-34.
49. Marzin L. Comparing dextranomer absorbent pads and dextranomer paste in the treatment of venous leg ulcers. *Journal of Wound Care* 1993;2(2):80--83.
50. Michiels I, Christiaens MR. Dextranomer (Debrisan) paste in post-operative wounds. A controlled study. *Clin Trials J* 1990;27(4):283-90.
51. Hersle K, Mobacken H. Uses of dextranomer absorbent pads after cryosurgery of cutaneous malignancies. *J Dermatol Surg Oncol* 1982;8(1):35-7.
52. Thomas S, Fear M. Comparing two dressings for wound debridement; results of a randomised trial. *Journal of Wound Care* 1993;2(5):272-274.
53. Colin D, Kurring PA, Yvon C. Managing sloughy pressure sores. *J Wound Care* 1996;5(10):444-6.
54. Sayag J, Meaume S, Bohbot S. Healing properties of calcium alginate dressings. *Journal of Wound Care* 1996;5(8):357-62.
55. Ljungberg S. Comparison of dextranomer paste and saline dressings for management of decubital ulcers. *Clin Ther* 1998;20(4):737-43.
56. Moberg S, Hoffman L, Grennert ML, Holst A. A randomized trial of cadexomer iodine in decubitus ulcers. *J Am Geriatr Soc* 1983;31(8):462-5.
57. Skog E, Arnesjo B, Troeng T, Gjores JE, Bergljung L, Gundersen J, et al. A randomized trial comparing cadexomer iodine and standard treatment in the out-patient management of chronic venous ulcers. *Br J Dermatol* 1983;109(1):77-83.
58. Ormiston MC, Seymour MTJ, Venn GE, Cohen RI, Fox JA. Controlled trial of Iodosorb in chronic venous ulcers. *Br. med. J.* 1985;291:308-310.
59. Harcup JWaS, P.A. A study of the effect of cadexomer iodine in the treatment of venous leg ulcers. *Br. J. clin. Pract.* 1986;40(9):360-364.
60. Lindsay G, Latta D, Lyons KGB, Livingstone ED, Thomson W. A study in general practice of the efficacy of cadexomer iodine in venous
leg ulcers treated on alternate days. *Acta ther.* 1986;12:141-148.
61. Kero M, Tarvainen K, Hollmen A, Pekanmäki K. A comparison of cadexomer iodine with dextranomer in the treatment of venous leg ulcers. *Curr. ther. Res.* 1978;42:761-767.

Polysaccharide beads
391

62. Laudanska H, Gustavson B. In-patient treatment of chronic varicose venous ulcers. A randomized trial of cadexomer iodine versus standard dressings. *The Journal of International Medical Research* 1988;16:428-435.

63. Holloway GA, Jr., Johansen KH, Barnes RW, Pierce GE. Multicenter trial of cadexomer iodine to treat venous stasis ulcer. *West J Med* 1989;151(1):35-8.

64. Danielsen L, Cherry GW, Harding K, Rollman O. Cadexomer iodine in ulcers colonised by Pseudomonas aeruginosa. *Journal of Wound Care* 1997;6(4):169-72.

65. Hansson C. The effects of cadexomer iodine paste in the treatment of venous leg ulcers compared with hydrocolloid dressing and paraffin gauze dressing. Cadexomer Iodine Study Group. *Int J Dermatol* 1998;37(5):390-6.

66. Apelqvist J, Ragnarson Tennvall G. Cavity foot ulcers in diabetic patients: a comparative study of cadexomer iodine ointment and standard treatment. An economic analysis alongside a clinical trial. *Acta Derm Venereol* 1996;76(3):231-5.

67. Bianchi J. Cadexomer-iodine in the treatment of venous leg ulcers: what is the evidence? *Journal of Wound Care* 2001;10(6):225-229.

14. Hydrogels and Xerogels

INTRODUCTION

A simple definition of a gel is a 'semi-rigid jelly-like colloid in which a liquid is dispersed in a solid'[1] and a hydrogel is therefore a gel in which the liquid constituent is water. An alternative description of a hydrogel, proposed by Schmidt, is 'a quasi-solid produced from a hydrocolloid (hydrosol) when the disperse solid phase is rendered continuous by some stimulus'.[2]

Hydrogels have been used in wound management for over 20 years. Originally conceived as alternatives to conventional absorbents in the treatment of chronic wounds such as leg ulcers, many hydrogels are now used for more specialised indications, facilitating wound cleansing and debridement.

Most hydrogel dressings are presented at least partially hydrated, but some are supplied in the dry state, and only formed into a true hydrogel by reconstitution immediately prior to administration to the wound; other products, applied to the wound in the dry state, subsequently form a gel as they absorb wound fluid. Such materials were described by Schmidt as 'Xerogels'.[2]

PROPERTIES OF HYDROGELS

Chemical and physical structure

Chemically, hydrogels consist of three-dimensional, water-swollen structures formed from hydrophilic synthetic or hemisynthetic homopolymers or copolymers. Some contain cross-linked networks which impart varying degrees of structural stability to the final product.

The strongest cross-links are formed by covalent bonds, these result in so-called *permanent* or *chemical* gels which have a defined structure and are often formed into thin sheets used for dressing relatively shallow surface wounds. Gels can also be formed from weaker bonds such as van der Waals forces, or hydrogen bonds,[3-4] these typically result in the formation of amorphous products with no defined structure. These are sometimes called *physical* or *pseudogels* which are generally used for dressing cavity wounds or sinuses.

Many amorphous hydrogels are produced from natural gel-forming agents such as alginates, carboxymethylcellulose and pectin. These together with polyvinylpyrrolidone (PVP) are polyelectrolytes - polymers whose repeating units bear an electrolyte group. These groups dissociate in aqueous solution, making the polymers electrically charged.

Polyelectrolytes have properties in common with both salts and polymers and can form viscous solutions or suspensions in water. These polymers may be anionic, cationic, amphipathic or neutral.

According to Hoffman,[5] examples of natural anionic polymers include: hyaluronic acid, alginic acid, carrageenan, chondroitin sulphate, dextran sulphate, and pectin.

Cationic polymers include chitosan and polylysine; amphipathic polymers include collagen (gelatin), carboxymethyl chitin and fibrin; neutral polymers comprise dextran, agarose, pullulan.

When a polyelectrolyte is combined with a multivalent ion of the opposite charge, it may form a physical hydrogel known as an *ionotropic* hydrogel, a familiar example of which is calcium alginate.

If polyelectrolytes of opposite charge are mixed together, they may gel or precipitate depending on their concentration and the ionic strength and pH of the solution. The products of these ion cross-linked systems are known as complex coacervates, or polyion complexes.

Some physical hydrogels can be formed by simply cooling polymer solutions made at elevated temperatures.

Chemical cross-links can be induced in a number of different ways, for example by exposure to ionising radiation, UV, or the use of chemical cross-linking agents such as dialdehydes or other reactive compounds. The various techniques available for producing hydrogels have been elegantly summarised by Hoffman,[5] and Rosiak,[4] and the chemistry and medical application for hydrogels have been also been reviewed previously.[4-7]

Uptake of fluid by hydrogels

Hydrophilic sites on the polymer chains interact with aqueous solutions enabling them to absorb and retain significant volumes of water. Typically, in the swollen state, the mass of water in a hydrogel is much higher than that of the polymer. When a dry hydrogel begins to absorb water, the first water molecules entering the matrix will hydrate the most polar hydrophilic groups. This is termed *primary bound water*. As the gel network swells and exposes more hydrophobic sites, these also interact with water molecules, leading to *hydrophobically-bound* water, or *secondary bound water*. Together these comprise the *total bound water*. Osmotic forces then draw further quantities of water into the gel causing further swelling which is opposed by the covalent or physical cross-links, leading to an elastic network retraction force resulting in an equilibrium swelling level. The additional water that is imbibed beyond the total bound water is called *free water* or *bulk water*.[5]

In a wound situation, the dissolved components of exudate also exert an osmotic effect which will tend to oppose or reduce the ability of a hydrogel dressing to take up or imbibe free water. Ions present in wound fluid may also affect a dressing's performance in this regard. This means that when testing such products in the laboratory, it is essential to use solutions which take account of both of these effects to avoid overestimating the fluid handling capacity of the product concerned.

Hydrogel sheets with a fixed three-dimensional structure do not change their physical form as they absorb fluid, although they may swell and increase in volume. Such products are defined in a European Standard, (BS EN 13726-1:2002)[8] as 'non-dispersible' hydrogels. In contrast as amorphous hydrogels absorb fluid they progressively decrease in viscosity and eventually take up the shape of the wound or vessel that contains them.

Amorphous gels can be further subdivided into 'soluble' gels that progressively lose all their cohesive properties upon dilution and simply form a solution in water, and 'dispersible' hydrogels that separate out on standing to form two distinct layers. A simple method that may be used to classify hydrogels in this way is described in BS EN 13726-1:2002.

If the network chains or cross-links which hold the structure together are degradable, the gel will begin to disintegrate and dissolve at a rate determined by its composition and the nature of the aqueous phase.

Most hydrogels contain microscopic pores which can vary both in size and the nature of the connections formed between them. The pore size of a gel can be of critical importance as it determines the ability of the matrix to allow or resist the penetration of molecules of varying size. Some polymers are homogeneous, containing no pores and in these gels the passage of water and low molecular solutes occurs by diffusion. The significance of the pore structure of hydrogels has been described in detail by Rosiak.[4]

Commercial applications for hydrogels

The fluid absorption properties of hydrogels are such that they find diverse applications such as thickening agents in food and medicines, moisture-retaining agents in horticulture, fluid retention aids in incontinence and feminine hygiene products and separation and diffusion gels in chromatography and electrophoresis. They are also widely used as dressings and as coatings for medical devices such as urinary catheters where they lower friction and increase lubricity. Some gels have pharmaceutical applications as drug delivery systems.

The potential value of hydrophilic polymers for medical applications such as the manufacture of implants, contact lenses and artificial arteries was first recognised by Wichterle and Lim,[9] who described a family of gels based upon glycolmethacrylates, the properties of which are governed by the nature of the monomers and the degree of cross-linking produced during their manufacture. They proposed that hydrogels for biological use should have significant water content, be inert to normal biological processes, and be permeable to metabolites; most important of all, they should be non-irritant when embedded into living tissue.

An early account of the use of hydrogels in wound management was provided by Yannas et al.[10] who described their application in the treatment of burns.

Smart hydrogels

Hydrogels as a group offer considerable potential in the medical field but some products, known as 'smart' gels, may prove to be of particular value as these can change their properties significantly in response to external stimuli such as temperature, pH, light, stress etc.

A pH-sensitive smart hydrogel, for example, may be used as a biomedical controlled release system, or for cell or enzyme immobilization. One gel made from a mixture of polyacrylic acid and poly(oxypropylene-co-oxyethylene) glycol is a liquid at room temperatures but as the temperature is increased to a preset threshold, typically that of the body surface, the polymers temporarily crosslink to form a network and the material changes from a liquid to a stable gel state. This is in marked contrast to other gel-forming polymers that tend to be liquid at high temperature forming a gel as they cool. This type of preparation has obvious potential in a wound-management context, as the reverse transition would enable the gel to be delivered or applied as a liquid, perhaps in the form of an aerosol, which rapidly solidifies into a solid gel structure that conforms precisely to the shape of its surroundings. The gel is also claimed to adhere well to mucous membranes, and therefore could be used as an ophthalmic sustained release system, or as a drug delivery system *via* the buccal, nasal, or vaginal routes.

A further novel formulation responds to environmental triggers such as pH changes by increasing in volume. This chemo-mechanical effect could be used for a number of medical applications. For example, a device consisting of dual chambers containing a pharmaceutical agent in one and a responsive hydrogel in the other, could be used as a drug delivery system which would be activated when a predetermined trigger, such as a pH change, caused the gel to swell and push the drug out of its chamber in a controlled manner.

An interesting practical application of hydrogel technology was reported by Suzuki *et al.*[11] who described the development of a hydrogel made from a succinylated polyvinyl alcohol that contained gentamicin bound to its structure through an enzymatically degradable peptide link. This link was particularly sensitive to hydrolysis by proteinases produced by *S. aureus* and *P. aeruginosa* with the result that the antibiotic was released from the gel in a controlled fashion in the presence of these organisms. According to the authors of this publication, when antibiotics or other medicaments are incorporated into conventional hydrogels they tend to be released very rapidly with the result that the local concentrations rapidly fall below therapeutically active levels; with this new development it was suggested that this problem was largely overcome.

Most hydrogels used in clinical practice either absorb exudate or donate moisture to dry tissue as appropriate. If the products concerned perform these functions in an acceptable manner, many clinicians give little attention to the chemical structure or composition of the gel itself. For this reason most hydrogels, but particularly the amorphous forms, are widely assumed to be equivalent and interchangeable in use. Eisenbud *et al.* in 2003[12] briefly reviewed the chemistry of hydrogels, the physiology of their interaction with the wound surface, and their role in patient care and concluded that although gels appear to offer advantages over conventional treatments in many areas, clinical evidence suggests that no particular hydrogel is significantly more efficacious than any other, implying that other factors such as cost and ease of use may guide clinician choice of product within this class of wound dressings.

In practice, however, this may be an unwarranted assumption, for it is difficult to believe that even simple gels, made from different chemical structures that vary in terms of their pH, osmotic characteristics and antimicrobial properties do not influence the healing of wounds in some subtle way. If the polymer, or one of the constituents of the gel, has a direct effect (positive or negative) on one or more of the cellular species or processes involved in the healing cascade, the potential for a particular dressing to facilitate or impair healing cannot be ignored.

In 1990 the effect of hydrogel composition was considered by Smetana et al.[13] who examined the influence of functional groups on cell behaviour. They showed in experimental studies that the presence of -OH, -CO-NH-, and $(CH_3)_2N$- groups on the molecule induced the spreading of macrophages on gel samples but gels containing -SO_3H and -COOH groups inhibited macrophage spread to a varying degree. They also found that functional groups had marked effects on macrophage development and postulated that the differences in the behaviour of the macrophages might be explained by electrostatic interaction between the hydrogel and the cellular membrane.

In 2002 Kirker et al. described the production of a glycosaminoglycan (GAG) hydrogel film prepared from hyaluronan and chondroitin sulphate which were first chemically manipulated then cross-linked to give a clear, soft hydrogel.[14] A solvent-casting method was then used to convert this into a hydrogel film. When compared with a control film in full-thickness wounds in mice, the new development was shown to provide a local environment which facilitated the production and assembly of other matrix components.

In 2004, the same group evaluated the film in a porcine model for donor-site autograft wounds,[15] and reported a statistically significant increase in epithelial coverage for GAG + Tegaderm-dressed wounds compared with Tegaderm alone at day three and day five post-surgery, leading the authors to conclude that the GAG hydrogel accelerated wound healing by enhancing reepithelialization.

In recent years 'biomimetic' hydrogels have been produced that are designed to mimic to a greater or lesser degree, the structure of and function of the highly sulphated glycosaminoglycans found on the surface of cells and in the extracellular matrix, a key part of the skin. These molecules have an important role as biological response modulators and the new hydrogels are believed to possess some properties which are similar to those of the naturally occurring molecules.

A family of new hydrogel dressings that include this type of technology has recently been introduced which are manufactured by First Water Ltd. They include Actiform Cool, marketed by Activa, together with more advanced developments currently identified as 'Pro-ionic' technology which are ionic polymers which are also capable of absorbing large volumes of wound fluid.

The potential advantages offered by wound dressings that possess functionality beyond that of simply providing physical protection and fluid management were discussed by Vachon and Yager[16] who described the development of a novel hydrophilic dressing material based on a sulfonated triblock polymer which was capable of binding and releasing a variety of therapeutic agents by means of an ion exchange reaction. In experimental studies prototype material was found to sequester the neutrophil proteases, elastase, and collagenase-2 (MMP-8) more effectively than a commercially available dressing marketed specifically for this purpose.

HYDROGEL SHEET DRESSINGS

Commercial preparations

Some examples of the numerous hydrogel sheet dressings available are described below. Where possible information on the composition of the various products is provided but in many cases this is simply not available.

Actiform Cool comprises a clear transparent, hydrogel sheet containing around 70% water, formed around a blue polyethylene matrix to impart strength and stability to the gel. On each side of the dressing as supplied is a flexible plastic liner. One of these is removed prior to application, but the other can either be removed or left *in situ* depending upon the amount of exudate produced by the wound.

Aqua-Gel is a transparent, flexible, elastic absorbent hydrogel sheet 3 - 4 mm thick, made from polyvinylpyrrolidone, polyethylene glycol and agar containing over 90% of water. The components are mixed together and formed into a cross linked gel by exposure to ionizing radiation. The dressing is said to be permeable to oxygen and moisture vapour but impermeable to bacteria.

Aquasorb is a non-adherent, water-based gel wafer supported by a fabric scrim bonded to a semipermeable polyurethane film. It is available without an adhesive border, with a transparent film border or a fabric tape border to eliminate adhesive taping.

ClearSite consists of 22% cross-linked polyvinylpyrrolidone polymer, 18% propylene glycol, and 60% water bonded to a semipermeable membrane bearing an imprinted grid. The dressing is also available as a bandage, or in the form of an island dressing with a film or foam adhesive border. The dressing was also marketed for a while by Baxter as NDM Gel-Syte.

Curagel a transparent sheet composed of 19% polyurethane gel, 73% water and 8% glycol as a humectant. The dressing is available both in a plain form and as an island dressing with a polyurethane top film surrounded by a border covered with polyethylene foam bearing an acrylic copolymer adhesive.

Elasto-Gel consists of a hydrogel sheet bonded to a polyurethane membrane. The gel contains 17.5% of a polyacrylamide polymer, 17.5% water and 65% glycerol, which acts as a humectant and bacteriostatic agent. The gel is relatively thick and is claimed to possess good protective and cushioning properties. Elasto-Gel Island dressing incorporates a polyurethane film backing layer with an adhesive border which facilitates dressing retention.

Flexderm, (Bertek Pharmaceuticals) is hydrogel sheet protected on both sides by polyethylene film.

Geliperm (Geistlich Pharma AG) introduced in 1977, was the first hydrogel sheet to be used in wound management and is therefore probably the best characterized. It consists of two different polymers interlaced together; a soft, relatively weak agar gel is supported by polyacrylamide, which imparts sufficient strength to make the final product suitable for use as a wound dressing. It is available in the form of a hydrated sheet, which contains about 96% water, 1% agar and 3% polyacrylamide. The dressing is strong, moist, flexible and totally transparent. If exposed to a dry, warm environment, however, it will gradually lose much of its water to form a thin, clear, semi-rigid transparent film. This formed the basis of a second presentation, a dry sheet form (now discontinued) which was chemically similar to the hydrated sheet with the exception of the addition of 35% glycerol as a humectant. When placed in an aqueous solution, the dry sheet rapidly absorbed liquid, taking up about 50 - 60% of its total fluid capacity in some 30 minutes. Thereafter, the rate of fluid uptake was reduced, as more than 24 hours was required to reach saturation.[17] A third preparation, Geliperm Granulated Gel, also now discontinued, consisted of the hydrated gel sheet reduced to an amorphous mass by a mincing process, which effectively increased the surface area and thus the rate of fluid absorption. The resultant granules were presented in a plastic tube with a short nozzle that could be used to introduce the gel into small wounds and cavities. There was a potential problem with this presentation; unlike normal amorphous dressings, the finely divided gel once introduced into a cavity would swell up and therefore not be easily flushed out with saline. This could theoretically result in residues of the gel becoming trapped within the depths of a wound although no problems of this nature were ever reported.

Hydrosorb (Hartmann) also known as **Aquaclear** in some markets, is an adhesive transparent hydrogel dressing consisting of an absorbent polyurethane gel containing around 60% water, covered with a gas-permeable polyurethane film which is impermeable to liquids and bacteria. Two presentations are available, a plain form, Hydrosorb, and an island dressing, Hydrosorb Comfort, which has a semipermeable film border. The dressing has a detachable foil backing marked with a grid upon which to record wound dimensions.

Iodozyme Iodozyme is a hydrogel dressing which, in common with other hydrogel sheet products, provides a moist environment that promotes autolytic wound debridement, reduces pain, and facilitates healing.

It also incorporates a biochemical system which increases the concentration of dissolved oxygen at the wound surface and liberates iodine from iodide ions present within the gel matrix.

It consists of two separate components, presented in individual aluminium pouches, which must be applied together as directed in order to activate the biochemical process. The first component, which is placed directly upon the wound surface, consists of a simple hydrogel sheet containing glucose. The second component is a smaller sheet of gel containing glucose oxidase, a naturally occurring enzyme which, in the presence of oxygen, catalyzes the oxidation of (beta)-D-glucose to D-gluconic acid and hydrogen peroxide. When the two gels are brought together, the glucose in the lower sheet diffuses into the other upper one. The hydrogen peroxide that is formed is released back into the gel and diffuses through the dressing, oxidizing any iodide ions it encounters to free iodine and liberating oxygen which remains in solution. Any peroxide that reaches the wound surface is immediately broken down to water and oxygen. The iodine it thought to exert a beneficial antimicrobial effect within the gel and also help to prevent the proliferation of microorganisms at the wound-dressing interface, whilst the dissolved oxygen is believed to have beneficial effects upon different aspects of cellular activity within the wound. The dressing therefore acts a little like a molecular pump, transporting dissolved oxygen through the dressing from the external environment and delivering it to the wound surface.

The dressing indicated for the treatment of dry to moderately exuding chronic wounds. It may also be used for the management of infected wounds under appropriate medical supervision.

Maxgel is a transparent sheet 3 - 4 mm thick made from polyvinyl pyrolidine, polyethylene glycol, and agar.

Novogel consists of a cross-linked polyacrylamide matrix that contains 17.5% water and 65% glycerin, which imparts a degree of bacteriostatic and fungistatic activity to the dressing and also prevents it from drying out on lightly exuding wounds. The gel sheet, which is backed with an outer layer of a four-way stretch cloth, can be cut to shape as required. It is also slightly adherent to dry skin but does not adhere at all to moist areas.

Oxyzyme is a hydrogel dressing which, in common with other hydrogel sheet products, provides a moist environment that promotes autolytic wound debridement, reduces pain, and facilitates healing.

Like Iodozyme it consists of two separate components which incorporate a biochemical system which increases the concentration of dissolved oxygen at the wound surface and liberates iodine from low levels (less than 0.04% w/w) of iodide ions present within the gel matrix.

The dressing indicated for the treatment of non-infected dry or lightly exuding chronic wounds. Although the iodine contained within the hydrogel imparts some protection against the growth of microorganisms, Oxyzyme is not indicated as a primary treatment for overtly infected wounds but it may be used in conjunction with systemic antimicrobial therapy where clinically indicated.

Vigilon also sold as Second Skin and Primskin, contains 96% water and consists of a radiation cross-linked, high molecular weight polyethylene oxide co-polymer. Because the gel has very little intrinsic strength, in the final dressing it is supported on a centered net of low-density polyethylene.

The dressing is presented in a sealed plastic pouch, enclosed in an aluminium outer cover. Inside the pack, the gel is covered on both sides with a sheet of polyester film. Immediately before use, one piece of film is removed and the gel is placed directly onto the skin or wound. The second sheet of plastic may be left in position or removed, as required - depending upon the amount of exudate that may be anticipated. On dry wounds, the sheet will help to conserve moisture in the dressing by reducing the loss of water vapour; on more heavily exuding lesions, it is usually appropriate to remove the backing layer, so that excess fluid may evaporate from the dressing at the maximum possible rate. The gel, with the plastic layers removed, is permeable to water vapour and gases, but impermeable to bacteria.

The manufacturers of Vigilon claimed that the dressing will absorb approximately 2 cm of fore, aft and lateral shear, and 360° of rotary shear, with a pressure of 30 kPa. It is suggested that this makes the dressing a useful covering for areas of tissue that are liable to frictional damage.

Physical properties

The principal factors that influence the acceptability of a hydrogel sheet used as a dressing are its water vapour permeability, adherence to the exposed wound surface, oxygen permeability, mechanical properties, impermeability to microorganisms and the ability to absorb exudate.[18]

Hydrogels also have potential value as a delivery system for antibiotics and antiseptic agents. One early study[19] showed that Geliperm could take up solutes with a molecular weight of up to about one million, although the rate of diffusion of these materials into and out of the gel was inversely proportional to their molecular weight. A comprehensive account of the chemical and physical properties of Geliperm was published by Kickhöfen[20] who also showed it to be non-immunogenic. Intramuscular, intraperitoneal and subcutaneous implantation studies in rats similarly showed Geliperm to be well tolerated when compared with other materials used as tissue implants.[21]

The potential value of Geliperm as a carrier for biologically active agents was investigated by Burgos,[22] who showed that PGFs incorporated in the gel stimulated granulation and epithelialization in chronic leg ulcers.

Microbiological properties

The effect of hydrogel dressings upon the growth of bacteria has been examined in a number of published studies and the ability of hydrogel sheets to act as bacterial barriers in experimental wounds in animals has also been investigated.

In an early laboratory study Geliperm was challenged with 100 different strains of bacteria and fungi.[23] Although the gel itself did not support the growth of clinically important microorganisms, in the presence of a growth medium containing suitable nutrients, bacteria could be cultured on the surface of the dressing after prolonged incubation. Under the conditions of test, however, no penetration or alteration of the structure of the gel by bacteria or fungi could be detected, leading the authors to conclude that the material should form an effective bacterial barrier under normal conditions of use. It was also suggested that Geliperm might reduce the concentration of bacterial exotoxins and enzymes in a wound, by absorption.

Mertz et al.[24] used two common skin pathogens, the non-motile S. aureus, and the motile P. aeruginosa, to challenge different dressings placed on partial-thickness wounds in swine. S. aureus was recovered from 100% of air-exposed wounds and from 50% of wounds treated with Vigilon or Opsite but was not isolated from Duoderm (Granuflex) covered wounds. P. aeruginosa was recovered from all air-exposed wounds and all wounds dressed with Vigilon or Opsite but from no wounds covered with Duoderm. The ability of the organism to enter the wound in this test probably reflects the nature of the adhesive bond that is formed between the dressing and the pigs' skin rather than by penetration through the dressing itself.

The same research group, some five-years later, compared the effect of these dressings upon pig wounds that had been deliberately inoculated with S. aureus, C. perfringens, B. fragilis, or P. aeruginosa.[25] Each wound was covered with one of three dressings, Duoderm, Opsite or Vigilon, or left exposed to air. Groups of wounds were sampled at 24, 48, and 72 hours when large numbers of S. aureus were recovered from beneath all of the dressings and from the air-exposed wounds. The numbers of C. perfringens and B. fragilis decreased in the air-exposed wounds and slightly reduced in the Opsite covered wounds but remained high in wounds dressed with Vigilon or the hydrocolloid. The numbers of P. aeruginosa were greatest in the Opsite and Vigilon covered wounds. On the basis of these results the authors suggested that occlusive dressings are not indicated in wounds that appear to be grossly contaminated or that may contain anaerobic organisms.

The results of this particular study should be considered in the context of results of a similar investigation using a rat model,[26] in which it was found that the deliberate introduction of large numbers of S. aureus and E. coli had no adverse effects upon healing even though bacterial counts within the wound increased up to the sixth day, falling back by day ten. In contrast, similar inoculums of P. aeruginosa caused wounds to deteriorate after about 10 days. These findings accord with those of an earlier investigation, which showed that although the continued use of a hydrogel sheet promoted granulation tissue production, infiltration of the wound by Pseudomonas sp. could delay healing.[27]

In an attempt to overcome the problems of bacterial proliferation under Vigilon, a new formulation was produced containing povidone iodine, an antimicrobial agent. The ability of this dressing to prevent the growth of S. aureus both in vitro and in vivo was subsequently examined by Mertz et al.[28] They showed that although the iodine impregnated dressing produced a significant reduction in the number of bacteria that could be recovered after 24 hours from pig wounds inoculated with low numbers of microorganisms, no reduction was detectable in wounds that received larger inoculums. They concluded that, although the addition of the antiseptic might increase the clinical value of the dressing, provided it was changed daily, it would probably be an inappropriate treatment for infected wounds.

The effects of two hydrogel dressings and a hydrocolloid dressing on bacterial proliferation in both an animal and laboratory model were investigated by Oliveria-Gandia et al.[29] who inoculated experimental burn wounds on pigs with 10^6 cfu of P. aeruginosa. Twenty-four hours after injury each wound was assigned to treatment with Duoderm, Clearsite or Elasto-Gel or left exposed to air. On days two, five, seven, and nine after the first treatment, quantitative microbiology was carried out on each wound using both a standard recovery medium to detect all viable bacteria, and a selective recovery medium for Pseudomonas that inhibited the growth of normal pig microflora. These results of these tests revealed that the number of Pseudomonas and other organisms recovered from wounds dressed with Elasto-Gel was significantly lower than from wounds dressed with the other two products but these differences were not reflected in the number of wounds that showed signs of clinical infection. All the occluded wounds, irrespective of the dressing applied, were judged clinically infected on days two and five, but this infection was eliminated by day nine in every case.

The authors then compared the same three dressings on the growth of *P. aeruginosa*, *E. coli. S. aureus* and *S. pyogenes* in an *in vitro* study in which they applied known numbers of each organism to small areas on an agar plates which they then covered with portions of the dressing under examination. After 24 hours the number of bacteria present both upon the agar and the dressing samples was determined. In each case it was found that compared with the other dressings examined, Elasto-Gel exhibited a marked inhibitory effect upon bacterial growth leading the authors to conclude that this product might be able to reduce the bacterial burden of a chronic colonised wound.

Animal studies

The effects of hydrogels on wound healing using an animal model have been investigated in several published studies. Using partial thickness wounds in pigs, Geronemus[30] found that wounds dressed with Vigilon healed 44% faster than untreated controls (2.5 *vs* 4.5 days). Wounds dressed with Bard Absorption Dressing, healed 24% faster than the controls in an average of 3.5 days. The authors theorised that both dressings promoted healing by preventing dehydration and crust formation thus allowing epidermal cells to migrate in an unobstructed manner across the wound surface.

Brennan *et al*.[31] used a hydrogel dressing (Geliperm) covered with an impermeable plastic sheet to provide occlusive conditions in a study of microangiogenesis in experimentally produced skin defects in 48 rats. They found that angiogenesis started earlier in the covered defects, and thereafter the covered wounds always had a smaller area of non-vascularised tissue than exposed wounds.

In a further study Gokoo and Burhop,[32] compared healing rates produced by Clearsite and Duoderm, on 32 full-thickness surgical wounds on the backs of four micropigs. Tracings and photographs of each wound site were made and computerised planimetry was performed to compare the rate of epithelialization. Histomorphometric measurements were also made to compare the effects of the dressing on the wounds at the cellular level.

The results indicated that wounds dressed with the gel healed 39% faster than those dressed with the hydrocolloid, and histopathology of the dermal component revealed that wounds dressed with the hydrocolloid contained larger numbers of foam cells, vacuoles and foreign body granulomas than wounds dressed with the hydrogel.

Carver *et al*.[33] compared Vigilon with two conventional dressing systems following the application of keratinocyte autografts to full thickness wounds on pigs. The dressing systems consisted of a knitted viscose fabric (Tricotex), backed with absorbent cotton gauze, or Tricotex used in conjunction with paraffin gauze and cotton gauze. No graft take was observed on any wound dressed with Tricotex at any time point, but after 16 days, 10 of 32 wounds dressed with Tricotex and paraffin gauze showed some evidence of epidermal growth.

At this point the wounds were redressed and examined at days 20 and 24 at which times a reduction in the area of tissue covered with epidermis was recorded due, at least in part, to adherence of the fragile tissue to the dressing. Wounds dressed with the hydrogel showed no evidence of an epidermal layer on day 10, but when these wounds were subsequently dressed with paraffin gauze and re-examined on day 13, islands of epidermis were visible on 11 of 16 wounds. This finding suggests that although the very wet environment beneath the gel sheet prevented the formation of a stable epidermal layer, the cells themselves had remained viable.

Fluid handling properties

In 1993, the physical properties and fluid handling characteristics of the two principal hydrogel available at that time, Geliperm and Vigilon, were compared in a laboratory-based study.[34] Geliperm, which was 2.3 mm thick and weighed 0.255 grams/cm^2, was approximately twice the weight and thickness of Vigilon, which was 1.2 mm thick, and weighed 0.133 grams/cm^2. A simple absorbency test, using deionised water at 25°C over a 96 hour period, revealed that Vigilon absorbed around 18 grams and Geliperm 54 grams per 100 cm^2. By 48 hours the uptake of water by Vigilon was substantially complete but Geliperm required substantially longer to achieve saturation.

The moisture vapour permeability of both dressings was determined using a Paddington Cup and the dynamic balance weighing method described in Chapter 7. The dressings were tested both in contact with liquid and with the cup inverted so that they were only in contact with water vapour. In order to examine the effect of temperature on permeability, the tests were also conducted at three different temperatures, 25°, 30° and 35°C. The results indicate that the permeability characteristics of the two dressings are very different. Moisture vapour passed through Vigilon at a constant rate that increased with temperature and when tested in the dry state, the dressing rapidly lost weight until it become totally dehydrated.

With Geliperm the MVTR was not constant but reduced with time. Interestingly, the rate at which the test system lost weight was initially similar in both the dry and wet state, indicating that the weight loss was actually due to the loss of water from the gel itself rather than the passage of liquid through it.

In a second study, the fluid handling properties of a number of hydrogel sheet dressings were compared using the standard Paddington Cup technique described in EN 13726-1:2002.[8] In all these tests the use of water as a test fluid instead of serum or a serum substitute, means that the absorbency values obtained for the dressings may not precisely predict the clinical performance of the dressings in this regard.

Figure 65 Effect of temperature on the permeability of hydrogel sheets

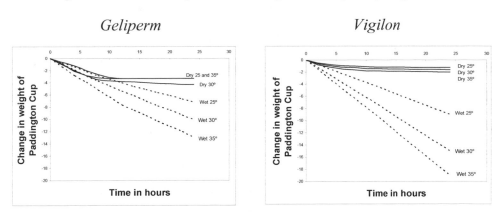

Figure 66: Effect of temperature on the fluid handling of hydrogel sheets

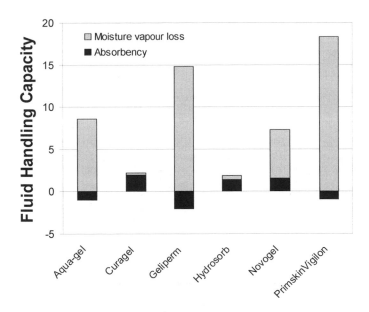

These results support those of the earlier study, for at 37°c Geliperm, together with Aqua-Gel and Primskin/Vigilon actually lost weight during the course of the test, despite the fact that that the Paddington cup contained an excess of test solution. Furthermore, compared with other wound management materials, the ability of all the products to absorb fluid was very limited, both in terms of the rate at which fluid was taken up and the total volume absorbed.

In the clinical situation, therefore, if the gels are applied to wounds that exude at a rate which exceeds the rate of uptake by the gel, pooling of fluid will occur on the wound surface, causing maceration and increasing the possibility of infection Conversely, the high MVTR of Vigilon and Geliperm in particular, means that if the dressings are applied to lightly exuding wounds, they will have a marked tendency to dry out. This will occur more quickly with Vigilon than Geliperm, but with Vigilon and similar products bearing a removable backing layer, the user has the option to leave the plastic film on the outer surface of the dressing to reduce moisture loss.

The results of these studies therefore suggests that the hydrogel sheets examined are only likely to be ideally suited to wounds which exude at a rate which is compatible with their fluid handling properties, for unlike products such as alginates, they are unable to transmit excess liquid from the wound surface into a secondary absorbent layer. Whilst it is possible to control the loss of water vapour from a gel sheet by covering it with a second semipermeable film dressing, for example, this only adds to the cost of the treatment and, in most instances, offers few advantages over the use of a film alone.

Clinical experience with hydrogel sheets

Provided that they are not allowed to dry out, hydrogels in sheet form can be applied and removed without causing pain and trauma. Once in place they are said to reduce pain and therefore have a high degree of patient acceptability and for this reason they sometimes find application in the treatment of minor burns. In appropriate cases, the dressings may be refrigerated before use, producing a cooling effect that further alleviates pain and irritation.

If the dressing is occluded, the cooling effect is transitory, lasting only until the gel warms up to body temperature, but if the outer surface of the gel is left exposed to the environment, the effect is enhanced or prolonged by evaporative cooling.[35]

As retention of a non-adhesive gel sheets can be a problem, they are sometimes used in conjunction with a piece of a self-adhesive retention material such as Mefix or Hypafix. Queen et al.[36] in a laboratory study, showed that the use of these products as secondary dressings reduced evaporative loss from the gel by 60-65%, to a more clinically appropriate level of around 4000 grams/m^2/24 hours.

Superficial cutaneous wounds

Because the ability of many of the first generation of hydrogel sheets to cope with large volumes of exudate is limited, they are best reserved for use on lightly exuding wounds. Being largely composed of water it might be supposed that they should be of value in the treatment of relatively dry epithelializing wounds or extensive superficial skin injuries provided that evaporation from the outer dressing surface could be controlled.

This was confirmed in 1982, by Mandy,[37] who recorded the use of Vigilon after 26 hair transplantations, ten dermabrasions, and 42 excisional surgeries. In this study, two of the dermabrasion patients each had half of their wound dressed with Vigilon, the other half with Adaptic, a commonly used dressing consisting of a petrolatum emulsion. For the purpose of this investigation the protective polyethylene film was only removed from the wound contact surface of Vigilon, the layer on the outer surface was left in place to reduce evaporative loss. The author reported that although Vigilon performed well in all three applications, it appeared to be most useful in situations where the epidermis was disrupted over a large area, as in the patients who had received dermabrasions. In the two patients whose wounds were dressed with two different dressings, those areas covered with Vigilon healed almost two days faster than those dressed with Adaptic, (4 - 5 *vs* 6 - 7 days). The use of the hydrogel also resulted in a noticeable relief of pain.

Fulton[38] compared Second Skin/Vigilon with the same dressing saturated with stabilised aloe vera extract following a full-face dermabrasion. One side of the subject's face was treated with the standard sheet, the other side with gel containing the extract. After 24 - 48 hours there was dramatic vasoconstriction and an accompanying reduction in oedema on the aloe-treated side. By the third to fourth day there was less exudate and crusting, and by the fifth to sixth day reepithelialization on the aloe-treated site was complete. Overall, healing was judged approximately 72 hours faster in wounds treated with the aloe extract and the author reported that the polyethylene oxide dressing provided an excellent matrix for the release of the active agent during the early part of the healing process.

Interestingly, the speed of healing resulting from the use of the standard Vigilon in this study was less impressive than that reported previously by Mandy, although it is possible that these differences could be explained by variations in dressing technique. For example, it is implied, although not specifically stated, that in this second study both layers of protective film were removed from the gel. In addition, every 12 hours the dressings were changed and 'vigorous water compresses' applied which kept the wound free of exudate.

According to Smith,[39] the introduction of hydrogels of various types revolutionised the management of skin following dermabrasion and similar procedures by accelerating healing and reducing pain. This view was supported by the results of a survey published in 1998 by Duke *et al.*,[40] which found that hydrogels sheets were used extensively both pre and post-laser resurfacing for photo damaged skin, rhytides and acne scarring.

Newman *et al.*[41] compared Second Skin/Vigilon with three other 'closed' (semipermeable) dressings in a randomized controlled trial in 40 patients who had undergone laser resurfacing of the face. They reported that although patients preferred not to continue with any of the dressings longer than necessary, usually stopping after 2-3 days, the use of all of the materials examined in the study decreased pain and reduced crust formation and pruritus compared with historical controls. There were no complications following treatment such as scarring, hyperpigmentation or prolonged erythema.

Hypertrophic scars

The moist environment provided by hydrogel sheets also may be of value in the treatment of hypertrophic scars. Ricketts *et al.*[42] compared Clearsite with a silicone gel sheet (Silastic) in the side-by-side treatment of 15 scars using both clinical and biochemical criteria. They suggested that silicone is not a necessary component of occlusive dressings used for the treatment of hypertrophic scars, and demonstrated that the hydrogel functioned by augmenting collagenolysis by enhancing the inflammatory process.

Surgical and traumatic wounds

Hydrogels have also been used in other conditions resulting in severe damage to large areas of the epidermis. In an early study, Knapp et al.[43] described the use of Geliperm following split skin grafting, suggesting that the use of the hydrogel sheet improved graft take. When the split skin sites of 23 patients were treated with Geliperm, good healing resulted in 22 cases in an average of 12.3 days.[44]

Vigilon was similarly evaluated in the treatment of 59 patients with partial or full-thickness burns, traumatic skin loss and skin graft donor sites.[45] Only one layer of protective film was removed from the hydrogel unless the wounds were exuding heavily. The dressings were initially changed every two or three days but this interval was subsequently extended to five to seven days. The authors reported that the dressing could be removed without causing pain, and that patients with partial thickness burns reported a modest reduction in discomfort when the dressing was applied. During this study hypergranulation occurred in four wounds and a similar number became infected. Although the gel was said to be useful in softening adherent eschar, it was said to be no better than standard dressings in the management of suppurating wounds and its value in promoting marginal epithelialization was also not known.

Mandy, in a second study, compared standard Vigilon with the gel containing povidone iodine.[46] Forty-five sutured surgical wounds were treated with either the standard gel or the product containing the antimicrobial agent. Three wound infections occurred in the control group but in the povidone iodine group no wound infections were recorded. The authors also reported that healing also appeared to take place more rapidly in wounds dressed with the medicated gel.

Burd[47] conducted a clinical evaluation of a sheet hydrogel dressing, Maxgel, in 50 burn-related wounds in 30 patients. The dressing was evaluated as a replacement for porcine and cadaver skin in the management of skin graft donor sites and acute partial-thickness burns, as well as a temporary dressing for excised full-thickness wounds, meshed autografts, and cultured cell applications. When used for donor sites, gauze was wrapped over the hydrogel, secured with a crepe bandage and tape and left undisturbed for ten days. Under these conditions although the gel sheet sometimes dried out, pain-free removal could be facilitated by rehydrating it with water or saline. All donor sites all healed within ten days, the normal range for the burn unit. In one patient with matched donor site wounds the dressing was compared with the alginate dressing, Kaltostat. Both dressings needed to be soaked before removal. Although slightly more difficult to apply than the calcium alginate dressing the hydrogel sheet appeared to be as effective as calcium alginate with respect to time to healing and ease of removal and was less expensive. The patient reported minimal pain with removal of both dressings. The use of the hydrogel was evaluated in 16 partial thickness wounds including a facial burn. Ten wounds were non-exuding and six exuding. In the case of the facial injury, the wound could be readily inspected through the dressing, and as the patient was unconscious and ventilated they required no retention dressing. The non-exuding wounds were all superficial partial-thickness wounds and all healed within ten days. The exuding wounds were deeper but all healed within 14 days following burn injury. In the treatment of full-thickness burns a widely meshed autograft was applied following excision and debridement and the gel was used in place of cadaver skin to prevent desiccation of the tissue in the interstices of the meshed graft. For the first few cases treated in this way, positive bacterial cultures, primarily for Pseudomonas sp., were isolated from the wound bed. This problem was overcome by the use of betadine or chlorhexidine-soaked gauze as a secondary dressing. Dressings were changed every two to three days and the wound bed remained healthy, viable, and non-infected, allowing further grafting once the first donor site wounds healed. The gel was also used with some success following the application of a suspension of cultured autologous keratinocytes cells in place of either cadaver skin or Mepitel. Symmetrical burns treated with either porcine skin or hydrogel sheets heal differently, with less inflammatory reaction and superficial scarring in the hydrogel treated wounds.

Based upon these experiences, the author concluded that despite some practical problems related to application and the lack of inherent antimicrobial activity, the sheet hydrogel represented a successful substitute for porcine and/or cadaver skin in a variety of burn and burn-related wounds.

Leg ulcers

Historically, hydrogel sheets have not proved highly successful in the treatment of exuding leg ulcers because of their inability to cope with large volumes of wound fluid but Hampton, in 2004,[48] reported how a new gel material, Actiform Cool, was used successfully for this indication following a simple uncontrolled product evaluation involving 20 wounds. Over a four-week period, two wounds healed completely, four were judged to be 90% healed and two were 80% healed. The overall average healing rate was 46% and during the study the average frequency of dressing changes reduced from 2.8 to 1.3 changes per week. Application of the dressing was found to reduce average pain scores from 8.65 to 3.75. Hampton also made reference to the pain reducing properties of Actiform Cool in a second publication in 2007,[49] and Moody in 2006 also reported a favourable outcome following the application of Actiform Cool to a longstanding painful leg ulcer.[50]

Pressure ulcers

In 1990, Biofilm, a hydrogel dressing manufactured by the Goodrich Company, was compared with Duoderm, in a randomized clinical trial involving 90 patients with 129 pressure ulcers.[51] Sixty-two wounds were treated with the hydrogel and 67 with the hydrocolloid for a maximum of 60 days. While 90% of hydrogel-treated wounds and 78% of those dressed with hydrocolloid improved during treatment, nearly twice as many of the hydrogel-treated wounds actually healed, (43% versus 24%) In addition, clinicians judged that the hydrogel dressings were easier to use, had superior fluid management capability, and demonstrated enhanced product integrity with minimal disruption to the healing wounds.

Kaya et al.[52] compared Elasto-gel with gauze soaked in povidone-iodine solution, in a prospective study involving 27 spinal-cord injury patients with a total of 49 pressure ulcers. Wounds were randomized to treatment and the primary outcome measure was the rate of wound healing calculated as cm^2 per day. Healing rates in the gel treated group were higher than those in the control group but this difference was not statistically significant. A statistically significant difference in favour of the hydrogel was detected in the number of wounds that healed in the two groups: 84% vs 54% (p = 0.04). The authors concluded that, compared with the more conservative wound management technique, the hydrogel dressing facilitated healing of pressure ulcers by promoting more rapid epithelialization.

Other wound types

The clinical performance and handling characteristics of Gel-Syte (Clearsite) were examined in a multicentre, open, non-comparative study involving 29 patients with 41 wounds.[53] Twenty patients with 28 wounds completed the study the duration of which ranged from 7 to 127 days depending upon the severity of their lesions. The authors concluded that the environment produced beneath the dressing promoted granulation and facilitated the autolytic removal of necrotic material. The dressing also appeared to have reasonable absorptive capacity, which made it suitable for application to exuding wounds.

Yamamoto et al.[54] recorded the advantages of using Clearsite following free-flap surgery, describing how the gel protected the wound from contamination whilst permitting visual assessment and Doppler examination to monitor patency of microvascular anastomoses. The disadvantages of the dressing related to its application to depressed (concave) areas and its inability to absorb exudate as well as other more conventional dressings.

Hydrogel dressings such as Clearsite and Flexderm (once distributed by Bertek Pharmaceuticals but now thought to be discontinued) were enthusiastically recommended by Cable et al.[55] for the treatment of nipple soreness and trauma associated with breast feeding, but when Elasto-gel, was compared with breast shells and lanolin cream in a randomized controlled trial involving of 42 breast-feeding women with sore nipples,[56] it was found that although both treatments were effective in reducing pain, statistically greater improvement was seen in the group using breast shells and lanolin. There were also significantly more infections in the gel dressing group, which resulted in early discontinuation of the study.

Contradictory results for the effect of hydrogel dressings on nipple infections were reported by Dodd and Chalmers[57] who comparing the use of polyurethane-based hydrophilic hydrogel pads, Maternimates, with lanolin ointment on nipple soreness experienced by lactating women in a multicentered, prospective, randomized controlled clinical trial involving 106 lactating mothers. Participants were randomized to either the lanolin ointment or the hydrogel dressings group and received instructions specific to their assignment. Subjects using the hydrogel dressing experienced less pain and discontinued treatment sooner than participants in the lanolin ointment group. Eight breast infections occurred in the lanolin treated group but none were reported by subjects using the hydrogel.

Compared with air exposure, a hydrogel dressing, in common with a hydrocolloid and semipermeable film, produced accelerated healing rates in experimentally induced partial thickness abrasions in volunteers,[58] leading the authors to conclude that 'occlusive dressings were more effective in healing than no dressing was' - a not unexpected observation given the amount of information that has been published on this subject previously.

A few studies have described the use of hydrogel sheets in the treatment of malignant wounds. Maund[59] employed Actiform Cool in the treatment of two patients with malodorous fungating wounds, and Strunk et al.[60] described the successful use of Vigilon for painful, slough-filled lesions in a patient undergoing radiotherapy for oesophageal carcinoma and concomitant corticosteroid therapy for cicatricial pemphigoid.

Small pieces of gel sheet are sometimes applied to the eyes of unconscious patients in intensive care units to keep the eyes closed and prevent them from becoming excessively dry.

In ultrasound therapy

In addition to their use as dressings for open wounds, hydrogel sheets have other potentially useful applications. Early studies with Geliperm suggested that it could be used as a coupling agent for ultrasound in the treatment of fractures,[61] and soft tissue injuries,[62] providing a sterile environment and physical protection to the skin whilst preventing problems of pin track infections. The gel sheet was moistened with saline and laid over the wound, ensuring that air bubbles were eliminated, and the transducer head was applied to the outer surface in the usual way. After treatment the gel was left in place as a dressing. Although it was suggested that wounds treated in this way healed more rapidly than usual, no attempt was made to conduct any type of controlled study to support this assertion.

The authors claimed that, under experimental conditions, Geliperm transmitted up to 95% of the incident power of the beam, but the methodology used in this early work to determine the transmission of sound energy through the gel was criticised by Klucinec et al.[63] who claimed that it did not reproduce normal clinical practice. They performed an in vitro study involving pig tissue in which they measured the amount of sound energy that could be transmitted through four different hydrogel sheets. Of the products examined, Nu-gel was found to have the greatest transmissivity (77.2%), followed by Clearsite (72%), Aquasorb Border (45.3%), and Carradress (42.8%). These differences were judged to have important implications for the effectiveness of ultrasound therapy.

The ability of 18 different dressings to transmit ultrasound for imaging purposes was investigated by compared by Kenney et al.[64] who showed that of the all the products examined the hydrogel sheet, Geliperm, was the most sonolucent; hydrocolloid dressings and dressings containing cellulose fibres were virtually opaque.

Current status of hydrogel sheet dressings

According to Corkhill *et al.*,[6] hydrogel sheet dressings appear to possess many of the properties of an ideal dressing, being flexible, non-antigenic, permeable to water vapour and metabolites but impermeable to bacteria.

Despite these theoretical benefits, the early hydrogel sheets failed to make a significant impact on mainstream clinical practice, because of their relatively poor fluid handling characteristics. Despite these deficiencies, because of their unique tactile properties, they do offer some advantages over conventional materials for specialist applications, reducing pain or discomfort in certain types of problem wounds.

More recently, however, developments in the hydrogel field may cause the role of hydrogel sheets to be reassessed, as products are now available with greatly enhanced absorbency which also offer other potential benefits by acting at a biochemical or molecular level within a healing wound.

AMORPHOUS HYDROGEL DRESSINGS

Commercial preparations

Amorphous hydrogel dressings were first introduced into wound management in the mid 1980s since which time there has been a virtual explosion in the number of products available. Although generally similar in appearance, these vary significantly in composition, and in many instances information on the constituents of the products concerned is hard to find, which makes informed choice difficult if not impossible.

The first amorphous hydrogel dressing to be launched was Scherisorb, initially marketed by Schering, but later purchased by Smith and Nephew. It consisted of a colourless to pale yellow, transparent, aqueous gel, based upon chemically modified cornstarch onto which hydrophilic side-chains had been grafted. These side-chains formed a T-shape with the basic starch molecules, for which reason the final structure was described as a graft T co-polymer. The dressing, which was presented in aluminium laminate sachets, contained 2% co-polymer, 78% water and 20% propylene glycol as a preservative and humectant.

When first produced, Scherisorb did not contain propylene glycol, and as a result it had to be changed daily as it showed a marked tendency to dry out or produce unpleasant odours. After reformulation, however, the gel could be left in position for up to three days with no apparent adverse effects upon wound healing.[65]

Soon after its acquisition by Smith and Nephew, Scherisorb gel was renamed Intrasite, and shortly after, in about 1993, it was reformulated, when the starch co-polymer was replaced by 3% carboxymethylcellulose.

Examples of commercially produced amorphous hydrogels are provided below, together with basic information on their composition where this information has been disclosed by the manufacturer.

- ActivHeal Hydrogel, contains 85% water and is claimed to be an effective moisture donating gel
- Aquaform, contains 3.5% of a modified starch co-polymer together with propylene glycol (20%) and water
- Askina Gel, contains a modified starch polymer
- Carrasyn Gel, contains acemannan, an extract of *aloe vera* claimed to possess beneficial wound healing properties
- Citrugel, contains carboxymethylcellulose and a high Grade modified pectin
- Curafil Gel, a clear amorphous hydrogel containing a preservative
- Cutimed Gel, a clear amorphous hydrogel, preservative free
- Flexigran Gel a clear colourless gel contains starch copolymer, glycerol, preservatives and water
- Gentell Hydrogel contains aloe vera extract
- Granugel, contains carboxymethylcellulose together with pectin, which is claimed to impart proteolytic activity to the dressing
- Hydrosorb Gel, a clear gel presented in a syringe
- Hypergel, a clear gel containing xanthan gum as a thickening agent together with 20% sodium chloride, which makes the gel hypertonic, a property that is claimed by the manufacturer to enhance its wound debridement properties
- Normlgel, contains xantham gum and 0.9% sodium chloride
- Nu-gel, contains 3% sodium alginate 70% water
- Purilon gel, contains carboxymethylcellulose and calcium alginate
- Solosite, a clear hydrogel made from water swellable polymers
- Sterigel, made from chemically modified starch (now discontinued)
- Skintegrity, contains aloes extract
- Suprasorb, clear gel presented in a syringe
- Tegagel, a preservative-free clear gel
- Wound'dres, contains collagen, panthenol, allantoin, tetra sodium EDTA, carbomer, citric acid, triethanolamine, methylparaben, imidazolidinyl urea, propylparabens

A number of companies have also introduced dressings consisting of a hydrogel impregnated into some form of open fabric, typically a nonwoven swab. This is said to facilitate application of the gel to the surface of large open wounds such as pressure ulcers or malignant wounds and reduce the problem of the gel being displaced from the surface of relatively shallow wounds, such as heels, when subjected to pressure or movement. Impregnated gauze dressings are also claimed to be useful for packing deep cavity wounds.

Examples include:

- Carragauze (contains acemannan from *Aloe vera*)
- Curafil
- Cutimed Sorbact Gel)
- Gentell Hydrogel (contains Aloe extract)
- Hydrosorb
- Intrasite Conformable
- Normlgel Impregnated Gauze
- Skintegrity

Animal studies

Despite the widespread use of hydrogel dressings, few papers have been published that record the results of animal studies involving these materials.

In one of the few published papers, Ågren[66] compared the effect of three amorphous hydrogels and a semipermeable film dressing (Tegaderm) on the healing of experimental wounds in pigs. The test materials were Intrasite gel, a poloxamer gel containing 3% hydrogen peroxide and 'Exgel' an experimental formulation produced by Coloplast (assumed to be Purilon), which consisted of sodium carboxymethylcellulose (NaCMC), calcium alginate and water.

A total of twelve wounds were treated with 2.0 mL of each type of hydrogel and covered with Tegaderm. Control wounds were dressed with Tegaderm alone. After 24 hours the wounds were photographed, cleansed and redressed with the same hydrogels.

Sixty-six hours after wounding the animals were killed and formalin-fixed, paraffin-embedded sections of the wounds were haematoxylin-eosin-stained and assessed morphometrically for epithelium coverage in a blinded fashion. The 66-hour point was chosen because by this time, such wounds when dressed with occlusive dressings are usually 50% covered with new epithelium. The authors reported that macroscopic examination of the wounds revealed that at 24 and 66 hours the Exgel remain virtually intact in contrast to the other hydrogels, which had dissolved. Exgel-dressed wounds had significantly increased epithelial coverage compared with the other treatments, 77.5% *vs* 55.4% for Intrasite ($p < 0.05$) and 62.0% for the Tegaderm control.

In vitro experiments performed upon the same formulations, showed that although Exgel, Polyoxamer gel, Intrasite and a corresponding concentration of propylene glycol, reduced keratinocyte proliferation, the inhibitory effect of Exgel was less than that of the other products examined. In a further study Exgel reduced the chemotactic effects of porcine wound fluid upon keratinocytes leading the authors to suggest that the gel sequesters these bioactive molecules but subsequently releases them at a rate that promotes epithelial migration *in vivo*. It should be noted, however, that Exgel contained alginate, a molecule that has been claimed by some to have a stimulatory effect upon wound healing.[67]

Fluid handling properties

As previously suggested, it is assumed that amorphous hydrogels promote debridement by increasing the moisture content of dead tissue or slough. This may be achieved either by reducing the loss of water vapour from the affected area, or by applying or donating water directly to the area by the application of a suitable dressing. Given the variation in the composition of the various hydrogels identified above, it is not unreasonable to assume that the ability of these products to donate or absorb liquid to or from a wound will also vary.

As previously In order to test this hypothesis, a simple test system was devised in which the material under examination was placed in contact with a series of gelatin gels of varying strength, representing dry wounds, and a series of agar gels representing moist or exuding wounds.[68] By measuring either the change in weight of the test sample or the gel to which it was applied, it is possible to measure how much liquid is donated or absorbed by a known weight of hydrogel. Using this technique, the fluid absorbing and donating properties of a number of hydrogel dressings were compared previously.[69-70]

The method was gradually refined and eventually became adopted as a British and European standard.[8] In final version of this test method, multiple 10 ± 0.1 gram samples of each gel are applied in turn to 10 ± 0.1 grams of test substrate consisting of 35% gelatin or 2% agar in modified 50/60 mL syringes from which the nozzle ends have been removed. The open ends of the cut off syringes are covered with an impermeable membrane to prevent evaporative loss and allowed to stand in a controlled environment for 48 hours. Prior to application of the test sample the syringes containing the agar or gelatin are weighed and reweighed again after 48 hours when the test sample is removed. From these values the percentage change in the weight of each gel sample can be calculated.

The results of a previously unpublished study[71] using the standard method to compare the performance of nine hydrogel dressings are shown in Figure 67 and Figure 68. In these figures the results represent the mean of five determinations, and the error bars the standard deviation in each case.

Figure 67: Percentage change in weight of samples applied to 2% agar

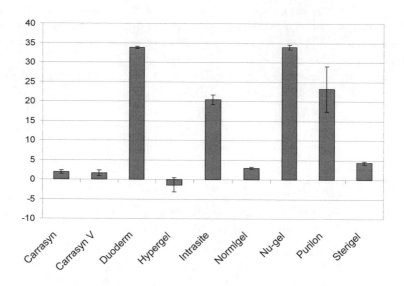

Figure 68: Percentage change in weight of samples applied to 35% gelatin

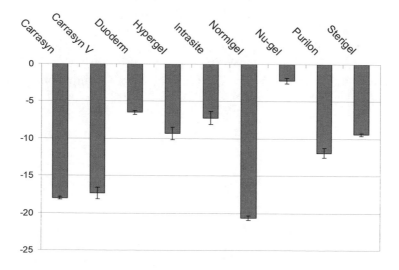

These results indicate that, as anticipated, differences exist in the performance of the various gels, which could have significant clinical implications. All of the products tested donated liquid to the relatively dry gelatin substrate and these therefore might reasonably be expected to facilitate rehydration of necrotic or sloughy tissue although perhaps at varying rates. Even products that donated relatively little fluid would, it is assumed, prevent further evaporative loss from a wound and thus increase the overall moisture content of the dead tissue.

The variation in the ability of the gels to take up fluid from the agar substrate may be rather more significant. It seems likely that when applied to moist or exuding wounds, products that have the greatest affinity for liquid in this test system should be capable of absorbing exudate thereby reducing the likelihood of maceration of periwound skin.

The aqueous nature of hydrogels suggests that they could usefully be employed as carriers for topical medicaments such as metronidazole powder in the treatment of fungating wounds and other malodorous lesions.[72] In a laboratory-based study the antimicrobial activity of Scherisorb gel containing 0.8% metronidazole was compared with Metrotop, a commercially available formulation of the same drug. When used systemically, metronidazole is indicated specifically for the treatment of anaerobic infections, but it was found that at the concentration used in the gel, metronidazole was also active against a range of aerobic microorganisms.[73]

As hydrogels are sometimes used to soften up necrotic tissue prior to the application of sterile maggots, a laboratory-based study was undertaken to compare the effects of different hydrogel residues on maggot survival and development. This revealed some interesting difference between the products most important of which was the fact that the presence of propylene glycol greatly inhibits maggot growth.[74] Somewhat bizarrely this finding subsequently caused the manufacturers of Purilon, the only gel examined at that time that did not contain propylene glycol, to describe their product as 'maggot friendly'.

Clinical experience with amorphous hydrogels

A key advantage of the amorphous hydrogels is that they may be introduced into narrow wounds or sinuses using an applicator tip, quill or syringe but perhaps more importantly, they can also be easily removed from such a wound by irrigation. Scherisorb gel was originally introduced as treatment for exuding wounds such as leg ulcers, but practical experience with the product soon revealed that the dressing was not well suited to this application as the gel rapidly decreased in viscosity and was thus lost from the wound. It was observed, however, that the gel was of value in the treatment of relatively dry wounds, particularly those covered with slough or black necrotic tissue that required debridement. It was therefore proposed that the gel promoted rehydration of dead tissue, and thus facilitated the normal autolytic processes that take place at the interface between this necrotic layer and the healthy tissue beneath.[75]

Numerous papers have since been published that describe the successful use of hydrogels to facilitate debridement in a variety of wound types and this has become the principal indication for these products, replacing solutions such as Eusol or hydrogen peroxide for this application.

Early publications described the use of Intrasite gel in sternal wounds,[76] a large infected wound following a radical vulvectomy,[77] multiple necrotic wounds on an arm,[78] an infected amputation wound,[79] pressure ulcers,[80] three surgical wounds,[81] Fournier's gangrene,[82] extensive areas of necrotic tissue on the abdomen of a baby,[83] necrotic wounds on the limbs of a infant suffering from homozygous protein C deficiency,[84] (a rare condition that affects the clotting cascade causing extensive tissue damage), and a degloving injury of the leg.[85]

Later publications described the use of an alternative hydrogel, Aquaform, in the treatment of a variety of wound types including three pressure ulcers and two fungating breast wounds.[86-88]

In 1987 Scherisorb was used to treat extravasation injuries in neonates,[89] a condition that can result in severe scaring or loss of function if managed inappropriately. The gel was applied liberally to the affected and the entire area enclosed in a sterile plastic bag, specially shaped to form a boot or glove. It was shown that the treatment offered a number of significant advantages over more traditional technique being painless to apply and remove, and - being transparent - permitting examination of the wound at all times. The high moisture content of the gel meant that dehydration and further loss of viable tissue was prevented, resulting in a healed wound with a highly acceptable cosmetic appearance. This technique, has since been widely adopted, using a number of different types of amorphous gels and is now regarded as a standard treatment for this condition.[90-91]

A similar approach was subsequently used with advantage in the treatment of necrotic lesions associated with meningococcal septicaemia.[92] It is in situations such as this, when the gels are applied inside plastic bags or beneath relatively impermeable plastic films, that their ability to promote rehydration without inducing maceration becomes important.

The first published clinical trial involving an amorphous hydrogel, compared the healing rates of leg ulcers dressed with Scherisorb with those of similar wounds dressed with the iodine-containing xerogel, Iodosorb.[93] This trial, which involved 98 patients, was carried out entirely in the community. No significant differences were detected between the two therapies in terms of healing rates, odour formation, or granulation tissue production. The authors concluded that, although an acceptable healing rate was achieved with both materials, Iodosorb was significantly more expensive in use. Furthermore, the presence of iodine in Iodosorb (as an antiseptic) did not appear to enhance the rate of healing.

A number of clinical studies have also been published that describe the use of hydrogels as wound debriding agents. The first of these, published in 1993, compared the original formulation of Intrasite gel (Scherisorb) with Debrisan paste in the management of sloughy pressure ulcers.[94] Forty patients with Grade III or Grade IV pressure ulcers containing significant amounts of slough were admitted to the study and randomized to treatment using a computer generated code. After 14 days treatment, eight wounds dressed with Intrasite and one dressed with Debrisan paste were fully cleansed, a statistically significant difference. During the next 14 days a further four wounds in the Debrisan paste group became free of slough, but there was no change in the number of cleansed wounds in the Intrasite group.

The eight wounds that were cleansed with Intrasite took an average of 11 days but the five wounds dressed with the paste took an average of 18.2 days. Overall 12 of 20 wounds (60%) dressed with paste and 16 of 19 wounds (85%) dressed with gel were judged to have improved during the course of the study. Leakage of exudate was reported with 18 of the 19 wounds dressed with gel and 10 of the 20 wounds dressed with paste, which was reflected in the mean interval between dressing changes (1.6 vs 1.9 days for gel and paste respectively), a difference that just failed to achieve statistical significance. Financial benefits also resulted from the use of the gel dressing. The results of this investigation suggested that a gel that contained 78% water was more effective at promoting debridement that the paste which contains 5.5% water.

In 1995 Flanagan[95] reported the results of a multicentre, prospective, non-comparative trial designed to assess the efficacy of the change in the formulation of Intrasite. Patients were considered eligible for inclusion if they presented with a wound of any aetiology 30% of the surface of which was covered with non-viable tissue. Patients were monitored for 21 days, or until the wounds were fully cleansed. Data from 47 patients were available for analysis and in each case the efficacy of the dressing was determined as the percentage reduction of non-viable tissue. A total of ten wounds (21%) were fully cleansed during the course of the study and the median percentage reduction in non-viable tissue at seven, 14 and 21 days was 14%, 41% and 75% respectively.

This was followed by a further, more formal investigation,[96] which took the form of a multicentre, parallel group, prospective randomized clinical trial involving 135 patients with pressure ulcers in which Intrasite gel was compared with Debrisan paste. As before, patients were monitored for 21 days or until the wounds were fully cleansed, and the primary outcome measure was the percentage reduction in the area of non-viable tissue during the 21-day study period. The median percentage reduction in the area of non-viable tissue at each of the weekly assessment points was 33%, 53% and 74% for Intrasite compared with 25%, 48%, and 62% for Debrisan paste but these differences were not statistically significant. A statistically significant difference was recorded for the two groups in the median reduction in wound area after 21 days treatment, 35% for the Intrasite group compared with 7% for the Debrisan paste group leading the authors to suggest that the amorphous gel provided an environment that facilitates healing.

Intrasite gel was compared with a second amorphous hydrogel, Sterigel, in a clinical trial reported by Bale et al.[97] Fifty patients with necrotic pressure ulcers, drawn from both the hospital and community setting, were randomized to treatment with the two primary dressings. A perforated plastic film dressing, Telfa, and a semipermeable polyurethane film were used as secondary dressings in both groups.

Dressings were replaced daily for the entire treatment period of 28 days and treatment was judged to be successful when 80% of the wound area was covered with granulation tissue and no necrotic tissue remained, although this end point was not defined prior to commencement of the study. Photographs of the wounds were taken at intervals, which were sent for computer analysis by an operator who was unaware of the treatment provided.

Complete debridement was achieved in 14 of the 21 patients treated with Sterigel who completed the study, compared with nine of the 17 patients treated with Intrasite. These differences were not statistically significant. No differences were detected between the treatment groups in terms of pain, odour production, or maceration of the surrounding skin.

Martin et al.[98] compared the wound cleansing properties of an enzymatic debriding agent, Varidase, (streptokinase and streptodornase) dispersed in a hydrogel (KY Jelly) with the hydrogel alone in the debridement of Grade IV pressure sores. Seventeen subjects with a total of 21 sores were studied, 11 of which were randomized to treatment with the enzyme. Somewhat unexpectedly, mean treatment times for patients in the hydrogel-only group were shorter that those treated with the enzyme/hydrogel combination (8.1 ± 1.8 vs 11.8 ± 2.9 days) but this difference did not achieve statistical significance. Nevertheless, the results suggest that the use of hydrogel alone may be a cost-effective alternative to the use of streptokinase/streptodornase and hydrogel in the treatment of these wounds.

Elta Hydrovase is an amorphous hydrogel that contains a combination of endopeptidase enzymes. In addition to the normal properties of hydrogels, the inclusion of the enzymes is claimed to facilitate the wound healing process by stimulating certain functions of macrophages and eosinophils. The gel possesses anti-bradykinin and anti-inflammatory activity, and it has been suggested that it in some way interacts with the immune system and cytokine pathways to enhance healing.

Parnell et al.[99] undertook a small study to evaluate the gel in the treatment of pressure ulcers in a 12-week prospective preliminary study involving ten nursing home patients with Stage II or III ulcers that had failed to respond to previous treatments. The study was uncontrolled but the healing rates achieved were said to be improved compared with those exhibited by the same wounds prior to inclusion in the trial. No adverse events associated with the product were reported and based upon their observations the authors concluded that additional studies were warranted to investigate the possible contribution of endopeptidase enzymes to wound healing .

The effect upon wound healing of an unnamed amorphous hydrogel dressing produced by Coloplast, assumed to be Purilon, was examined by Matzen et al.,[100] who compared it with a conventional treatment (wet saline compress) on the healing time of 32 pressure ulcers, represented by a reduction in wound volume, determined by measuring the amount of water required to fill the cavity. All patients were followed for 12 weeks or until the ulcer had healed. Relative volumes of hydrogel-dressed wounds at the end of the study period were significantly less than those of saline treated wounds, 26% vs 64% respectively ($p < 0.02$). The saline-treated wounds also required more frequent debridement.

In a small study involving 17 evaluable patients,[101] the cost of debriding wounds containing at least 75% dry adherent eschar with Hypergel, covered with a polyurethane film, were compared with those of treating similar wounds with saline moistened gauze, the standard wet-to-dry technique. Wounds were dressed twice daily for four weeks or until 50% of eschar was removed (the transition point). The wounds of all nine patients dressed with the hydrogel reached the transition point in an average of 10.9 days, but only three wounds dressed with the saline gauze reached this point by the end of four weeks. Two wounds still required further treatment and two were removed from the study because of infection. In a second publication, the authors compared the treatment costs involved during this study and found that although the daily cost of treatment with the hydrogel was slightly greater than that of the saline gauze, it was much more cost-effective overall. They concluded that the choice of treatment should be dictated jointly by cost and the time taken to achieve the desired effect for neither individual cost nor daily cost of a material may necessarily dictate overall cost-effectiveness.[102]

Hydrogel dressings are very widely used and well tolerated by patients, rarely causing any adverse effects. The most common problem tends to be maceration of the periwound skin, which can occur if the dressings are left in place too long on heavily exuding wounds. There is also a possibility that propylene glycol, which is present in many amorphous hydrogels, may cause skin reactions in some patients although this problem is not commonly encountered in clinical practice. Nevertheless, in one study,[103] when 36 patients with chronic venous insufficiency were patch tested, 3 (8.3%) were found to be sensitive to Intrasite and this was shown to be due to the presence of propylene glycol.

Like the hydrogel sheet dressings, amorphous hydrogels are sometimes used for the treatment or prevention of radiation-induced skin lesions. In a laboratory-based study, Roberts and Travis compared severity of radiation-induced acute skin reactions in mice following the application of two commercial preparations consisting of a 'personal lubricating gel' and a 'healing ointment' with Carrasyn Gel with acemannan extract.[104]

To determine the optimum time for the application of each gel, it was applied beginning on day -7, 0, or +7 relative to the day of irradiation, and application was continued for one, two, three, four, or five weeks thereafter. The average peak skin reactions of the wounds dressed with the aloe extract were reduced compared with those of the untreated mice but the average peak skin reactions for mice treated with personal lubricating jelly or healing ointment were similar to irradiated control values. The greatest benefit resulted from applying the gel immediately after irradiation and continuing treatment for at least two weeks. No benefit was noted if gel was applied only before irradiation or if treatment was commenced one week after irradiation.

When Carrasyn gel was subsequently compared with moist saline gauze in 30 patients with pressure sores, no difference between the two therapies was detected in wound healing rates.[105]

Macmillan et al.[106] in a randomized controlled clinical trial, compared the hydrogel dressing, Intrasite covered with a simple knitted viscose dressing, Tricotex, with Tricotex alone on the time to healing of moist desquamation after radiotherapy to the head-and-neck, breast, or anorectal areas. A total of 357 patients were randomized to treatment prior to radiotherapy and instructed to use their dressings from the onset of moist desquamation, if it occurred. Of the 357 patients, 100 (28%) developed moist desquamation. In the patients assigned to gel dressings, the time to healing was significantly prolonged and no evidence was found that gel dressings had a significant impact on subjectively reported skin symptoms. The authors concluded that based upon the results of their study the routine use of hydrogels in the care of patients with moist desquamation cannot be supported - a finding that might have been predicted from the animal studies described by Macmillan et al.[106]

Gollins et al.[107] compared a hydrogel dressing with gentian violet for radiotherapy-induced moist desquamation in a prospective randomized trial in 30 patients undergoing radiotherapy to the breast or head and neck region, who had developed moist desquamation in the radiotherapy field. Patients were randomized to treatment with 0.5% aqueous gentian violet (GV) (n = 16) or the hydrogel dressing (n = 14). The area of desquamation was regularly measured until healing or withdrawal from the study. The speed of healing with the hydrogel was shown to be statistically much greater than with GV. (The median time to healing for hydrogel treated areas was 12 days but this had not been achieved following GV treatment in 30 days). Ten of 16 patients treated with GV withdrew from the study, due to stinging in five, and failure to heal in five others compared with two of the 14 treated with hydrogel. Hydrogel dressings were therefore judged to be more likely to heal radiotherapy-induced moist desquamation and be better tolerated than GV.

XEROGELS

Commercial preparations

Xerogels be produced in the form of sheets, granules, fibres, beads, flakes and pastes which, when fully rehydrated, form either amorphous gels or products with a defined structure. The first xerogels to be widely used in wound management were the fibrous alginate dressing, but other examples include the polysaccharide bead dressings Debrisan and Iodosorb, and products such as Comfeel Powder and Granuflex granules (now discontinued).

A further example of a xerogel is Bard Absorption Dressing (BAD), now thought to be discontinued, a base-hydrolyzed polysaccharide prepared from cornstarch which is presented in the form of dry flakes that have to be reconstituted prior to use by the addition of five parts by weight of water to one part of powder. The reconstituted gel, which has been described as having the consistency of finely crushed ice, does not flow but is easily moldable and in this condition is, arguably, one of the first amorphous hydrogel dressings. When placed upon a wound or brought into contact with liquid, the gel absorbs more fluid, further increasing in volume as it does so.

Results of clinical studies

After some initial veterinary studies in which the gel was used to treat some 40 skin ulcers in dogs and horses, clinical trials were undertaken on 148 human patients, all of whom suffered from pressure ulcers or venous ulcers. It was reported that, without exception, all wounds treated in this way responded favourably to the treatment. Interestingly, however, the authors stressed that BAD was not a substitute for surgical debridement, stating necrotic tissue was always removed prior to the application of the gel.[108]

Montgomery[109] described how a patient with a huge wound that extended from the perineum and left groin down to the medial and lateral aspects of the left knee, was treated daily with about 140 grams of BAD. After a week of this therapy the patient suffered an acute episode of hyperkalaemia. Subsequent investigations revealed that the gel contained a significant amount of potassium, and it was proposed that this could have been at least partially responsible for the patient's condition. When blood levels of

30 other patients treated with BAD were monitored, raised potassium levels were recorded in approximately one half of those examined These findings led the author to propose that that the composition of all dressings should be declared on the literature or packaging, and information on potential side effects and advice on maximum usage should also be provided by the manufacturer. Regrettably, this recommendation has been ignored and the composition of many of the products on the market remains unknown.

The suggestion that Bard Absorption Dressing had been responsible for the episode of hyperkalaemia, was vigorously contested by Jeter *et al.*[110] who suggested that it was more likely to be caused by other factors such as reduced renal function or an electrolyte shift associated with tissue destruction. They supported their view of the safety of the gel by describing their experience with more than 40 patients, including five with problem wounds, which comprised pressure ulcers, a dehisced abdominal wound, and a necrotic lesion following a Pirogoff amputation of the foot. They reported that the gel cleansed the wounds, encouraged the formation of granulation tissue, reduced wound odour, and produced dramatic wound healing in some instances, concluding that the benefits of the treatment far outweighed any known risks. As far as is known, however, these authors did not measured blood potassium levels in patients undergoing treatment and were therefore not in a position to state categorically that this problem would not occur following the repeated application of very large amounts of gel to extensive wounds on a daily basis. Further published case studies described the use of Bard Absorption Dressing in the management of a large abdominal wound[111] and a sternal wound.[112]

The possibility that BAD could exert some form of biochemical effect on the wound healing process was investigated by Chung *et al.*[113] Using a nitroblue tetrazolium reduction assay, they demonstrated that, in common with other products such as Granuflex and Comfeel powder, Bard Absorption Dressing displayed superoxide scavenging activity. They proposed that, in addition to the dressing providing a moist wound-healing environment, this activity might contribute to the establishment and maintenance of the reducing environment necessary for energy production and hence cell division, thus enhancing the gel's ability to promote a favourable wound healing environment.

REFERENCES

1. Makins M, editor. *Collins English Dictionary*. Third ed. Glasgow: Harper Collins, 1995.
2. Turner TD, Schmidt RJ, Harding KG, editors. Xerogel dressings - an overview. Advances in Wound Care; 1985; Cardiff. John Wiley.
3. Peppas NA, Mikos AG. Preparation methods and structure of hydrogels. In: Peppas NA, editor. *Hydrogels in medicine and pharmacy,*. Florida: CRC Press, 1986.
4. Rosiak JM. *Radiation formation of hydrogels for biomedical applications.* Institute of Applied Radiation Chemistry, Technical University of Lodz, 2002 http://www.mitr.p.lodz.pl/biomat/raport/book_index.html
5. Hoffman AS. Hydrogels for biomedical applications. *Ann N Y Acad Sci* 2001;**944**:62-73.

6. Corkhill PH, Hamilton CJ, Tighe BJ. Synthetic hydrogels. VI. Hydrogel composites as wound dressings and implant materials. *Biomaterials* 1989;**10**(1):3-10.
7. Williams D. Hydrogels: Are they keeping their heads above water. *Medical Device Technology*, 1995:8-11.
8. BS EN 13726-1:2002 Test methods for primary wound dressings - Part 1: Aspects of absorbency. 2002.
9. Wichterle O, Lim D. Hydrophilic gels for biological use. *Nature* 1960;**185**:117-118.
10. Yannas IV, Lee E, Orgill DP, Skrabut EM, Murphy GF. Synthesis and characterization of a model extracellular matrix that induces partial regeneration of adult mammalian skin. *Proc Natl Acad Sci U S A* 1989;**86**(3):933-7.
11. Suzuki Y, Tanihara M, Nishimura Y, Suzuki K, Kakimaru Y, Shimizu Y. A novel wound dressing with an antibiotic delivery system stimulated by microbial infection. *Asaio J* 1997;**43**(5):M854-7.
12. Eisenbud D, Hunter H, Kessler L, Zulkowski K. Hydrogel wound dressings: where do we stand in 2003? *Ostomy Wound Manage* 2003;**49**(10):52-7.
13. Smetana K, Jr., Vacik J, Souckova D, Krcova Z, Sulc J. The influence of hydrogel functional groups on cell behavior. *J Biomed Mater Res* 1990;**24**(4):463-70.
14. Kirker KR, Luo Y, Nielson JH, Shelby J, Prestwich GD. Glycosaminoglycan hydrogel films as bio-interactive dressings for wound healing. *Biomaterials* 2002;**23**(17):3661-71.
15. Kirker KR, Luo Y, Morris SE, Shelby J, Prestwich GD. Glycosaminoglycan hydrogels as supplemental wound dressings for donor sites. *J Burn Care Rehabil* 2004;**25**(3):276-86.
16. Vachon DJ, Yager DR. Novel sulfonated hydrogel composite with the ability to inhibit proteases and bacterial growth. *J Biomed Mater Res A* 2006;**76**(1):35-43.
17. Wokalek H. Theoretical aspects and clinical experience on a new hydrogel wound dressing material,. In: Woods HF, Cottier D, editors. *Geliperm: A Clear Advance in Wound Healing, Proceedings of a Conference,.* Oxford, 1983:3-33.
18. Gilbert EC, Schenk WN. Hydrogel dressings 1: Physical attributes of a new absorbent wound dressing with unique fluid management characteristics. *Wounds* 1989;**1**:198-208.
19. Butcher G, Woods HF. Geliperm as a molecular carrier. In: Woods HF, Cottier D, editors. *Geliperm: A Clear Advance in Wound Healing, Proceedings of a Conference,.* Oxford, 1983:77-87.
20. Kickhöfen B, Wokalek H, Scheel D, Ruh H. Chemical and physical properties of a hydrogel wound dressing. *Biomaterials* 1986;**7**(1):67-72.
21. Taylor DEM, Penhallow J. Biotolerance of Geliperm: a six-week implantation study in the rat. In: Woods HF, Cottier D, editors. *Geliperm: A Clear Advance in Wound Healing, Proceedings of a Conference.* Oxford, 1983:63-75.
22. Burgos H. Incorporation and release of placental growth factors in synthetic medical dressings. *Clin. Mat* 1987;**2**:133-139.
23. Barzokas CA. Microbiological studies on Geliperm. In: Woods HF, Cottier D, editors. *Geliperm: A Clear Advance in Wound Healing, Proceedings of a Conference,.* Oxford, 1983:39-47.
24. Mertz PM, Marshall DA, Eaglstein WH. Occlusive wound dressings to prevent bacterial invasion and wound infection. *J Am Acad Dermatol* 1985;**12**(4):662-8.
25. Marshall DA, Mertz PM, Eaglstein WH. Occlusive dressings. Does dressing type influence the growth of common bacterial pathogens? *Arch Surg* 1990;**125**(9):1136-9.
26. Leaper DJ, Brennan SS, Simpson RA, Foster ME. Experimental infection and hydrogel dressings. *J Hosp Infect* 1984;**5 Suppl A**:69-73.

27. Brennan SS. Infection and healing under hydrogel occlusive dressings. In: Woods HF, Cottier D, editors. *Geliperm: A Clear Advance in Wound Healing, Proceedings of a Conference,*. Oxford, 1983:49-62.
28. Mertz PM, Marshall DA, Kuglar MA. Povidone-iodine in polyethylene oxide hydrogel dressing. Effect on multiplication of Staphylococcus aureus in partial-thickness wounds. *Arch Dermatol* 1986;**122**(10):1133-8.
29. Oliveria-Gandia M, Davis SC, Mertz PM. Can occlusive dressing composition influence proliferation of bacterial wound pathogens. *Wounds; A compendium of clinical research and practice* 1998;**10**(1):4-11.
30. Geronemus RG, Robins P. The effect of two new dressings on epidermal wound healing. *J. derm. Surg. Oncol.* 1982;**8**:850-852.
31. Brennan SS, Foster ME, Leaper DJ. A study of microangioneogenesis in wounds healing by secondary intention. *Microcirc Endothelium Lymphatics* 1984;**1**(6):657-69.
32. Gokoo C, Burhop K. A comparative study of wound dressings on full-thickness wounds in micropigs. *Decubitus* 1993;**6**(5):42-3, 46, 48 passim.
33. Carver N, Navsaria HA, Green CJ, Leigh IM. The effect of backing materials on keratinocyte autograft take. *Br J Plast Surg* 1993;**46**(3):228-34.
34. Thomas S. Examining the properties and uses of two hydrogel sheet dressings. *Journal of Wound Care* 1993;**2**(3):176-179.
35. Coats TJ, Edwards C, Newton R, Staun E. The effect of gel burns dressings on skin temperature. *Emerg Med J* 2002;**19**(3):224-5.
36. Queen D, Evans JH, Gaylor JD, Courtney JM, Reid WH. The physical effects of an adhesive dressing top layer on burn wound dressings. *Burns Incl Therm Inj* 1986;**12**(5):351-6.
37. Mandy SH. A new primary wound dressing made of polyethylene oxide gel. *J Dermatol Surg Oncol* 1983;**9**(2):153-5.
38. Fulton JE, Jr. The stimulation of postdermabrasion wound healing with stabilized aloe vera gel-polyethylene oxide dressing. *J Dermatol Surg Oncol* 1990;**16**(5):460-7.
39. Smith R. Dermabrasion. Is it an option? *Aust Fam Physician* 1997;**26**(9):1041-4.
40. Duke D, Grevelink JM. Care before and after laser skin resurfacing. A survey and review of the literature. *Dermatol Surg* 1998;**24**(2):201-6.
41. Newman JP, Koch RJ, Goode RL. Closed dressings after laser skin resurfacing. *Arch Otolaryngol Head Neck Surg* 1998;**124**(7):751-7.
42. Ricketts CH, Martin L, Faria DT, Saed GM, Fivenson DP. Cytokine mRNA changes during the treatment of hypertrophic scars with silicone and nonsilicone gel dressings. *Dermatol Surg* 1996;**22**(11):955-9.
43. Knapp U, Rahn HD, Schauwecker F. Clinical experiences with a new gel-like wound dressing after skin transplantation. *Aktuelle Traumatol* 1984;**14**(6):275-81.
44. Sattler G, Hagedorn M. Wound management with split skin flaps--Donor sites. Covering with the moist gel Geliperm. *Fortschr Med* 1990;**108**(5):94-6.
45. Yates DW, Hadfield JM. Clinical experience with a new hydrogel wound dressing. *Injury* 1984;**16**(1):23-4.
46. Mandy SH. Evaluation of a new povidone-iodine-impregnated polyethylene oxide gel occlusive dressing. *J Am Acad Dermatol* 1985;**13**(4):655-9.
47. Burd A. Evaluating the use of hydrogel sheet dressings in comprehensive burn wound care. *Ostomy Wound Manage* 2007;**53**(3):52-62.
48. Hampton S. A small study in healing rates and symptom control using a new sheet hydrogel dressing. *J Wound Care* 2004;**13**(7):297-300.
49. Hampton S. A focus on ActiFormCool in the reduction of pain in wounds. *Br J Community Nurs* 2007;**12**(9):S37-42.

50. Moody A. Use of a hydrogel dressing for management of a painful leg ulcer. *Br J Community Nurs* 2006;**11**(6):S12, S14, S16-7.

51. Darkovich SL, Brown-Etris M, Spencer M. Biofilm hydrogel dressing: a clinical evaluation in the treatment of pressure sores. *Ostomy Wound Manage* 1990;**29**:47-60.

52. Kaya AZ, Turani N, Akyuz M. The effectiveness of a hydrogel dressing compared with standard management of pressure ulcers. *J Wound Care* 2005;**14**(1):42-4.

53. Fowler E, Papen JC. A new hydrogel wound dressing for the treatment of open wounds. Gel-Syte wound care dressing evaluation see comments. *Ostomy Wound Manage* 1991;**37**:39-45.

54. Yamamoto Y, Minakawa H, Yoshida T. A transparent dressing in free-flap surgery. *J Reconstr Microsurg* 1994;**10**(4):235-6.

55. Cable B, Stewart M, Davis J. Nipple wound care: a new approach to an old problem. *J Hum Lact* 1997;**13**(4):313-8.

56. Brent N, Rudy SJ, Redd B, Rudy TE, Roth LA. Sore nipples in breast-feeding women: a clinical trial of wound dressings vs conventional care. *Arch Pediatr Adolesc Med* 1998;**152**(11):1077-82.

57. Dodd V, Chalmers C. Comparing the use of hydrogel dressings to lanolin ointment with lactating mothers. *J Obstet Gynecol Neonatal Nurs* 2003;**32**(4):486-94.

58. Beam JW. Occlusive dressings and the healing of standardized abrasions. *J Athl Train* 2008;**43**(6):600-7.

59. Maund M. Use of an ionic sheet hydrogel dressing on fungating wounds: two case studies. *J Wound Care* 2008;**17**(2):65-8.

60. Strunk B, Maher K. Collaborative nurse management of multifactorial moist desquamation in a patient undergoing radiotherapy. *J ET Nurs* 1993;**20**(4):152-7.

61. Breuton RN. The effect of ultrasound on the repair of a rabbit's tibial osteotomy held in rigid external fixation. *Bone and Joint Surgery* 1987;**69**:494.

62. Breuton RN, Campbell B. The use of Geliperm as a sterile coupling agent for therapeutic ultrasound. *Physiotherapy* 1987;**73**(12):653-654.

63. Klucinec B, Scheidler M, Denegar C, Domholdt E, Burgess S. Effectiveness of wound care products in the transmission of acoustic energy. *Phys Ther* 2000;**80**(5):469-76.

64. Kenney IJ, Delves NJ. The effect of wound dressings on diagnostic ultrasound imaging. *Journal of Wound Care* 1997;**6**(3):117-20.

65. Cherry G, Ryan TJ, Garaint M, Johnson K. Scherisorb gel investigated. *Care Sci. Pract.* 1985;**(Special Edn)**:Dec-14.

66. Agren MS. An amorphous hydrogel enhances epithelialisation of wounds. *Acta Derm Venereol* 1998;**78**(2):119-22.

67. Thomas S. Alginate dressings in surgery and wound management - part 3. *Journal of Wound Care* 2000;**9**(4):163-166.

68. Thomas S, Hay NP. Assessing the hydro-affinity of hydrogel dressings. *Journal of Wound Care* 1994;**3**(2):89-92.

69. Thomas S, Hay P. Fluid handling properties of hydrogel dressings. *Ostomy Wound Manage* 1995;**41**(3):54-6, 58-9.

70. Thomas S, Hay NP. In vitro investigations of a new hydrogel dressing. *Journal of Wound Care* 1996;**5**(3):130-131.

71. Thomas S, Fram P. Hydrogel testing, Data on file. Bridgend: SMTL, 1999:1-14.

72. Gomolin IH, Brandt JL. Topical metronidazole therapy for pressure sores of geriatric patients. *J. Am Geriat. Soc.* 1984;**31**:710-712.

73. Thomas S, Hay NP. The antimicrobial properties of two metronidazole medicated dressings used to treat malodorous wounds. *Pharmaceutical Journal* 1991;**March 2**:264-266.

74. Thomas S, Andrews AM. The effect of hydrogel dressings on maggot development. *Journal of Wound Care* 1999;**8**(2):75-77.
75. Thomas S. Milton and the treatment of burns. *Pharmaceutical Journal* 1986;**236**:128-129.
76. Regan MB. The use of intrasite gel in healing open sternal wounds. *Ostomy Wound Manage* 1992;**38**(3):15, 18-21.
77. Roberts KJ, Rowland CM, Benbow ME. Managing a patient's infected wound site after a radical vulvectomy. *Journal of Wound Care* 1992;**1**(4):14-17.
78. Benbow M. The treatment of a patient with infected arm wounds. *Journal of Wound Care* 1993;**2**(6):326-329.
79. Platt L, Benbow M. Care of a patient's foot after amputation of toes. *Journal of Wound Care* 1992;**1**(4):18-20.
80. Spooner R. Managing a patient's multiple pressure sores. *Journal of Wound Care* 1993;**2**(3):139-141.
81. Krasner D. Treating postoperative wounds with an amorphous hydrogel. *Journal of Wound Care* 1993;**2**(3):148-150.
82. Cooper L, Benbow BA. Management of a patient with Fournier's gangrene. *Journal of Wound Care* 1993;**2**(5):266-268.
83. Riggs RL, Bale S. Management of necrotic wounds as a complication of histiocytosis X. *Journal of Wound Care* 1993;**2**(5):260-261.
84. Benbow M, Pearce C. The care of an infant with homozygous protein C deficiency. *Journal of Wound Care* 1994;**3**(1):21-24.
85. Price A, Thomas S. Care of a patient after a degloving of the leg injury. *Journal of Wound Care* 1994;**3**(3):129-130.
86. Thomas S, Jones H. Clinical experiences with a new hydrogel dressing. *Journal of Wound Care* 1996;**5**(3):132-133.
87. Shutler SD, Jones M, Thomas S. Management of a fungating breast wound. *Journal of Wound Care* 1997;**6**(5):213-4.
88. Trudgian J. Investigating the use of Aquaform Hydrogel in wound management. *Br J Nurs* 2000;**9**(14):943-8.
89. Thomas S. A new approach to the management of extravasation injury in neonates. *Pharm. J.* 1987;**239**:584-585.
90. Irving V. Managing extravasation injuries in preterm neonates. *Nursing Times* 2001;**97**(35):40-46.
91. Lehr VT, Lulic-Botica M, Lindblad WJ, Kazzi NJ, Aranda JV. Management of infiltration injury in neonates using duoderm hydroactive gel. *Am J Perinatol* 2004;**21**(7):409-14.
92. Thomas S, Humphreys J, Fear-Price M. The role of moist wound healing in the management of meningococcal skin lesions. *Journal of Wound Care* 1998;**7**(10):503-507.
93. Stewart AJ, Leaper DJ. Treatment of chronic leg ulcers in the community; a comparative trial of Scherisorb and Iodosorb. *Phlebology* 1987;**2**:115-121.
94. Thomas S, Fear M. Comparing two dressings for wound debridement; results of a randomised trial. *Journal of Wound Care* 1993;**2**(5):272-274.
95. Flanagan M. The efficacy of a hydrogel in the treatment of wounds with non-viable tissue. *Journal of Wound Care* 1995;**4**(6):264-267.
96. Colin D, Kurring PA, Quinlan D, Yvon C. Managing sloughy pressure sores. *Journal of Wound Care* 1996;**5**(10):444-446.
97. Bale S, Banks V, Haglestein S, Harding KG. A comparison of two amorphous hydrogels in the debridement of pressure sores. *Journal of Wound Care* 1998;**7**(2):65-8.
98. Martin SJ, Corrado OJ, Kay EA. Enzymatic debridement for necrotic wounds. *Journal of Wound Care* 1996;**5**(7):310-1.

99. Parnell LK, Ciufi B, Gokoo CF. Preliminary use of a hydrogel containing enzymes in the treatment of stage II and stage III pressure ulcers. *Ostomy Wound Manage* 2005;**51**(8):50-60.
100. Matzen S, Peschardt A, Alsbjorn B. A new amorphous hydrocolloid for the treatment of pressure sores: a randomised controlled study. *Scand J Plast Reconstr Surg Hand Surg* 1999;**33**(1):13-5.
101. Mulder GD, Romanko KP, Sealey J, Andrews K. Controlled randomized study of a hypertonic gel for the debridement of dry eschar in chronic wounds. *Wounds* 1993;**5**(3):112-115.
102. Mulder GD. Cost-effective managed care: gel versus wet-to-dry for debridement. *Ostomy Wound Manage* 1995;**41**(2):68-70, 72, 74 passim.
103. Gallenkemper G, Rabe E, Bauer R. Contact sensitization in chronic venous insufficiency: modern wound dressings. *Contact Dermatitis* 1998;**38**(5):274-8.
104. Roberts DB, Travis EL. Acemannan-containing wound dressing gel reduces radiation-induced skin reactions in C3H mice. *Int J Radiat Oncol Biol Phys* 1995;**32**(4):1047-52.
105. Thomas DR, Goode PS, LaMaster K, Tennyson T. Acemannan hydrogel dressing versus saline dressing for pressure ulcers. A randomized, controlled trial. *Adv Wound Care* 1998;**11**(6):273-6.
106. Macmillan MS, Wells M, MacBride S, Raab GM, Munro A, MacDougall H. Randomized comparison of dry dressings versus hydrogel in management of radiation-induced moist desquamation. *Int J Radiat Oncol Biol Phys* 2007;**68**(3):864-72.
107. Gollins S, Gaffney C, Slade S, Swindell R. RCT on gentian violet versus a hydrogel dressing for radiotherapy-induced moist skin desquamation. *J Wound Care* 2008;**17**(6):268-70, 272, 274-5.
108. Spence WR, Bates I. New absorption dressing for secreting ulcers. *Texas Medical Association Annual Session*. Texas, 1981.
109. Montgomery BA. Product ingredients: important ramification. *J. enterostom. Ther.* 1985;**12**:203-204.
110. Jeter KF, Chapman RM, Tintle T, Davis A. Comprehensive wound management with a starch-based copolymer dressing. *J Enterostomal Ther* 1986;**13**(6):217-25.
111. Brown M, Myers RB, Rideout BK. A non-traditional approach to abdominal wound closure. *Ostomy and Wound Management* 1991;**34**(May/June):37-43.
112. Radford KA. Wound complications after cardiac surgery: a new approach to healing by secondary intention. *J Cardiovasc Nurs* 1993;**7**(4):82-7.
113. Chung LY, Schmidt RJ, Andrews AM, Turner TD. A study of hydrogen peroxide generation by, and antioxidant activity of, Granuflex (DuoDERM) Hydrocolloid Granules and some other hydrogel/hydrocolloid wound management materials. *Br J Dermatol* 1993;**129**(2):145-53.

15. Honey and sugar dressings

INTRODUCTION

Although honey has been used medicinally for thousands of years, it was not until the later part of the 20th Century that it began to be used widely in Western medicine. It is perhaps no coincidence that it was around his time that sugar (sucrose) also began to be used as a dressing for in some instances at least, sugar was regarded as a cheaper more convenient alternative to honey as it was assumed, incorrectly, that the two agents are so similar in composition and function, that for wound management applications they can be considered equivalent in performance terms. In practice, however, there are marked differences between the two products in their mode of action and spectrum of activity,[1] as will be discussed later.

SUGAR AS A WOUND DRESSING

Historical use of sugar

In an early account of the use of sugar published in 1973,[2] it was reported that, over a five-year period, an 80% healing rate was achieved in pressure ulcers dressed with granulated sugar packed very tightly into the wound and covered with an 'air-tight' dressing, a treatment that the author claimed 'arose out of sheer frustration' after other modalities had proved unsuccessful. Thomlinson in 1980[3] described how icing sugar was applied to the malodorous malignant breast ulcers of four patients every twelve hours using a teaspoon or salt cellar. In all four cases, the smell from the wound was greatly reduced, no adverse effects were recorded, and as a result patients were able to manage their wounds at home.

A larger comparative study was performed by Knutson *et al.*,[4] who dressed 605 wounds of various types with granulated sugar alone or sugar combined with povidone iodine solution or ointment. The healing rates of sugar treated wounds were compared with those of a further 154 patients who were treated with other unspecified therapies. The study was not well controlled but overall the wounds treated with sugar were said to heal faster than those in the control group.

Scientific basis for use

The scientific basis for the use of granulated sugar was discussed by Chirife *et al.*[5-7] in 1982 and 1983 who also measured the effects of increasing sugar concentrations upon the growth of *S. aureus*, an organism particularly resistant to osmotic effects. They demonstrated that a level of 195 g of sugar per 100 g of water produced complete inhibition of growth, with the number of viable organisms declining steadily throughout the incubation period. They concluded that granulated sugar could act as a 'universal antimicrobial agent' for the treatment of infected wounds and other superficial lesions, and suggested that 'on grounds of safety, economy and availability this therapeutic use of sugar may have widespread applicability, even in emergencies and disasters.'

These enthusiastic conclusions were challenged by Forrest,[8] who considered that the osmotic pressure of partially dissolved sugar could have harmful or undesirable effects, tending to dehydrate epithelial cells, macrophages and fibroblasts and thus delay healing. He also questioned the description of sugar as a 'universal antimicrobial agent' on the basis of tests carried out on a single organism, and doubted the possibility of sustaining the required concentration of sugar at the wound surface for any length of time. Bose[9] was also unconvinced of the merits of sugar, and considered that honey offered a number of practical advantages. Nevertheless, favourable reports on sugar continued to find their way into the literature.

Results of animal studies

The effects of sugar on wound healing were compared with those of gauze soaked in a variety of topical preparations in an animal model.[10] Full thickness wounds on pigs, up to 9 mm deep, were treated with the substances under test and covered with a semipermeable film dressing, Opsite. Other wounds were dressed with Opsite alone as a control. The experiment was terminated after seven days when the whole wound, complete with dressing, was excised for histological examination. Wounds covered with Opsite alone and those treated with sugar paste under Opsite were found to be filled with granulation tissue over which epidermal migration was taking place. Wounds packed with gauze to which had been added chlorhexidine gluconate 0.2%, Irgasan 0.2%, povidone iodine 0.8% or half-strength Eusol, showed delayed healing in that less infilling had taken place over the same time period. This delay was attributed to the nature of the chemicals used and/or the influence of the gauze packing. Healing appeared to be most affected by chlorhexidine and least affected by Eusol. No toxic effects were observed with sugar paste which, the authors suggested, may be preferable to antiseptics for the management of dirty or infected wounds.

Pharmaceutical considerations

Normal commercial sugar is not always sterile, and may contain calcium phosphate, sodium aluminium silicate or other permitted agents to prevent caking upon storage.[11] A paste made from additive-free caster and icing sugar, polyethylene glycol 400 and hydrogen peroxide was developed in 1985, and its use reported by Gordon et al.[12] and Middleton and Seal.[13] Two versions were produced, a thin form for instillation into abscesses (as an alternative to ribbon gauze packing), and a thicker form for the treatment of large open wounds. The thin paste, particularly, was found to be effective in situations where traditional Eusol packs had failed, and the authors concluded that both formulations had many advantages over conventional materials.

The ability of a number of formulations containing sucrose or xylose along with polyethylene glycol 400 and hydrogen peroxide to inhibit growth of a number of pathogenic organisms was investigated by Ambrose et al.[14]

The pastes, which were chemically stable for six months if stored at 2 to 8 degrees C, were shown to be bactericidal even when diluted up to 50% with serum. Of the organisms tested, *S. aureus* proved the least susceptible to the bactericidal effects of these pastes, and Candida sp. and Gram-negative organisms proved the most susceptible. Pastes containing hydrogen peroxide were more rapidly bactericidal than without. Polyethylene glycol 400 was also shown to possess considerable antimicrobial activity.

Clinical experience with sugar

Rahal[15] described how 42 patients with infected wounds were treated with common sugar their infections cleared within five to 30 days and in 1985, Trouillet *et al.*[16] described the results of an uncontrolled trial of the use of sugar in 29 patients with acute post-operative mediastinitis. In this study, 11 patients were initially treated with gauze soaked in povidone-iodine, which was replaced two days later by granulated sugar packed tightly into the wound. The wounds were cleansed and repacked twice daily and fresh sugar was added at intervals of three to four hours as required. The remaining patients had their wounds subjected to continuous irrigation with a weak solution of povidone-iodine. All patients in both groups also received systemic antibiotic therapy. Eight of the patients treated with povidone-iodine alone failed to respond favourably, and were therefore changed to the sugar treatment. Debridement and granulation tissue production occurred within five to nine days in the majority of the 19 wounds that were dressed with sugar - only three required surgical debridement. Overall, 17 of the 19 wounds responded well to the treatment but two patients had severe acute haemorrhage from exposed vascular sutures which required immediate surgery. Four patients died of unrelated causes and 13 patients were eventually discharged completely healed.

Similar encouraging results were reported by Quatraro *et al.*,[17] following the treatment of 15 diabetic patients 13 of whom had dystrophic or ischaemic ulcers of the lower limbs. One of the remaining patients had a 'suppurative process of the feet'; the other had a burn upon the hand. All the wounds were packed with sugar and covered with gauze, and more sugar was added every 3-4 hours. Granulation tissue formed within 5-6 days and all wounds were completely healed in 9-12 days.

Tanner[18] used a sugar and polyethylene glycol paste to treat 20 patients with chronically infected abdominal and perineal wounds that had failed to respond to conventional forms of treatment. Complete healing was achieved in 19 patients. The paste was claimed to be especially effective in the treatment of large abscess cavities with small external openings whilst being inexpensive and easy to prepare and painless to apply.

Although the topical use of sugar appears to be relatively free of adverse effects, osmotic nephrosis resulting in acute renal failure was reported in one patient - after the extensive use of granulated sugar in a deep infected pneumonectomy wound in the right chest of a 64-year-old male. The sugar was removed from the cavity; when urine flow resumed on the second day, it was found to contain large amounts of sucrose.[19] However, Archer *et al.*[20] questioned whether this nephrotoxity might have been related, at least in part, to the use of gentamicin (which was applied to the wound in the form of an irrigation before the application of sugar).

When the value of sugar in wound healing was reviewed by Keith and Knodel in 1988,[21] they concluded that 'based upon available information the use of sugar as the sole treatment of wounds cannot be recommended, when used alone sugar has not been shown to be effective in hastening wound healing in controlled clinical testing.' But this conclusion simply reflected the lack of well controlled studies rather than a problem with the treatment itself - a common occurrence with systematic reviews in wound management!

Sugar and sugar paste were used to treat surgical wound infections in patients who had undergone cardiac surgery. In one prospective study[22] involving 1164 patients, postoperative mediastinitis occurred in 15 individuals (1.3%). Ten were treated by closed mediastinal irrigation and in five cases the treatment was effective. Granulated sugar was applied to the wounds of the five cases where the closed treatment had failed, and also in four cases of advanced mediastinitis and sternum osteomyelitis. The wounds were filled with granulated sugar twice a day, which resulted in rapid granulation tissue formation in all patients. Of the nine patients treated with granulated sugar three died before discharge, but none of the deaths were due to wound complications. The rest of the patients were discharged with healed wounds after an average of 91.6 ± 8.0 days. During subsequent follow up period, no wound-related problems occurred in patients treated with sugar, but two of the five patients whose wounds were closed by mediastinal irrigation had to undergo a further operation after a few months because of the formation of sternal fistulae. Based upon these experiences, the authors considered granulated sugar to be an effective treatment for obstinate and advanced mediastinal infections.

Additional support for the use of sugar for this indication was provided by De Feo et al.[23] In 2000 they described the use of granulated sugar in the treatment of nine patients with postoperative mediastinitis which had proved refractory to a closed irrigation system. All patients were febrile with leukocytosis and yielded positive wound cultures of S. aureus (n = 6), S. epidermidis (n = 2), and Pseudomonas sp. (n = 1).

Wounds were debrided and filled with granulated sugar four times a day. Three patients also received hyperbaric therapy. Fever ceased within 4.3 ± 1.3 days from the beginning of treatment and white blood counts returned to normal after 6.6 ± 1.6 days. Complete wound healing was achieved in 58.8 ± 32.9 days, with three patients receiving pectoralis muscle flaps.

Their second publication,[24] described a retrospective review of historical clinical data designed to determine whether a staged approach to treatment could reduce morbidity and mortality following a post-cardiotomy deep sternal wound infection. Analysis of patients' records from 1979 to 2000 revealed that 14,620 individuals had undergone open heart surgery and that mediastinitis developed in 124 individuals (0.85%). In 62 patients treated in 1979 to 1994, (Group A) conservative antibiotic therapy was attempted followed by surgical intervention in the case of failure. For the 62 patients in 1995 to 2000, (Group B) the treatment was staged in three phases: The wound was first debrided, all wires and sutures were removed and closed irrigation provided for ten days. In the 11 patients in whom this treatment proved unsuccessful, their wounds were treated with sugar and hyperbaric therapy. In the case of three patients, with further delayed healing and negative wound cultures, plastic reconstruction was undertaken. Analysis of the data revealed that the incidence of mediastinitis was higher in Group B that Group A, (1.3% *vs* 0.7% respectively) but the mean interval between diagnosis and treatment was shorter in Group B (18 ± 6 days) than in Group A (38 ± 7 days) (P = 0.001). Hospital mortality was higher in Group A than in Group B (31% *vs* 1.6%) (P = 0.001). In Group B complete healing was observed in all the 61 survivors: 47 cases (76%) after Stage 1, 11 (18%) after Stage 2; three (4.8%) after Stage 3. The authors concluded that despite the fact that the two patient groups related to different decades, this study showed that an aggressive therapeutic approach can significantly reduce morbidity and mortality of deep sternal wound infection.

In a third publication,[25] using historical data they compared clinical outcomes and perioperative data for patients treated with granulated sugar versus early muscle flap surgery in the management of recurrent postoperative Staphylococcal mediastinitis.

Between January 1995 and January 2002, 25 patients with severe recurrent staphylococcal mediastinitis were treated either with granulated sugar wound dressing (Group A) or with wound debridement, v-shape sternectomy and associated muscle flap surgery (Group B). A complete cure was achieved earlier in Group A than in Group B and the length of hospital stay was also reduced. A statistically significant difference was found in hospital mortality (16% overall) in favour of patients in Group A (p = 0.039). In patients with the most serious preoperative profile (haemodialysis, tracheostomy, inotropic support) surgical treatment produced worse results than the sugar dressing method (p = 0.048). Once again the authors concluded that the use of granulated sugar proved a safe effective treatment option for severely compromised patients.

The free availability of sugar, and its relatively limited cost, makes it a potentially useful treatment in countries where healthcare resources are limited. In 1988 Topham[26] described the use of sugar pastes on the island of Zanzibar and concluded that they offered a cheap and chemically pure aid to wound healing.

Grauwin et al.[27] described how, at the Leprosy Institute of Dakar, sugar could was used to treat to treat bone infections in open wounds following surgical debridement. They reported that the hyperosmolar environment produced by the dressing kills or inhibits bacterial growth and facilitates the development of granulation tissue over the debrided nude bones. In total 36 cases of osteitis and septic arthritis were treated in this way during a two year period from March 1995 to March 1997. All wounds healed in an average of 44 days and the treatment was said to be easy to apply and very cheap.

A less favourable view of sugar was reported by Bajaj et al.[28] who conducted a randomized controlled trial comparing Eusol and sugar in the treatment of traumatic wounds and found Eusol to be more effective in cleaning and promoting healing.

Chiwenga et al.[29] reviewed treatment outcomes for 71 patients with malodorous, painful wounds that were treated with sugar dressings in Lilongwe Hospital, Malawi, to assess the effects of the dressings on pain and odour. Mean patient odour scores reduced from 5.45 (out of 10) on application, to 2.94 at ten days: mean patient discomfort scores reduced from 6.73 on application to 3.87 at ten days. They concluded that the cheap treatment provided reproducible benefits as part of an appropriate protocol for use in developing world hospitals with limited resources and nursing care.

Commercial preparations made from sugar which incorporate povidone iodine have also been described.[26,30] The effect of a commercial preparation consisting of 70% sugar and 3% povidone iodine (U-Pasta Kowa Co., Ltd. (Nagoya, Japan) on various functions of cultured human keratinocytes and fibroblasts was examined by Nakao et al.[31] who concluded that the mixture is likely to act on wounds not only as an antiseptic agent, but also as a modulator for keratinocytes and fibroblasts.

Shi et al.[32] examined the effect of this paste on full thickness wounds on diabetic mice that were infected with methicillin-resistant Staphylococcus aureus (MRSA). The paste was applied to the closed wounds for eight days after which the wounds were assessed. They found that compared to a non-treated control group, the paste significantly accelerated reepithelialization ($P < 0.01$) and decreased the number of organisms isolated from the wounds ($P < 0.05$).

HONEY AS A WOUND DRESSSING

Historical use of honey

It is not known when honey was first used to treat wounds, but an early Sumerian clay tablet clearly shows that it has been used for this purpose for at least 4000 years, describing the production of a wound salve thus;

> 'Grind to a powder river dust . . . and then knead it in water and honey, and let oil and hot cedar oil be spread over it.'

It was also routinely used in ancient Egypt; Case Number ten of the Edwin Smith Papyrus, circa 1700 BC, describes a treatment for a wound in the top of a man's eyebrow which penetrates to the bone as follows:

> 'You should palpate his wound and draw together his gash for him with stitching. After you have stitched it you should bind fresh meat upon it the first day. If you find that the stitching of the wound has come loose, you should draw it together for him with two strips (of plaster) and you should treat it with grease and honey every day until he recovers.'

Honey has a long history in Chinese medicine, and was known to other civilizations as diverse as the ancient Greeks, eastern African tribes and American Indians. Honey is frequently mentioned in the Bible, although not in the context of wound management, but the medicinal properties of honey are recorded in the Quran.[33-34] An interesting summary of the history of honey in medicine and wound management has been provided by Blair[35]

The addition of an oily or greasy material to honey to render it less sticky, as described in the Egyptian text, has also been a common practice: residents of Shanghai used a mixture of honey and lard to treat their wounds during the Second World War.

A reference to the use of honey and fat combined in this way was published in 1954,[36] and a mixture of honey and cod liver oil was used to treat ulcers, burns, fistulas and boils in Germany.[37] In the 1970s a tulle dressing containing cod liver oil and honey, M & M Tulle, Malam Laboratories, was sold commercially in the UK.

In the 1960s and 70s, a few publications described the clinical use of honey, including one on the treatment of surgical wounds following carcinoma of the vulva,[38] but it was not until the late 80s and early 90s that honey began to be more widely used in mainstream wound care.

The increasing popularity of honey was influenced by a number of factors: scientific papers published around that period, later comprehensively summarised by Molan in 1999,[39] described the antimicrobial properties of honey, suggesting that the material offered an attractive alternative to the use of antibiotics and other chemotherapeutic agents for the treatment of wound infections. This was opportune at a time when the emergence of antibiotic strains of bacteria were beginning to cause real concern[40-41] following an outbreak of MRSA in London in 1980/81.[42]

Honey also capitalised upon the increasing enthusiasm of large sections of the population for 'natural' treatments and complementary medicine, and as result it gained considerable publicity in the media including television and radio, the tabloid press, and various women's and health-related magazines.

The upsurge in interest in the use of honey led to the introduction of a number of different honey-containing products some of which have been enthusiastically adopted for all types of wounds and skin conditions.

A further bee product, propolis, a resinous mixture that honey bees collect from tree buds, sap flows, or other botanical sources and which is used by them as a sealant for unwanted open spaces in the hive was also known to the ancient world and used in medicine.

According to Golder[43] more than 15 Greek and Roman authors made reference to the use of this preparation, chiefly for the preparation of ointments and plasters for the management of surgical and other types of wounds and minor injuries.

Composition of honey

Honey is essentially a super-saturated solution principally comprising a mixture of sugars together with small quantities of enzymes and amino acids, vitamins, minerals, organic acids and aromatics responsible for its flavour and odour, although the exact composition varies widely, according to the geographical source and the plants upon which the bees have been feeding.

An analysis of 490 samples of American floral honey reported that the average concentrations of the principal components were as follows: moisture 17.2%, fructose 38.2%, glucose 31%, maltose 7.35%, and sucrose 1.3%. Small quantities of other higher sugars and oligosaccharides were also present.[44]

In addition to the carbohydrate components, honey contains the enzymes invertase, which converts sucrose to glucose and fructose; amylase, which breaks down starch; glucose oxidase, which converts glucose to hydrogen peroxide and gluconolactone, which in turn yields gluconic acid; catalase, which breaks down the peroxide formed by glucose oxidase to water and oxygen; and acid phosphatase, which removes inorganic phosphate from organic phosphates.

Other minor components include trace amounts of B vitamins, calcium, iron, zinc, potassium, phosphorous, magnesium, selenium, chromium and manganese and antioxidants such as flavonoids ascorbic acid, and catalase.

Also present are organic acids such as acetic, butanoic, formic, citric, succinic, lactic, malic, pyroglutamic and gluconic acids which together are responsible for the low pH (3.5-6). The main acid present is gluconic acid, formed in the breakdown of glucose by glucose oxidase.[44]

According to Perez et al.[45] the amino acid content of honey is attributable both to the bees and plant sources. The former group are common to many honeys, while the second group depend on the botanical and geographical origin of the honey. The amount of total free amino acids in honey varies between 10 and 200 mg/100 g with proline as the major constituent representing about 50% of the total.

Antimicrobial activity of honey

According to an informative review published by Molan in 1992,[46] the first report of honey possessing antibacterial activity was made by a Dutch scientist Van Ketel in 1882. Initially this was assumed to be entirely due to its high osmotic pressure, a property known to prevent the growth of microorganisms. This theory was later shown to be incorrect when in 1919 it was demonstrated that the antibacterial activity of some of types of honey increased upon dilution.

Subsequently it was found that this unexplained activity was largely due to the formation of hydrogen peroxide produced by the enzyme glucose oxidase which only becomes active as the honey is diluted: the addition of catalase to honey eliminates this activity.

The rate at which hydrogen peroxide was produced by different honeys upon dilution, was measured in eight samples from six different floral sources by Bang et al.[47] The highest level of hydrogen peroxide recorded in the diluted honeys ranged from 1 - 2 mmol/L when diluted to between 30% and 50% by volume, with at least 50% of the maximum levels recorded occurring at dilutions of 15-67%. The authors calculated this to be equivalent to a 10×10 cm dressing containing 20 mL of honey absorbing 10 to 113 mL of wound exudate.

More recent studies have identified that a third component contributes to the antimicrobial activity of some types of honey which is independent of both hydrogen peroxide production and the osmotic effects previously described. This 'non-peroxide' activity persists in the presence of catalase, and was originally assumed to be associated with bioactive molecules such as phenolics and flavenoids[48] derived from the plants upon which the bees forage.

This activity is almost exclusively found in honey produced by bees that feed upon nectar from the flowers of the manuka bush, *Leptospermum scoparium*, a plant native to New Zealand which grows wild throughout the country. Honey from this botanical source has the unusual property that it is thixotropic. Jellybush honey, which also has thixotropic properties which give it its name, is non-peroxide containing Australian honey produced from Leptospermum sp.[49]

The non-peroxide activity can be measured and characterized in a bioassay in which dilutions of phenol (carbolic acid) are included as reference standards. The activity is then expressed as the equivalent percentage concentration of phenol which produces the same antimicrobial effect. This activity has been described as the Unique Manuka Factor (UMF), a term that became the trademark of the Active Manuka Honey Industry.

In a comprehensive experimental study which formed the subject of a PhD thesis, summarised in the New Zealand Beekeeper,[50] apparent differences in the UMF of different so-called manuka honeys were detected from samples collected from different geographical sources.

Measurement of the rheological properties of these materials indicated that some contained varying amounts of nectar collected from species other than *L. scoparium* but by using these rheological measurements it was possible to estimate the proportion of Manuka honey in each sample and thus adjust the UMF estimate accordingly.

It was concluded that honey which contains a reasonable proportion of *L. scoparium* nectar will inevitably contain UMF activity, from which it follows that a honey described as 'Manuka', which does not possess a reasonable UMF value, must be either adulterated or misnamed. For example, viscosity measurement of samples with very low UMF values (< 4 UMF units) suggested that these materials contained less than 30% *L. scoparium* nectar.

Even after adjustments were made to the recorded UMF values of the honey samples included in the study described previously, some variation in UMF activity remained although all possessed an activity > 8 UMF units.

Upon further examination it was established that, contrary to what had previously been suspected, this variation was not greatly influenced by environmental changes but rather the existence and hybridisation of different varieties of *L. scoparium* notably *L. scoparium* vars. *incanum* and *linifolium* (high UMF) and *L. scoparium* var. *myrtifolium* (Low UMF).

A classification system was therefore adopted by the industry consisting of the initials UMF followed by a number indicating the strength of the UMF property. In accordance with this rating, a minimum UMF rating of ten was originally proposed for medical applications but this could rise to 25 in some batches.

Unfortunately, according to Molan,[51] for a variety of reasons this classification system has been abused and devalued as a result of deliberate misrepresentation concerning botanical source, inappropriate claims for antimicrobial activity and poor experimental technique and laboratory practices utilised in the assay process. These have lead to legal disputes in New Zealand which involve several of the major honey producers and processers. Molan therefore proposes that an unambiguous claim be used in its place stating for example that, when tested in accordance with a validated method, the sample contains 'non-peroxide antibacterial activity equivalent to that of 12% phenol'

The agent at least partly responsible for this additional activity of manuka honey was identified by Mavric *et al.*,[52] who showed it is due to methylglyoxal (MGO) a molecule that is also formed in very low concentrations in a wide range of other foodstuffs following processing, cooking or prolonged storage. MGO levels in

European and non Manuka honeys ranged from 0-10 mg/Kg, but Manuka honeys ranged from 20 - 800+ mg/Kg.

According to Henle, one of the authors of the paper cited previously,[52] a minimum MGO concentration of about 100 mg/Kg is required in honeys used for medical applications and based upon these findings, a classification system has been developed by one supplier, whose products are labelled with the minimum MGO content.

MGO has been shown to be formed during storage of honey, from dihydroxyacetone which is present in the nectar of manuka flowers in varying amounts.[53] MGO levels are also known to increase significantly in some plants in response to stress caused by drought and cold which might explain in part the variability in UMF values recorded over time.

Adams et al.,[54] in an elegant study, examined the relationship between MGO content and the UMF value of the honey when they assayed the MGO content of 83 different honeys and determined the UMF of each.

Of 34 non-manuka honey samples examined only five showed any antimicrobial activity and none of these contained sufficient MGO to account for this activity, leading the authors to speculate that the activity of these honeys could might be due to plant derived phenolics and flavenoids as previously thought.

Unfortunately the relationship between MGO content and the antimicrobial activity of honey is not linear, certainly in honeys with low levels of antibacterial activity, which means that doubling the concentration of MGO does not result in a similar increase in the UMF values determined microbiologically. Conversely extrapolation of methylglyoxal concentration back to zero in the graph prepared by Adams[54] still appears to leave a substantial amount of unexplained activity present in the honey.[55]

Molan has proposed the existence of a synergistic effect between the MGO and some other component(s) of honey and strongly argued that for the this reason it is not acceptable to quote the MGO content of a honey sample to describe its antibacterial properties, suggesting that this is likely to mislead the consumer.[56-57] This issue remains to be resolved.

There is little doubt that the non-peroxide activity of honey is potentially very important when honey is used as a wound dressing. Catalase occurs naturally in wound and tissue fluids[58] and therefore there exists a real possibility that honeys which rely heavily on the production of hydrogen peroxide to exert an antimicrobial activity will be much less effective *in vivo* than is predicted from the results of laboratory tests undertaken in the absence of catalase. The high concentrations of MGO found in some honeys also means that these can be diluted by up to 20 times by exudate present within a wound, but still retain significant antimicrobial activity.[55]

The low pH of honey also contributes to its antimicrobial activity. According to Gethin et al.,[59] chronic non-healing wounds frequently have an elevated pH. They postulated that this may be lowered by the application of honey which in turn would potentially reduce protease activity, increase fibroblast activity and oxygen release, although the likely duration of such an effect is unknown. They therefore undertook a small non-randomized prospective study to investigate the relationship between honey and wound pH involving 17 patients with 20 wounds of which ten were leg ulcers of venous origin, seven leg ulcers of mixed aetiology, two were arterial leg ulcers and one was a pressure ulcer.

The area of each wound was measured by planimetry and the pH determined on admission to the study and following two weeks treatment with a manuka honey.

Reduction in wound pH after two weeks was statistically significant ($p < 0.001$). Wounds with pH ≥ 8.0 did not decrease in size but wounds with pH ≤ 7.6 decreased in area by 30%. A reduction in 0.1 pH unit was associated with an 8.1% reduction in wound size ($p < 0.012$). The authors considered that surface wound pH measurements may contribute to objective wound assessments, but proposed that further research was required to confirm this possibility.

The possibility that the use of sub-lethal doses of honey could lead to the development of resistance was investigated by Blair et al.[60] Using E. coli macroarrays, they showed that resistance to honey could not be induced under conditions that rapidly induced resistance to antibiotics. They also found that the pattern of gene expression differed to that reported for other antimicrobial agents, indicating that honey acts in a unique and multifactorial way leading them to conclude that honey is an effective topical antimicrobial agent that could help reduce some of the current pressures that are promoting antibiotic resistance.

Importance of geographical source

The activity of honey from different locations has been evaluated in numerous publications. Unfortunately these studies have used different microbiological techniques which can make interpretation of the results difficult.

The potency of each of 345 different honey samples was compared with that of phenol solution using a standard agar well diffusion technique.[61] In New Zealand honeys, potency ranged from the equivalent of $< 2\%$ to 58% phenol. The addition of catalase eliminated the activity from all but two of the honeys tested - L. scoparium (manuka honey) and Echium vulgare (viper's bugloss).

Willix et al.[62] compared the activity of manuka honey with that of a normal peroxide-producing variety against seven potentially pathogenic organisms. No significant differences between the two types of honey were detected overall, but marked differences were detected in the rank order of sensitivity of the seven bacterial species. The non-peroxide antibacterial activity of manuka honey completely inhibited the growth of S. aureus at a honey concentration of 1.8% v/v during incubation for eight hours. The growth of all seven species was completely inhibited by both types of honey at concentrations below 11% v/v.

Wilkinson and Cavanagh[63] compared the activity of 13 honeys, including three which were marketed as 'antibacterial honeys', at four concentrations from 1.0% to 10% w/v against E. coli and P. aeruginosa using a standard well diffusion method. These were compared with corresponding dilutions of an 'artificial' honey, a solution containing the principal sugars found in honey at the appropriate concentrations. All samples were also tested in the presence of catalase to eliminate the antibacterial effects of hydrogen peroxide.

The results of this investigation were subjected to statistical analysis which confirmed that artificial honey had no measurable effect upon *E. coli* but inhibited the growth of *P. aeruginosa* at 10% and 5%. All true honeys inhibited the growth of *E. coli* and *P. aeruginosa,* to varying extents, and all were more effective than the artificial honey at 5% and 10%. Only one (Patterson's curse honey) demonstrated significant activity against E coli at 2.5%. Five honeys inhibited growth of *P. aeruginosa* at 5% and three at 2.5%. No honey was active at 1% against either organism. A Bulgarian lavender honey was found to produce the largest zones of inhibition against *P. aeruginosa* and although this activity was not statistically different from that of rosemary or lavender honey, it was significantly greater that all the other honeys examined, including the manuka honeys. In the presence of catalase manuka and four lavender honeys were found to exhibit antibacterial action.

The authors of this paper emphasised the importance of a statistical approach to the analysis of data used to compare the effectiveness of different types of honeys, and on this basis called into question the validity of the conclusions of two earlier studies,[61,64] which are described later, when they subjected the published data to statistical analysis and showed that the MIC for pasture honey and manuka honey against clinical isolates of *P. aeruginosa* were not significantly different, even though the authors of the original paper had not made any particular claims about the difference in the activities of these samples.

However, whilst the application of statistical method to this subject area must be welcomed, it must be remember that failure to demonstrate significance does not of itself mean that a difference does not exists. This failure could be due to an inadequate sample size or too few replicate tests (a Type II error), a particular problem with biological assays.

Forty two Canadian honeys were compared against *E. coli* and *Bacillus subtilis* using a broth micro-dilution assay.[65] The importance of hydrogen peroxide on was determined by measuring the concentration before and after the addition of catalase and correlating these results with the observed levels of antibacterial activity.

The Canadian honeys were found to possess moderate to high antibacterial activity against both bacterial species. The honeys exhibited selective inhibitory activity against *E. coli*, which was strongly influenced by endogenous hydrogen peroxide. *B. subtilis* activity was marginally significantly correlated with hydrogen peroxide content. The removal of hydrogen peroxide by catalase reduced the honeys' antibacterial activity, but the enzyme was unable to completely decompose endogenous peroxide. The 25% - 30% 'leftover' was significantly correlated with the honeys' residual antibacterial activity against *E. coli*. The authors therefore suggested that hydrogen peroxide levels in honey are a strong predictor of its antibacterial activity.

Using a broth dilution method, Basson *et al.*[66] compared the antibacterial activity of different types of South African honey including that produced from the blossoms of *Eucalyptus cladocalyx* (Bluegum) trees, an indigenous South African plant *Leucospermum cordifolium* (Pincushion), and a mixture of wild heather shrubs, mainly Erica species (Fynbos), with that of a *L. scoparium*, manuka, honey. Although some inhibitory effects were noted, the activity present in the in the South African honeys was not considered sufficiently high to confer 'medical grade' status.

The antimicrobial activity of each of 25 honey samples acquired in Costa Rica was tested over a range of dilutions against *S. aureus*, *S. epidermidis*, *P. aeruginosa*, *E. coli*, *Salmonella enteritidis*, *Listeria monocytogenes* and *Aspergillus niger*. Of the 25 samples examined, 24 inhibited the growth of *S. aureus* in a 25% v/v dilution but *A. niger* was not inhibited by any of the samples tested.[67]

Lusby et al.[68] compared the antimicrobial activity of three types of local honey with three commercial 'therapeutic' honeys, using thirteen bacteria and the yeast *C. albicans* in an *in vitro* study that did not include the addition of catalase. All honey samples were tested at concentrations ranging from 0.1% to 20% using an agar dilution method. Under the conditions of test, 12 of the 13 bacteria were inhibited by all the samples included in the study with only *Serratia marcescens* and the yeast *C. albicans* remaining unaffected. Little or no antibacterial activity was seen at honey concentrations < 1%, with minimal inhibition at 5%.

No honey was able to produce complete inhibition of bacterial growth at the concentration used by this method. *L. scoparium (*manuka) had the overall best activity but the locally produced honeys had equivalent inhibitory activity for some, but not all, bacteria. Had catalase been included, the results might have been somewhat different.

When the antimicrobial properties of manuka honey from Australia, heather honey from the United Kingdom, and locally marketed Indian honey were compared against 152 isolates of *P. aeruginosa*, the Indian, khadikraft, honey was said to have the greatest inhibitory effect but it not thought that catalase was included in this test protocol.[69]

Tan et al.[70] compared the antibacterial profile of manuka honey and Malaysian tualang honey using a broth dilution method to determine their minimum inhibitory concentrations (MIC) against 13 different microorganisms. Minimum bactericidal concentrations (MBC) were determined by a plating technique. MIC values for both honey types typically ranged from about 9-25%. The lowest MBC for tualang honey was 20% compared with 11.25% for manuka honey. The authors concluded that Tualang could be used as an alternative to manuka honey for certain therapeutic indications.

For a comprehensive review of the mode of action of all aspects of honey see Molan.[51]

Given the potential clinical and commercial importance of identifying the geographical source of a given batch of honey, various techniques have been described by which this can be achieved. Pollen analysis is one way, but this is time consuming and requires considerable expertise. Other methods that have been evaluated include amino acid analysis, as described by Perez et al.[45] and determining the relationship between dilution and the pH and electrical conductivity of honey as described by Acquarone et al.[71]

Spectrum of activity

The activity of different types of honey against clinical isolates and potentially pathogenic organisms has been compared in numerous studies.

Samples provided by apiarists and honey packers were tested against wound commensals in the undiluted form and in varying dilutions down 10% w/v. Most undiluted samples inhibited the growth of a number of test organisms to varying degrees. Some honey provided by apiarists completely inhibited *S. aureus* and *S. epidermidis* and also inhibited the growth of *S. aureus* at 50% dilution. No inhibition of *Micrococcus luteus* and *Enterococcus faecalis* growth was detected. Activity of honey samples provided by apiarists was greater than that of honey provided by honey packers.[72]

Cooper *et al.* in several studies compared the activity of manuka honey with pasture honey against clinical strains of different organisms in the absence of catalase. The minimum inhibitory concentration (MIC) of honey against Pseudomonas species isolated from swabs taken from 20 infected wounds was 6.9 ± 1.3%. and 7.1 ± 1.0% for manuka honey and pasture honey respectively.[73] A further 17 strains isolated from infected burns were all inhibited by honey concentrations below 10% v/v.[64]

When 58 clinical strains of coagulase-positive *S. aureus*[74] were examined, little variation was detected between the isolates in their sensitivity to honey, MICs were all between 2% and 3% v/v for the manuka honey and 3% and 4% for the pasture honey.

Similar results were achieved when 18 clinical isolates of coagulase-negative staphylococci were examined,[75] as the honeys were inhibitory at dilutions down to 3.4 ± 0.5% and 3.6 ± 0.7% for the manuka honey and pasture honey respectively. An 'artificial honey', sugar syrup of equivalent osmolarity to honey, produced an MIC of 29.9 ± 1.9%. These results indicate that honey is typically about eight times more potent that sugar solution if bacterial inhibition was due to osmolarity alone, and suggest that honey with this level of antibacterial activity could be expected to remain effective in preventing the growth of microorganisms *in vivo* even if it were to become diluted more than ten-fold by wound exudate. However, as the test method did not include the addition of catalase, the results may well have tended to overestimate the potential clinical activity of some pasture honey.

Honey also kills antibiotic resistant strains of microorganisms. Manuka honey successfully inhibited the growth of 18 strains of methicillin-resistant *S. aureus* and seven strains of vancomycin-sensitive enterococci isolated from infected wounds, and 20 strains of vancomycin-resistant enterococci isolated from hospital environmental surfaces.[76] For all of the strains tested, the MIC values against manuka and pasture honey were below 10% v/v, but concentrations of artificial honey at least three times higher were required to achieve equivalent inhibition *in vitro*.

George and Cutting compared the sensitivity of 130 Gram-positive and Gram-negative clinical isolates, some of which possessed multiple antibiotic resistance, to a Leptospermum honey, Medihoney.[77] They reported that the growth of the *S. aureus* and MRSA was inhibited by 4% honey but the Gram-negative enterobacter including vancomycin resistant organisms required concentrations of 6-8% to inhibit growth. *P. aeruginosa* was the most resistant organism examined requiring 12-14% honey to inhibit bacterial development.[77]

All these laboratory studies may actually represent a very conservative assessment of the antimicrobial properties of honey when used as a wound dressing. Honey is often applied to a wound in much higher concentrations than those used in the laboratory and therefore its ability to kill microorganisms may be much greater than the studies suggest. At the highest concentrations, although the production of hydrogen peroxide may initially be inhibited, as the honey becomes diluted by the absorption of exudate, the hydrogen peroxide concentration will increase but this in turn will be broken down by catalase present in wound tissue and exudate.

Most studies which have investigated the antimicrobial properties of have concentrated upon its antibacterial activity, but Irish and her colleagues[78] examined the effects of four honeys and an artificial honey consisting of a number of sugars in water on three clinical isolates of Candida species. The honeys selected were; an unprocessed Jarrah honey; Medihoney Antibacterial Honey Barrier (a proprietary blend of Leptospermum and hydrogen peroxide honeys) and Comvita Wound Care 18+ (a manuka honey). The results varied according the species of Candida. Only Jarrah honey was significantly more active than the artificial honey against all three species. The remaining honeys were only marginally more effective, with MICs around 40% suggesting that most of the products depended principally on their high osmotic pressure to influence the growth of the fungi. Nevertheless, the authors concluded that these levels were achievable clinically provided that honey was applied in a concentrated form, and suggested that the results supported the case for conducting a formal clinical trial.

The ability of honey to kill common dermatophytes which cause skin infection (tineas) in man was invested by Brady et al.[79] Manuka and pasture honey (with a high degree of peroxide activity) were tested against clinical isolates including Epidermophyton, Microsporum and Trichophyton species and found to be active against all the organisms tested at concentrations ranging from 5-20%. The addition of catalase eliminated the activity of the pasture honey but the Manuka honey retained significant activity in the presence of the enzyme, suggesting that studies to assess the effectiveness of honey in the treatment of skin conditions caused by these organisms were indicated to confirm this effect in vivo.

The antibacterial properties of honey have been reviewed by Molan,[39,46,80,81] Cooper,[49,82] and Blair.[55]

Cytotoxicity of honey

The cytotoxicity of honey to human skin keratinocytes and dermal fibroblast in culture was compared with that of silver-impregnated dressings. Small dressing implants of monofloral, medicinal honey (L-Mesitran) and nanocrystalline silver (Acticoat) were placed in test wells and co-cultured with each of the two cell lines. Morphological changes, including cell toxicity, were assessed using standard techniques. Untreated cultures consisting of both keratinocytes and fibroblasts (group 1) were established in 90% of all cases. Cultures exposed to honey-impregnated implants, remained viable for extended periods (two and four months) but marked toxicity was observed in cultures exposed to the silver containing product ($p < 0.05$).

Effect of honey on biofilm formation

A major contribution to the development of infection by some species of bacteria is the formation of a biofilm, an aggregate of microorganisms in which individual cells become bound to a surface and to each other within a complex matrix of extracellular polymeric substances. Biofilm formation may be initiated by many factors, including specific or non-specific attachment sites on a surface or the presence of sub-inhibitory concentrations of antibiotic.

Biofilm formation commences with the attachment of free-floating microorganisms to a surface. These facilitate the arrival of other cells, a process which may be facilitated by quorum sensing, communication between the cells facilitated by signalling molecules such as oligopeptides in Gram-positive bacteria and N-Acyl Homoserine Lactones (AHL) in Gram-negative bacteria. Microbial cells growing in a biofilm are physiologically distinct from those of the same organism which exist in a liquid medium, and once in this form they become much harder to kill with antibiotics or antiseptics. It is for this reason that that the topic has attracted so much attention in recent years.

Laboratory studies have shown, however, that honey is effective against biofilms formed by a number of bacterial species including *P. aeruginosa*, *S. aureus*, (both antibiotic resistant and sensitive strains) and *K. pneumoniae*,[83-84] an observation which may help to explain the reported antimicrobial activity of honey when used as a topical wound dressing.

The possible reasons for this activity were investigated by Lerrer *et al.*[85] who showed that biofilm formation by *P. aeruginosa* is inhibited by fructose in honey, and mannosylated glycoproteins present in royal jelly. These molecules competitively blocked the activity of a lectin, PA-IIL, a key molecule involved in biofilm production.

The potential clinical benefits of topically applied honey are not limited to its antimicrobial properties however. It has been suggested that, following the use of honey, infection is rapidly cleared, inflammation, swelling, pain and odour are reduced, sloughing of necrotic tissue is induced, granulation and epithelialization are hastened, and healing occurs rapidly with minimal scarring.[51,86] Possible explanations for some of these effects are considered below.

Effect upon free radicals

A major cause of tissue damage in chronic wounds is thought to be the presence of free radicals, highly reactive molecules produced from superoxide anions generated by cells such as activated polymorphonuclear neutrophils (PMNs).

Henriques *et al.*[87] examined various types of honey for free radical production and quenching effects using electron paramagnetic resonance (EPR) spectroscopy and a superoxide quenching assay. The honeys examined were manuka, pasture, and commercial heat processed non-antibacterial honey. All samples tested had antioxidant potential, with manuka able to completely quench added radicals within five min of spiking. Only one peroxide-producing honey was found to form radicals on dilution.

The authors suggested that this superoxide quenching activity might contribute to the demonstrated ability of some types of honey to reduce inflammation in chronic wounds.

According to van den Berg et al.,[88] the major constituents of buckwheat honey, responsible for reducing levels of reactive oxygen species (ROS) by activated human PMNs 'in vitro' are phenolic constituents. These are present in relatively large but variable amounts, with the highly active honey exceeding the activities of samples with minor effects by factors of 4 to 30. The authors postulated that these phenolic compounds may also contribute to their antibacterial activity.

Pérez et al.[45] have suggested that the amino acid content of honey may have a previously underestimated role in determining its antioxidant properties of honey, perhaps even more important than that of the polyphenols.

Growth promoting action

The mechanisms responsible for the reported ability of honey to actively stimulate wound healing have been investigated in a number of studies including those published by Tonks et al. In their first publication they showed that release of tumour necrosis factor-alpha (TNF-alpha), a major factor in the control of the inflammatory process, is enhanced by honey in a monocytic cell line, Mono Mac 6 (MM6)[89]

In a second publication they compared the effect of each of three honeys (manuka, pasture and jelly bush) and a sugar syrup control (artificial honey) on the release of important inflammatory cytokines from the same cell line using specific ELISA assays for tumour necrosis factor-alpha (TNF-alpha) and interleukin (IL)-1beta and IL-6. All honeys significantly increased the TNF-alpha, IL-1beta and IL-6 release from MM6 cells when compared with untreated and artificial-honey-treated cells, suggesting that the effect of honey on wound healing may in part be related to the stimulation of inflammatory cytokines from monocytic cells.[90]

Conflicting views have been expressed about the identity of the agent(s) responsible for this activity. In their third paper, Tonks et al.[91] found that cytokine production did not correlate with endotoxin levels in honey and was not inhibited by polymyxin B an agent known to inhibit the effects of endotoxins. They also found that the activity was reduced significantly following heat treatment, indicating that component(s) other than endotoxins were responsible for the stimulatory activity of manuka honey. They then separated honey into fractions of different molecular weight, and upon further analysis showed the active fraction contained a number of components of varying molecular weights including a 5.8-kDa component, which stimulated production of TNF-alpha via TLR4

Timm et al.[92] also investigated the stimulatory effects of honey and like Tonks et al., showed that they induce interleukin-6 release from MM6 cells in culture, as well as the release of reactive oxygen species from all-trans retinoic acid (ATRA) differentiated HL-60 cells. However, in contrast to findings of Tonks, they reported that the immunomodulatory component of the natural honeys was heat stable, had a molecular weight greater than 20 kDa. Its activity was also eliminated by the addition of polymyxin B, leading them to conclude that it was in fact due to the presence of endotoxins.

The immunomodulatory properties of honey have been discussed in detail elsewhere,[93] in a review which also describes how manuka honey appears to increase prostaglandin E_2 (PGE$_2$) from monocytic cells. PGE$_2$ is involved in the inflammatory process and is known to increase sensitivity to pain which might explain the increased pain reported by some patients following the application of topical honey, although there is some evidence to suggest that pain associated with the use of honey may also be associated with its low pH.

Results of animal studies

Wound healing studies

Several studies have examined the effect of honey on wound healing using animal models. In one early study commercial unboiled honey was applied topically to open wounds on 12 mice. Twelve other mice had wounds dressed with saline to act as controls. Wound healing was judged histopathologically by measuring the speed of formation of granulation tissue and new epithelium. In this study wounds of the honey-treated animals healed much faster than the wounds of the control animals ($p < 0.001$).[94]

The effect of honey on healing rates of cutaneous wounds in rabbits was monitored by histopathological and biochemical changes. A three cm incision made was in the skin of the left thigh of each of 40 rabbits and the wounds of half the animals were treated twice daily treated with a topical application of five mL pure unheated honey, the other wounds remained untreated as controls. Honey treated wounds healed faster and developed greater strength days 14 and 21 than the controls.[95]

Similar benefits for the use of honey have been reported following its use in experimental wounds in rats. Osuagwu *et al.* divided twenty adult animals with excisional wound surgically inflicted on their sides into two groups. The experimental group had their wounds dressed with honey while the control group had normal saline dressing. Honey dressed wounds showed evidence of accelerated wound contraction, a key features of wound healing.[96]

Iftikhar *et al.* also reported an increase in the speed of wound healing in experimental incision, excision, burn and dead-space wounds in that were dressed with Acacia honey using in different formulations and dosages. Increases were reported in the area of epithelization which was followed by an increase in wound contraction, skin-breaking strength, and tissue granulation. The hydroxyproline content also increased in animals treated with higher doses of honey compared to control, indicating an increase in collagen formation.[97]

Less positive outcomes for the use of honey were recorded when it was compared with mafenide acetate in the treatment of experimental auricular burns in rabbits as the incidence of chondritis in honey-treated wounds was significantly raised compared with those dressed with mafenide.[98]

Infected wounds

When honey was applied to infected experimental wounds on rats inoculated with *S. aureus* or Klebsiella sp., and used to treat bacterial conjunctivitis induced by *E. coli*,

Proteus sp., *S. aureus*, Klebsiella sp., and *P. aeruginosa*, it was found to eliminate infection and accelerate healing in the infected wounds, and reduced redness, swelling, pus discharge and the time taken to eradicate bacterial infections in bacterial conjunctivitis. In all instances its potency was judged to be comparable to that of topical antibiotics.[99]

Surgical wounds

Several papers have described possible application for honey during surgical procedures following two separate animal studies in which the effect of honey was investigated on tumour implantation (TI) and the development of adhesions following peritonitis.

Tumour implantation development in surgical wounds is a potentially important consequence of cancer surgery. Particular attention has been given to trocar site recurrence following the growth of laparoscopic surgery. The effect of honey of TI was investigated in an animal study in which 60 mice, divided into two groups, were wounded in the posterior neck area. Mice in group one formed the control group, and those in group two had their wounds coated with honey before and after inoculation with transplantable Ehrlich ascites tumour. The presence of TI was confirmed in the wounded area by histopathological examination on the 10th day. Tumour implantation occurred in all the control animals but in only 8 of 30 mice in the honey treated group ($p < 0.001$). It was postulated that the physiological and chemical properties of honey protected wounds against TI and it was suggested that the use of honey could be considered as a wound barrier against TI during oncological surgery.[100]

To examine the effect of honey on the formation of peritoneal adhesions, 40 rats divided into two equal groups had adhesions surgical induced in the caecum and terminal ileum. In the control group, the adhesion areas were subsequently washed with saline solution five mL of which was left in the peritoneal cavity.

In the rats in the other group the surgical site was covered with honey and five mL of honey was left in the peritoneal cavity of each animals. Ten days later the rats were sacrificed and the adhesions were graded according to their degree of severity. The difference between the groups was found to be highly significant in favour of the honey treatment ($p < 0.001$). The authors concluded that although the mechanism of action is not clear, intra-peritoneal honey administration reduces peritoneal adhesion formation.[101]

In a similar study, bacterial peritonitis was induced in 18 rats by caecal ligation and puncture. The rats were randomly assigned to receive intraperitoneal injections of honey, 5% dextrose or no fluid or medicine intraperitoneally one day after surgery. Animals were sacrificed 14 days later to assess the adhesion score. Intraperitoneal honey was found to decrease the formation of postoperative intra-abdominal adhesions and reduce oxidative stress during peritonitis.[102]

The effects of honey on intestinal morphology, postoperative adhesions, and the healing of colonic anastomoses were also examined.[103] Colonic resection and anastomosis were performed on 36 rats divided into three equal groups. All the animals were given a standard diet, supplemented in one group by honey 10 g/kg/day or an artificial honey supplement with the same caloric content as honey. The third group received an unmodified diet.

The animals were sacrificed and adhesion scores, bursting pressures and histopathological examinations were undertaken. The colonic bursting pressures of the honey group were significantly higher than those of the control and artificial honey groups. On histological examination honey treated animals showed more advanced healing and a statistically significant reduction in adhesion scores compared with the artificial honey and control groups, indicating that honey has a protective role against intra-abdominal adhesions and anastomotic dehiscence.

Reports also exist of honey being used in veterinary practice. In one it was used to manage a bite wound in a stumptail macaque (*Macaca arctoides*) where it produced rapid healing and reduced the need for sedation for frequent bandage changes.[104]

Allen and Molan examined the sensitivity of organisms responsible for the formation of mastitis in cows, and showed that six organisms were inhibited by 5% manuka honey, only one, *Klebsiella pneumoniae*, was able to survive under these conditions although this was killed by a 10% honey solution and on this basis suggested that a clinical study was warranted to investigate the effectiveness of intramammary honey for mastitis.[105]

Burns

Medical honey of defined activity was compared with sugar and silver sulphadiazine (SSD) in deep dermal experimental burns in pigs.[106] Wounds treated with the materials under examination were biopsied on days 7, 14, 21, 28, 35 and 42. Wounds treated with SSD were fully epithelialized after 28-35 days, whereas those treated with honey or sugar were closed in 21 days. Upon histological examination at day 21, compared with sugar treated wounds, those dressed with honey showed 'quiet granulation', inconspicuous inflammation and a decrease in actine staining in myofibroblasts, leading the authors to conclude that honey offered advantages over sugar for this application.

Wijesinghe et al.[107] undertook a systematic review and meta-analysis of randomised controlled trials which compared the efficacy of honey with a comparator dressing treatment in the management of burns. They identified eight studies involving a total of 624 subjects. Despite the poor quality of the studies, the fixed effects odds ratio for healing at 15 days was 6.1 (95% CI 3.7 to 9.9) in favour of honey having a superior effect. The random effects pooled odds ratio was 6.7 (95% CI 2.8 to 15.8) in favour of honey treatment. The authors concluded that although the available evidence indicated that honey was superior to alternative dressing treatments (typically gauze impregnated with SSD) for superficial or partial thickness burns, the limitations of the studies restricted the clinical value of their findings.

Pharmaceutical considerations

Bioburden of natural honey

Raw honey can be contaminated with microorganisms such as fungi and bacteria, including anaerobic spore forming organisms, the presence of which is particularly undesirable in a substance used as a wound dressing. According to Yoon and Newlands,[108] historically the bioburden of honey has been found to vary from < 100 colony forming units (cfu)/g to > 50,000 cfu/g.

When the bioburden of 25 honey samples acquired in Costa Rica were determined using standard laboratory techniques, only 9% produced counts >10 cfu/g and *C. botulinum* was not isolated from any samples.

For both legal and clinical reasons, honey used as a dressing is required to be sterile. As heating adversely affect its antimicrobial properties, an alternative method of sterilization is required to eliminate this contamination.

Sterilization of honey

The possible use of ionizing radiation was investigated by Postmes *et al.*,[109] who examined the effects of increasing doses of gamma irradiation ranging from 6 to 25 kGy on six batches of honey spiked with *C. botulinum* or *B. subtilis* at a concentration of approximately 10^6 spores per 50 grams of honey.

Even at the highest dose the antibacterial activity remained unaltered and all batches honey proved to be sterile after irradiation with a dose of 25 kGy.

Molan and Allen[110] compared the antibacterial activity of two honeys with activity due to hydrogen peroxide and three manuka honeys before and after commercial sterilization using gamma irradiation. They found no significant change in potency, even when the dose of radiation was doubled from 25 kGy to 50 kGy and confirmed that 25 kGy of gamma-irradiation was sufficient to achieve sterility in honey seeded with *C. tetani* and *C. perfringens* at a concentration of 1,000 and 10,000 spores per gram of honey of respectively.

An International Medical Device requirement is that the bioburden of materials to be sterilised by irradiation must be < 500 cfu/g, to ensure that the process successfully inactivates all viable organisms present.

This means that all possible efforts must be made to ensure that production, collection and manipulation of honey is conducted as cleanly as possible. The practical problems and quality standard relating to the production of honey intended for medical use have been described by Yoon and Newlands[108] and Molan and Hill[111].

Combining honey with different ointment bases was shown to markedly influence its stability and bioavailability.[112]

Commercial sources of honey dressings

Numerous companies supply honey-based products for use as wound dressings although precise details of the nature of the honey used in the production of these products is not always clearly indicated on the label or contained in their supporting literature. Users of honey based products should, in the first instance, be guided by product claims on the packaging and the 'Instructions for Use' (IFU) leaflet, as it is these claims that determine regulatory approval. Some honeys claim a specific level of antimicrobial activity and so any potential user should therefore ensure that they are familiar with the properties of the various products available and select one that contains the required level of activity. Honey containing dressings are supplied by numerous companies as follows.

Advancis Medical is owned by Brightwake Ltd and use *L. scoparium* (manuka) honey, with the brand name of 'Activon'. Preparations containing this honey are:

- Activon Tube, 25 grams of honey in a plastic tube
- Activon Tulle, a low-adherent knitted viscose primary wound dressing impregnated with honey
- Actilite, a low-adherent knitted viscose primary wound dressing impregnated with a mixture of Activon honey and manuka oil which is claimed to enhance its antimicrobial properties
- Algivon, a calcium alginate fleece impregnated with Activon

Aspen Medical, previously Unomedical, market the Mesitran range of honey dressings manufactured by Triticum. Unlike Medihoney (see later) which is marketed as an 'antibacterial honey', the Mesitran range is promoted by Aspen Medical principally for debridement and odour control. No information on the source of the honey is provided in the relevant literature. The honey is simply described as 'medical Grade' and is available in a number of forms:

- Mesitran is a hydrogel sheet approximately one mm thick attached to a semipermeable polyurethane membrane by means of a thin fibrous bonding layer. The hydrogel, which is capable of absorbing seven times its own weight of wound fluid, contains 30% of medical Grade honey
- Mesitran Border consists of a piece of Mesitran gel the backing layer of which extends past the margin of the hydrogel to form an island dressing
- Mesitran Mesh consists of an open net-like structure coated with Mesitran hydrogel which allows wound exudate to pass into a secondary absorbent dressing
- Mesitran Ointment, an ointment containing 47% honey
- Mesitran Ointment S, an ointment containing 40% honey for patients with 'sensitive wounds'

Dermagenics BV, a subsidiary of Greystone Pharmaceuticals, produces Melmax a sterile, non-adherent wound dressing composed of buckwheat honey which the manufacturers claim contains a rich source of phenolic compounds that have been shown to provide antioxidant activity and an anti-bacterial effect

ERAS produces 'Wound Honey' made from active manuka honey, *Aloe vera* extract and D-panthenol.

Manuka Honey USA is an importer of a range of New Zealand honey products to the USA. These include:
- Wound Care 18+, pure manuka honey
- Meloderm Ointment which consists of 40% manuka honey (UMF16+), white soft paraffin, Purified Honey BP, cetyl stearyl alcohol, acetylated lanolin alcohol, sorbitan sesquioleate, caprylic/capric triglyceride, 2-bromo-2-nitropropane, 1,3 diol, dichlorobenzyl alcohol in 50 gram tubes

Medihoney brand is owned by Comvita Ltd (NZ). The product is available in a number of formulations and contains a blend of honey predominantly from *Leptospermum* sp. including Jellybush honey.
- Medihoney Medical Honey, 20 or 50 grams of honey in a plastic tube (primarily used for fistulas and sinuses)
- Medihoney Antibacterial Wound Gel consists of 80% Medihoney and plant waxes, used for general wound care.
- Medihoney Antibacterial Gel Sheet consists of Medihoney mixed with alginate powder to form a cohesive layer (also called Honeycolloid)
- Medihoney Antibacterial Tulle, is a low-adherent knitted viscose primary wound dressing impregnated with Medihoney
- Medihoney Calcium Alginate, is a fleece of alginate fibre impregnated with Medihoney
- Medihoney Barrier Cream contains 30% honey with other natural ingredients

Mediprof in the Netherlands produces Honeysoft, a low adherent dressing made of ethylene vinyl acetate impregnated with a multifloral honey harvested in the pre-Andes mountains of Chili (1500 m).

Sanomed produces Sanoskin Melladerm, and Melladerm Plus, both honey based ointment/gels presented in 50 gram tubes. No information on composition or the nature of the honey is freely available.

Triticum Exploitatie BV, produces the Mesitran range marked by Aspen Medical, also sells a similar range of products under the brand name L-Mesitran:
- L-Mesitran Hydro is a hydrogel sheet approximately one mm thick attached to a semipermeable polyurethane membrane by means of a thin fibrous bonding layer. The hydrogel, which is capable of absorbing seven times its own weight of wound fluid, contains 30% of medical Grade honey
- L-Mesitran Border consists of a piece of Mesitran gel the backing layer of which extends past the margin of the hydrogel to form an island dressing
- L-Mesitran Active, small pieces of L-Mesitran Border for use in the consumer market as first aid dressings
- L-Mesitran Mesh consists of an open net-like structure coated with the Mesitran hydrogel which allows wound exudate to pass into a secondary absorbent dressing
- L-Mesitran Ointment, an ointment containing 47% honey together with medical Grade lanolin, cod liver oil (claimed to stimulate epidermal cell

growth), Sun flower oil as a scavenger of free radicals, Calendula Mari Gold, a product attributed with 'inflammatory properties', Aloe Vera, vitamins E and C as antioxidants, and zinc oxide

- L-Mesitran Soft, an ointment containing 47% honey together with medical Grade lanolin, Polyethylene Glycol, a humectant and preservative and vitamins E and C as antioxidants

Clinical experience with honey

Unlike most dressings, which pass through predetermined stages of development and testing prior to clinical use in order to ensure consistency and demonstrate safety and efficacy, honey was being applied to wounds for many millennia before any attempt was made to standardize or characterize it in any way.

As result, unlike with most dressings, where it is possible to make comparisons between clinical results achieved with a specific product, the variable nature of honey either precludes such comparisons or greatly reduces their value. For example, many of the early studies utilised honey obtained from sources which have since been shown in laboratory studies to possess little or no non-peroxide activity and it is therefore unwise to assume that these will necessarily perform in a similar way to products with high levels of non-peroxide antibacterial activity.

Miscellaneous wounds

Much of the early use of honey was in Africa where it was used for treating wounds of all types because it was cheap and freely available. It was one of the agents used in Ghana to treat 25 patients with sickle cell disease over a three year period,[113] although a subsequent study comparing honey with a hypochlorite solution, Edinburgh University solution of lime (EUSOL) in 20 patients with this condition found no significant difference in healing rates between the treatment groups.[114]

A rather more positive outcome for honey compared with EUSOL was reported following a randomized controlled trial involving the treatment of 32 Nigerian children with 43 abscesses caused by pyomyositis, a serious infection of skeletal muscle. All subjects had their wounds incised and drained and were given a 21-day course of antibiotics. The wounds were packed twice-daily with either honey or EUSOL-soaked gauze. Honey-treated wounds healed significantly faster than those packed with EUSOL and the length of hospital stay was significantly shorter.[115]

In Burandi honey was used to treat 40 patients with various wounds, producing healing in 88% of cases.[116]

In an early report of the use of honey in the treatment of patients with longstanding ulcers in Nigeria published in 1988,[117] 58 of 59 wounds showed remarkable improvement, only one case, later diagnosed as a Buruli ulcer, failed to respond; wounds that were initially free of contamination remained so until healed, whilst the bioburden of infected wounds and ulcers was virtually eliminated within one week of the application of honey. Honey debrided wounds rapidly, replacing slough with granulation tissue. It also promoted rapid epithelialization, and absorption of oedema from around the ulcer margins.

In an early Phase II feasibility study featuring 21 patients with chronic wounds, 23 with complicated surgical wounds and or 16 with acute traumatic wounds, honey was found easy to apply, helpful in cleaning the wounds, and without side effects in all but one patient.[118]

Equally positive results were reported following an evaluation of a sterile, non-adherent dressing impregnated with manuka honey in 20 patients with a variety of wounds.[119]

Honey has been compared with a variety of other dressings in numerous studies, the results of which have generally favoured the honey. In one, 40 patients with open or infected wounds were randomized to receive either honey or sugar dressings. In 22 honey treated patients the number who had positive wound cultures fell from 55% at the start of treatment to 23% after one week. In the 18 sugar treated wounds the corresponding figures were 52% and 39% respectively. The median rate of healing in the first two weeks of treatment was 3.8 vs 2.2 cm^2 and after three weeks of treatment 86% of patients treated with honey had no pain during dressing changes, compared with 72% treated with sugar. The authors concluded that honey appears to be more effective than sugar in reducing bacterial contamination, promoting wound healing, and is less painful than sugar during dressing changes and motion.[1]

In a prospective, randomized, double-blind controlled trial, honey was compared with Intrasite Gel for the treatment of shallow wounds and abrasions incurred by goldmine workers. No evidence of a real difference between the two treatments was detected in terms of healing rates but honey was a fraction of the price of the hydrogel and therefore judged to be extremely cost effective in use.[120]

Ahmed et $al.$[118] described the results of a phase II feasibility study in which they assessed a honey impregnated dressing, Honeysoft, in the treatment of 60 patients with a variety of non healing wounds. One patient withdrew because of pain, but healing was achieved in 57 of the remaining 59 subjects in an average treatment time of three weeks (range 1 - 28 weeks).

Fournier's gangrene

In 1993 Efem[121] described treatment outcomes for 41 cases of Fournier's gangrene. Twenty one patients were given standard treatment consisting of wound debridement and excision, secondary suturing, and in some cases scrotal plastic reconstruction. The remaining 20 cases were managed conservatively with the topical application of unprocessed honey. Both groups were given systemic antibiotic therapy.

Even though the average duration of hospitalization was slightly longer in the honey treated patients, 4.5 vs 4 weeks, the honey treatment showed distinct advantages over the orthodox method. No deaths occurred in patients treated with honey but three deaths occurred in the conventionally treated group. Furthermore by the use of honey the need for anaesthesia and expensive surgical operation was obviated and a favourable response to treatment accelerated.

Tahmaz et $al.$ conducted a similar study involving 33 patients.[122] As in the previous study, 21 patients were given broad-spectrum antibiotics, surgical debridement, exhaustive cleaning, and split-thickness skin grafts or delayed closure as appropriate.

The remaining 12 patients were treated with unprocessed honey, 20 - 50 mL daily and antimicrobial therapy without debridement. The wounds were inspected daily and the honey was reapplied after cleaning with normal saline. The patients' scrotum and penis were then covered with their own new scrotal skin. The mean duration of hospital stay was 41 ± 10.5 days (range 14 - 54).

Two patients given traditional treatment treated died from severe sepsis. There were no deaths in the honey treated group. Clinical and cosmetic results were judged to be superior in honey treated wounds leading the authors to conclude like those of the previous paper that 'unprocessed honey might revolutionise the treatment of this dreadful disease by reducing its cost, morbidity, and mortality'

Hejase et al.[123] and Gurdal et al.[124] also used honey in the treatment of patients with Fournier's gangrene but only as an adjunct to conventional treatment.

Abdominal wall dehiscence

Phuapradit and Saropala[125] assessed the value of honey as a method of managing abdominal wound dehiscence in fifteen patients whose wounds had broken down after a Caesarean section. The wounds were dressed with honey application and the wounds edges brought together using surgical tape instead of resuturing. Excellent results were achieved in all cases with complete healing within two weeks.

The use of honey for this indication was investigated more formally in 50 patients having postoperative wound infections following caesarean sections or total abdominal hysterectomies. Twenty-six patients were treated with 12 hourly applications of crude honey and 24 patients were treated with local antiseptics which included povidone-iodine. Both groups received appropriate systemic antibiotic cover. Infections were eliminated after 6 ± 1.9 days in honey-treated wounds and 14.8 ± 4.2 days in those dressed conventionally ($p < 0.05$). Antibiotic usage was also greatly reduced 6.88 ± 1.7 days vs 15.45 ± 4.37 days ($p < 0.05$) as was the length of hospital stay. Complete healing was achieved in 10.73 ± 2.5 days vs 22.04 ± 7.33 days ($p < 0.05$). Closure without wound disruption or a need for re-suturing was achieved in 22/26 (84.4%) of honey-treated patients and only four patients showed mild dehiscence. In the control group only 12/24 (50%) of patients healed uneventfully, 12 patients developed wound dehiscence and six required re-suturing under general anaesthesia. The quality of the healed wounds was also improved following honey treatment, resulting in smaller scars, 3.6 ± 1.4 mm using topical honey and 8.6 ± 3.8 mm with local antiseptics ($p < 0.05$).[126]

Infections caused by antibiotic-resistant bacteria

Honey has also been used successfully to treat antibiotic-resistant strains of microorganisms in vivo,[127] when full healing was achieved in seven consecutive patients whose wounds were either infected or colonized with methicillin-resistant S. aureus that had failed to respond to other forms of treatment.

Paediatric wounds

Honey was used to dress the wounds of nine infants with large, open, infected wounds that failed to heal with conventional treatment. All infants had their wounds dressed with 5 - 10 mL of fresh unprocessed honey twice daily and after five days of treatment all showed marked clinical improvement. By 21 days the wounds of all infants were closed, clean and sterile.[128]

In an unusual case, honey was used to treat an 11-day-old baby who presented with necrotizing fasciitis of the scalp from which *E. coli* was cultured. Treatment consisted of administration of parenteral broad-spectrum antibiotics and debridement. Skin grafting of the resulting scalp defect was not permitted by the parents. The wound healed with scar tissue over a three month period.[129]

Simon *et al.*[130] described how Medihoney was successfully used, often in conjunctions with systemic antibiotics, for treating a variety of different wounds in immunosuppressed paediatric patients receiving chemotherapy in Department of Paediatric Oncology, Children's Hospital, University of Bonn for three years.

Surgical wounds

The successful use of honey was reported as part of a treatment regimen which also involved the use the maggots and vacuum assisted closure to achieve closure of an extensive wound to the lower abdomen on a patient undergoing chemotherapy for the treatment of mantle cell lymphoma.[131]

Eight patients who had undergone coronary artery bypass who had developed wound dehiscence in their leg wounds following removal of veins for grafting were successfully treated with Medihoney Antibacterial Gel.[132]

Radiotherapy wounds

It is generally believed that honey may be of value in the treatment of radiation induced dermatitis. This possibility was investigated in a small randomized control trial in which a honey gauze (Honeysoft) was compared with a paraffin gauze dressing in 24 evaluable patients.[133] The results of the study revealed a non significant trend towards more rapid healing in favour of the honey dressing.

In a second study, four patients who had previously undergone radiotherapy that left them with fragile friable areas of damaged skin that did not respond to conventional treatment had the affected areas dressed with honey. The wounds of two healed in 2.5 weeks, and the other two showed marked improvement at the time of the patients' death. The authors suggested that prospective, randomized, controlled clinical studies were needed to confirm their initial observations.[134]

The possibility that honey could be used with good effect as a prophylactic treatment to prevent radiochemotherapy-induced mucositis was investigated in a randomised study involving 40 patients diagnosed with head and neck cancer who were receiving concomitant chemotherapy and radiotherapy and in whom a significant area of directly visible oral and/or oropharyngeal mucosa was included in the radiation field.[135] No patients in the group treated with honey developed grade four mucositis and only three patients (15 per cent) developed grade three mucositis. In the control group, 13 patients (65 per cent) developed grade three or four mucositis (p < 0.05). Candida colonisation was found in 15 per cent of the treatment group and 60 per cent of the control group, either during or after radiotherapy (p = 0.003). Positive cultures for aerobic pathogenic bacteria were observed in 15 per cent of the treatment group and 65 per cent of the control group, during or after radiotherapy. The results of this investigation strongly support the proposition that the prophylactic use of pure natural can reduce mucositis in this patient group.

Epidermolysis Bullosa

Epidermolysis bullosa (EB) represents a particular challenge to those responsible for patients who suffer from this distressing condition. One report described how a honey impregnated dressing successfully achieved closure in a 20 year lesion in just 15 weeks.[136] A second report described the use of honey in a 45-year-old man with this condition.[137]

Diabetic ulcers

Honey dressings were compared with povidone iodine followed by normal saline for treating for Wagner Grade-II diabetic foot ulcers following surgical debridement. Appropriate antibiotic cover was also provided to all patients. The mean healing time for 30 patients in the povidone iodine group was 15.4 days (range 9 - 36) compared with to 14.4 days (range 7 - 26) in the honey group (p < 0.005).[138]

Ophthalmology

The effect of honey on the ocular flora of patients with tear deficiency and meibomian gland disease, which leads to an overgrowth of bacteria on the surface of the eye, was investigated in a prospective, open label pilot study. A total of 66 subjects with dry eye and 18 non-dry eye subjects were recruited as controls, all of whom had not worn contact lenses for at least three months before entering the study.

Sterile cotton-tipped applicators were used to swab the surface of the eye and the lid margin and the total number of colony forming units present determined using standard microbiological techniques. Each subject was then instructed to apply Medihoney ophthalmic ointment to the eye three times daily for three months. Initially the number of colony forming units isolated from each of the dry eye subjects was significantly greater than that isolated from the non-dry eye subjects, but following the use of the honey there was a progressive decrease in number so that by the end of three months the number in the two groups was not statistically different suggesting that honey has a potential role in the treatment of chronic ocular infections.[139]

Catheter infections

The ability of a manuka honey, Medihoney, to prevent catheter-associated infections in catheter exit sites was compared with that of mupirocin in a randomized, controlled pilot study involving 101 patients who were receiving haemodialysis via tunnelled, cuffed central venous catheters. Both treatment groups were given thrice-weekly applications of the appropriate agent and the incidences of catheter-associated bacteraemias in both were comparable: no exit-site infections occurred. It was concluded that the use of the standardized honey appeared to be was a safe, cost-effective treatment for this indication but that much larger studies would be required to demonstrate therapeutic equivalence.[140]

Toenail surgery

One study, which did not result in a particularly favourable outcome for honey, compared it with paraffin gauze in a double-blind randomized controlled trial in 100 patients who had undergone with matrix phenolization for toenail removal. Fifty two participants were randomly assigned to receive active manuka honey dressing and 48 a paraffin-impregnated tulle gras. The mean healing times for all honey treated wounds compared with paraffin gauze were 40.3 ± 8.2 days vs 40.0 ± 25.4.

Following partial avulsion, wounds healed statistically significantly faster ($p = 0.01$) with paraffin tulle, 19.6 ± 9.31 vs 31.8 ± 18.8 days but no significant difference ($p = 0.21$) was found following total avulsion when comparing honey 45.28 ± 8.03 vs 52.03 ± 21.3.[141]

Burns

The use of honey in the treatment of burns in the Indian subcontinent has been described in a number of publications by Subrahmanyam, who compared it with several other forms of treatment in the management of partial thickness burns with generally positive results. In the first study involving 46 patients, honey-impregnated gauze was compared with a semipermeable film dressing, Opsite when the mean healing times for the two treatments were found to be 10.8 vs 15.3 days respectively.[142]

In a similar study involving 64 patients, honey-impregnated gauze was compared with amniotic membrane. The 40 honey treated wounds healed in mean of 9.4 days compared with 17.5 days for wounds dressed with amnion ($p < 0.001$). The quality of healing was also superior with honey with residual scarring noted in 8% of honey-treated patients compared with 16.6% of those treated with amnion ($p < 0.001$).[143]

Honey was also found to be superior to another natural product, boiled potato peel, in a randomized controlled trial involving 100 patients. The wounds of 90% of the 50 patients treated with honey became 'sterile' within seven days but in those treated with potato peel persistent infection was noted. All honey treated wounds healed within 15 days but only 50% of wounds treated with boiled potato peel healed during this time. The mean healing times for the two treatments were 10.4 vs 16.2 days respectively.[144]

Honey also appeared to offer benefits over a more modern conventional treatment, silver sulfadiazine (SSD), when compared in two groups of 25 randomly allocated patients. By day seven 84% of honey treated wounds had epithelialized compared with 72% of those treated with SSD. After three weeks all honey treated wounds had healed compared with 84% of patients treated with SSD. Histological examination of the wounds showed that in honey treated burns acute inflammatory changes subsided relatively rapidly but in the SSD treated wounds sustained inflammatory reaction was noted even on epithelialization.[145]

Much less favourable results were obtained when honey was employed to treat more serious (deeper) burns. Fifty patients were randomized to early tangential excision and skin grafting, or the application of honey dressings with delayed skin grafting as necessary. Patients in both groups were well matched in terms of wound area and burn severity. In the surgical group, the skin graft take rate was $99 \pm 3\%$ but in the 11 patients in the honey group who required grafting the graft take rate was $74 \pm 18\%$ ($p < 0.01$). Treatment outcomes were also better in the surgically treated group. Three patients treated with honey died from sepsis but only one patient died in the control group due to status asthmaticus. After three months 92% of the surgical patients had 'good' to 'excellent' functional and cosmetic results compared with 55% of those treated with honey, three of whom had significant contractures.

The only advantage associated with the use of the honey treatment was that less blood was required, an important consideration as the availability of suitable allogenic blood was considered to be a potential logistical problem. The mean percentage of blood volume replaced was $35 \pm 12\%$ in the surgical patients compared with $21 \pm 15\%$ in those treated with honey, ($p < 0.01$). The authors concluded that in patients with moderate burns, early tangential excision and skin grafting was clearly superior to the use of topical honey.[146]

A review of all patients with burn injuries admitted to hospital over a 5-year period in Ilesha, Nigeria, revealed that about 70% of the 156 patients had major burns or scalds. In about 90% of cases, silver sulphadiazine was used as a topical antimicrobial agent while natural honey was used on the rest. Wound infection occurred in 24.4% of wounds and the mortality rate was recorded in 7.7% of cases.[147]

Skin grafts

One publication has described a pilot study involving 11 patients in which a honey dressing was successfully used to help retain split thickness skin grafts.[148]

Leg ulcers

A potentially important indication for the use of honey is the treatment of leg ulcers, and the literature contains numerous case studies describing its use for this application with varying degrees of success.[149-151] One study described how, without cessation of hydroxyurea or cyclosporine therapy, manuka honey eliminated MRSA and successfully promoted healing in an immunosuppressed patient who developed a hydroxyurea-induced leg ulcer.[152]

In another, eight cases of leg ulceration of differing aetiology were dressed weekly with manuka honey for four weeks during which the mean wound area decreased from 5.6 to 2.25 cm^2, odour was eliminated and pain reduced.[153]

Forty patients with ulcers that had previously failed to respond to three months compression therapy were dressed with Medihoney for a further 12 weeks.[154] During this time 12 patients dropped out and one died. The average wound area of the remaining patients decreased steadily, and seven ulcers healed completely. A significant reduction was recorded in the size of the 20 ulcers which had not closed by the end of the study, but the size of the wounds of the surviving patients who dropped out remained static.

In this trial, honey also appeared to have marked effect upon wound pain. Eleven patients reported an increase in wound pain (6 of whom dropped out of the study), 20 reported that their pain decreased and in five patients pain levels remained unchanged. The presence of pain was found to be inversely related to healing. Only those patients who had no pain or a decreasing pain showed a substantial reduction in wound size.

The use of honey as a dressing following split-skin grafting in six patients with chronic venous leg ulcers and a 'less than ideal blood supply' was investigated by Schumacher et al.[155] He recorded that healing times in this group of patients, whom he regarded as being at a higher than normal risk of graft failure, appeared to be similar to those in patients free of the additional risk factors.

Emsen[148] also reported good results when he used honey as a retention dressing following split thickness skin grafting in 11 patients .

Honey has also been used as a donor site dressing during skin grafting. Misirlioglu et al.[156] compared the effectiveness of honey-impregnated gauze, hydrocolloid dressings, paraffin gauze and saline-soaked gauze as dressing for donor sites in a non-randomized, prospective, open-label study.

Eighty-eight patients who underwent skin grafting were split into two groups. In the first group, the donor site was divided into two equal halves. One half of each wound was treated with honey-soaked gauze and the other half with paraffin gauze, a hydrocolloid dressing, or saline-soaked gauzes. In the second group, two separate donor sites were formed, one of which was treated with honey-impregnated gauze and the other with one of the alternative products.

In both groups honey-impregnated gauze produced more rapid healing and reduced pain than paraffin gauze and saline-soaked gauze. No significant difference was detected between the honey-impregnated gauze and the hydrocolloid dressing.

Honey has also been compared with phenytoin or a phenytoin/honey mixture in 50 patients with leg ulcers. The overall reduction in the area of honey treated wounds was less than that achieved with phenytoin although the difference was not statistically significant. Four wounds dressed with phenytoin progressed to complete healing by the end of four weeks leading the authors to conclude that phenytoin may be superior to honey as a topical agent in the treatment of chronic ulcers.[157]

At least three large-scale studies have investigated the use of honey in the treatment of leg ulcers, two of which compared it with current best practice and one with a hydrogel.

In a community-based open-label randomized trial,[158] 187 patients with a venous ulcer were randomized to treatment with a calcium alginate dressing impregnated with manuka honey, and 181 to 'usual care'. All participants received compression bandaging. After 12 weeks, 104 ulcers (55.6 percent) in the honey-treated group and 90 (49.7 percent) in the usual care group had healed but this difference was not significant (p = 0.258). Wounds treated with honey also achieved a 9.6% greater reduction in area compared to baseline and 23% fewer episodes of infection although neither parameter achieved statistical significance.

The application of honey was found to result in increased pain compared with traditional treatments, 47 *vs* 18, (p = 0·001). In the honey treated group, the wounds of 19 patients deteriorated compared with nine in the standard therapy but this difference was failed to reach significance (p = 0·061). Patients allocated to honey treatment spent a total of ten patient-days in hospital compared with 40 patient-days for those treated conventionally, but the authors dismissed this finding suggesting that it was probably due to 'random variation'. When the treatment costs were compared, overall there was a financial advantage in favour of honey if the cost of hospitalization was included in the calculation but this was reversed if the hospital costs were omitted.

The authors concluded that although the use of honey appeared to produce some beneficial effects upon healing and infection rates, these were was insufficiently robust to support the proposition that honey-impregnated dressings significantly improved venous ulcer healing at 12 weeks compared with usual care. They also stated that treatment with honey was probably more expensive and statistically likely to be associated with more adverse events (p = 0.013).

In the second study,[159] a standardised medical Grade honey (Medihoney) was compared with conventional treatments on the healing rates of wounds healing by secondary intention in a single centre, open-label randomized controlled trial in which patients were randomized to receive either a conventional wound dressing or honey. The median time to healing in the honey group was 100 days compared to 140 days in the control group. The healing rate at 12 weeks was equal to 46.2% in the honey group compared to 34.0% in the conventional group, but this difference in the healing rates failed to reach significance (p = 0.321).

Although not specifically addressed in this study it is likely that the reduction in healing times had implications for treatment costs (consumables and nursing time) and also improved the quality of life of the patients concerned.

Whilst the data strongly suggests that healing times following treatment with honey are reduced compared with conventional treatment, and the results are of clinical significance (median of 100 compared to 140 days respectively), as with the Jull study,[158] insufficient patients were included for this to reach statistical significance.

The ability of manuka honey (WoundCare 18+) to promote debridement in leg ulcers was compared with that of Intrasite Gel in a prospective, multicentre, open label randomized controlled trial. One hundred and eight patients with venous leg ulcers having ≥ 50% of the wound area covered in slough were recruited. The treatment was applied weekly for four weeks and follow-up was made at week 12. After four weeks the mean percentage reduction in slough was 67% *vs* 52.9% for honey and hydrogel respectively (p = 0.054). The mean area of the wound covered in slough similarly reduced, 29% *vs* 43%, respectively (p = 0.065). The median percentage reduction in wound area was 34% *vs* 13% (p = 0.001). By three months 44% of honey dressed wounds had healed compared with 33% dressed with hydrogel (p = 0.037). Infection developed in six of the honey treated patients compared with 12 in the hydrogel group. This difference was judged to be 'clinically but not significantly significant'.[160]

In a second publication prepared from data obtained during this study, the same authors compared the qualitative bacteriological changes that occurred within the wounds dressed with the two products during the four week treatment period. *S. aureus* was the most common isolate, being identified in 41 wounds (38%). At baseline, methicillin-resistant *S. aureus* was identified in 16 wounds (ten honey *vs* six hydrogel). After four weeks MRSA had been eradicated from 70% (n = 7) of the manuka-honey treated wounds versus 16% (n = 1) of the hydrogel treated wounds. *P. aeruginosa* was reported in 14% (n = 16) of all wounds at baseline. After four weeks this organism was eliminated from 33% (n = 2) honey treated wounds and 50% (n = 5) of wounds treated with the hydrogel. The number of wounds at baseline (n = 11) and at week 4 (n = 15) with ≥ 3 bacterial species remained constant over the four weeks.[161]

The results of these three studies provide some further support for the proposition that there are clinical benefits associated with the use of honey in the management in leg ulcers in clinical practice.

Meningococcal lesions

Dunford provided an impressive account of the benefits of a honey in the treatment of a young male patient with partial amputations and long-standing areas of extensive skin loss resulting from meningococcal septicaemia. The wounds on his legs were heavily infected with a number of organisms including *S. aureus*, pseudomonads and enterococcus sp. Conventional treatment, including skin grafts, had proved unsuccessful, but a change of therapy to a Manuka honey dressing resulted in a rapid, marked improvement in all treated wounds within a few days enabling them to be grafted successfully.[162]

Current status of honey in wound care

Several systematic reviews have been undertaken on the clinical use of honey. Moore *et al.*[163] in 2001 in a review entitled 'Systematic review of the use of honey as a wound dressing' reported that 'Confidence in a conclusion that honey is a useful treatment for superficial wounds or burns is low' but admitted 'There is biological plausibility.'

Bardy *et al.*[164] in 2008 in their review 'A systematic review of honey uses and its potential value within oncology care' were a little more positive, suggesting that 'Honey was found to be a suitable alternative for wound healing, burns and various skin conditions and to potentially have a role within cancer care.'

Jull *et al.*[165] concluded that 'Honey may improve healing times in mild to moderate superficial and partial thickness burns compared with some conventional dressings. Honey dressings as an adjuvant to compression do not significantly increase leg ulcer healing at 12 weeks. There is insufficient evidence to guide clinical practice in other areas'.

Kingsley[166] also adopted a cautious stance, suggesting that not all the expected beneficial effects of honey are always realised in practice.

The studies included in these reviews involved the use of honey from widely different sources with, it is assumed, very different levels of antimicrobial activity. The value of these systematic reviews is therefore open to question. Only clinical data generated using honeys of known potency should be combined in this way, particularly in relation to the management of infected wounds. To do otherwise is not to compare like with like. Furthermore, future clinical trials should only be conducted using materials the properties of which have been fully characterized.

Rather more favourable views on the value of honey have been expressed by others in more general and less structured reviews. Many of these authors have concluded that despite the absence of data from large-scale randomized controlled trials, clinical experience with honey appears to suggest that it does have a role to play in the management of infected or sloughy wounds.[167-175] A further group of authors whilst sharing this opinion stressed the need for more clinical studies.[176-179] Practical advice on use of honey offered by Betts,[180] and White.[181]

In 1989 Zumla and Lulat[34] said that 'Although honey has been used for commercial and domestic uses for thousands of years, much of the literature is only descriptive. Further evaluation and application of the healing properties of honey in other clinical and laboratory situations is warranted.'

In the intervening 20 years, much additional work has been undertaken although some questions still remain unanswered. Nevertheless, it is difficult not to have some sympathy with the position of Molan[182] who, in 2006, produced an excellent comprehensive summary of published data on the use of honey available at that time. In total he identified 17 randomized controlled trials involving a total of 1965 participants, and five clinical trials of other forms involving 97 participants treated with honey and 16 trials on a total of 533 wounds on experimental animals. Given this wealth of information, he expressed his astonishment that there appears to be a lack of universal acceptance of honey as a wound dressing, and invited clinicians to compare the amount of data available on honey with that available to support other much more widely used products.

Perhaps the most up to date assessment of the value of honey in the treatment of problems wounds, particularly leg ulcers, is that provided by Bolton,[183] who undertook a review of recent controlled studies and concluded that published evidence suggests that although there is reliable evidence to confirm the safety of honey used in wound management, and some evidence to support claims for efficacy of Manuka honey as a primary dressing on chronic venous ulcers, currently insufficient evidence exists upon which to base a conclusion concerning the efficacy of manuka honey on non-venous ulcers or of honey from other sources on any types of leg ulcers.

Medical applications of other bee products

Royal jelly (RJ), which is also harvested from bee hives, has generated some interest in the medical field. Royal jelly is secreted from the hypopharyngeal glands in the heads of young worker bees and is used as one of the nutrient sources for all of the larvae in the colony, including those destined to become workers. However, a larva chosen to become a queen will be fed exclusively on large quantities of this material which trigger the development of queen morphology. Royal jelly consists principally of water, crude protein, simple sugars, and fatty acids together with many trace minerals, some enzymes, antibacterial and antibiotic components, and trace amounts of vitamin C.

In a study originally designed to detect any possible insulin-like activity in royal jelly, diabetes was induced in a group of rats by the administration of a single i.v.

injection of streptozotocin. They were then administered oral RJ administered at a dose of 10, 100 and 1000 mg/kg/day. Although no insulin-like activity was found, RJ exhibited some interesting anti-inflammatory properties and reduced the healing time of skin lesions.[184]

The antimicrobial activity of royal jelly was investigated both on its own and in conjunction with honey using *P. aeruginosa* as the test organism.[185] The minimum inhibitory concentration of honey and royal jelly were first determined independently then inhibitory concentrations of both materials combined were evaluated.

When tested separately, the MIC of the four varieties of honey ranged from 12 - 18% v/v, and that of RJ was 4% v/v. When tested in combination with RJ, each honey variety tested showed a greater than 90% reduction in the MIC with 3% RJ, a 66.6% reduction with 2% RJ, and a 50% reduction with 1% RJ.

The MIC of RJ decreased by 75% when used with a 50% dilution of honey that alone provides the MIC. A strong linear correlation was shown between the MIC drop of each variety of honey and RJ. The authors suggested the development of antibiotic-resistant bacteria may renew interest in the use of both honey and royal jelly in wound management.

The wound healing properties of three bee products, honey, propolis, and royal jelly were compared using an animal model. Oral mucositis was induced on the cheek pouch of hamsters by a combination of 5-fluorouracil and mild abrasion. Varying concentrations of the three test materials were applied to the lesions and their effects upon healing determined by measuring the rate of change in the size of the mucositis. Honey (1%, 10% and 100%) and propolis (0.3%, 1% and 3%) ointments did not reduce the size of the mucositis compared with a Vaseline-treated control group, but all concentrations of the royal jelly ointment significantly improved healing in a dose-dependent manner.[186]

The potential value of an ointment prepared from royal jelly and panthenol in the treatment of patients with limb-threatening diabetic foot infections was investigated in a preliminary study conducted by Abdelatif *et al.*[187] Sixty patients presenting with limb-threatening diabetic foot infections were categorised into three groups based on the severity of the lesions: full-thickness skin ulcer (Wagner Grades 1 and 2), deep tissue infection and suspected osteomyelitis (Wagner Grade III) and gangrenous lesions (Wagner Grades 4 and 5). The ulcers were cleansed and surgically debridement if required and covered with the dressings. No other topical treatment was given. Patients were followed for six months or until full healing occurred. All of the ulcers in the first group healed, as did 92% of those in the second group. All patients in the third group also healed following surgical excision, debridement of necrotic tissue and conservative treatment with the ointment. The authors suggested that further controlled trials were required to confirm these promising findings.

REFERENCES

1. Mphande AN, Killowe C, Phalira S, Jones HW, Harrison WJ. Effects of honey and sugar dressings on wound healing. *J Wound Care* 2007;16(7):317-9.

2. Anon. Sugar sweetens the lot of patients with bed sores. *Jama* 1973;223:122.
3. Thomlinson RH. Kitchen remedy for necrotic malignant breast ulcers,. *Lancet* 1980(ii):594.
4. Knutson RA, Merbitz LA, Creekmore MA, Snipes HG. Use of sugar and povidone-iodine to enhance wound healing: five year's experience. *South Med J* 1981;74(11):1329-35.
5. Chirife J. In-vitro study of bacterial growth inhibition in concentrated sugar solutions: microbiological basis for the use of sugar in treating infected wounds. *Antimicrob. Ag Chemother* 1983;23:766-773.
6. Chirife J, Herszage L. Sugar for infected wounds. *Lancet* 1982;2(8290):157.
7. Chirife J, Scarmato G, Herszage L. Scientific basis for use of granulated sugar in treatment of infected wounds. *Lancet* 1982;1(8271):560-1.
8. Forrest RD. Sugar in the wound. *Lancet* 1982;1(8276):861.
9. Bose B. Honey or sugar in treatment of infected wounds? *Lancet* 1982;1(8278):963.
10. Archer HG, Barnett S, Irving S, Middleton KR, Seal DV. A controlled model of moist wound healing: comparison between semi- permeable film, antiseptics and sugar paste. *J Exp Pathol (Oxford)* 1990;71(2):155-70.
11. Addison MK, Walterspiel JN. Sugar and wound healing, (letter) *Lancet* 1985;2:665.
12. Gordon H. Sugar and wound healing, (letter) *Lancet* 1985;2:663-664.
13. Middleton KR, Seal D. Sugar as an aid to wound healing. *Pharm. J.* 1985;235:757-758.
14. Ambrose U, Middleton K, Seal D. In vitro studies of water activity and bacterial growth inhibition of sucrose-polyethylene glycol 400-hydrogen peroxide and xylose-polyethylene glycol 400-hydrogen peroxide pastes used to treat infected wounds. *Antimicrob Agents Chemother* 1991;35(9):1799-803.
15. Rahal F, Mimica IM, Pereira V, Athie E. Sugar in the treatment of infected surgical wounds. *Int Surg* 1984;69(4):308.
16. Trouillet JL, Chastre J, Fagon JY, Pierre J, Domart Y, Gibert C. Use of granulated sugar in treatment of open mediastinitis after cardiac surgery. *Lancet* 1985;2(8448):180-4.
17. Quatraro A. Sugar and wound healing, (letter) *Lancet* 1985;2:664.
18. Tanner AG, Owen ER, Seal DV. Successful treatment of chronically infected wounds with sugar paste. *Eur J Clin Microbiol Infect Dis* 1988;7(4):524-5.
19. Debure A, Gachot B, Lacour B, Kreis H. Acute renal failure after use of granulated sugar in deep infected wound. *Lancet* 1987;1(8540):1034-5.
20. Archer H, Middleton K, Milledge J, Seal D. Toxicity of topical sugar. *Lancet* 1987;1(8548):1485-6.
21. Keith JF, Knodel LC. Sugar in wound healing. *Drug Intell. clin. Pharm, .* 1988;22 409-411.
22. Szerafin T, Vaszily M, Peterffy A. [Topical treatment using granulated sugar in advanced mediastinitis following open heart surgery]. *Orv Hetil* 1990;131(13):691-5.
23. De Feo M, Gregorio R, Renzulli A, Ismeno G, Romano GP, Cotrufo M. Treatment of recurrent postoperative mediastinitis with granulated sugar. *J Cardiovasc Surg (Torino)* 2000;41(5):715-9.
24. De Feo M, Gregorio R, Della Corte A, Marra C, Amarelli C, Renzulli A, et al. Deep sternal wound infection: the role of early debridement surgery. *Eur J Cardiothorac Surg* 2001;19(6):811-6.
25. De Feo M, De Santo LS, Romano G, Renzulli A, Della Corte A, Utili R, et al. Treatment of recurrent staphylococcal mediastinitis: still a controversial issue. *Ann Thorac Surg* 2003;75(2):538-42.

26. Topham JD. Sugar paste in the treatment of pressure sores, burns and wounds. *Pharm. J.* 1988;241:118-119.

27. Grauwin MY, Cartel JL, Lepers JP. [How does one treat the osteitis and osteoarthritis of the extremities in older leprosy patients using granulated table sugar?]. *Acta Leprol* 1999;11(4):147-52.

28. Bajaj G, Karn NK, Shrestha BP, Kumar P, Singh MP. A randomised controlled trial comparing eusol and sugar as dressing agents in the treatment of traumatic wounds. *Trop Doct* 2009;39(1):1-3.

29. Chiwenga S, Dowlen H, Mannion S. Audit of the use of sugar dressings for the control of wound odour at Lilongwe Central Hospital, Malawi. *Trop Doct* 2009;39(1):20-2.

30. Topham J. Sugar paste and povidone-iodine in the treatment of wounds. *Journal of Wound Care* 1996;5(8):364-5.

31. Nakao H, Yamazaki M, Tsuboi R, Ogawa H. Mixture of sugar and povidone--iodine stimulates wound healing by activating keratinocytes and fibroblast functions. *Arch Dermatol Res* 2006;298(4):175-82.

32. Shi CM, Nakao H, Yamazaki M, Tsuboi R, Ogawa H. Mixture of sugar and povidone-iodine stimulates healing of MRSA-infected skin ulcers on db/db mice. *Arch Dermatol Res* 2007;299(9):449-56.

33. Ali ATMM. The pharmacological charcacterization and the scientific basis of the hidden miracles of honey. *Saudi Med J* 1989;10(3):177-179.

34. Zumla A, Lulat A. Honey-a remedy rediscovered. *Journal of the Royal Society of Medicine* 1989;8:384-385.

35. Blair S. An introduction to the medicinal use of honey. In: Cooper R, Molan P, White R, editors. *Honey in modern wound management product.* Aberdeen: Wounds UK Publishing, 2009:1-6.

36. Ivakhnenko GS. [Treatment of thermal burns with an emulsion of honey & fat.]. *Vestn Khir Im I I Grek* 1956;77(2):83-8.

37. Bansal V, Medhi B, Pandhi P. Honey – A remedy rediscovered and its therapeutic utility. *Kathmandu University Medical Journal* 2005; 3(11):305-309.

38. Cavanagh D, Beazley J, Ostapowicz F. Radical operation for carcinoma of the vulva. A new approach to wound healing. *J Obstet Gynaecol Br Commonw* 1970;77(11):1037-40.

39. Molan PC. The role of honey in the management of wounds. *Journal of Wound Care* 1999;8(8):415-8.

40. Law MR, Gill ON, Turner A. Methicillin-resistant Staphylococcus aureus: associated morbidity and effectiveness of control measures. *Epidemiol Infect* 1988;101(2):301-9.

41. Boyce JM. Methicillin-resistant Staphylococcus aureus. Detection, epidemiology, and control measures. *Infect Dis Clin North Am* 1989;3(4):901-13.

42. Townsend DE, Ashdown N, Bradley JM, Pearman JW, Grubb WB. "Australian" methicillin-resistant Staphylococcus aureus in a London hospital? *Med J Aust* 1984;141(6):339-40.

43. Golder W. [Propolis. The bee glue as presented by the Graeco-Roman literature]. *Wurzbg Medizinhist Mitt* 2004;23:133-45.

44. White JW, Doner LW. *Bee keeping in the United States.* Washington,: U.S. Government Printing office, 1980.

45. Perez RA, Iglesias MT, Pueyo E, Gonzalez M, de Lorenzo C. Amino acid composition and antioxidant capacity of Spanish honeys. *J Agric Food Chem* 2007;55(2):360-5.

46. Molan PC. The antibacterial activity of honey 1.The nature of the antibacterial activity. *Bee World* 1992;73(1):5-28.

47. Bang LM, Buntting C, Molan P. The effect of dilution on the rate of hydrogen peroxide production in honey and its implications for wound healing. *J Altern Complement Med* 2003;9(2):267-73.

48. Havsteen BH. The biochemistry and medical significance of the flavonoids. *Pharmacol Ther* 2002;96(2-3):67-202.

49. Cooper R. The antimicrobial activity of honey. In: White R, Cooper R, editors. *Honey: A modern wound management product*. Aberdeen: Wounds UK Publishing, 2005:24-32.

50. Stephens J, Molan P. The explanation of why the levels of UMF varies in Manuka honey. *The New Zealand Bee Keeper,* 2008(March):17-21.

51. Molan P. Why honey works. In: Cooper R, Molan P, White R, editors. *Honey in modern wound management product*. Aberdeen: Wounds UK Publishing, 2009:7-20.

52. Mavric E, Wittmann S, Barth G, Henle T. Identification and quantification of methylglyoxal as the dominant antibacterial constituent of Manuka (Leptospermum scoparium) honeys from New Zealand. *Mol Nutr Food Res* 2008.

53. Adams CJ, Manley-Harris M, Molan PC. The origin of methylglyoxal in New Zealand manuka (Leptospermum scoparium) honey. *Carbohydr Res* 2009;344(8):1050-3.

54. Adams CJ, Boult CH, Deadman BJ, Farr JM, Grainger MN, Manley-Harris M, et al. Isolation by HPLC and characterisation of the bioactive fraction of New Zealand manuka (Leptospermum scoparium) honey. *Carbohydr Res* 2008;343(4):651-9.

55. Blair S. Antibacterial activity of honey. In: Cooper R, Molan P, White R, editors. *Honey in modern wound management product*. Aberdeen: Wounds UK Publishing, 2009:21-46.

56. Molan P. An explanation of why the MGO level in Manuka honey does not show the antimicrobial activity *The New Zealand Bee Keeper,* 2008(March):17-21.

57. Molan P. Why using the level of the active component in manuka honey to replace the UMF rating is misleading. *The New Zealand Bee Keeper,* 2008(March):17-21.

58. Gaetani GF, Ferraris AM, Rolfo M, Mangerini R, Arena S, Kirkman HN. Predominant role of catalase in the disposal of hydrogen peroxide within human erythrocytes. *Blood* 1996;87(4):1595-9.

59. Gethin GT, Cowman S, Conroy RM. The impact of Manuka honey dressings on the surface pH of chronic wounds. *Int Wound J* 2008;5(2):185-94.

60. Blair SE, Cokcetin NN, Harry EJ, Carter DA. The unusual antibacterial activity of medical-grade Leptospermum honey: antibacterial spectrum, resistance and transcriptome analysis. *Eur J Clin Microbiol Infect Dis* 2009;28(10):1199-208.

61. Allen KL, Molan PC, Reid GM. A survey of the antibacterial activity of some New Zealand honeys. *Journal of Pharmacy and Pharmacology* 1991;43:817-822.

62. Willix DJ, Molan PC, Harfoot CG. A comparison of the sensitivity of wound-infecting species of bacteria to the antibacterial activity of manuka honey and other honey. *J Appl Bacteriol* 1992;73(5):388-94.

63. Wilkinson JM, Cavanagh HM. Antibacterial activity of 13 honeys against Escherichia coli and Pseudomonas aeruginosa. *J Med Food* 2005;8(1):100-3.

64. Cooper RA, Halas E, Molan PC. The efficacy of honey in inhibiting strains of Pseudomonas aeruginosa from infected burns. *J Burn Care Rehabil* 2002;23(6):366-70.

65. Brudzynski K. Effect of hydrogen peroxide on antibacterial activities of Canadian honeys. *Can J Microbiol* 2006;52(12):1228-37.

66. Basson NJ, Grobler SR. Antimicrobial activity of two South African honeys produced from indigenous Leucospermum cordifolium and Erica species on selected micro-organisms. *BMC Complement Altern Med* 2008;8:41.

67. Estrada H, Gamboa Mdel M, Arias ML, Chaves C. [Evaluation of the antimicrobial action of honey against Staphylococcus aureus, Staphylococcus epidermidis, Pseudomonas aeruginosa,

Escherichia coli, Salmonella enteritidis, Listeria monocytogenes and Aspergillus niger. Evaluation of its microbiological charge]. *Arch Latinoam Nutr* 2005;55(2):167-71.

68. Lusby PE, Coombes AL, Wilkinson JM. Bactericidal activity of different honeys against pathogenic bacteria. *Arch Med Res* 2005;36(5):464-7.

69. Mullai V, Menon T. Bactericidal activity of different types of honey against clinical and environmental isolates of Pseudomonas aeruginosa. *J Altern Complement Med* 2007;13(4):439-41.

70. Tan HT, Rahman RA, Gan SH, Halim AS, Hassan SA, Sulaiman SA, et al. The antibacterial properties of Malaysian tualang honey against wound and enteric microorganisms in comparison to manuka honey. *BMC Complement Altern Med* 2009;9:34.

71. Acquarone C, Buera P, Elizalde B. Pattern of pH and electrical conductivity upon honey dilution as a complementary tool for discriminating geographical origin of honeys *Food Chemistry* 2006;101(2):695-703.

72. Basualdo C, Sgroy V, Finola MS, Marioli JM. Comparison of the antibacterial activity of honey from different provenance against bacteria usually isolated from skin wounds. *Vet Microbiol* 2007;124(3-4):375-81.

73. Cooper R, Molan P. The use of honey as an antiseptic in managing Pseudomonas infection. *Journal of Wound Care* 1999;8(4):161-4.

74. Cooper RA, Molan PC, Harding KG. Antibacterial activity of honey against strains of Staphylococcus aureus from infected wounds. *J R Soc Med* 1999;92(6):283-5.

75. French VM, Cooper RA, Molan PC. The antibacterial activity of honey against coagulase-negative staphylococci. *J Antimicrob Chemother* 2005;56(1):228-31.

76. Cooper RA, Molan PC, Harding KG. The sensitivity to honey of Gram-positive cocci of clinical significance isolated from wounds. *J Appl Microbiol* 2002;93(5):857-63.

77. George NM, Cutting KF. Antibacterial Honey(Medihoney™): in-vitro Activity Against Clinical Isolates of MRSA, VRE, and Other Multiresistant Gram-negative Organisms Including Pseudomonas aeruginosa. *Wounds* 2007;19(9):231 - 236.

78. Irish J, Carter DA, Shokohi T, Blair SE. Honey has an antifungal effect against Candida species. *Med Mycol* 2006;44(3):289-91.

79. Brady NF, Molan PC, Harfoot CG. The sensitivity of dermatophytes to the antimicrobial activity of Manuka honey and other honey. *Pharmaceutical Sciences* 1996;2:471-473.

80. Molan PC. Honey as an antimicrobial agent. In: Mizrahi A, Lensky Y, editors. *Bee Products Properties, Applications and Apitherapy*. New York: Plenum Press, 1996:27-37.

81. Molan PC. The antibacterial activity of honey 2. Variation in the potency of the antibacterial activity. *Bee World* 1992;73(2):59-76.

82. Cooper RA, Molan PC. Honey in wound care. *J Wound Care* 1999;8(7):340.

83. Alandejani T, Marsan J, Ferris W, Slinger R, Chan F. Effectiveness of honey on Staphylococcus aureus and Pseudomonas aeruginosa biofilms. *Otolaryngol Head Neck Surg* 2009;141(1):114-8.

84. Merckoll P, Jonassen TO, Vad ME, Jeansson SL, Melby KK. Bacteria, biofilm and honey: a study of the effects of honey on 'planktonic' and biofilm-embedded chronic wound bacteria. *Scand J Infect Dis* 2009;41(5):341-7.

85. Lerrer B, Zinger-Yosovich KD, Avrahami B, Gilboa-Garber N. Honey and royal jelly, like human milk, abrogate lectin-dependent infection-preceding Pseudomonas aeruginosa adhesion. *ISME J* 2007;1(2):149-55.

86. Tonks A. Immunomodulatory components of honey. In: Cooper R, Molan P, White R, editors. *Honey in modern wound management product*. Aberdeen: Wounds UK Publishing, 2009:189-198.

87. Henriques A, Jackson S, Cooper R, Burton N. Free radical production and quenching in honeys with wound healing potential. *J Antimicrob Chemother* 2006;58(4):773-7.
88. van den Berg AJ, van den Worm E, van Ufford HC, Halkes SB, Hoekstra MJ, Beukelman CJ. An in vitro examination of the antioxidant and anti-inflammatory properties of buckwheat honey. *J Wound Care* 2008;17(4):172-4, 176-8.
89. Tonks A, Cooper RA, Price AJ, Molan PC, Jones KP. Stimulation of TNF-alpha release in monocytes by honey. *Cytokine* 2001;14(4):240-2.
90. Tonks AJ, Cooper RA, Jones KP, Blair S, Parton J, Tonks A. Honey stimulates inflammatory cytokine production from monocytes. *Cytokine* 2003;21(5):242-7.
91. Tonks AJ, Dudley E, Porter NG, Parton J, Brazier J, Smith EL, et al. A 5.8-kDa component of manuka honey stimulates immune cells via TLR4. *J Leukoc Biol* 2007;82(5):1147-55.
92. Timm M, Bartelt S, Hansen EW. Immunomodulatory effects of honey cannot be distinguished from endotoxin. *Cytokine* 2008;42(1):113-20.
93. Cooper R, Jones K, Morris K. Immunomodulatory properties of honey that may be relevant to wound repair. In: White R, Molan P, editors. *Honey: A modern wound management product*. Aberdeen: Wounds UK Publishing, 2005:143-148.
94. Bergman A, Yanai J, Weiss J, Bell D, David MP. Acceleration of wound healing by topical application of honey. An animal model. *Am J Surg* 1983;145(3):374-6.
95. Oryan A, Zaker SR. Effects of topical application of honey on cutaneous wound healing in rabbits. *Zentralbl Veterinarmed A* 1998;45(3):181-8.
96. Osuagwu FC, Oladejo OW, Imosemi IO, Aiku A, Ekpos OE, Salami AA, et al. Enhanced wound contraction in fresh wounds dressed with honey in Wistar rats (Rattus Novergicus). *West Afr J Med* 2004;23(2):114-8.
97. Iftikhar F, Arshad M, Rasheed F, Amraiz D, Anwar P, Gulfraz M. Effects of acacia honey on wound healing in various rat models. *Phytother Res* 2009.
98. Hashemi B, Bayat A, Kazemei T, Azarpira N. Comparison between topical honey and mafenide acetate in treatment of auricular burn. *Am J Otolaryngol* 2009.
99. Al-Waili NS. Investigating the antimicrobial activity of natural honey and its effects on the pathogenic bacterial infections of surgical wounds and conjunctiva. *J Med Food* 2004;7(2):210-22.
100. Hamzaoglu I, Saribeyoglu K, Durak H, Karahasanoglu T, Bayrak I, Altug T, et al. Protective covering of surgical wounds with honey impedes tumor implantation. *Arch Surg* 2000;135(12):1414-7.
101. Aysan E, Ayar E, Aren A, Cifter C. The role of intra-peritoneal honey administration in preventing post-operative peritoneal adhesions. *Eur J Obstet Gynecol Reprod Biol* 2002;104(2):152-5.
102. Yuzbasioglu MF, Kurutas EB, Bulbuloglu E, Goksu M, Atli Y, Bakan V, et al. Administration of honey to prevent peritoneal adhesions in a rat peritonitis model. *Int J Surg* 2009;7(7):54-57.
103. Gollu A, Kismet K, Kilicoglu B, Erel S, Gonultas MA, Sunay AE, et al. Effect of honey on intestinal morphology, intraabdominal adhesions and anastomotic healing. *Phytother Res* 2008;22(9):1243-7.
104. Staunton CJ, Halliday LC, Garcia KD. The use of honey as a topical dressing to treat a large, devitalized wound in a stumptail macaque (Macaca arctoides). *Contemp Top Lab Anim Sci* 2005;44(4):43-5.
105. Allen KL, Molan PC. The sensitivity of mastitis-causing bacteria to the antibacterial activity of honey. *New Zealand Journal of Agricultural Research* 1997;40:537-540.

106. Postmes TJ, Bosch MMC, Dutrieux R, van Baare J, Hoekstra MJ. Speeding up the healing of burns with honey. In: Mizrahi A, Lensky Y, editors. *Bee Products: Properties, Applications and Apitherapy* Ney York: Plenum Press, 1996.

107. Wijesinghe M, Weatherall M, Perrin K, Beasley R. Honey in the treatment of burns: a systematic review and meta-analysis of its efficacy. *N Z Med J* 2009;122(1295):47-60.

108. Yoon YM, Newlands C. Quality standards of medical grade manuka honey. In: White R, Cooper R, editors. *Honey: A modern wound management product*. Aberdeen: Wounds UK Publishing, 2005:89-102.

109. Postmes T, van den Bogaard AE, Hazen M. The sterilization of honey with cobalt 60 gamma radiation: a study of honey spiked with spores of Clostridium botulinum and Bacillus subtilis. *Experientia* 1995;51(9-10):986-9.

110. Molan PC, Allen KL. The effect of gamma-irradiation on the antibacterial activity of honey. *J Pharm Pharmacol* 1996;48(11):1206-9.

111. Molan P, Hill C. Quality standards for honey. In: Cooper R, Molan P, White R, editors. *Honey in modern wound management product*. Aberdeen: Wounds UK Publishing, 2009:63-69.

112. Zaghloul AA, el-Shattawy HH, Kassem AA, Ibrahim EA, Reddy IK, Khan MA. Honey, a prospective antibiotic: extraction, formulation, and stability. *Pharmazie* 2001;56(8):643-7.

113. Ankra-Badu GA. Sickle cell leg ulcers in Ghana. *East Afr Med J* 1992;69(7):366-9.

114. Okany CC, Atimomo CE, Akinyanju OO. Efficacy of natural honey in the healing of leg ulcers in sickle cell anaemia. *Niger Postgrad Med J* 2004;11(3):179-81.

115. Okeniyi JA, Olubanjo OO, Ogunlesi TA, Oyelami OA. Comparison of healing of incised abscess wounds with honey and EUSOL dressing. *J Altern Complement Med* 2005;11(3):511-3.

116. Ndayisaba G, Bazira L, Habonimana E, Muteganya D. [Clinical and bacteriological outcome of wounds treated with honey. An analysis of a series of 40 cases]. *Rev Chir Orthop Reparatrice Appar Mot* 1993;79(2):111-3.

117. Efem SE. Clinical observations on the wound healing properties of honey. *Br J Surg* 1988;75(7):679-81.

118. Ahmed AK, Hoekstra MJ, Hage JJ, Karim RB. Honey-medicated dressing: transformation of an ancient remedy into modern therapy. *Ann Plast Surg* 2003;50(2):143-7; discussion 147-8.

119. Stephen-Haynes J. Evaluation of a honey-impregnated tulle dressing in primary care. *Br J Community Nurs* 2004(Suppl):S21-7.

120. Ingle R, Levin J, Polinder K. Wound healing with honey--a randomised controlled trial. *S Afr Med J* 2006;96(9):831-5.

121. Efem SE. Recent advances in the management of Fournier's gangrene: preliminary observations. *Surgery* 1993;113(2):200-4.

122. Tahmaz L, Erdemir F, Kibar Y, Cosar A, Yalcyn O. Fournier's gangrene: report of thirty-three cases and a review of the literature. *Int J Urol* 2006;13(7):960-7.

123. Hejase MJ, Simonin JE, Bihrle R, Coogan CL. Genital Fournier's gangrene: experience with 38 patients. *Urology* 1996;47(5):734-9.

124. Gurdal M, Yucebas E, Tekin A, Beysel M, Aslan R, Sengor F. Predisposing factors and treatment outcome in Fournier's gangrene. Analysis of 28 cases. *Urol Int* 2003;70(4):286-90.

125. Phuapradit W, Saropala N. Topical application of honey in treatment of abdominal wound disruption. *Aust N Z J Obstet Gynaecol* 1992;32(4):381-4.

126. Al-Waili NS, Saloom KY. Effects of topical honey on post-operative wound infections due to gram positive and gram negative bacteria following caesarean sections and hysterectomies. *Eur J Med Res* 1999;4(3):126-30.

127. Blaser G, Santos K, Bode U, Vetter H, Simon A. Effect of medical honey on wounds colonised or infected with MRSA. *J Wound Care* 2007;16(8):325-8.

128. Vardi A, Barzilay Z, Linder N, Cohen HA, Paret G, Barzilai A. Local application of honey for treatment of neonatal postoperative wound infection. *Acta Paediatr* 1998;87(4):429-32.

129. Ameh EA, Mamuda AA, Musa HH, Chirdan LB, Shinkafi MS, Ogala WN. Necrotizing fasciitis of the scalp in a neonate. *Ann Trop Paediatr* 2001;21(1):91-3.

130. Simon A, Sofka K, Wiszniewsky G, Blaser G, Bode U, Fleischhack G. Wound care with antibacterial honey (Medihoney) in pediatric hematology-oncology. *Support Care Cancer* 2006;14(1):91-7.

131. Dunford CE. Treatment of a wound infection in a patient with mantle cell lymphoma. *Br J Nurs* 2001;10(16):1058, 1060, 1062, 1064-5.

132. Bateman S, Graham T. The use of Medihoney Antibacterial Wound Gel on sugical wounds post CABG. *Wounds UK* 2007;3(3):76-83.

133. Moolenaar M, Poorter RL, van der Toorn PP, Lenderink AW, Poortmans P, Egberts AC. The effect of honey compared to conventional treatment on healing of radiotherapy-induced skin toxicity in breast cancer patients. *Acta Oncol* 2006;45(5):623-4.

134. Robson V, Cooper R. Using leptospermum honey to manage wounds impaired by radiotherapy: a case series. *Ostomy Wound Manage* 2009;55(1):38-47.

135. Rashad UM, Al-Gezawy SM, El-Gezawy E, Azzaz AN. Honey as topical prophylaxis against radiochemotherapy-induced mucositis in head and neck cancer. *J Laryngol Otol* 2009;123(2):223-8.

136. Hon J. Using honey to heal a chronic wound in a patient with epidermolysis bullosa. *Br J Nurs* 2005;14(19):S4-5, S8, S10 passim.

137. Alese OB, Irabor DO. Pyoderma gangrenosum and ulcerative colitis in the tropics. *Rev Soc Bras Med Trop* 2008;41(6):664-7.

138. Shukrimi A, Sulaiman AR, Halim AY, Azril A. A comparative study between honey and povidone iodine as dressing solution for Wagner type II diabetic foot ulcers. *Med J Malaysia* 2008;63(1):44-6.

139. Albietz JM, Lenton LM. Effect of antibacterial honey on the ocular flora in tear deficiency and Meibomian gland disease. *Cornea* 2006;25(9):1012-1019.

140. Johnson DW, van Eps C, Mudge DW, Wiggins KJ, Armstrong K, Hawley CM, et al. Randomized, controlled trial of topical exit-site application of honey (Medihoney) versus mupirocin for the prevention of catheter-associated infections in hemodialysis patients. *J Am Soc Nephrol* 2005;16(5):1456-62.

141. McIntosh CD, Thomson CE. Honey dressing versus paraffin tulle gras following toenail surgery. *J Wound Care* 2006;15(3):133-6.

142. Subrahmanyam M. Honey impregnated gauze versus polyurethane film (OpSite) in the treatment of burns--a prospective randomised study. *Br J Plast Surg* 1993;46(4):322-3.

143. Subrahmanyam M. Honey-impregnated gauze versus amniotic membrane in the treatment of burns. *Burns* 1994;20(4):331-3.

144. Subrahmanyam M. Honey dressing versus boiled potato peel in the treatment of burns: a prospective randomized study. *Burns* 1996;22(6):491-3.

145. Subrahmanyam M. A prospective randomised clinical and histological study of superficial burn wound healing with honey and silver sulfadiazine. *Burns* 1998;24(2):157-61.

146. Subrahmanyam M. Early tangential excision and skin grafting of moderate burns is superior to honey dressing: a prospective randomised trial. *Burns* 1999;25(8):729-31.

147. Adesunkanmi K, Oyelami OA. The pattern and outcome of burn injuries at Wesley Guild Hospital, Ilesha, Nigeria: a review of 156 cases. *J Trop Med Hyg* 1994;97(2):108-12.

148. Emsen IM. A different and safe method of split thickness skin graft fixation: medical honey application. *Burns* 2007;33(6):782-7.

149. Alcaraz A, Kelly J. Treatment of an infected venous leg ulcer with honey dressings. *Br J Nurs* 2002;11(13):859-60, 862, 864-6.

150. van der Weyden EA. Treatment of a venous leg ulcer with a honey alginate dressing. *Br J Community Nurs* 2005(Suppl.):S21, S24, S26-7.

151. Sare JL. Leg ulcer management with topical medical honey. *Br J Community Nurs* 2008;13(9):S22, S24, S26 passim.

152. Natarajan S, Williamson D, Grey J, Harding KG, Cooper RA. Healing of an MRSA-colonized, hydroxyurea-induced leg ulcer with honey. *J Dermatolog Treat* 2001;12(1):33-6.

153. Gethin G, Cowman S. Case series of use of Manuka honey in leg ulceration. *Int Wound J* 2005;2(1):10-5.

154. Dunford CE, Hanano R. Acceptability to patients of a honey dressing for non-healing venous leg ulcers. *Journal of Wound Care* 2004;13(5):193-7.

155. Schumacher HH. Use of medical honey in patients with chronic venous leg ulcers after split-skin grafting. *J Wound Care* 2004;13(10):451-2.

156. Misirlioglu A, Eroglu S, Karacaoglan N, Akan M, Akoz T, Yildirim S. Use of honey as an adjunct in the healing of split-thickness skin graft donor site. *Dermatol Surg* 2003;29(2):168-72.

157. Oluwatosin OM, Olabanji JK, Oluwatosin OA, Tijani LA, Onyechi HU. A comparison of topical honey and phenytoin in the treatment of chronic leg ulcers. *Afr J Med Med Sci* 2000;29(1):31-4.

158. Jull A, Walker N, Parag V, Molan P, Rodgers A. Randomized clinical trial of honey-impregnated dressings for venous leg ulcers. *Br J Surg* 2008;95(2):175-82.

159. Robson V, Dodd S, Thomas S. Standardized antibacterial honey (Medihoney) with standard therapy in wound care: randomized clinical trial. *J Adv Nurs* 2009;65(3):565-75.

160. Gethin G, Cowman S. Manuka honey vs. hydrogel--a prospective, open label, multicentre, randomised controlled trial to compare desloughing efficacy and healing outcomes in venous ulcers. *J Clin Nurs* 2009;18(3):466-74.

161. Gethin G, Cowman S. Bacteriological changes in sloughy venous leg ulcers treated with manuka honey or hydrogel: an RCT. *J Wound Care* 2008;17(6):241-4, 246-7.

162. Dunford C, Cooper R, Molan P. Using honey as a dressing for infected skin lesions. *Nurs Times* 2000;96(14 Suppl):7-9.

163. Moore OA, Smith LA, Campbell F, Seers K, McQuay HJ, Moore RA. Systematic review of the use of honey as a wound dressing. *BMC Complement Altern Med* 2001;1(1):2.

164. Bardy J, Slevin NJ, Mais KL, Molassiotis A. A systematic review of honey uses and its potential value within oncology care. *J Clin Nurs* 2008;17(19):2604-23.

165. Jull AB, Rodgers A, Walker N. Honey as a topical treatment for wounds. *Cochrane Database Syst Rev* 2008(4):CD005083.

166. Kingsley A. The use of honey in the treatment of infected wounds: case studies. *Br J Nurs* 2001;10(22 Suppl):S13-6, S18, S20.

167. Dunwoody G, Acton C. The use of medical grade honey in clinical practice. *Br J Nurs* 2008;17(20):S38-44.

168. Eddy JJ, Gideonsen MD, Mack GP. Practical considerations of using topical honey for neuropathic diabetic foot ulcers: a review. *WMJ* 2008;107(4):187-90.

169. Lay-flurrie K. Honey in wound care: effects, clinical application and patient benefit. *Br J Nurs* 2008;17(11):S30, S32-6.

170. Dunford C, Cooper R, Molan P, White R. The use of honey in wound management. *Nurs Stand* 2000;15(11):63-8.

171. Molan PC. Potential of honey in the treatment of wounds and burns. *Am J Clin Dermatol* 2001;2(1):13-9.

172. Molan PC. The potential of honey to promote oral wellness. *Gen Dent* 2001;49(6):584-9.

173. Lusby PE, Coombes A, Wilkinson JM. Honey: a potent agent for wound healing? *J Wound Ostomy Continence Nurs* 2002;29(6):295-300.

174. Molan PC. Re-introducing honey in the management of wounds and ulcers - theory and practice. *Ostomy Wound Manage* 2002;48(11):28-40.

175. Simon A, Traynor K, Santos K, Blaser G, Bode U, Molan P. Medical Honey for Wound Care Still the 'Latest Resort'? *Evid Based Complement Alternat Med* 2008.

176. Fox C. Honey as a dressing for chronic wounds in adults. *Br J Community Nurs* 2002;7(10):530-4.

177. Namias N. Honey in the management of infections. *Surg Infect (Larchmt)* 2003;4(2):219-26.

178. Bell SG. The therapeutic use of honey. *Neonatal Netw* 2007;26(4):247-51.

179. Pieper B. Honey-based dressings and wound care: an option for care in the United States. *J Wound Ostomy Continence Nurs* 2009;36(1):60-6; quiz 67-8.

180. Betts J. The clinical application of honey in wound care. *Nurs Times* 2008;104(14):43-4.

181. White R. The benefits of honey in wound management. *Nurs Stand* 2005;20(10):57-64; quiz 66.

182. Molan PC. The evidence supporting the use of honey as a wound dressing. *Int J Low Extrem Wounds* 2006;5(1):40-54.

183. Bolton L. Leg ulcers and honey: a review of recent controlled studies. In: Cooper R, Molan P, White R, editors. *Honey in modern wound management product.* Aberdeen: Wounds UK Publishing, 2009:139-152.

184. Fujii A, Kobayashi S, Kuboyama N, Furukawa Y, Kaneko Y, Ishihama S, et al. Augmentation of wound healing by royal jelly (RJ) in streptozotocin-diabetic rats. *Jpn J Pharmacol* 1990;53(3):331-7.

185. Boukraa L. Additive activity of royal jelly and honey against Psuedomonas aeruginosa. *Altern Med Rev* 2008;13(4):331-4.

186. Suemaru K, Cui R, Li B, Watanabe S, Okihara K, Hashimoto K, et al. Topical application of royal jelly has a healing effect for 5-fluorouracil-induced experimental oral mucositis in hamsters. *Methods Find Exp Clin Pharmacol* 2008;30(2):103-6.

187. Abdelatif M, Yakoot M, Etmaan M. Safety and efficacy of a new honey ointment on diabetic foot ulcers: a prospective pilot study. *J Wound Care* 2008;17(3):108-10.

16. Silver Dressings

INTRODUCTION

Historical use of silver

Silver is about the sixty-sixth most abundant element in the Earth's crust and is found both as the native metal and in ores such as argentite, a form of silver sulphide. Silver is also present in mixed ores in association with other metals including lead, copper and mercury.

The first recorded use of metallic silver was in Mesopotamia sometime in the Ubaid period, which extended from 5000 to 3500 B.C. This silver is believed to have come from Asia Minor where it was extracted from galena, an ore of lead, which contained up to 600 ounces of silver to a ton of lead.

Silver was also highly prised in ancient Egypt, but because the country had no deposits of her own, all supplies had to be imported. As a result it is thought that at one stage silver metal was more highly valued than gold. Evidence for this may be obtained by comparing the thinness of the silver bracelets of the 4th Dynasty queen Hetepheres (*c.*2600 B.C.) with the more extravagant construction of her gold jewellery!

The antimicrobial properties of metallic silver were used empirically for thousands of years, long before the existence of microorganisms was first suspected. For example, Aristotle advised Alexander the Great (335 B.C.) to store his water in silver vessels and boil it before use, and Burrell[1] has described how early American settlers placed silver dollars in their wooden water barrels to preserve the water. The ability of silver to keep water potable is still utilised today as water tanks on spacecraft are lined with silver to prevent bacterial growth.[2]

According to Russell,[3] the biocidal properties of silver ions were first investigated by Ravelin in 1869, followed by Von Behring who, in 1887, showed that 0.25% and 0.01% silver nitrate solutions were effective against typhoid and anthrax bacilli.[1] In 1893 Naegeli found that silver ions at a concentration of 9.2×10^{-9} molar (0.0000001%) would kill the freshwater algae Spirogyra, and at a concentration of 5.5×10^{-6} molar (0.00006%) they prevented the germination of *Aspergillus niger* spores.[3]

Chemistry of silver

Silver exhibits three valance/oxidation states: Ag^+, Ag^{++} and Ag^{+++} although the most common is the cation Ag^+. Metallic silver, Ag^o, is inherently stable but in the presence of moisture it oxidizes very slowly to form silver oxide which in turn can lead to the formation of the monovalent Ag^+ ion. The rate of this reaction is determined by the surface area of the exposed metal, and this may explain, at least in part, the marked antimicrobial activity of dressings coated with metallic silver with a particle size less than 20 nm as found in so called 'nanocrystalline' silver dressings such as Acticoat.[1]

In fact, the explanation for the observed antimicrobial activity of nanocrystalline silver is actually likely to be far more complex than this. According to Nadworny and Burrell,[4] single crystals of silver, equivalent in size to those present in Acticoat have no demonstrable antimicrobial activity; similarly dressings with crystallite sizes greater than 32 nm are relatively inactive. They therefore suggested that the antimicrobial activity associated with the nanocrystalline dressings is due to the formation of higher oxidation states of silver and 'unstable crystallite surfaces and grain boundary atoms' and postulated that the highly energetic and active surface of the nanocrystalline silver may produce complex metastable silver hydroxide compounds at the surface of the crystals which are capable of forming biological interactions that typical silver compounds cannot produce.

Burrell[1,5] also suggested that nanocrystalline silver releases metallic silver, Ag^0, in the form of a 'cluster structure' which he suggests also has marked biological activity, also this possibility is strongly disputed by others.[6] Evidence for the activity of silver nanoparticles in suspension was presented by Pal et al.,[7] who compared the antibacterial properties of differently shaped crystals against E. coli in both in liquid systems and on agar plates, concluding that these appear to undergo a shape-dependent interaction with the bacterium. They speculated that the mode of action of these particles is similar to that of the silver ion; when in contact with a nanoparticle a bacterial cell takes in silver ions which inhibit a respiratory enzyme(s) to facilitate the generation of a reactive oxygen species which then causes damage to the cell. As this work was conducted on silver particles prepared by a totally different method from that used to produce nanocrystalline silver dressings, it cannot be assumed, however, that the two preparations necessarily share a common mode of action.

The silver ion is extremely reactive, able to form numerous organic and inorganic complexes, although Ag^{++} complexes are less stable than those of Ag^+ and Ag^{+++}. Silver ions bind readily to thiol groups on proteins (including albumins and metallothioneins) and interact with trace metals in metabolic pathways. If ingested, for example in the form of a colloidal solution, regarded by some as an agent with useful medicinal properties, silver can be deposited in the skin in the form of silver sulphide, producing a slate-gray permanent skin discoloration known as argyria.

Most silver containing dressings and topical preparations function by liberating Ag^+ on contact with aqueous solutions. The mechanisms responsible for the antimicrobial activity of silver have been described in some detail by Lansdown previously,[8] but essentially it is believed that the silver cations bind to bacterial cell walls and intracellular and nuclear membranes, disrupting them, thereby causing leakage of the cells' contents. They also inactivate enzymes, interfere with DNA synthesis and inhibit the respiratory burst through their very strong oxidizing potential.[9]

Lansdown[8] also suggested that the microbiocidal action of low concentrations of silver ions does not necessarily reflect any remarkable effect of comparatively small number of ions on the cell but rather the ability of microorganisms to take up and concentrate silver from very dilute solutions. He further proposed that bacteria killed by silver may contain 10^5-10^7 Ag^+ ions per cell, the same order of magnitude as the estimated number of enzyme-protein molecules in the cell.

In a wound environment, the marked reactivity of the silver ion presents a practical problem because it is rapidly inactivated, both by the formation of relatively insoluble silver chloride and by combining with proteins present in wound exudate or in the base of the wound itself. The interaction between silver and the exudate and cellular debris present in chronic wounds was investigated in a further study by Lansdown.[10] He examined the release patterns of silver from selected dressings and considered the protective role played by proteins in inactivating or sequestering free silver ions which otherwise might induce some form of toxic response. Using atomic absorption spectrometry he measured the silver content of wound exudate and wound scale collected from seven patients and found that silver accumulation in wound exudate correlated well with its viscosity and protein content and approximated to the silver released from the dressings. In the same study he also examined the bactericidal action of the products concerned and showed that following silver therapy the bacterial bioburden was controlled but not eliminated. He therefore concluded that silver dressings appeared to be safe to use in the treatment of chronic wounds.

Burrell[1] suggested that the reactivity of the silver ion impairs its ability to penetrate the wound bed, and that this in turn might limit its ability to treat established soft tissue infections.

The effect of chloride ions on silver concentration was discussed by Nadworny and Burrell.[4] They reported that although the concentration of Ag^+ in an aqueous solution of silver chloride is around 1.4 mg/L, in the presence of excess chloride ions at the concentrations found clinically, or in a bacterial culture medium, the concentration of Ag^+ falls to around 0.3 µg/L (0.0003 mg/L) due to the common ion effect (Le Chatelier's Principle).

As the Ag^+ ion is responsible for the antimicrobial activity of silver, it follows that the activity of a dressing containing silver chloride will be greatly reduced in simulated wound fluid compared with that exhibited in a plain aqueous environment.

This was illustrated by Nadworny and Burrell,[4] who described the results of a previously published study which showed that the minimum inhibitory concentrations of silver nitrate solution for a selected test organism was 0.003 mg/L in a buffered system with no organic material present. Upon the addition of serum this rose to around 8 mg/L, a 2500 times increase in the required silver concentration caused by the interaction between the silver ion and the serum. For this reason the concentration of silver ions required to exert a bactericidal effect within a wound is very much higher than that required under normal experimental conditions, typically 30 - 50 mg/L.[9]

As Nadworny and Burrell emphasised,[4] when developing or evaluating silver-containing dressings, it is therefore important to consider the quantity of bioavailable silver ions not just the total silver content of the product.

Problems with the availability of silver ions exist even with a soluble silver salt such as silver nitrate. The application to a wound of a gauze pad soaked in silver nitrate solution will initially deliver a high concentration of silver ions but this will rapidly fall as a result of interaction with the chloride ions and proteins in wound exudate.

Silver nitrate soaks are also associated with other practical problems in that they require frequent replacement, can cause electrolyte imbalances and produce staining of tissues. It is for these reasons that numerous different formulations of silver-containing dressings have been developed, designed to deliver clinically effective levels of silver ions over an extended period.

Antimicrobial activity of silver

Silver has a broad spectrum of action and in numerous studies has been shown to be active against bacteria, yeast, filamentous fungi, and viruses although marked variations between different types of organisms have been reported.

Development of silver containing dressings

Several excellent reviews have been published on the antimicrobial properties of silver, which include information on the mechanism of action, development of bacterial resistance, toxicity, clinical indications, and the historical background to its use.[1-3,8,11-13] These describe how early observations concerning the antimicrobial properties of silver and its salts led to its use in a variety of topical preparations for preventing or treating soft tissue infections.

In the 17th Century for example, silver nitrate was used to treat venereal buboes and chancres, to open abscesses and reduce proud flesh and sores. In the 19th Century dilute solutions instilled into the conjunctival sac were used to treat postpartum eye infections including gonorrhoeal ophthalmia, also known as ophthalmia neonatorum. This procedure was somewhat controversially claimed to reduce infection rates from 10.8% to 0.2%.[8] Silver in various forms, sometimes associated with arsenic, was also used systemically in the form of an injection for the treatment of gonorrhoea.

Since the beginning of the 20th Century, there has been considerable interest in the medicinal use of colloidal silver, a liquid suspension of microscopic particles of metallic silver. Colloidal silver preparations containing 30 ppm or less are typically manufactured by electrolysis, but where higher concentrations are required the silver is usually bound to a protein. Scientific opinion on the medicinal value of colloidal silver is very mixed and there appears to be little independent published evidence to support its use.

Until well into the 20th Century, silver nitrate solution was also employed in the treatment of burns, until it was largely superseded for this indication by silver sulphadiazine (SSD), a complex formed from silver nitrate and sodium sulphadiazine.

SSD was developed by Fox in 1967 who subsequently published numerous articles describing its use, particularly for wounds infected with Pseudomonas sp,[14-18] although according to Morin et al.,[9] SSD is actually regarded as a rather poor agent for the treatment of infections caused by this organism.

Despite the recognised limitations of SSD, the results of a recent international survey published by Hermans,[19] revealed that it remains the most frequently used topical preparation for the treatment of both superficial and deep partial thickness burns. The survey also revealed that although some new silver dressings are gaining acceptance for this indication, they are currently much less popular than SSD despite the fact that, in the view of the author of the survey at least, they offer practical benefits in use in terms of reduced pain and accelerated healing.

Silver ions generated by electrolysis were shown in laboratory studies to possess marked antibacterial and antifungal properties at concentrations below 5 µg/mL,[20-21] and in 1978 Becker[22] described how silver ions generated in this way were used practically an as adjunctive therapy in the management of chronic osteomyelitis in fifteen wounds, twelve of which responded favourably to treatment.

In a second study,[23] the wounds of patients with active chronic osteomyelitis were surgically debrided then given daily applications of electrically activated silver dressings. Sixteen of 25 patients (64%) treated in this fashion achieved healing, but the remainder required persistent drainage or amputation.

An alternative approach to the delivery of silver ions in the prevention or treatment of orthopaedic infections was described by Spadaro *et al.*[24] They incorporated low concentrations of inorganic silver compounds into polymethyl-methacrylate bone cement and showed in laboratory studies that these retained antimicrobial activity over extended periods without compromising the performance or biocompatibility of the cement.

The possibility of incorporating silver into commercial wound dressings was first investigated in 1987 by Deitch *et al.*[25] They evaluated the antimicrobial activity of two silver-nylon fabrics and showed them to be microbiocidal *in vitro* against *S. aureus*, *P. aeruginosa*, and *C. albicans*. They also demonstrated that this activity could be significantly augmented by passing a weak DC current through the material, which increased the rate of release of silver ions.

Chu[26] also used silver coated nylon dressings as part of an electrical circuit in the treatment of experimental full-thickness scald injuries in a rat model which were subsequently inoculated with a lethal dose of *P. aeruginosa*. When used as the anode, the silver nylon was therapeutic at currents between 0.4 and 40 microamps, but when used as a cathode, the dressing was not effective. Nylon cloth without a silver metal coating was ineffective with or without applied current, but silver nylon dressings without applied current were effective, although less so than when the dressing was used as an anode. Silver nylon without an electric current was also found to provide a protective barrier to infection if applied to the wound before the bacterial culture, leading the authors to conclude that silver nylon dressings may be a valuable antimicrobial dressing.

A silver chloride coated nylon wound dressing, which was said to possess marked antimicrobial activity against five common wound pathogens, was described by Adams *et al.*,[27] and Ersek and Denton described how silver impregnated into aldehyde cross-linked skin,[28] or a porcine xenograft,[29] could be used to decontaminate and promoting healing of massive and chronically contaminated longstanding wounds.

The first commercially successful silver dressing was Actisorb Plus, now Actisorb Silver 220, developed from an earlier product called Actisorb, also formed from activated charcoal but which contained no silver. This dressing was shown by Frost *et al.*[30] in experimental studies to adsorb bacteria from suspension, an effect which was claimed to offer potential benefits within an infected wound. Further tests showed, however, that although these organisms were held firmly by the dressing, they still remained viable. Silver was therefore added to the cloth prior to carbonisation to provide a degree of antimicrobial activity.

Commercial silver dressings

Early studies such as those described by Deitch and his colleagues,[25] eventually resulted in the development of a large number of silver-containing dressings examples of which are summarized in Table 20.

Most of these dressings employ one of a relatively small range of silver compounds to exert an antimicrobial effect. These include simple inorganic molecules such as silver chloride and silver sulphate or silver complexes which are available in a number of forms. The most commonly used is silver sodium hydrogen zirconium phosphate a ceramic ion-exchange resin produced under the brand name of Alphasan (Milliken Chemicals) but others include silver sulphadiazine, silver alginate, and a silver-containing 'bioactive glass' or 'biologically active glass', an inorganic glass material formed from silver-calcium-sodium phosphates which is capable of breaking down and releasing silver in the presence of physiological fluids.

Some products are formed from fibres produced from silver-sodium carboxymethylcellulose or silver-calcium alginate produced by means an ion-exchange process where sodium is replaced by silver. When these materials are used in wound care, sodium in the wound exudate binds to the dressing, causing a release of silver from the dressing fibres. Other products utilise silver in the metallic state either as silver coated fibres or deposited over the entire surface the dressing. One product includes colloidal silver (very finely divided particles of silver) suspended in an aqueous medium.

Irrespective of their composition, all of these preparations share a common function in that they represent a source of silver cations which are released into the wound over time. In the case of metallic silver this is only very sparingly soluble in water and only releases ions on contact with water through an oxidation process although the rate at which this occurs can be enhanced by increasing the surface area of metal exposed to the aqueous environment. The nature and concentration of the silver contained in each of the commercially available products is summarised in Table 25.

Table 20: Commercial silver dressings

Product	Description
Actisorb Silver 220	Previously known as Actisorb Plus, the dressing consists principally of activated carbon impregnated with metallic silver produced by heating a treated fine viscose fabric under carefully controlled conditions. The carbonised fabric is enclosed in a spun-bonded non-woven nylon sleeve sealed along all four edges to facilitate handling and reduce particle and fibre loss.
Acticoat	Acticoat Silver consists of two layers of a high-density polyethylene mesh that has been coated with silver by magnetron sputtering, a vapour deposition process. This results in the formation of microscopic 'nanocrystals' of metallic silver less than 1 μm thick,[31] (Silcryst technology). Between the two silver-coated polyethylene layers is a single layer of an apertured non-woven fabric of rayon and polyester. These three elements are ultrasonically welded together to maintain the dressing's integrity during use. Acticoat is described as an 'antimicrobial barrier dressing' which will remain active for up to three days.
Acticoat 7	Acticoat 7 is similar in appearance to Acticoat but the inner core consists of two layers of an apertured non-woven fabric made from rayon and polyester. Between the two layers of non-woven fabric is an additional layer of the silver coated polyethylene mesh. All five layers are ultrasonically welded together as before and this presentation has a projected wear time of up to seven days.
Acticoat Absorbent	Acticoat Absorbent is a single ply dressing made from Type 1 calcium alginate fibre that has been coated on both surfaces with nanocrystalline silver and so combines the absorbency of the alginates with the antimicrobial properties of silver.
Acticoat Moisture Control	Acticoat Moisture Control consists of an apertured polyurethane membrane coated with nanocrystalline silver forming a low-adherent wound contact layer, bonded to a sheet of polyurethane foam bearing a blue semipermeable film backing layer. This presentation combines the fluid handling and moisture retaining properties of a foam dressing with the antibacterial activity of silver.
AFM Ag	AFM Ag, previously called 'Selectsilver' is described by the manufacturer as a multi-component textile substrate which contains ionic silver in a controlled-release form.

Table 21: Commercial silver dressings (continued)

Product	Description
AFM Ultra Ag	AFM Ultra Ag comprises a polyurethane foam sheet with a semipermeable film backing layer. The foam has a textile wound contact layer designed to promote uniform fluid uptake by the foam. The dressing contains ionic silver in a controlled-release form.
Algicell Ag	Algicell Ag is a fibrous silver-containing dressing prepared by blending alginate fibres rich in mannuronic acid (high gelling) with others rich in guluronic acid to ensure that the dressing gels well while maintaining its physical integrity to facilitate removal.
Algidex Ag	See Calgitrol Ag
Allevyn Ag	Allevyn Ag comprises a silver containing absorbent foam layer sandwiched between a perforated wound contact layer and an outer waterproof semipermeable film layer. An adhesive island version is also available.
Altreet Ag	See Physiotulle Ag
Arglaes	Arglaes consists of a mixture of an alginate powder and an inorganic silver polymer. In the presence of moisture the alginate absorbs liquid to form a gel and the silver complex breaks down in a controlled fashion to liberate ionic silver into the wound.
Aquacel Ag	Aquacel Ag consists of a fleece of silver-sodium carboxymethyl-cellulose fibres containing ionic silver. In the presence of exudate, the dressing absorbs liquid to form a gel, binding sodium ions and releasing silver ions.
Aquacel Ag with strengthening fibre	Aquacel Ag with strengthening fibre, a ribbon dressing for packing wounds, has the same composition as standard Aquacel Ag ribbon dressing, but is stitch bonded for added strength.
Atrauman Ag	Atrauman Ag is silver coated wound contact layer impregnated with a low adherent ointment containing triglycerides (see chapter on low adherent dressings).
Avance	Avance consists of a polyurethane foam-film dressing containing silver zirconium phosphate.
Biatain Ag	Previously called Contreet Ag Foam, Biatain Ag is a polyurethane foam dressing containing ionic silver which is released as the foam absorbs liquid.

Table 22: Commercial silver dressings (continued)

Product	Description
Contreet	Contreet, previously called Comfeel Ag, is a hydrocolloid dressing which is based on the original Comfeel with the addition of silver.
Calgitrol Ag/Algidex Ag	Calgitrol Ag consists of an absorbent polyurethane foam sheet which is coated on one surface with an alginate matrix containing ionic silver. In the presence of exudate the silver alginate matrix forms a soft gel allowing the slow extended release of silver ions.
Cellosorb Ag	Cellosorb Ag, also known as Urgocell Ag, is a three layered dressing comprising a low-adherent wound contact layer made of a non-occlusive polyester mesh impregnated with hydrocolloid, petroleum jelly and silver particles bonded to an absorbent foam pad with a semipermeable film backing layer.
Contreet Foam	See Biatain Ag.
Granufoam	Granufoam is a polyurethane foam to which is bonded metallic silver which is used as a component of the VAC system in the treatment of infected wounds.
Maxorb Extra Ag	Maxorb Extra Ag is an absorbent silver containing primary dressing made from a blend of carboxymethylcellulose fibres and calcium alginate fibres.
Mepilex Ag	Mepilex Ag is an absorbent silver-containing polyurethane foam dressing. The outer surface of the foam is bonded to a vapour-permeable polyurethane membrane and the wound contact surface is coated with a layer of soft silicone that does not stick to the wound surface or cause trauma to delicate new tissue upon removal.
Miro-Silversorb	A multilayered silver containing absorbent dressing comprising polyester and alginate fibres together with silver in an ionic form
Polymem Silver	The foam contains silver and a non-ionic surfactant together with a humectant and a starch copolymer to enhance the fluid handling properties of the foam.
Physiotulle Ag	Physiotulle Ag is a non-adherent, moist wound healing contact layer containing hydrocolloid particles, petrolatum and silver. Physiotulle Ag should be used in conjunction with a secondary dressing the nature of which is determined by the amount of exudate produced.

Table 23: Commercial silver dressings (continued)

Product	Description
Promogran Prisma	A matrix composed of 55% collagen, 44% oxidised regenerated cellulose and 1% silver. In the presence of exudate the dressing forms a biodegradable gel which binds with and inactivates proteolytic enzymes
Release Ag	See Silvercel
Reliamed	Reliamed is an absorbent silver containing primary dressing made from a blend of carboxymethylcellulose fibres and calcium alginate fibres.
Seasorb Ag	Seasorb Ag is an absorbent silver containing primary dressing made from a blend of carboxymethylcellulose fibres and calcium alginate fibres
Selectsilver	See AFM Ag
Silvercel	Silvercel, also known as Release Ag, is a non-woven pad composed of high tensile strength alginate, carboxymethylcellulose (CMC) and silver coated nylon fibres.
Silverlon	Silverlon, is a knitted fabric dressing, which has been silver-plated by means of a proprietary autocatalytic electroless chemical (reduction-oxidation) plating technique which coats the entire surface of each individual fibre from which the dressing is made, resulting in a very large surface area for the release of ionic silver. This technology is used in the production of large numbers of dressing products.
Silvasorb	Silversorb, Medline, is composed of a synthetic, polyacrylate hydrophilic hydrogel matrix in which is dispersed or suspended microscopic silver-containing particles. On exposure to moisture the silver is released into the wound in a controlled fashion.
Sorbsan Silver	An absorbent silver-containing primary dressing made from calcium alginate fibres rich in mannuronic acid, available as sheet dressings and rope.
Sorbsan Silver	Sorbsan Silver Plus is a multi-component dressing. The wound contact layer consists of a layer of silver-containing alginate fibre bonded to a thin layer of absorbent viscose fibres. Sorbsan Silver Plus SA is a self adhesive dressing in which the absorbent pad is located centrally on a thin cream-coloured polyurethane foam sheet which extends past the edges of the pad to form an island dressing.
Suprasorb A +Ag	An absorbent silver containing primary dressing made from fibres of calcium alginate rich in mannuronic acid

Table 24: Commercial silver dressings (continued)

Product	Description
Urgocell Ag	See Cellosorb
Urgosorb Silver	Urgosorb Silver is an absorbent silver-containing primary dressing made from a blend of fibres of carboxymethylcellulose fibres and alginic acid with a high guluronic acid content.
Urgotul SSD	A low-adherent silver containing wound contact layer made of a non-occlusive polyester mesh impregnated with hydrocolloid petroleum jelly and silver sulphadiazine.
Urgotul Silver	A low-adherent silver containing wound contact layer made of a non-occlusive polyester mesh impregnated with hydrocolloid and petroleum jelly.
Urgotul Duo Silver	A two component silver containing dressing in which a low-adherent wound contact layer made of a non-occlusive polyester mesh impregnated with hydrocolloid, and petroleum jelly is bonded to a thin absorbent lining.
Vliwaktiv Ag	The dressing consists of activated carbon impregnated with metallic silver produced by heating a specially treated fine viscose fabric under carefully controlled conditions. The carbonised fabric is enclosed in a spun-bonded non-woven nylon sleeve sealed along all four edges, to facilitate handling and reduce particle and fibre loss.

PROPERTIES OF SILVER DRESSINGS

Silver content

The silver content of many of the silver dressings in current use is contained in Table 25. These data have been drawn from a number of sources including published papers containing the results of independent laboratory analyses, information provided directly by the manufacturers of the products concerned, and values abstracted from other published sources, the accuracy of which cannot be guaranteed.

The data set is divided into two groups. The majority of results are expressed as silver content per unit area (mg/100 cm^2), the most relevant way to express silver content. In other instances this information is not available and the silver content is expressed as a percentage of the dressings' weight.

Table 25: Silver content of dressings

Proprietary Name	Ag$^+$ content (mg/100cm^2)	Form of silver
Silverlon	546[†]	Metallic silver
Calgitrol Ag/Algidex Ag	96-222*, 141[†]	Ionic silver
Suprasorb A +Ag	195$^\Omega$	n/a
Acticoat 7	148$^\Omega$	Metallic nanocrystalline silver
Mepilex Ag	120$^\Omega$	Silver sulphate
Acticoat Moisture Control		Metallic nanocrystalline silver
Acticoat Absorbent	104[‡]	Metallic nanocrystalline silver
Silvercel/Release Ag	113[‡]	Metallic silver
Acticoat (standard)	109H	Metallic nanocrystalline silver
Biatain Ag/ Contreet foam	95*,85§, 77[‡]	SSHZP
Allevyn Ag	90$^\Omega$	Silver sulphadiazine
Maxorb Extra Ag	51$^\Omega$	SSHZP
Reliamed	51$^\Omega$	SSHZP
Atrauman Ag	50$^\Omega$	Metallic silver
AFM Ag	38$^\Omega$	n/a
Contreet Hydrocolloid	30*, 32[†]	SSHZP

Table 26: Silver content of dressings (continued)

Proprietary Name	Ag^+ content (mg/100cm^2)	Form of silver
Physiotulle Ag	30*	Silver sulphadiazine
Cellosorb Ag/ Urgocell Ag	17*	Silver sulphate
Urgotul Duo Silver	17*	Silver sulphate
Urgotul Silver	17*,14 [‡]	Silver sulphate
Urgotul SSD	14*	Silver sulphate
Sorbsan Silver	13.8*	Silver alginate
Sorbsan Silver Plus	13.8*	Silver alginate
Polymem Silver	12[Ω],13[‡]	Metallic nanocrystalline silver
Aquacel Ag	8.3[†], 9[‡]	Silver-sodium carboxymethylcellulose
Seasorb Ag	7*	SSHZP
Urgosorb Silver	6.0*	Silver alginate
Silvasorb	5.3[†], 5.4[‡]	Silver chloride
Vliwaktiv Ag	3.6[Ω]	Metallic silver
Actisorb Silver 220	2.9[†], 3.3*	Metallic silver
Avance	1.6[†]	SSHZP
Promogran Prisma	1.6*	Silver oxidised regenerated cellulose
Silversorb	0.9*	SSHZP
Arglaes powder	6.9%[†]	Silver glass
Algicell Ag	1.4%*	Silver alginate
Granufoam	10%*	Metallic silver

Key to table

[†] Thomas S, McCubbin P. Journal of Wound Care 2003;12(8):305-8.
§ Thomas S, Ashman P. Journal of Wound Care 2004;13(9):392-393.
[‡] Parsons D, Bowler PG, Myles V, Jones S. Wounds 2005;17(8):222-232.
* Data provided by manufacturer
[Ω] Data from unverified source
SSHZP = Silver sodium hydrogen zirconium phosphate

Whilst the total silver content of a dressing is clearly important, the factor that ultimately determines the biological activity and safety of a silver-containing dressing is the number of bioavailable silver cations that are released into solution and the rate at which these are produced. This depends upon a number of factors that will be discussed later.

Antimicrobial activity

Although the antimicrobial properties of silver dressings have been examined in numerous published studies, these have employed a range of different test organisms and experimental techniques which effectively prevents meaningful comparison of the published data. Some studies have used more than one type of test, arguing that by so doing it is possible to simulate the different clinical conditions under which the dressings may eventually be used. Others have concentrated upon the importance of the composition of the test solution with particular regard to its sodium and chloride content. The full range of test systems that can be employed to compare the antimicrobial properties of dressings, including those containing silver, were comprehensively described by Nadworny and Burrell[4] but for convenience the techniques most commonly described in the literature are summarised below together with the principal advantages and disadvantages of each.

Zone of inhibition method

Arguably, the simplest technique, in essence it simply involves placing a piece of the dressing under examination upon the surface of an agar plate previously seeded with a test organism. Following incubation the bacteria multiply to form a visible layer upon the agar surface and any antimicrobial activity inherent in the test sample is indicated by the formation of a transparent zone or halo around the dressing margin.

If required, the dressing sample may be removed from the incubated plate and placed upon a second seeded plate which is subsequently incubated to detect the presence of any remaining activity, a process which can be repeated as often as necessary. However, this technique has several potential limitations.

If a dressing sample is particularly absorbent it will withdraw moisture from the agar and thus inhibit the ability of the active agent to migrate in the reverse direction to exert its antimicrobial effect. This problem can be addressed by pre-moistening the dressing sample with an appropriate volume of a suitable solution. Alternatively a 'well' technique may be employed. This involves seeding an agar plate as before than cutting a hole in the agar to form a chamber into which the test sample is placed together with a suitable quantity of an appropriate test solution to extract the active from the dressing which is then free to diffuse into the surrounding agar and kill or prevent the growth of the bacteria present upon the surface.

A further feature of this type of test is that it only provides evidence of activity if the active agent is both soluble in water and free to migrate out of the dressing, i.e. one which is not locked or bound into the structure in some way. This ability to differentiate between potentially mobile and immobile active antimicrobial agents can in itself, however, be regarded as a positive attribute of the technique.

Finally there is a real possibility that as the active agent migrates out of the dressing and into the agar it may react with one or more of the components of the gel which will reduce or eliminate its antimicrobial activity.

Gallant-Behm *et al.*[32] compared seven silver-containing dressings and two non-silver-containing topical agents against 17 clinically relevant microorganisms using zone of inhibition assays and time-kill kinetic assays (described below) in complex media. They found no correlation between the two systems and proposed that this was due to the silver interacting with the media in the zone of inhibition test, thus invalidating the results of this test. They therefore concluded that zone of inhibition data generated for silver-containing dressings is of little value and that time-kill assays are of greater use. This view was echoed by Nadworny and Burrell,[4] who considered them to be 'clearly inappropriate' and supported the view of Gallant-Behm *et al.*,[32] that 'it is a basic tenet of diffusion based test assays that the test compound cannot interact with the test medium or the test is invalidated.'

This statement is regarded as something of an oversimplification. Whilst it is true of an assay system that is designed to quantify the concentration or strength of an active agent present in a test sample, it is not necessarily the case when the test method is intended to function not as an assay, but to determine or predict how a product is likely to perform during normal clinical use. If the interactions that take place in the test system, such as the combination of silver ions with chloride ions or proteins, are precisely those which will occur *in vivo,* it can be argued that the test does bear some relevance to clinical practice.

It is therefore suggested that zone of inhibition technique does have a role to play as part of a battery of tests as it is quick and easy to perform and provides some indication of the release characteristics of the active agent from the dressing. Furthermore, although the technique may theoretically produce a false negative result, it cannot lead to a false positive outcome, so although a product which performs poorly in such a test may, or may not, function more effectively clinically, a product that performs well may reasonably be expected to function similarly *in vivo.* A further advantage of the method is that it also permits a piece of dressing to be reused several times to examine its release characteristics over time.

Challenge testing/logarithmic reduction assays

In its simplest form, this technique involves incubating a piece of dressing with a suspension of a test organism containing a known quantity of viable cells. At predetermined intervals, small aliquots are removed from the suspension and the number of viable organisms present determined using a standard microbiological technique. As before test it is usual to pre-moisten the test sample to ensure that it simply does not absorb all the suspension that is added to it.

This type of test addresses some of the problems associated with the zone of inhibition method in that it ensures that the active agent is exposed to a relatively large volume of solution to facilitate extraction. Furthermore, if the sample is shaken or agitated continuously throughout the test, it also ensures that the bacteria come into intimate contact with the test material and any antimicrobial agent bound within its structure which is not released into solution. If required, the test may be modified by the addition of a fresh bacterial suspension at different time points to simulate a more stringent challenge.

This method is also not without some disadvantages. It does not differentiate between bound and unbound antimicrobials and the possibility also exists that microorganisms will become bound to the structure of the dressing and so effectively be taken out of suspension, resulting in an overestimate of the test sample's true antimicrobial activity. This second problem may be addressed, at least in part, by running appropriate controls using unmedicated versions of the same dressings if these are available, or alternatively by washing or extracting the dressing sample with water or some suitable solvent in an attempt to recover any organisms taken up by the dressing in this way. This later procedure requires that individual test samples must be prepared for each assessment point as it is not possible to use each one more than once.

Whichever method is used, the number of surviving organisms may be converted to a logarithm and compared to the logarithmic equivalent of the initial inoculum. The difference between these two values is termed the log reduction. If this value is greater than three, then the agent is deemed to be bactericidal in nature. If the difference is less than three it may be regarded as bacteriostatic. In the context of testing silver dressings, in all of these tests the chemical composition of the test extract is once again likely to be very important.

For the reasons given above, however, it is by no means certain that this technique used alone will actually predict the ability of a silver-containing dressing to exert a significant clinical effect.

Bacterial transfer test

This test, which developed specifically for this type of study, examines the ability of bacteria to survive on the surface of a dressing and thus predict, for example, if it would permit organisms to move laterally out of a contaminated wound onto the surrounding skin, or migrate from the intact skin into the wound itself.

Using a sterile scalpel a strip of agar is removed from a standard agar plate leaving two areas of agar separated by a narrow channel. A second strip of agar is then removed on the outer side of one of these areas producing a small chamber, effectively forming the adjacent agar block into an island in the Petri dish.

This island is inoculated with a bacterial suspension, and after a short drying period, three strips of one the dressings under test, each approximately 10 mm wide and 50 mm long are placed across the two remaining agar areas forming a bridge.

The chamber on the outer side of the agar island is then carefully filled with sterile test fluid taking care not to wet the dressing or flood the surface of the agar. The plate is then incubated in the upright position for 24 - 48 hours. During this period the agar slowly absorbs some of the added solution which in turn is taken up by the dressing strip and distributed throughout its length, carrying with it bacteria drawn up from the surface of the agar 'island'. In the absence of any significant antimicrobial activity within the dressing, these microorganisms eventually reach the second area of agar where they grow to form colonies around the margin of the end of the test sample. If the dressing contains an active antimicrobial agent the movement of organisms in this way is prevented and no growth is detected upon the previously sterile agar island. This simple test provides very clear evidence of the ability of a dressing to permit or prevent the growth of microorganisms upon its surface.

Results of published laboratory studies

The antimicrobial properties of Actisorb Plus (now Actisorb Silver 220) were compared with those of the original Actisorb in an elegant series of tests undertaken in 1994 by Furr et al.[33] Using a zone of inhibition technique, they showed that Actisorb Plus, but not Actisorb, was able to inhibit the growth of a range of different bacteria growing on the surface of Diagnostic Sensitivity Test Agar (DST). Inhibition of this activity by the sulphydryl compound sodium thioglycollate, confirmed that this antimicrobial action was due to the release of low concentrations of silver ions from the dressing into the agar.

The ability of this dressing to remove bacterial cells from a suspension was examined by Addison and Rennison,[34] using the technique first described by Frost some 20 years earlier. They compared the performance of Actisorb Silver with that of two other dressings, Contreet Hydrocolloid dressing and Avance, in a log_{10} reduction assay. Over a three-hour period they found that Actisorb produced five log reductions and Contreet Hydrocolloid dressing four log reductions; no significant antimicrobial effect could be demonstrated with Avance. It is likely, however, that this experiment was comparing the ability of dressings to remove organisms from suspension, not necessarily measuring their bactericidal effect.

Muller et al.[35] subsequently demonstrated that not only could Actisorb Silver 220 take up and kill P. aeruginosa, it could do so without releasing endotoxins into the environment, leading them to speculate that this effect might be beneficial in the treatment of wounds infected with this and other organisms.

Wright in a laboratory-based study,[36] compared the antimicrobial properties of Acticoat with a solution of silver nitrate and a cream containing silver sulfadiazine against eleven antibiotic multi-resistant clinical isolates. He showed that of the three preparations Acticoat was the most effective, killing all the organisms examined. Based upon these results, he suggested that silver products could be used as an alternative to antibiotics to curb the spread of antibiotic-resistant bacteria.

In a subsequent study,[37] Wright compared the activity of the same three dressings against a spectrum of common burn wound fungal pathogens and showed that the Acticoat provided the fastest and broadest-spectrum fungicidal activity.

Yin et al.[38] compared the antimicrobial activity of Acticoat with silver nitrate, silver sulfadiazine and mafenide acetate using different test systems to determine their minimum inhibitory concentration (MIC), minimum bactericidal concentration (MBC) and zone of inhibition. They showed that although the mafenide acetate produced the greatest zone of inhibition, the MBC of the product was much higher than its MIC indicating that it had a bacteriostatic rather than a bactericidal action. In contrast the

MICs and MBCs of the silver-containing products were very similar, indicating that their activity is essentially bactericidal. They also showed that although the MIC values for the three silver preparations were comparable in terms of their silver content, the speed of action of Acticoat was more rapid than the other two products. They suggested that the metallic silver on the surface of the dressing forms a reservoir of silver ions that are released continuously and therefore always available for bacterial uptake. Because of the apparent differences provided by the various test systems used, the authors concluded that a single susceptibility test such as an MIC or zone of inhibition test does not provide a comprehensive profile of antimicrobial activity of a topical agent or dressing and recommended that a combination of tests is desirable when comparing the performance of such preparations.

Fraser et al.[39] compared the antimicrobial activity of Acticoat with 1% SSD and Silvazine, a cream containing 1% SSD and 0.2% chlorhexidine digluconate, against eight common burn wound pathogens. Samples of each product were inoculated with bacterial growth medium to which had been added aliquots of a suspension of the chosen bacterial isolates containing approximately 10^4 - 10^5 organisms. The samples were then incubated and aliquots removed at specified intervals for examination. The combination of 1% SSD and 0.2% chlorhexidine digluconate proved to be most effective biocide; SSD and Acticoat performed similarly against a number of isolates, but Acticoat appeared to be only bacteriostatic against E. faecalis and MRSA. Also E. cloacae and P. mirabilis could still be recovered after 24 hours.

The antimicrobial properties of Aquacel Ag were investigated in a further study conducted by Jones et al.[40] using a zone of inhibition technique and by Bowler et al.[41] who used both a zone of inhibition technique and a form of repeat challenge test against recognised burn pathogens in a simulated wound fluid. Dressing samples were inoculated with the challenge organisms at time zero and then reinoculated on days 4 and 9 to mimic the worst-case clinical scenario. The dressing maintained its activity throughout the 14 day test period.

Castellano et al.[42] compared eight commercially available silver-containing dressings: Acticoat 7, Acticoat Moisture Control, Acticoat Absorbent, Silvercel, Aquacel Ag, Contreet F, Urgotol SSD and Actisorb, against three commercially available topical antimicrobial creams, a non treatment control, and a topical silver-containing antimicrobial hydrogel, Silvasorb. Zone of inhibition and quantitative testing was performed by standard methods using E. coli, P. aeruginosa, E. faecalis and S. aureus. Silver-containing dressings with the highest concentrations of silver exhibited the strongest bacterial inhibitive properties. Sulfamylon and gentamicin sulphate, and the topical antimicrobial gel Silvasorb exhibited superior bacterial inhibition and bactericidal properties, essentially eliminating all bacterial growth at 24 hours.

A more unconventional approach to assessing the antimicrobial activity of two silver dressings was reported by O'Neill et al.[43] who used the technique of isothermal microcalorimetry to compare the antimicrobial efficacy of Aquacel Ag and Acticoat 7. According to the authors, this technique allows non-invasive and non-destructive analysis to be performed directly on a test sample, regardless of whether it is homogeneous or heterogeneous in nature. Both dressings were tested against S. aureus and *P. aeruginosa* and found to have the capacity to kill organisms within one to two hours of contact.

The same technique was subsequently used by the same authors,[44] in a study in which the growth of *P. aeruginosa* was monitored in the presence and absence of Aquacel Ag. They found that 10 mg of dressing was sufficient to ensure no detectable growth of the test organism in 2.5 mL of medium containing 10^6 cfu/mL. This was equivalent to a silver load of 1.1×10^{-6} moles, equivalent to 4.4×10^{-4} M, in the volume of medium used in the experiment.

When the experiment was repeated with silver nitrate solution in place of the dressing the concentration required to prevent growth was 1×10^{-4} M. The authors suggested that this difference was due to the fact that not all the silver in the dressing was bioavailable, at least over the lifetime of the experiment and suggested that this may either reduce the possibility of silver toxicity or prolong the useful life of the product.

Ip *et al.*[45] compared the antibacterial activities of five silver dressings: Acticoat, Aquacel Ag, Contreet, Polymem Silver and Urgotul SSD, against nine common burn-wound pathogens using a broth culture method. They and found that although all were bactericidal against Gram-negative bacteria, including Enterobacter species, Proteus species and *E. coli*, there were differences between the products in terms of their speed and spectrum of activity. Acticoat and Contreet performed well and had a broad spectrum of bactericidal activities against both Gram-positive and Gram-negative bacteria. Contreet was characterized by a very rapid bactericidal action and achieved a reduction of $\geq 10,000$ cfu/mL in the first 30 min for *E. cloacae*, *P. vulgaris*, *P. aeruginosa* and *Acinetobacter baumanii*. Other dressings demonstrated a narrower range of bactericidal activities and Aquacel Ag and Polymem performed poorly against some of the test organisms, particularly the Gram-positive *S. aureus*. This study was subsequently criticised by Nadworny and Burrell,[4] because the large volumes of extract applied to each dressing sample were greatly in excess of that to which the dressings would be exposed in normal clinical practice.

The ability of a silver-containing dressing, Acticoat, to form a bacterial barrier was demonstrated in the laboratory by Holder *et al.*[46] in 2003, and subsequently by Edwards-Jones[47] who compared the ability of five dressings, three silver donating and two non-silver-donating, in this regard. The dressings were applied to the moist surface of blood agar plates covered with 10^6 colony-forming units of the respective strain of MRSA. The plates were incubated for different time periods and the upper and lower surfaces of the dressings were subcultured to detect residual growth. The silver donating Acticoat dressings were effective as a barrier from one hour until the study was terminated at 72 hours as neither organism penetrated through the dressings. Evidence of antimicrobial activity beneath the dressing was also detected throughout this time. The remaining dressings failed to function as an effective barrier and only produced limited antimicrobial activity after 24 hours

The antimicrobial properties of various silver containing dressings were compared using several different test systems in two laboratory-based studies reported by Thomas and McCubbin.[48-49] The results of the zone of inhibition tests undertaken in these studies indicated that Acticoat, Aquacel Ag, Calgitrol, Contreet hydrocolloid dressing and Silverlon exhibited the most activity. This activity could be demonstrated over several days by applying the same test sample to a series of plates. Arglaes and Silvasorb also showed some activity but no zones of inhibition could be detected with Actisorb and Avance.

The second test, a microbiological challenge test, compared the speed at which each product was able to kill microorganisms applied to it in the form of a suspension. To portions of each dressing were added aliquots of a log phase culture of each test organism. The inoculated dressings were then incubated for 2 hours after which they were transferred into 10 mL of 0.1% peptone water and vortexed to remove any viable organisms remaining in the dressings. Serial dilutions were performed in triplicate on each extract and the number of viable organisms present in each determined using a standard surface counting technique.

If viable organisms were recovered during this process the test was repeated as before using a 4-hour contact period then again with a 24-hour contact period. If no organisms were detected in a particular dressing after two hours, in subsequent tests the dressing was not extracted with peptone water but placed in 10 mL of tryptone soya broth (TSB) to detect very low levels of residual contamination – effectively a form of sterility test. As no inactivator for silver was used during this test, there is a possibility that low concentrations of silver ions could be carried over in the dilutions which could prevent the recovery of these organisms. It is also possible that some organisms remained bound to the dressings which would further overestimate the killing ability of the various products.

The results of this comprehensive comparison suggest that although Acticoat produced the most rapid kill, other products also exhibited considerable activity following more prolonged incubation. Significant differences were also detected between the activities of the dressings on the two different bacterial strains (Table 27).

There are apparent inconsistencies between some of the results of these tests and those reported by Addison and Rennison[34] which suggested that after 3 hours incubation Actisorb Silver reduced the number of viable organisms in suspension from 10^5 to virtually undetectable levels. It is likely, however, that in their tests, Addison and Rennison were simply observing what Frost had demonstrated previously, specifically that the Actisorb was removing the organisms from suspension and binding them to the surface of the charcoal fibres. The results from the present study suggest that these organisms remain viable for many hours until they are progressively inactivated by the silver ions incorporated into the dressing.

When the dressings were examined by the bacterial transfer test, evidence of transmission of bacteria was clearly visible with all three samples of Avance. Actisorb produced mixed results in that one test strip out of three examined permitted bacterial transfer with both *S. aureus* and *E. coli*. When only the central core of the Actisorb dressing was tested in this way, however, no evidence of transmission was seen, suggesting that although the inner core that contains the silver forms an effective barrier, the outer nylon sleeve does not. These results suggest that at least some of the organisms recovered from the Actisorb during the challenge test may have been associated with the outer sleeve. All the other test samples prevented the transfer of the test organisms.

Table 27: Summary of microbial challenge test results

	S. aureus	E. coli	C. albicans
Products that demonstrated marked antibacterial activity after 2 hours incubation	Acticoat Calgitrol Ag	Acticoat Calgitrol Ag Contreet Ag Silverlon	Acticoat Calgitrol Ag Contreet Ag Silverlon
Products that demonstrated marked antimicrobial activity after 4 hours incubation	Silverlon	Contreet H Aquacel Ag Silversorb	
Products that demonstrated marked antimicrobial activity after 24 hours incubation.		Actisorb	
Products that demonstrated limited evidence of antimicrobial activity after 24 hours incubation.	Aquacel Ag Contreet H Contreet Ag Silvasorb		Contreet H Aquacel Ag Silvasorb
Products that demonstrated no convincing evidence of antimicrobial activity even upon prolonged incubation	Actisorb Avance	Avance	Actisorb Avance

Despite the shortcomings of the individual test systems they identified major differences in the properties of the dressings examined, and even the zone of inhibition technique, which has been heavily criticized by Nadworny and Burrell,[4] revealed marked differences in the performance of the dressings, particularly in their ability to function over an extended period.

The effect of test solution composition on antimicrobial activity

Following the publication of their first two studies,[48-49] Thomas and McCubbin discussed the problems of conducting clinically-relevant laboratory-based studies designed to compare the antimicrobial properties of different types of silver containing dressings.[50] They acknowledged that Biatain Ag (previously called Contreet Foam), one of the dressings examined in their earlier study, might not have achieved its full antimicrobial potential because the silver ions in the product in question are not available to exert an antimicrobial effect until they are released from the dressing by contact with sodium ions - information that had not been previously made available by the manufacturer.

A small supplementary study was therefore undertaken to examine the effect of the ionic composition of test solutions on dressing with particular reference to the presence of sodium and calcium ions.[51] Circular samples of dressing, 15 mm in diameter, were prepared and moistened with deionised water, a solution containing sodium and calcium ions at equivalent concentrations to those found in human serum (Solution A), or foetal calf serum. These circular samples were then placed onto the surface of tryptone soya agar plates, previously seeded with a log-phase culture of S. aureus. Further samples, prepared in an identical fashion, were introduced into wells about 18 mm in diameter cut into agar plates previously seeded with S. aureus followed by sufficient test solution added to nearly fill each well. All the plates were incubated overnight at 33°c and any zones of inhibition were measured to provide an indication of the amount of active silver released from each product. The results of these tests are shown in Table 28

Table 28: Effect of test solution upon microbiological activity

Test method	Test sample	Zone diameter (mm)		
		Water	Solution A	Serum
Surface method	Acticoat	2-3	1-2	1-2
	Contreet	0	0-1	0
Well method	Acticoat	<2-3	<1	<1
	Contreet	0	2-3	1-2

In second experiment samples of both dressings each measuring 40×40 mm were extracted with either 10 mL of sterile water or a similar volume of Solution A for 24 and 48 hours. Aliquots of each extract were then added to wells cut into agar plates bearing the test organism and after 24 hours incubation the diameters of any zones of inhibition measured, (Table 29).

Table 29: Effect of test solution upon microbiological activity (well method)

Test method	Test sample	Zone diameter (mm)	
		Water extract	Solution A extract
24 hours extract	Acticoat	3-4	0
	Contreet	0	2-3
48 hour extract	Acticoat	3-4	0
	Contreet	0	1-2

The results confirm that the choice of extractant can have important implications for the performance of the products under the test conditions described. The activity of an extract of Acticoat made with Solution A or serum is significantly reduced or inhibited compared with that made in an identical fashion with deionised water, due it is assumed to the precipitation of insoluble silver chloride. These findings are consistent with the instructions for use provided by the manufacturer, which suggests that the dressing must be moistened with water not saline prior to use.

They are also consistent with the observations of Walker et al,[52] who measured the release of silver from Aquacel Ag and Acticoat. When the dressings were hydrated with water, the amount of silver released from Acticoat was 50 - 60 times that released from Aquacel Ag ($p < 0.005$) but when saline was used as the hydration medium, the release rates were low for both dressings and not significantly different, approximately 1 µg/mL - the solubility limit of silver chloride.

The observation that antimicrobial activity was detected in the extract of Acticoat made with Solution A in the first experiment, but not in the second, may be explained by the fact that in the former case a portion of dressing was placed in the well and the vast reservoir of silver present released sufficient silver ions to overwhelm the relatively low number of chloride ions in solution.

In the second experiment only the extract was tested and in this case there were insufficient free silver ions present to exert a significant effect as these were removed from solution by the formation of the virtually insoluble silver chloride. The results also support the statement made by the manufacturer of Contreet that the product requires activation by sodium ions to exert a significant effect. It is unfortunate that this information was not placed in the public domain at an earlier stage.

The differing requirements of the two dressings make the development and general adoption of a standard test system extremely difficult, creating something of a dilemma. Specifically it raises the question whether they should be tested using the solutions recommended by the manufacturers of the products concerned, making reasonable attempts to prevent or minimise inactivation of silver ions, or should they be tested using a wound exudate substitute such as serum, accepting that any inactivation that occurs is simply reflecting the clinical environment. Variations in the choice of test solutions used in published studies undoubtedly contribute to the variability of test results recorded in the literature.

The importance of the choice of test solution was recognised by Parsons *et al.*[53] who undertook a study in which they compared the characteristics of seven silver-containing antimicrobial dressings: three fibrous products, Aquacel Ag, Acticoat Absorbent, and Silvercel; two foam dressings, Contreet Foam/Biatain Ag and Polymem Silver; an impregnated gauze dressing, Urgotul SSD; and a hydrogel coated product, Silvasorb.

The total silver content of each dressing was determined by atomic absorption spectrophotometry following acid digestion and was found to range from 6 to 113 mg/100 cm^2. Silver content was greatest in Acticoat Absorbent and Silvercel and least in Urgotul SSD and Silvasorb. The amount of silver released by each dressing into deionised water in a temperature-controlled environment over seven days was also determined. Weighed samples of each product were suspended in water in the ratio of 1:100 by weight; aliquots were removed at timed intervals, filtered, diluted as appropriate, and analyzed by atomic absorption spectrometry. Measured silver values ranged from 17 to 111 mg/100 cm^2 for the majority of dressings after 48 hours.

Antibacterial activity of the dressings was assessed in repeat-challenge assays over a seven day period against *S. aureus* and *P. aeruginosa*. To make the test as clinically relevant as possible, a simulated wound fluid (SWF) was prepared consisting of 50% foetal calf serum and 50% maximum recovery diluent containing 0.1% w/v peptone (beef protein extract) and 0.9% w/v sodium chloride. Portions of the dressings under examination were added to a suitable volume of SWF containing a standard number of microorganisms and incubated at 35°C. Aliquots were removed at 4, 24, 48, 72, and 96 hours and on Day 7 in order to determine the total number of viable organisms remaining in suspension. At the 48-hour time point, each test sample was re-inoculated with approximately 1×10^6 cfu/mL of the original challenge organism.

The three fibrous products, Aquacel Ag, Acticoat Absorbent, and Silvercel and the impregnated gauze Urgotul Ag demonstrated the greatest overall antibacterial activity, reducing bacterial counts for both test organisms from > 10^6 colony-forming units per mL (cfu/mL) of SWF (< 500 cfu/mL) within 48 hours. Acticoat Absorbent reduced the number of *S. aureus* to below the limit of detection (< 10 cfu/mL) by 24 hours. Aquacel Ag and Acticoat Absorbent were both highly effective against *P. aeruginosa*, reducing the viable microbial count below the limit of detection by 24 hours and both remained highly active when rechallenged with bacteria 48 hours after the start of the test. Impregnated gauze (which contains silver sulfadiazine) and Silvercel were also active against both organisms but were less effective against *P. aeruginosa* when rechallenged.

The two foam dressings and the hydrogel coated dressing showed only limited antibacterial activity against the selected organisms in this test system, (

Table 30).

Table 30: Comparison of silver content, rate of silver release and antibacterial activity [†]

	Ag content (mg/100cm^2)	Silver released in deionised water (µg/100cm^2)		Antibacterial activity in SWF after rechallenge
		After 3 h	After 48 h	
Aquacel	9	3.2	17	+++
Acticoat Absorbent	104	555	3,011	+++
Silvercel	113	0.07	64	++
Biatain Ag/Contreet foam	77	4.6	102	+
Polymem Silver	13	0.00	70	+
Urgotul SSD	14	0.53	49	++
Silvasorb	6	5.4	111	+

[†]*Table constructed from data contained in Parsons D, Bowler PG, Myles V, Jones S. Wounds 2005;17(8):222-232.*

No correlation was found between silver release and silver content as the amount of silver released from Acticoat Absorbent was approximately 50-fold greater than that released from Silvercel despite the fact that the dressings have a similar total silver content. An even greater difference (180-fold) was recorded in the amount of silver released into water after 48 hours by Acticoat Absorbent and Aquacel Ag; once again these differences did not correlate with the antibacterial activity of the dressings. The authors stressed that it is important to remember that these measurements of aqueous silver concentrations fail to distinguish between active ionic silver (Ag+) and inactive silver in solution.

The dissolution results and the antimicrobial results may be partly explained by consideration of the mechanisms and rate of the formation of ionic silver. With some dressings, although they actually contain relatively high levels of silver, the concentration of silver ions produced in deionised water is principally determined by the chemical nature or form of the silver. In the case of Acticoat for example, it is assumed that the silver ion is formed from the metallic silver crystals by oxidation followed by the formation of the hydroxide ion. The maximum solubility of silver in this form is around 14,000 µg/L[9] although this will be reduced by if carbon dioxide is also present in solution. This value is not inconsistent with that found experimentally

---

[9] http://www.silver-colloids.com/Papers/Solubility_Products.PDF

described in the table above. Silvasorb contains silver chloride, which has a solubility of 1400 μg/L and therefore it might be predicted that this would produce approximately one tenth of the concentration of silver ions produced by Acticoat. Once again this is not inconsistent with the experimental data.

A second important factor that determines the rate of formation of silver ions in deionised water is the nature of the product itself. Silvercel actually contains more silver that Acticoat but because the surface area of the silver is much less, the rate of oxidation and ion formation is reduced. Similarly if the silver containing compound is contained in the structure of the dressing the rate at which test solution or exudate moves into and out of the product may be a rate limiting factor determining the release of silver ions.

In the presence of chloride ions, the situation changes for under these conditions the silver ions in solution react with the chloride to form the insoluble silver chloride which then precipitates out. Similar interactions occur with soluble proteins. In the clinical situation, therefore, it might be expected that most silver-releasing dressings would perform in a similar way, because irrespective of their ability to release silver ions, the concentration of the active species would always be limited by the solubility of silver chloride, assuming of course that the number of silver ions produced exceed the solubility product of silver chloride.

In practice, however, this is not found to be the case, for marked differences between the activities of various dressings have been shown in the microbiological studies described previously. The reason for these differences is by no means clear but it may be related to the rate of formation of the silver ions. Within the wound environment the situation is not static as the chloride ions which react with the silver ions are constantly replaced by more ions present in fresh wound fluid which is produced on a continuous basis. Similarly there is an enormous excess of protein material present in wound fluid which also will also tend to 'mop up' the relatively small numbers of silver ions released by some dressings. For this reason the rate of silver ion production may become an important factor in determining activity. This issue, with particular emphasis on the importance of the rate of kill by silver ions was debated in the literature by Burrell and Parsons.[1,5-6]

Brett[54] in a review which was subsequently criticised for lack of objectivity in some areas,[55] suggested that the differences reported in the literature for the performance of different silver dressings might be explained in part by variations in the sensitivity of different strains of particular microorganisms to silver ions. According to Parsons et al,[53,55] optimal activity is observed for dressings that can produce and maintain the highest concentration of ionic silver permitted by the total wound environment, but they argued that is it is difficult to assess each the performance of a dressing in this regard accurately by chemical measurements, a direct measure of antibacterial activity provides a more accurate predictor of potential clinical activity than simply comparing silver content or silver release into an unrealistic solution such as water.

The test systems so far described involved free-living or planktonic bacteria. Percival et al.[56] described a test in which they compared the sensitivity of a range of antibiotic-sensitive and antibiotic-resistant bacteria grown on agar with those grown on a poloxamer gel which they suggested encourages microorganisms to exhibit a more clinically relevant biofilm phenotype. The organisms were challenged with two silver dressings, Aquacel Ag and Acticoat, using a zone-of-inhibition test system. They reported that when grown on agar (presenting a quasi-sessile state of each organism), the antibiotic-susceptible microorganisms were generally more susceptible to Aquacel Ag than Acticoat. When grown on poloxamer gel, (presenting the biofilm state of each organism) the same group of microorganisms were less susceptible to both dressings. Aquacel was most effective against strains of *P. aeruginosa*, *C. albicans* and *S. aureus*, but Acticoat was most effective against strains of *K. pneumoniae*, *E. faecalis* and *E. coli*. Nine of the ten antibiotic-resistant bacterial strains grown on agar were more susceptible to Aquacel than Acticoat.

The effect of dressing design on antimicrobial activity

As previously identified, although total silver content is important, there are other factors that influence the ability of a silver-containing dressing to kill microorganisms. These include:

- The location of the silver within the dressing, whether it is present as a surface coating or dispersed through the structure.
- The chemical and physical form of the silver, whether it is present in the metallic, bound, or ionic state.
- The affinity of the dressing for moisture – a prerequisite for the release of active agents in an aqueous environment.

Products which contain silver in an ionic form, particularly those which have the silver content concentrated on the surface of the dressing rather than 'locked up' within its structure, tend to perform well in laboratory tests, particularly those involving zone of inhibition testing.

Aquacel Ag, for example, contains ionic silver in a hydrophilic fibrous fleece made from CMC fibre. The affinity of this material for liquid is such that it is readily capable of drawing fluid out of the agar, which then releases the silver ions from the dressing. This enables the dressing to exert significant antimicrobial activity on extended incubation despite the relatively modest silver content. Silvasorb, which also contains a relatively low concentration of ionic silver, shows broadly similar activity to Aquacel, due to the hydrophilic nature of its structure and its location on the dressing surface.

White and Cutting[12] also stressed the importance of dressing conformability, specifically its ability to conform to the wound bed to eliminate dead spaces where bacterial-rich exudate can accumulate, particularly for those products which have the ability to take up bacterial cells and remove them from suspension.[30,34,57]

The distance between the source of the silver ions and the wound bed is also important, the smaller the space, the greater the chance of achieving clinically effective concentrations of silver ions at this location.

Considerable caution must be exercised, however, when extrapolating the results of any laboratory-based wound-management studies to the clinical situation, as there may be factors which influence the acceptability or clinical effectiveness of a dressing which are not identified in a simple laboratory study.

For example, Avance, which performed very poorly in all these tests, is claimed to provide a moist wound healing environment that promotes wound healing. Similarly Actisorb Silver 220 appears to offer little prospect of killing bacteria within the wound itself but there is good evidence to suggest that the dressing is capable of removing microorganisms from wound exudate and sequestering them until the silver within the charcoal fibres subsequently inactivates them. The results of clinical studies involving Actisorb Silver 220 also appear to suggest that dressing is more effective clinically than appears to be predicted by the laboratory results (Chapter 17).

It has also been suggested that the presence of silver ions within a wound may have properties unrelated to their antimicrobial activity that could influence the wound-healing cascade.[11] If the concentration of silver required is below that necessary to produce an antimicrobial effect, it is theoretically possible, although not considered likely, that *all* of the dressings examined may liberate sufficient quantities of silver to initiate these effects. Conversely it is also possible that excessive silver delivered to a wound could have a deleterious effect and thus delay wound healing; further work is required to address all of these issues

Miscellaneous properties of silver dressings

Effect on proteolytic enzymes

The ability of silver ions to combine with proteins, including enzymes, suggests that in some situations, this property may impart clinical benefits to silver dressings that are not related to their antimicrobial activity.

One area where this reactivity may be important is in controlling excessive proteinase activity, a problem which is sometimes encountered in chronic wounds. Four silver-containing products, Aquacel Ag, Acticoat, Silvercel and a 0.5% w/v aqueous solution of silver nitrate together with a freeze-dried composite of collagen and oxidised regenerated cellulose (Promogran) were examined *in vitro* by Walker *et al.*[58] who compared their effect on selected members of an important group of enzymes, the matrix metalloproteinases (MMPs) which include collagenases, elastase, and gelatinases produced both by human tissue and bacteria.

For the purpose of their study they used MMP-2 and MMP-9 sourced from *ex vivo* dermal tissue and blood monocytes respectively. All the dressings and the solution were shown to sequester both enzymes, but Aquacel Ag showed significantly greater sequestration of MMP-2 at six and 24 hours ($p < 0.001$) compared with other treatments. For MMP-9, both Aquacel Ag and Promogran achieved significant sequestration when compared to the other treatments at 24 hours ($p < 0.001$), which was maintained to 48 hours ($p < 0.001$).

The authors concluded that these results suggested that silver-containing dressings are effective in sequestering or inactivating MMPs and that this can be achieved without the use of a sacrificial protein such as collagen.

Further evidence for this effect was published by Wright *et al.*[59] following a study in which they showed that when full-thickness wounds in pigs, previously contaminated with an inoculum of *P. aeruginosa*, Fusobacterium sp. and a coagulase-negative staphylococci, were dressed with Acticoat, reduced levels of MMPs were detected compared with control wounds. This activity also appeared to be associated with more rapid healing.

Anti-inflammatory properties

Nadworny et al.[60] showed that nanocrystalline silver possessed anti-inflammatory properties using a porcine model of contact dermatitis. An inflammatory reaction was induced by the application of dinitrochlorobenzene and this was subsequently treated daily with Acticoat dressings, 0.5% silver nitrate, or saline.

After 72 hours the appearance of the skin of the animals treated with the silver dressings had virtually returned to normal in terms of erythema and oedema, an observation supported by histological examination, but the skin of the remaining animals remained inflamed. The decreased inflammation was associated with increased inflammatory cell apoptosis, a decreased expression of proinflammatory cytokines, and decreased gelatinase activity. Silver nitrate treatment induced apoptosis in all cell types, delaying wound healing.

The authors argued persuasively that their results provide further support for the existence of Ag^0 clusters, comparing their anti-inflammatory effect with that of gold Au^0, known to suppress the activity of interleukin-6 and tumour necrosis factor-α (TNF- α).

Use of silver dressings in a magnetic resonance environment

Given the widespread use of silver dressings it is not unlikely that these will be in use on some patients scheduled to receive an MRI scan. Current package inserts recommend removal of these dressings prior to any MRI procedure, although there is no clear evidence to support this recommendation. Chaudhry et al.[61] in an experimental study using limbs removed from pigs applied three standard silver wound dressings and obtained images with both dry and wet dressings. Skin temperature was assessed before and during MRI by probes inserted between the dressing and skin, and images were independently reviewed for distortion. None of the dressings exhibited significant temperature increases nor produced significant distortion, leading the authors to conclude that the removal of these dressings is not warranted for clinical MRI examinations.

Results of animal studies

The effects of silver-containing dressings on animal wounds have been examined in a number of studies. Burrell et al.[62] found that mean percent survival in an experimentally infected group of animals treated with Acticoat was 85%, compared with 0% in a control group treated with silver nitrate solution.

Heggers et al.[63] compared three silver dressings, Acticoat, Silverlon and Silvasorb, on 20% TBSA burns in rats whose injuries were infected with cultures of *P aeruginosa* and *S. aureus*. The dressings remained on the wounds for 10 days after which the mean bacterial counts of untreated controls ranged from 1.2×10^5 to 6.5×10^5 for *P. aeruginosa* and *S. aureus* respectively. Acticoat-treated wound counts for both organisms were 0 and 1.8×10^3, Silvasorb counts were 0 and 6.3×10^3 and those of Silverlon 1.5×10^4 and 7.4×10^4. Acticoat and Silvasorb were both significantly lower ($p < 0.05$) than the control for *P. aeruginosa*, and Acticoat was significantly lower ($p < 0.05$) than the control for *S. aureus*. Although counts for Silvasorb were lower than the controls for *S. aureus*, this failed to achieve significance.

Ulkur *et al.*[64] also used a rat model to compare Acticoat with a tulle containing chlorhexidine acetate 0.5%, and silver sulfadiazine 1% in burns infected with *P. aeruginosa*. Compared with untreated controls, all treatments were shown to be effective against this organism. Viable counts conducted on burn eschar did not differ significantly between Acticoat and chlorhexidine acetate treated wounds, but those treated with silver sulfadiazine contained fewer organisms than the other treated wounds, indicating that silver sulfadiazine eliminated *P. aeruginosa* more effectively from the tissues than did the other two agents although all treatments prevent the organism from invading underlying muscle tissue or causing systemic infection.

In a second study using the same wound model, the same authors compared Acticoat, chlorhexidine acetate 0.5%, and a fusidic acid 2% in full-thickness burns inoculated with a clinical strain of MRSA.[65] This organism was subsequently recovered from the eschar of all wounds except those treated with fusidic acid. Once again significant differences were recorded between treated and control group but the mean bacterial counts obtained from the eschar did not differ significantly between the Acticoat and chlorhexidine acetate groups although but there were significant differences between the fusidic acid treated group and the other treatment groups. No systemic spread was seen in the treatment groups, but it was seen in six animals in the control group. The authors suggested that based upon these data, fusidic acid remains the most effective agent in the treatment of burn wounds contaminated with MRSA, but suggested that Acticoat should be regarded as the treatment of choice because of the reduced requirement for dressing changes.

Bell *et al.*[66] used a partial-thickness excisional wound model in the pig to compare Aquacel Ag and Silvercel dressings in terms of their fluid handling properties, stability on exposure to exudate, and adherence to wound tissues. They also examined the extent to which dressing residues were retained in the wound and recorded their ability to induce tissue reactions. They concluded that, according to their criteria, Silvercel was more effective in managing wound exudate than Aquacel Ag, maintaining its shape and mechanical strength as Aquacel Ag formed a fluid (semi-fibrous) gel, with minimal mechanical integrity and variable retention at the wound site. However, Silvercel was significantly more adherent to wound tissues than Aquacel Ag leading the authors to propose that further development of absorbent fibre-based dressings should be directed at maximising exudate management, minimising dressing adherence and preventing dressing-debris entrapment. During the course of this investigation the authors apparently discounted the possibility that the moist environment produced under the CMC dressing might be contributing to wound healing.

The antibacterial activity and wound-healing effects of commercially available silver-coated or silver-impregnated wound dressings were compared by Lee *et al.*[67] in a laboratory-based study involving MRSA-infected full thickness wounds in 108 rats.

The rats were divided into six groups and their wounds dressed with either Acticoat, Aquacel Ag, Medifoam silver, PolyMem silver, Ilvadon, or Betadine. As part of the experimental procedure the authors recorded changes in wound sizes, histological findings, and bacterial colony counts for the groups. In a separate exercise they also compared the inhibition zones produced by the dressings on Mueller-Hinton agar plates inoculated with MRSA. The efficacy of the dressing, as represented by the rate at which the wounds decreased in size, was found to be in the order:

Acticoat > Aquacel Ag > PolyMem silver > Medifoam silver > Ilvadon > Betadine.

Histological examination of tissue samples revealed that the Acticoat showed more reepithelialization and granulation tissue formation and less inflammatory cell infiltration than the other materials. A reduction in bacterial numbers was noted in all groups with the exception of the Medifoam silver group, a finding that was generally consistent with the results of zone of inhibition testing which produced results which showed that the relative sizes of the zones were as follows:

Acticoat > Aquacel-Ag > Ilvadon > PolyMem silver > Betadine >Medifoam silver.

TOXICITY OF SILVER DRESSINGS

The toxicity of silver to mammals and mammalian cells was discussed in detail by Lansdown[11] who differentiated its potential effects into four areas: the skin surface, the wound or wound bed, dermal tissues and hypodermal tissues. He also suggested that low levels of silver appear to advance wound repair, an effect possibly due in part to their observed ability to induce metallothioneins (MT-1 and MT-2) in epithelial cells at the wound margin. These molecules are involved in the uptake and metabolism of zinc and copper in proliferating cells and therefore may have an indirect mitogenic effect at some concentrations. Evidence of a stimulatory effect of silver dressings upon wound healing was also presented by Ring et al.[68] who showed that silver ions, released to striated skin muscle from two silver-containing dressings in a mouse wound model, appeared to increase functional blood vessel density in the early stages of treatment. Unfortunately, not all studies on silver-containing dressings result in such a positive outcome as will be seen in the following overview of published accounts of the toxicity of silver in cell culture and animal models.

Local effects

Cytotoxicity

Cultured skin substitutes (CSS) are increasingly being used to treat extensive burns, but these have the disadvantage that they remain susceptible to microbial destruction longer than split-thickness skin grafts. This problem can be addressed by the use of topical antimicrobial agents to protect the wound and the newly applied cells, but these solutions must not be toxic to the cultured skin.

Cell culture systems of various types are frequently used to assess the toxicity of antimicrobials. Lam et al.[69] adopted this approach to assess the effect of Acticoat on a subconfluent layer of human keratinocytes cultured on a hyaluronate-derived membrane using dermal fibroblasts as the feeder layer. After 30 minutes incubation at 37° C, the inhibitory effect of the nanocrystalline silver on keratinocyte growth was measured by an MTT assay which showed that the cell layer was totally nonviable; leading the authors to conclude that the dressing is cytotoxic to cultured keratinocytes and should not be applied as a topical dressing on cultured skin grafts. Similar results were reported by Poon et al.[70] when they examined the cytotoxic effects of silver on keratinocytes and fibroblasts using both silver nitrate solution and Acticoat dressings as the source of the metal ions. The toxic dose for skin cells ranged from 7×10^{-4} to 55×10^{-4} percent, values comparable with those known to be toxic to bacteria.

Extracts of four different silver containing dressings together with other non-silver containing products were included in an in vitro study to compare their effect on keratinocyte survival and proliferation.[71] Keratinocyte cultures were exposed for 40 hours to extracts of Acticoat, Aquacel Ag, Aquacel, Algisite M, Avance, Comfeel Plus transparent, Contreet H, Hydrasorb, and Seasorb. Extracts of the silver-containing dressings: Acticoat, Aquacel Ag, Contreet-H, and Avance, were found to be the most cytotoxic; Hydrasorb extracts were less cytotoxic but markedly affected keratinocyte proliferation and morphology. Extracts of the alginate dressings, Algisite M, Seasorb, and Contreet H demonstrated high calcium concentrations which markedly reduced keratinocyte proliferation and affected keratinocyte morphology. Aquacel and Comfeel Plus transparent extracts induced small but significant inhibition of keratinocyte proliferation. The authors concluded, based upon these results, that silver-based dressings are cytotoxic and should not be used in the absence of infection.

Le Duc et al.[72] compared the toxicity of twelve topical preparations using two different human skin substitutes: autologous reconstructed epidermis on fibroblast-populated human dermis and an allogenic reconstructed epidermis on a fibroblast-populated rat collagen gel. Results obtained with these test substrates were compared with those obtained using a conventional full-thickness autograft.

In each case, the test materials were applied to the outer surface of the stratum corneum for 24 hours, taking care that no leakage occurred around the edges. In this way the products under examination could only exert a cytotoxic effect after penetrating through the epidermal barrier layer. Evidence of cytotoxicity was indicated by changes in histology, metabolic activity (MTT assay) and RNA staining of tissue sections. When compared as described test materials exhibited varying degrees of cytotoxicity. Acticoat, Aquacel Ag, Dermacyn, Fucidin, 0.5% silver nitrate solution and chlorhexidine digluconate were not found to be cytotoxic for either the HSS or autograft preparations. Flamazine and zinc oxide cream resulted in moderate cytotoxicity but Betadine, cerium-silver sulfadiazine cream, silver sulfadiazine cream with 1% acetic acid and Furacine resulted in a substantial decrease in cell viability and a detrimental effect on tissue histology when applied to autograft and especially to HSS. However, it must be stressed that because in this study the materials under examination were applied to an intact layer of stratum corneum, the results should not be considered be indicative of their toxicity when introduced to an open wound.

Whilst there is a sustainable argument for avoiding potentially cytotoxic agents in a normally healing wound, if infection is present or suspected then the potential or theoretical adverse effects resulting from the use of a topical antimicrobial are likely to be far less significant than those caused by the presence of pathogenic microorganisms.

The benefits of silver-containing dressing in the presence of infection were demonstrated in a laboratory study in which Contreet Hydrocolloid (Contreet H) was compared with an unmedicated hydrocolloid when the two dressings were applied to reconstituted human epithelium (RHE) infected with *C. albicans* or MRSA. Contreet H induced no major morphological changes in the control cell system and although both dressings reduced the growth of microorganisms, only Contreet H prevented major morphological changes in the monolayer leading the authors to conclude that delivering silver to infected keratinocytes in a moist healing environment improves the benefit/risk ratio compared to the use of similar unmedicated products.[73]

Fredriksson *et al.*[74] in an elegant study prepared a laboratory wound healing model using waste human skin from an abdominoplasty to compare the effects of different silver-containing dressings upon healing. From pieces of skin from which fatty tissue had previously been removed, standard circular samples were prepared using an 8-mm biopsy punch. A dermal wound about one mm deep was then produced in the centre of each using as three mm diameter punch. The discs were then transferred to tissue culture plates and various dressing materials added into the central well of each in accordance with the instructions provided by the relevant manufacturer. After 14 days the wounds were fixed and examined histologically. Wounds in the positive control group (not exposed to dressings) had epithelialized completely by this time but wounds dressed with Acticoat, Silverlon, Silvasorb or silver nitrate showed no signs of epithelialization. Wounds dressed with silver sulphadiazine and Polymem Silver showed some limited evidence of epithelialization but only wounds dressed with Aquacel Ag showed significant evidence of epithelial growth. Black discoloration or particle deposits or both were seen throughout the tissue in all wounds treated with silver containing products except for Polymem Silver and Silvasorb. Acticoat produced the most deposits and was the only dressing to cause a black discoloration of the keratinocyte layer. Aquacel Ag caused the second most deposits followed by Silverlon, SSD and Silvasorb. Some of these deposits were around structures identified as blood vessels causing the authors to consider the possibility that silver particles deposited in this way could find their way into the systemic circulation and thus form protein complexes elsewhere in the body. The authors stressed, however, that the conditions produced in this test system cannot be assumed to be typical of those which exist *in vivo*.

Whilst cell culture and other *in vitro* methods undoubtedly have a role to play in assessing the toxicity of medical devices, when used in isolation they frequently produce results which predict that products may induce adverse effects which are not actually subsequently encountered during normal clinical use of the materials concerned. For this reason animal studies arc often undertaken to determine if these predicted effects actually occur *in vivo*.

Burd *et al.*[75] compared the cytotoxicity of five silver-containing dressings, Acticoat, Aquacel Ag, Contreet Foam, Polymem Silver, Urgotul SSD in a monolayer cell culture system, a tissue explant culture model, and a mouse excisional wound model. They found that Acticoat, Aquacel Ag, and Contreet Foam, when pretreated with specific solutes, were likely to produce the most significant cytotoxic effects on both cultured keratinocytes and fibroblasts; Polymem Silver and Urgotul SSD demonstrated the least cytotoxicity. Perhaps not surprisingly, cytotoxicity correlated with the silver concentration produced in the culture medium. In the tissue explant culture model, in which the epidermal cell proliferation was evaluated, all silver dressings resulted in a significant delay of reepithelialization. In the mouse excisional wound model, Acticoat and Contreet Foam indicated a strong inhibition of wound reepithelialization on the seventh day after wounding. The authors suggested that these finding might explain clinical observations that delayed wound healing or inhibition of wound epithelialization may occur following the use of certain topical silver dressings and urged caution when using silver-based dressings in clean superficial wounds such as donor sites and superficial burns and also when cultured cells are being applied to wounds.[75]

Supp et al.[76] examined the effects of Acticoat dressing both on cultured skin substitutes (CSS) in vitro and following application to full-thickness wounds in athymic mice. In the cell culture model, cellular viability in the CSS was determined by MTT conversion on days zero, one and seven following Acticoat exposure. In the animal model wounds were traced, and areas of healing CSS were calculated by image analysis one, two, three and four weeks after grafting. Also at four weeks, wound biopsies were evaluated and scored for engraftment of human cells. In a subsequent study, wounds were inoculated with P. aeruginosa before the application of CSS or inoculated onto the surface of Acticoat. After four weeks, swab cultures were collected from the surface of CSS and examined for the presence of the organism. Their results revealed that although exposure of CSS to Acticoat in vitro produced a cytotoxic effect within one day, one week of exposure in vivo did not injure CSS or inhibit wound healing. Contaminated wounds treated with Acticoat healed similarly to control treatments, with comparable rates of engraftment. The test organism was isolated from only one graft. The authors therefore proposed that Acticoat was a useful treatment for reducing environmental contamination of CSS, if used in conjunction with additional antimicrobials.

Nadworny and Burrell in a comprehensive review,[77] summarised the various animal and tissue based methods used for assessing the biological activity of silver and silver dressings. They concluded that tissue explant models and murine excisional models described above are not predictive of wound healing outcomes but suggested that in vivo porcine models are appropriate for determining biological efficacy in terms of inflammation or healing and are thus predictive of clinical outcomes. Murine models they also considered to offer valuable insights into antimicrobial activity that may be predictive of clinical outcomes.

The possibility of developing silver impregnated materials capable of exerting an antimicrobial effect without causing significant cytotoxicity was investigated by Agarwal et al.[78] who described the results of an initial study of thin films of polyallylamine hydrochloride and polyacrylic acid loaded with approximately $0.4\,\mu g/cm^2$ to approximately $23.6\,\mu g/cm^2$ of silver nanoparticles. S. epidermidis, a bacterium known to be very susceptible to the antibacterial activity of silver was selected as a test organism. Although films containing high loadings of silver were toxic to a murine fibroblast cell line, those containing low levels of silver, approximately 0.4 $\mu g/cm^2$, were not toxic and allowed attachment and growth of the mammalian cells.

Skin changes

In addition to its potential to induce local toxic effects, silver is also known to be capable of inducing systemic effects such as Argyria, a clinical condition in which excessive administration and deposition of silver as silver sulphide causes a permanent irreversible gray-blue discoloration of the skin or mucous membranes. Once silver particles are deposited in this way they remain immobile and may accumulate during the aging process. Argaria must be differentiated from the transient skin staining resulting from the topical application of silver salts such as silver nitrate.

The ability of two silver-containing dressings, Aquacel Ag and Acticoat, to cause skin staining was investigated by Walker et al,[52] who applied the dressings to human skin samples taken from electively amputated lower limbs. They found that when the dressings were hydrated with saline, silver deposition from both dressings was minimal and concluded that controlling the amount of silver released from silver-containing dressings should help reduce excessive deposition of silver into wound tissue and minimise staining.

Trop et al.[79] described a case in which in a previously healthy 17-year-old boy with 30% mixed depth burns developed hepatotoxicity and argyria-like symptoms, after one week of local treatment with Acticoat. When Acticoat treatment was discontinued both the clinical symptoms and liver enzymes returned to normal, leading the authors to suggest that silver levels in plasma and/or urine should be monitored during treatment of large exuding wounds. These conclusions were subsequently questioned by Parkes[80] who argued that the evidence presented in their original paper did not support their conclusions that the changes in liver function were silver-related, for all available research suggests that the liver is not a target organ for silver toxicity. Parkes also questioned the validity of the diagnosis of argyria as this would not normally be expected to resolve in a short period of time as described in the original publication.

Systemic effects

In an informative review White and Cutting[12] discussed the possible development of silver toxicity in which they identified factors which might be significant in this regard. Specifically they highlighted the degree of absorption (a function, at least in part, of the formulation and solubility of the silver molecule), the ability of the silver ion to bind with important biological sites, and the degree to which absorbed silver is sequestered or metabolized and ultimately excreted.

Wan et al.[81] reported in subjects without industrial or medicinal exposure to silver produced blood levels of < 2.3 $\mu g/L$ and that 2 $\mu g/day$ were excreted in urine. Liver and kidney levels were around 0.05 $\mu g/g$ of wet tissue but all these levels could increase dramatically following the use of silver sulphadiazine cream, rising to 50 $\mu g/L$ within six hours of application and reaching a maximum of 310 µg/L depending upon the size and nature of the wound. In patients treated with SSD who died of renal failure after eight days of treatment, silver levels of 970 µg/g, 14 µg/g, and 0.2 µg/g were present in the cornea, liver and kidney respectively. In the case study reported by Trop et al.,[79] after one week of local treatment with Acticoat silver, plasma levels reached 107 µg/kg and urine 28 µg/kg.

The toxicity of Acticoat on the hepatic and renal function of patients with burns was determined in a comparative study in which 26 burn patients with partial thickness burn covering 6-12% TBSA were compared with a control group comprising 30 healthy adult volunteers.[82] The burns were dressed with Acticoat for five days and the silver content of the serum and urine measured at different time points before and after the application of the dressing using atomic absorption. The hepatic and renal function of all participants was monitored on the seventh and 14th post treatment days (PTD). The silver content of tissue samples from the wound and wound edge 14 days after treatment was also determined. The silver content of the serum and urine in silver treated patients increased on the third and fifth PTD, but returned to the normal level on the 14th PTD. Mild hepatic dysfunction was noted in seven cases on the seventh PTD, but renal function remained normal. The tissue mass percentage of silver in burn wound and wound edge was $0.7 \pm 0.1 \times 10^{-6}$, but no silver deposition in tissue could be detected by transmission electron microscope. The authors concluded that no safety issues were associated with the application of the silver dressing to small to medium sized partial thickness burn wounds. Dunn and Edwards-Jones similarly concluded that Acticoat produced no evidence of resistance or cytotoxicity when used of in the treatment of burns.[83]

Vlachou et al.,[84] in a prospective, open-label study, determined the systemic absorption of silver in 30 patients with relatively small burns (circa 12% TBSA) that required skin grafting. Serum silver levels were measured before, during and after cessation of Acticoat treatment then again after three and six months following completion of treatment. Prior to treatment patients who had been treated with an alternative silver product prior to enrolment had a plasma silver reading of 5.0 µg/L (range 0 - 53 µg/L) For patient not previously treated with silver the corresponding readings were 0.4 µg/L (range 0 - 48.1 µg/L)

The median maximum serum silver level, achieved after nine days, was 56.8 µg/L. By six months this had dropped to 0.8 µg/L. No haematological or biochemical indicators of toxicity associated with the absorption of silver observed were noted during the study.

Hoekstra[85] reviewed the evidence for the possible adverse effects resulting from the use of nanoparticles of silver such as those present in Acticoat. He stated that unlike silver ions, these particles can enter the body via a wound, circulate in the blood stream to be eventually excreted in the same form. He also cited a couple of publications which suggested that nanoparticles induce a concentration-dependent effect in some cellular and animal models and concluded that these early published studies 'contribute to the growing concern that the use of products containing silver nanoparticles may have detrimental effects upon human health and the environment'. In the second part of his review he considered Aquacel Ag, and concluded that this 'can be used without serious risk to human health or the environment.'

CLINICAL EXPERIENCE WITH SILVER DRESSINGS

Publications describing the various silver dressings on the market are reviewed below. Where these relate to a single type of dressing these reviews are grouped together by brand, but if they involve two or more silver-containing dressings they are described in a separate section.

Acticoat

Early clinical experience with Acticoat was reported by Tredget et al. in 1998,[31] who also described its use in a randomized, prospective clinical study involving thirty patients each of whom had two burns that were comparable in size, depth and anatomical location. The wounds in each pair were randomized to treatment with Acticoat or a standard therapy that consisted of fine mesh gauze soaked in 0.5% silver nitrate solution when remoistened every two hours. The frequency of burn wound sepsis, $> 10^5$ organisms per gram of tissue, was less in Acticoat-treated wounds than in those treated with silver nitrate (5 vs 16). Secondary bacteraemias arising from infected burn wounds were also less frequent with Acticoat than with silver nitrate-treated wounds (1 vs 5). No differences were detected between the groups in the proportion of successful skin grafts when examined on the fifth postoperative day; the rate of spontaneous healing in both groups was also comparable.

Acticoat was also reported to be less painful in use than silver sulfadiazine when applied to partial-thickness burns following a randomized controlled trial in which the mean visual analog pain scores for wounds treated with Acticoat and silver sulfadiazine were 3.2 and 7.9, respectively (p < 0.0001).[86]

The use of Acticoat as a dressing for donor sites was similarly evaluated, both in a pig model,[87] where it was compared with petrolatum gauze, and in humans,[88] where it was compared with a foam dressing, Allevyn. In the animal study, which involved 72 dermatome wounds on the backs of six young pigs, the wounds dressed with Acticoat were completely reepithelialized in 70% of the time taken by wounds dressed with petrolatum gauze. The results of the human study were less favourable. Sixteen paired sites in 15 patients (3 female, 12 male) were studied. Donor sites dressed with Allevyn were > 90% reepithelialized in a mean of 9.1 ± 1.6 days while donor sites dressed with Acticoat required a mean of 14.5 ± 6.7 days to achieve > 90% reepithelialization (p = 0.004). There were no significant differences in the incidence of positive bacterial cultures between dressings at any time point examined. Donor sites dressed with Acticoat had significantly worse scars after one and two months but this difference resolved by three months. The authors concluded that their findings did not support the use of Acticoat as a skin graft donor site dressing.

Acticoat was compared with Silvazine cream, in two 'before and after' patient care audits conducted in 2000 and 2002 in order to compare clinical effectiveness and treatment costs for in-patient treatment of early burn wounds.[89] The main outcome variables were the formation of cellulitis, antibiotic use and cost of treatment. The first audit in 2000 reflected the then standard treatment which involved twice daily showers or washes with 4% chlorhexidine soap followed by the application of Silvazine cream (n = 51). The second audit reflected the outcomes of the standard 2002 treatment which consisted of daily showers of the burn wound using 4% chlorhexidine soap followed by the application of an Acticoat dressing (n = 19). Costs were examined using a sample of matched pairs (n = 8) of current and previous patients. With the use of Acticoat the incidence of infection fell from 55% (28/51) in 2000 to 10.5% (2/19) in 2002. Antibiotic use fell from 57% (29/51) to 5.2% (1/19) in the same period. Treatments costs, excluding antibiotics, staffing and surgery, for those treated with Silvazine were $109,357, and for those treated with Acticoat $78,907. The average duration of hospital stay was 17.25 days for the Silvazine group and 12.5 days for the Acticoat group - a difference of 4.75 days. The authors concluded that compared to Silvazine, in the treatment of early burn wounds the use of Acticoat reduced the incidence of cellulitis, antibiotic use and overall cost.

The clinical efficacy and safety of Acticoat in the treatment of burns was assessed in 98 patients with 166 residual burn wounds in a multicenter randomized trial. One group had Acticoat applied to their wounds, the other silver sulfadiazine. The average healing time was 12 ± 5 days with Acticoat, and 16 ± 6 days for silver sulphadiazine, (p = 0.005).

A method for treating burns to the hand with Acticoat described by Kok et al.[90] who used a customised Acticoat glove.

The safety and efficacy of Acticoat when uses to treat burns and other injuries in premature neonates was investigated by Rustogi et al.[91] Eight premature neonates ranging from 23 to 28 weeks gestation who sustained burn injuries and other cutaneous injuries from various agents were treated with the dressing which was changed every three to seven days. Wounds were assessed for infection and blood cultures were taken where sepsis was suspected. Serum silver levels were measured in three infants. Total burned body surface area ranged from 1% to 30% and miscellaneous injuries included: alcoholic chlorhexidine, alcoholic wipes, electrode jelly, extravasated intravenous fluids, artery illuminator, temperature probe and adhesive tape removal. All wounds had healed by day 28 and scar management was not required. There were no wound infections or positive blood cultures during the treatment period but there were four mortalities secondary to problems associated with extreme prematurity. Measured serum silver levels ranged from 0 to 1 μmol/L.

Peters and Verchere[92] following a review of historical data reported the time spent in hospital by 30 children treated with Acticoat was 0.83 days compared with 13.85 days for 73 matched historical controls dressed with silver sulphadiazine (p < 0.001). Sixty seven percent of all wound observations revealed that the MRSA load had reduced following the use of the dressing and in 11% of cases the organisms was eliminated altogether.

Acticoat and silver sulphadiazine were compared in a randomized comparative trial involving 98 patients with 166 burn wounds and patients were observed for up to 20 days. Acticoat-treated wounds healed in 12.4 ± 5.4 days, nearly 3.4 days earlier than the wounds treated with silver sulphadiazine.[93]

The value of Acticoat Absorbent as a dressing for surgical sites following lower limb surgery was assessed by Childress et al.[94] in a cohort study in which they compared treatment outcomes for all infrainguinal revascularization cases involving leg incisions at a single centre over a 39 month period. During the first 15 months wounds were dressed with conventional materials; from the 16th month onwards they were dressed with Acticoat and a film dressing. The number of wound-related complications fell from 14% (17/118), to 5% (7/130) (p = 0.016) following the introduction of Acticoat treatment.

The successful use of Acticoat has also been reported in a case of toxic epidermal necrolysis involving 90% body surface area of a paediatric patient,[95] and an MRSA colonised wound following complex knee surgery in a patient with generalised psoriasis.[96]

The ability of Acticoat to form an effective barrier against MRSA was examined prospectively in both the laboratory and clinical setting by Strohal et al.[97] The laboratory data indicated that the dressing exhibited a sustained antimicrobial effect, effectively preventing MRSA penetration. The clinical relevance of this finding was subsequently assessed in a double-centre clinical trial in which the dressing was used to cover ten MRSA colonised wounds in seven patients. The MRSA load on the upper side of the dressing and the wound bed was determined each time the dressing was changed after 1, 24, 48 and 72 hours. These results indicated that in 95% of instances, the dressing provided a total barrier to the penetration and therefore potential dissemination of the organism.

Eight patients with ulcers associated with chronic lower limb lymphoedema were treated with Acticoat as a primary dressing supported by an alginate and a polyurethane foam dressing under multilayer short-stretch compression bandaging. All ulcers completely healed after one to nine weeks of treatment.[98]

Sibbald et al.[99] conducted a small pilot-scale evaluation of Acticoat 7, in 15 patients with non-healing venous leg ulcers. Bacteriological analysis of biopsies taken at baseline, and at an average of study week 6.5 revealed a significant reduction in the log_{10} total bacterial count. (p = 0.011) Heavy neutrophilic infiltration in skin biopsies at week 6.5 was associated with high bacterial counts and delayed healing (p = 0.037) but elevated numbers of lymphocytes were associated with an increased reduction of ulcer size at week 6.5 and final assessment at week 12 (p < 0.05). Serum silver levels increased slightly, but values were within the normal range.

Gravante et al.[100] performed a meta-analysis on data from randomized trials in burn patients to assess the potential advantages of nanocrystalline silver (NC) versus older silver formulations including silver sulfadiazine and silver nitrate. The primary outcome was the evaluation of differences in the infection rate of burns. Secondary outcomes were the eventual differences in the pain experienced during medications, the length of hospitalization (LOS) and costs. The five articles that met the inclusion criteria described the treatment of 285 patients. Compared with the SS group, the NC group had a significant lower incidence of infections, 9.5% vs 27.8% (p < 0.001), with a 2.9-fold decrease of the risk. Available data also suggested reduced costs for NC treated patients. ($946 vs $1533) and also decreased pain values while contrasting results were obtained for LOS.

Actisorb Plus

Actisorb, and subsequently Actisorb Plus, were originally marketed as odour-absorbing dressings for the management of malignant and infected wounds,[101] but early clinical experience with the dressings suggested that they also appeared to have beneficial effects upon infection and healing rates of wounds such as pressure sores and leg ulcers.[102-103] Actisorb has also been used prophylactically to dress percutaneous enterostomal gastrostomy (PEG) sites to prevent infection[104]

In 2002, Cassino et al., reviewed treatment outcomes for 75 chronic skin lesions showing local signs of infection that were treated with Actisorb Plus, and compared them with 75 wounds dressed with moist gauze or alginate on patients receiving systemic antibiotic therapy.

They found that although the Actisorb Plus treatments tended to be longer, 14 days compared with 10 days for systemic antibiotics, there was no statistical difference in effectiveness between the two treatments. A particularly interesting finding was that 30-day recurrence rates were much higher in the antibiotic treated group (12% vs 1.3%). Major cost savings were also reported for the Actisorb Plus treated wounds.

The most comprehensive account of the use of Actisorb yet published described the combined results of five observational studies undertaken between 1996 and 2000 as part of the German regulatory process.[105] These studies involved patients with a total of 12,444 chronic wounds of all types, many of which initially contained signs of infection. During the course of the study wounds were monitored for exudate production, odour, the presence of necrotic tissue, fibrinous deposits and the formation of new granulation or epithelial tissue. Other recorded parameters included changes in infection rates, healing characteristics and dressing tolerability. After initiating treatment with Actisorb, it was reported that 96% of wounds improved and 41% healed completely. Infection rates fell from 65% to 6%, and 80% of patients did not require additional medication. Dressing tolerability was also rated as excellent. Like Cassino et al., Stadler[105] concluded that Actisorb plus was very effective on infected or colonised chronic wounds with the potential to limit the use of other local antiseptics or antibiotics. It also had a highly favourable benefit/risk-ratio.

The effect of Actisorb on the bioburden of chronic wounds was investigated by Verdu Soriano et al.[106] Patients were randomly assigned to the intervention or control group and monitored for two weeks. Bacterial counts were obtained at baseline and then after 15 days of treatment. After two weeks, 85.1% (57/67) of the wounds in the intervention group exhibited a reduction in the number of bacteria present in the wound compared with 62.1% (36/58) in the control group (p = 0.003).

Allevyn Ag

The results of a multi-centre clinical evaluation of 126 patients conducted to assess the performance of Allevyn Ag for a range of clinical indications was reported by Kotz et al.[107] The study included the adhesive, non adhesive and sacral presentations and clinicians rated the products as acceptable for use in various wound types in 88% of patients. The majority of clinical signs of infection reduced between the initial and the final assessment of dressing usage and the condition of wound tissue and surrounding skin was judged to have improved. There was also significant evidence of a reduction in the level of exudate from initial to final assessment (p < 0.001).

Aquacel Ag

An early favourable account of the use of Aquacel Ag was provided by Vanscheidt et al.[108] following a multicenter, noncomparative, non-randomized, pilot trial involving 18 subjects conducted in France and Germany in 2001 which was undertaken to collect preliminary data on the safety and performance of the dressing in the management of chronic leg ulcers. This was followed soon after by an account of the use of the dressing in the management of partial-thickness wounds following a phase II trial in superficial, mid dermal, and mixed partial-thickness burns.[109] Despite the noncomparative nature of the study the authors judged speed of reepithelialization to be similar to that they had previously experienced with silver sulphadiazine. Dressing conformability and general ease of use and were also rated very positively.

The effect of four weeks application of Aquacel on chronic non-healing wounds was examined in a single centre, open-label study which included a total of 30 evaluable participants with wounds of varying aetiology.[110] All the wounds were stalled or had the signs and symptoms consistent with critical colonisation, but all participants had adequate vascular supply, indicating that they possessed the potential to heal. Once the underlying medical problem had been addressed, Aquacel was applied to each for a period of four weeks. The majority of wounds treated (70%), decreased both in size and exudate production. They also became less purulent and a resolution of surface slough was noted in 75% accompanied by an increase in the quality and quantity of healthy granulation tissue. Periwound maceration was noted in 54% of participants at baseline, but the problem resolved in 85% of these following the use of the dressing.

An early assessment of Aquacel Ag in the treatment of burns of varying aetiology was undertaken by Lohana and Potokar,[111] who recorded its use in the treatment of 22 patients. The dressing was covered with one or two layers of gauze and a crepe bandage. Although the outer dressing layers were replaced regularly, the primary dressing was left for 14 ± 3 days or until it separated spontaneously. Successful healing was achieved in 16/22 patients in a mean of 11.6 days.

Aquacel Ag was compared with or silver sulphadiazine in the management of 84 partial-thickness burns covering 5% to 40% body surface area, in a controlled trial lasting up to 21 days.[112] The use of the dressing resulted in fewer dressing changes, each requiring less nursing time. Pain and anxiety during use and at dressing changes was also less with Aquacel Ag but the silver sulphadiazine cream was associated with greater flexibility and ease of movement. Adverse events, including infection, were comparable between treatment groups. Aquacel Ag treatment cost less than the cream, $1040 vs $1180, and produced an enhanced rate of reepithelialization, 73.8% vs 60.0%.

Paddock et al. in two separate publications reviewed Burn Registry Data from a large Children's Hospital for two eight month periods in successive years. In the first period paediatric inpatients with partial-thickness burns were treated with silver sulfadiazine cream, in the second period Aquacel Ag. They found that on average, the use of Aquacel Ag reduced the time spent in hospital from 8.4 to 4.5 days (p = 0.002).[113] Total charges and direct costs were also significantly lower for Aquacel Ag-treated patients.[114]

Aquacel Ag was compared with paraffin gauze dressing in the management of 20 split-thickness skin graft (STSG) donor sites by Lohsiriwat and Chuangsuwanich.[115] The mean initial areas of the treated wounds were 145.5 cm^2 and 135.8 cm^2 for Aquacel and paraffin gauze respectively. Mean healing times for the two groups were 7.90 and 11.20 days respectively (p = 0.031). The average pain scores at rest were 0.74 and 0.80 (ns) but the average pain score at dressing removal were 3.12 and 4.70, respectively (p = 0.027). There was no infection or seroma in both groups. The authors concluded that, compared to paraffin gauze dressing, the use of Aquacel Ag reduced STSG donor site pain and promoted re-epithelization.

A similar study was reported by Lohsiriwat et al.[116] who also compared the Aquacel Ag with paraffin gauze dressings in the treatment of 20 donor sites of similar size. Epithelialization was found to be complete on days 7.90 and 11.20 for the two treatment groups respectively (p = 0.031). The average pain score at rest were 0.74 and 0.80 and on dressing removal were 3.12 and 4.70, respectively (p = 0.027). No infection or seroma was noted in either group. From these observations it was concluded that compared with paraffin gauze, Aquacel Ag dressing can reduce STSG donor site pain and enhance reepithelization.

The use of Aquacel Ag has also been recorded in the treatment of the diabetic foot. In a prospective, multicentre study, 134 out-patients with Type 1 or 2 diabetes mellitus and non-ischaemic foot ulcers classified as Wagner Grade 1 or 2 were stratified by antibiotic use on enrolment and randomly assigned to similar protocols including off-loading and the use of Aquacel Ag or an alginate dressing, Algosteril, together with secondary foam dressings. Each patient was followed for a maximum of eight weeks or until healing was achieved. The mean time to healing was 53 days for ulcers treated with Aquacel and 58 days for alginate-treated ulcers (p = 0.34). Wounds treated with the silver dressing reduced in depth nearly twice as much as alginate-treated ulcers, 0.25 cm vs 0.13 cm (p = 0.04). Ulcer treated with the silver dressing improved more than alginate treated subjects (p = 0.058), particularly in the subset initially using antibiotics (p = 0.02). The authors concluded that when added to standard care with appropriate off-loading, ulcers treated with Aquacel Ag produced more favourable clinical outcomes than those treated with alginate dressings.[117] Further anecdotal support for the use of Aquacel Ag for this indication was provided by Stang.[118]

Aquacel Ag was compared with povidone-iodine gauze for the management of open surgical and traumatic wounds in a prospective randomized clinical trial in which patients were monitored for up to two weeks. By the end of the study 8/35 (23%) of wounds in the Aquacel Ag group had healed compared with 3/32 (9%) of those in the povidone-iodine gauze (ns). The use of Aquacel Ag was also associated with significant less pain and discomfort when assessed using a visual analogue scale.[119]

Following a review of the literature on the use of Aquacel Ag, Barnea et al.[120] concluded that although the results of in vitro studies suggest that the cytotoxicity of ionic silver to keratinocytes and fibroblasts can delay wound re-epithelialization, clinical studies confirm that the dressing is an effective and safe treatment for a variety of wound types, both acute and chronic. Incorporation of ionic silver appears to reduce local pain and dressing changes, and provides significant broad-spectrum antimicrobial properties, with no delay in wound healing.

Atrauman Ag

Atrauman Ag was shown in laboratory studies to be capable of killing a range of bacterial species including both skin commensals and pathogenic strains while demonstrating only limited cytotoxicity to keratinocytes. In a clinical study involving 86 patients with traumatic and non-healing wounds of varying aetiology the dressing was shown to be associated with a reduction in slough, increased granulation tissue and enhanced epithelialization. The authors suggested that the relatively low rate of silver release enabled the dressing to exert significant antimicrobial activity without impacting greatly upon wound-healing mechanisms.[121]

Avance

The literature on Avance is limited to two publications that describe a handful of case studies recording the successful use of the dressing in different problem wounds.[122-123] In none of the case histories presented, however, was there any evidence to suggest that the benefits associated with the use of the dressing were related to the antimicrobial action of the silver.

Biatain Ag/Contreet Foam

The effect of Contreet Foam on the wounds of 25 patients with moderate to heavily exuding chronic venous leg ulcers was assessed on a weekly basis by Karlsmark et al.[124] who paid particular attention to the appearance of the wound-bed, degree of odour and pain, dressing performance and the dressings' effect on the peri-ulcer skin. Blood samples were also analyzed for silver content. Twenty three patients completed the four week study during which time mean ulcer area reduced by 56% from 15.6 cm^2 to 6.9 cm^2. There was also an overall improvement in the appearance of the wound bed and a marked reduction in odour. Mean dressing wear time was 3.1 days, and there were only minimal incidences of leakage. Serum silver levels did not exceed reference values.

In a multicentre, open, randomized, controlled study lasting 4 weeks, the silver-containing Contreet foam was compared with Allevyn in 129 patients with critically colonised venous leg ulcers that exhibited delayed healing.[125] Ulcer area and healing were assessed weekly but odour, maceration, absorption capacity and leakage were evaluated at each dressing change. After four weeks there was a significantly greater reduction in ulcer area in the Contreet Foam group than in the Allevyn group, 45% vs 25% respectively. After one and four weeks, odour was present in significantly fewer of the ulcers in the Contreet Foam group, 17% and 19% respectively, compared with the Allevyn group, 47% and 39% respectively. Problems of leakage and maceration were also reduced in the Contreet group, suggesting that dressings that deliver sustained release of silver may offer advantages in the treatment of critically colonised chronic wounds.

In the largest study reported to date, the effect of the silver-releasing Contreet Foam was compared with local best practice (LBP) on delayed healing ulcers.[126] A total of

619 patients with ulcers of varying aetiologies were treated for four weeks with either the silver foam dressing or LBP. Wounds treated with the silver foam decreased in area by 50% compared with 34% for LBP. Use of the foam dressing was also associated with reduced slough and maceration and a faster reduction in exudate production. Mean wear time was longer for the silver foam than for LBP (3.1 vs 2.1 days). The authors concluded that the silver foam dressing outperformed all of the competitors, and judged that it supports faster healing of wounds showing delayed healing.

The importance of the silver component of Contreet Foam on healing was investigated by Dimakakos et al.[127] who compared the effectiveness of the silver containing foam with the original material which is identical in structure but contains no silver. Forty-two patients with infected venous ulcers were included in the study and randomized into two treatment groups. There were no significant differences between patients or their wounds in the two groups. In both groups, ulcer size and depth, intensity of pain, wound exudation, bacterial load, side effects of both materials, and ulcer healing were documented and compared. After nine weeks treatment, 81% (17/21) of wounds treated with the silver dressing had healed compared with 48% (10/21) of those dressed with standard foam. This difference was significant (p = 0.02). Pain intensity was also significantly less in silver treated wounds.

The value of Biatain Ag/Contreet Foam was assessed in the treatment of 27 diabetic patients with Grade I or II foot ulcers over a six week period. Following a one week run-in period in which the wounds were dressed with unmedicated Biatain, each patient was treated for four weeks' with the Biatain Ag/Contreet foam. The dressing showed good exudate management properties and was considered easy to use. Four ulcers (56%) healed during the four-week treatment and two developed an infection during the study.[128]

Calgitrol Ag

Calgitrol Ag was compared with Algosteril, an unmedicated alginate dressing, in 42 patients with locally infected acute wounds or chronic wounds (pressure ulcers, venous or mixed aetiology leg ulcers, diabetic foot ulcers) in a prospective, open-label, controlled and randomized trial over a two-week period.[129] Wounds were monitored for local signs of infection, using a clinical score ranging from 0 to 18, and the change in the bacteriological status of each was determined by bacteriological examination of two biopsies performed on days one and 15. A three-point scale (deterioration, unchanged, improvement) was used for this purpose. The general acceptability, usefulness and tolerance of the treatments were also assessed. Most of the forty-two patients had chronic wounds such as pressure ulcers (57%) or venous or mixed aetiology leg ulcers and diabetic foot ulcers (29%); few had acute wounds (14%). Initial clinical scores of infection were comparable in both groups, 8.9 ± 2.4 and 8.6 ± 3.2 in the Calgitrol Ag group and the Algosteril group respectively (n.s). These decreased significantly in both groups by day 15, falling to 3.8 ± 2.9 in the Calgitrol Ag group (p = 0.001) and 3.8 ± 3.4 in the Algosteril group (p = 0.007). No differences between the treatment groups were observed for the local tolerance, acceptability and usefulness of the dressings.

Granufoam silver

Gerry *et al.*[130] described the successful use of Granufoam Silver in conjunction with topical negative pressure in the treatment of two patients with longstanding venous stasis ulcers that had persistent purulent drainage. Based on their experiences they proposed that this combination may be of value for cleansing wounds when standard therapies have failed.

Mepilex Ag

Mepilex Ag has been described in two published studies. The first consisted of a single-centered, non-randomized prospective study to assess the effects of the dressing on wound infection, wound related pain, and progress towards healing.[131] Thirty patients with a variety of wound types showing signs of infection were enrolled and followed for four weeks or until wound closure, which ever came first. By the end of the study clinical signs of infection had been eliminated from 27/30 patients. The condition of all wounds improved and 16 achieved closure in the allocated time frame. Pain scores also showed a highly significant improvement. The second publication,[132] consisted of a short series of three case reports which broadly supported the findings of the previous study.

Physiotulle Ag

Physiotulle Ag was evaluated in the treatment of 30 chronic venous leg ulcers with delayed healing and signs of critical colonization in an open prospective non-comparative multicentre clinical study. Patients were treated for four weeks with the dressing which was covered by Alione as a secondary layer. One ulcer healed after three weeks of treatment and the mean relative ulcer area reduced by 55% after four weeks. The mean amount of healthy granulation tissue increased from 26% to 62%, and the mean amount of fibrin decreased from 63% to 32%. Upon inclusion to the study 50% of wounds were judged to be malodorous but after one week this had fallen to 20% and by four weeks to 3%.[133]

In open non-comparative study involving 24 patients the combined use of Physiotulle Ag and Biatain-IBU, an ibuprofen-releasing foam, was assessed in the treatment painful, exuding and locally infected non-healing leg ulcers. General pain and pain at dressing change were monitored using an 11-point numerical scale. Note was also taken of the appearance of the wound bed and exudate handling ability, reduction in wound area and the concentration of ibuprofen in the exudate Details of any adverse effects were also recorded. During the study period, the mean persistent wound pain score decreased from 6.3 ± 2.2 to 3.0 ± 1.7 after 12 hours and remained low thereafter. Pain at dressing change also decreased and remained low. Forty-eight hours after the first dressing application, the mean concentration of ibuprofen in the wound exudate reached a constant level of 35 ± 21 µg /mL. After 31 days, the relative wound area had reduced by 42% and the number of patients malodorous wounds decreased from 37% to 4%. The authors concluded that the combined use of the ibuprofen-releasing foam dressing and silver-releasing contact layer reduced wound pain and promoted healing without compromising safety.[134]

Silvercel

The ability of Silvercel to prevent the development of infection in colonized chronic wounds was examined in a randomized open-label multicentre comparative two-arm parallel-group study. Thirteen centres recruited 99 patients with either a venous leg ulcer (n = 71), or a pressure ulcer (n = 28). None of the wounds required systemic antibiotics but had to exhibit at least two of a list of symptoms to be included in the study. These were: continuous pain, erythema, oedema, heat, and moderate to high levels of serous exudate. Patients were allocated to treatment with a silver-releasing alginate dressing, Silvercel, or a standard calcium alginate dressing, Algosteril. All wounds were initially assessed daily for 14 days then weekly for two additional weeks. Fifty-one and 48 patients were randomized to the test and control groups respectively. Four out of 38 (10.5%) patients who completed the trial in the control group were treated with systemic antibiotics at the final visit but none of the 40 in the test group were so treated (p = 0.053). The healing rate was statistically greater in the test group than the control, 0.32 ± 0.57 vs 0.16 ± 0.40 cm^2/day, (p = 0.024). There was also a greater decrease in the wound severity score at week four in the silver alginate treated wounds, -5.6 ± 3.2 vs -4.1 ± 4.3 (p = 0.063). The authors considered that the results suggest that the use of the silver-releasing alginate may offer some clinical benefits but that further work was required to confirm this effect.[135]

Silverlon

Epstein[136] described a retrospective analysis of patient data to determine whether the substitution of an iodine or alcohol-based swab and dry 4×4 gauze by a silver-impregnated dressing, Silverlon, reduced the risk of superficial or deep infection after lumbar laminectomy with instrumented fusion. Analysis of data from the first 128 patients who were dressed conventionally was compared with that from 106 patients who were dressed with the silver dressing. Of the 128 conventionally treated patients, three developed deep postoperative wound infections and 11 patients developed superficial infection/irritation. Seven of these patients required oral antibiotics alone and four were referred to plastic surgeons for superficial wound revision. None of the 106 patients in the silver treated group developed deep or superficial wound infections. The authors acknowledged that the number of cases in each series was small, but stated that there appeared to be a positive trend toward a reduction in postoperative wound infection using the silver dressing.

An equally positive outcome was reported following a similar study to determine the effect of Silverlon on mediastinitis rates in postoperative cardiac sternotomy incisions.[137] Infection rates recorded in 1,235 patients treated with the standard gauze collected retrospectively from 24 months of infection control records were compared with those determined in the prospective treatment arm of the study when the wounds of 365 consecutive surgical patients were covered with a silver nylon dressing. During the three week postoperative period, 13 patients in the control group (1%) and none of the patients in the treatment group developed mediastinitis (p < 0.05).The authors concluded that these findings justified the conduct a large, prospective, controlled clinical study to confirm the effects of these dressings on mediastinitis, resultant morbidity, and costs of care.

Urgocell Silver

Urgocell Silver was evaluated in a prospective multicentre non-comparative phase III clinical trial involving 45 leg ulcers. The wounds were assessed weekly for up to four weeks to record the presence of one or more signs of critical colonization: severe spontaneous pain between dressing changes, erythema, oedema, malodour and heavy exudate. The mean number of these signs present at baseline was 3.6 ± 0.7, which decreased to 1.2 ± 1.2 by the end of the fourth week, an average reduction of 2.3 ± 1.3 ($p < 0.001$). Ulcer area reduced by $35.0 \pm 58.0\%$ ($p < 0.001$) after the four weeks treatment and the area of the wounds covered with granulation tissue increased from 41% to 77% during this period suggesting that the test dressing had a favourable influence on the wound progress to healing.

Urgotul SSD

The efficacy of Urgotul SSD dressing in the treatment of second-degree burns was examined in a four week multicentre phase III non-comparative open-label prospective study involving 41 subjects with second-degree thermal burns in which treatment with silver sulphadiazine was indicated. Of the 41 patients, 24 healed within a mean of 10.8 days and 13 had a skin graft on the study burn within a mean of 11.5 days. Mean dressing wear time was 1.73 days. There were four premature study withdrawals. None of the subjects acquired a secondary infection and examination of 121 bacteriological samples revealed that only one wound was colonized with *S. aureus*.[138]

Urgotul SSD was evaluated in a more formal fashion in a study involving 68 patients who had partial thickness burn wound less than 15% total body surface area who were divided into two groups and treated with either Urgotul SSD or 1% silver sulfadiazine. Treatment costs were 52 ± 38 for Urgotul SSD *vs* 45 ± 34 US for the silver sulfadiazine treated group. Time of wound closure was significantly shorter in the Urgotul SSD treated group, 10 ± 4 days *vs* 12 ± 6 ($p < 0.05$). Average pain scores and pain medication in Urgotul SSD treated group was significantly lower than 1% silver sulfadiazine treated group, 3 ± 1 *vs* 6 ± 2 ($p < 0.05$).[139]

Urgotul Silver

The influence of the silver present in the dressing was determined in a multicenter, open-label, randomized, controlled clinical trial.[140] Patients with venous leg ulcer ulcers who exhibited at least three of five specific clinical signs identified previously were randomly allocated to be treated for four weeks either with Urgotul Silver or standard Urgotul which contains no silver and therefore acted as a control. After the fourth week, patients in the silver group had their treatment changed to the standard material and both groups were followed to complete healing or for a maximum of four additional weeks to a total of eight weeks. Blood samples were taken from patients in the silver group at baseline and at week four to determine blood silver levels. A total of 51 patients were treated with the silver dressing and 48 with the control. Twenty eight subjects failed to complete the study, eight of whom were in the silver group and 20 in the control group. Wounds were assessed at weekly intervals until week four and every two weeks thereafter until week eight.

By week four, ulcer area had decreased on average by 6.5 ± 13.4 cm^2 in the silver group and by 1.3 ± 9.0 cm^2 in the control group (p = 0.023). Following the change in treatment, the wounds of patients in the silver group continued to decrease in size. At week eight the median absolute wound surface reduction was 5.9 cm^2 and 0.8 cm^2 in the silver and control groups respectively (p = 0.002) corresponding to a percentage reduction (relative to baseline) of 47.9% and 5.6%. (p = 0.036). By the end of the follow-up period, 55% of the silver-treated wounds had decreased by 40% or more compared to 35% for wounds receiving only the non silver releasing dressing throughout the study period (p = 0.051). Blood silver levels determined at baseline and at week four in ten patients in the silver treated group. In seven patients these values remained lower than 1.62 μg/mL, the limit of detection of blood silver with the selected method, and in the remaining three patients, less than 3.7 μg/mL. The results of this study strongly suggest that the presence of the silver had a positive effect upon healing by, it is assumed, reducing the bioburden of the treated wounds. This benefit appeared to persist even after cessation of the treatment.

Clinical comparisons of silver dressings

Unfortunately, little comparative data on the clinical performance of different silver dressings is available to guide practice, and some of the limited number of papers that have been published consists of retrospective reviews rather than prospective studies.

In the first of these,[141] four commonly used venous leg ulcer treatment were compared in a health-economic analysis reflecting the UK treatment practice and cost structure which suggested that use of Contreet Foam in preference to the alternative dressings, Aquacel Ag, Actisorb Silver and Iodoflex, could produce savings of 2.2 - 4.4 million UK pounds per year.

In a second retrospective review,[142] data from a cohort of 2687 clients who received 3716 episodes of care between September 2005 and January 2006 was analysed to determine the length of time for which clients received care from community nurses for each wound and the number of visits required. The median number of visits was statistically significantly higher for the silver-dressing users than for users of other dressings, 31 *vs* 11 (p < 0.0001), while the median treatment duration was also greater, 97 *vs* 39 days (p < 0.0001). The interval between visits was also significantly shorter in the silver dressing group (p < 0.001). The authors suggested that these results call into question the effectiveness of silver dressing materials in the management of chronic wounds in a community care setting but acknowledge that they need to be substantiated by prospective randomized controlled clinical trials to produce more reliable evidence. It is possible, for example, that silver dressings were used selectively for infected or chronic, hard to heal wounds which would inevitably introduce considerable bias into the data.

A similar approach was adopted by Cuttle *et al.*[143] who undertook a retrospective cohort study to determine whether changing to Acticoat from Silvazine enhanced the care provided to paediatric patients with burns. Data collected from 328 patients treated with Silvazine from January 2000 to June 2001 was compared with that obtained from

241 patients treated with Acticoat from July 2002 to July 2003. In the Silvazine-treated group, 25.6% of children required grafting compared to 15.4% in the Acticoat group (p=0.001). When patients requiring grafting were excluded, the time taken for reepithelialization in the Acticoat group was significantly less than that for the Silvazine group, 14.9 vs 18.3 days respectively (p = 0.047). Only one positive blood culture was recorded in each group, indicating that both products are potent antimicrobial agents. The authors concluded that the replace of Silvazine by Acticoat had dramatically changed clinical practice as the vast majority of patients could be treated on an outpatient basis and this contributed to the financial savings associated with the use of Acticoat compared with Silvazine.

Jester[144] compared the use of two silver containing products in a retrospective cohort study involving two groups of 20 paediatric patients with burns treated with Urgotul SSD and Contreet Ag to evaluate both dressing performance and amount of pain during the dressing changes, a process that was continued until the wounds were healed or grafted. In total seventy dressing changes were evaluated in the Contreet Ag group and 67 dressing changes in the Urgotul group. Every dressing change was assessed in terms of exudate handling, adherence, bleeding, ease of dressing application/removal, and pain. Pain was 'absent or slight' in 61 (92%) dressing changes with Urgotul SSD, and in 60 (85%) of the dressing changes with Contreet Ag. As might be expected, Contreet Ag was more absorbent than Urgotul which rated 'very good' in 60 (85%) and 34 (51%) of changes respectively. However, Urgotul was found to be slightly easier to apply than Contreet. The authors concluded that both dressings provided nearly painless wound management, and were therefore well accepted by the patients and nursing staff alike.

Three silver dressings were compared in a prospective clinical trial described by Gago et al.[145] A total of 75 patients with venous ulcers, pressure ulcers, diabetic foot ulcers or traumatic ulcers displaying at least three out of a standard series of clinical signs indicative of local infection, pain, redness, heat, oedema, and/or purulent exudate were enrolled to the study.

Patients were not randomized to treatment but were allocated in a block fashion. The first 25 patients enrolled were allocated to treatment with Acticoat, the second 25 to treatment with Biatain Ag (n = 16) or Contreet Hydrocolloid (n = 9), and the third group to treatment with Aquacel Ag. (The reason that two different types of dressings were used in group 2 was caused by confusion over dressing nomenclature). All three medicated products were used until the signs of infection were judged to have disappeared after which the silver-containing dressings were replaced by a non-medicated version of each product or a foam sheet as appropriate.

During the study all clinical signs of infection resolved significantly faster in patients treated with Acticoat compared to the other two groups (p < 0.05). The percentage of wounds showing no signs of clinical infection at weeks one, two, three and four for each treatment was as follows: For Acticoat 28%, 60%, 60%, 100%; for Biatain Ag/Contreet 0%, 4%, 8%, 100% and for Aquacel 0%, 8%, 12%, 100%.

Time to complete healing was also significantly less in Acticoat treated wounds compared to the other groups after adjusting for baseline wound area variations

($p < 0.05$). Patients treated with Acticoat were also nearly three times more likely to heal at any time during the study than patients treated with alternative products.

Despite some methodological shortcoming, the study appeared to demonstrate clear advantages associated with the use of Acticoat compared with the other silver dressings evaluated.

A recent paper described a pragmatic, prospective randomised controlled trial designed to examine the effectiveness and cost-effectiveness of a variety of antimicrobial silver-donating dressings in the treatment of venous leg ulcers compared with simple non-adherent, also known as low-adherent, dressings.[146] Two hundred and thirteen patients with active ulceration of the lower leg that had been present for a period of greater than six weeks were randomised to receive either a silver-donating or non-silver low-adherent dressing applied in conjunction with graduated compression although the choice of primary dressing within these groups was left to clinician preference. A non-randomised observational group consisting of 91 patients was also recruited. The primary outcome measure was complete ulcer healing at 12 weeks but secondary measures were treatment costs and quality-adjusted life-years (QALYs), cost-effectiveness, time to healing, and recurrence rate at 6 months and 1 year. No significant difference was detected between the two treatment groups for the primary outcome measure of proportion of ulcers healed at 12 weeks (59.6% for silver and 56.7% for control dressings). The overall median time to healing was also not significantly different between the two groups ($p = 0.408$). Compared with the control group, the antimicrobial group had an incremental cost of £97.85 and an incremental QALY gain of 0.0002, resulting in an incremental cost-effectiveness ratio for the antimicrobial dressings of £489,250. The authors concluded that these results clearly do not provide support for the routine use of silver dressings for this indication either on clinical or financial grounds but a potential criticism of this study must be their failure to standardise on a particular silver dressing given the well-recognised variation in silver content and performance of the different dressings identified in other laboratory and clinical investigations.

RESISTANCE TO SILVER DRESSINGS

The first report of resistance to silver was reported in 1975 in a strain of *Salmonella typhimurium* isolated sequentially from three patients in a burns unit who wounds were treated with 0.5% w/v silver nitrate solution.[147] The organism was found to be resistant not only to silver nitrate but also mercuric chloride, ampicillin, chloramphenicol, tetracycline, streptomycin, and sulphonamides. It was shown that this pattern of multiple resistance could be transferred *in vitro* by a plasmid to sensitive recipient strains of *E. coli* and *S. typhimurium* and thereafter between different strains of E. coli.

However, in 2005 Percival *et al.*,[148] when discussing the possible development of bacterial resistance to silver, concluded that despite a rapid increase in the use of silver-containing products, concerns that this might lead to a serious problem may well have been overstated.

Brett in 2006[54] identified a number of potential pathogens that had been isolated from clinical and environmental sources that were resistant to silver including strains of

P. aeruginosa, *Pseudomonas stutzeri*, *E. coli* and *K. pneumoniae*. He also discussed the mechanisms by which bacteria might develop resistance to silver, and referenced previous studies that described how silver resistant organisms had been developed in the laboratory by exposing bacteria to sub-lethal concentrations of silver using a 'multiple step exposure protocol'. In this way a strain of *E. coli* was produced that was resistant to silver at a concentration of silver in excess of 1000 ppm. He concluded, however, that resistance to silver was unlikely to occur in a single step but intimated that the use of silver dressings that liberated low concentrations of silver ions could possibly lead to the development of silver resistance.

Chopra,[149] in a brief review published in 2007, stated that at that time there were less than 20 published reports of silver resistance in bacteria and in only a small number of these was any data provided relating to the mechanism by which this occurs, such as plasmid acquisition and gene mutation. Irrespective of the mechanism of resistance, he concluded that products that release low levels of silver are likely to be more dangerous in terms of selection for resistance, especially if the silver ion concentration is sublethal. Faster acting dressings he proposed will prevent less risk because organisms are more likely to be killed, thereby eliminating the possibility of enrichment of the resistant population.

Nadworny and Burrell[4] proposed that in order to prevent the development and selection of silver-resistant mutant cells, dressings should produce concentrations of silver ions in complex media significantly in excess of 1 mg/L in order to comfortably exceed the MIC of potential pathogens.

Percival *et al.*,[150] in a second publication, described an *in vitro* investigation to assess the prevalence of silver resistance genes in 112 bacterial isolates obtained from ulcers of patients attending a diabetic foot clinic in the UK. They used a polymerase chain reaction to screen for three silver-resistance transcriptional units and identified two silver-resistant bacteria, both strains of *E. cloacae*, an organism rarely implicated as a primary pathogen in chronic wounds. Despite the evidence of genetic resistance to silver, the organisms were killed following a maximum of 48 hours of exposure to the dressings. Encouragingly, none of the 24 *S. aureus* isolates or nine *P. aeruginosa* isolates was found to contain silver-resistant genes. The authors concluded that the presence of silver resistance genes is rare and that genetic resistance does not necessarily translate to phenotypic resistance to silver.

CONCLUSIONS

According to one report,[146] in 2006–2007, the UK National Health Service (NHS) spent over £100 million on wound dressings and that expenditure on silver-containing dressings accounted for a quarter of this sum. In the light of the evidence presented above, there can be little doubt that this does not represent good value for money. Whilst it may be possible to make a case for the short term use of some silver-containing dressings where infection is known to be present or is strongly suspected, on the basis of the evidence currently available, the practice of using silver dressings as a first line treatment for all types of wounds including leg ulcers, for example, cannot be supported either on clinical or economic grounds.

REFERENCES

1. Burrell RE. A scientific perspective on the use of topical silver preparations. *Ostomy Wound Manage* 2003;**49**(5A Suppl):19-24.
2. White RJ. An historical overview of the use of silver in modern wound management. *British Journal of Nursing* 2002;**10**((15 silver supplement)):3-8.
3. Russell AD, Hugo WB. Antimicrobial activity and action of silver. In: Ellis GP, Luscombe DK, editors. *Progress in Medinical Chemistry*: Elsevier Science, 1994:351-369.
4. Nadworny PL, Burrell RE. A review of assessment techniques for silver technology in wound care. Part I: *In Vitro* methods for assessing antimicrobial activity *Journal of Wound Technology* 2008;**1**(2):6-13.
5. Burrell RE. Polishing the information on silver (letter reply). *Ostomy Wound Manage* 2003;**49**(8):11-2, 14, 16
6. Parsons D, Bowler PG, Walker M. Polishing the information on silver (letter). *Ostomy Wound Manage* 2003;**49**(8):10-1.
7. Pal S, Tak YK, Song JM. Does the antibacterial activity of silver nanoparticles depend on the shape of the nanoparticle? A study of the Gram-negative bacterium Escherichia coli. *Appl Environ Microbiol* 2007;**73**(6):1712-20.
8. Lansdown AB. Silver. I: Its antibacterial properties and mechanism of action. *Journal of Wound Care* 2002;**11**(4):125-30.
9. Morin RJ, Tenenhaus M, Granick MS. A review of silver in the management of burns. *Journal of Wound Technology* 2008(2):28-32.
10. Lansdown AB, Williams A, Chandler S, Benfield S. Silver absorption and antibacterial efficacy of silver dressings. *J Wound Care* 2005;**14**(4):155-60.
11. Lansdown AB. Silver. 2: Toxicity in mammals and how its products aid wound repair. *Journal of Wound Care* 2002;**11**(5):173-7.
12. White R, Cutting K. Exploring the Effects of Silver in Wound Management—What is Optimal? *Wounds* 2006(11).
13. Leaper D. Sharp technique for wound debridement. *World Wide Wounds* 2002;**http://www.worldwidewounds.com/2002/december/Leaper/Sharp-Debridement.html**.
14. Fox CL, Jr. Silver sulfadiazine--a new topical therapy for Pseudomonas in burns. Therapy of Pseudomonas infection in burns. *Arch Surg* 1968;**96**(2):184-8.
15. Fox CL, Jr., Rappole BW, Stanford W. Control of pseudomonas infection in burns by silver sulfadiazine. *Surg Gynecol Obstet* 1969;**128**(5):1021-6.
16. Fox CL, Jr., Sampath AC, Stanford JW. Virulence of Pseudomonas infection in burned rats and mice. Comparative efficacy of silver sulfadiazine and mafenide. *Arch Surg* 1970;**101**(4):508-12.
17. Fox CL, Jr., Modak SM. Mechanism of silver sulfadiazine action on burn wound infections. *Antimicrob Agents Chemother* 1974;**5**(6):582-8.
18. Fox CL, Jr. Silver sulfadiazine for control of burn wound infections. *Int Surg* 1975;**60**(5):275-7.
19. Hermans MHE. A survey: Silver is still the gold standard in burn care. *Journal of Wound Technology* 2008(2):56-57.
20. Spadaro JA, Berger TJ, Barranco SD, Chapin SE, Becker RO. Antibacterial effects of silver electrodes with weak direct current. *Antimicrob Agents Chemother* 1974;**6**(5):637-42.

21. Berger TJ, Spadaro JA, Bierman R, Chapin SE, Becker RO. Antifungal properties of electrically generated metallic ions. *Antimicrob Agents Chemother* 1976;**10**(5):856-60.

22. Becker RO, Spadaro JA. Treatment of orthopaedic infections with electrically generated silver ions. A preliminary report. *J Bone Joint Surg Am* 1978;**60**(7):871-81.

23. Webster DA, Spadaro JA, Becker RO, Kramer S. Silver anode treatment of chronic osteomyelitis. *Clin Orthop* 1981(161):105-14.

24. Spadaro JA, Webster DA, Becker RO. Silver polymethyl methacrylate antibacterial bone cement. *Clin Orthop Relat Res* 1979(143):266-70.

25. Deitch EA, Marino AA, Malakanok V, Albright JA. Silver nylon cloth: in vitro and in vivo evaluation of antimicrobial activity. *J Trauma* 1987;**27**(3):301-4.

26. Chu CS, McManus AT, Pruitt BA, Jr., Mason AD, Jr. Therapeutic effects of silver nylon dressings with weak direct current on Pseudomonas aeruginosa-infected burn wounds. *J Trauma* 1988;**28**(10):1488-92.

27. Adams AP, Santschi EM, Mellencamp MA. Antibacterial properties of a silver chloride-coated nylon wound dressing. *Vet Surg* 1999;**28**(4):219-25.

28. Ersek RA, Denton DR. Cross-linked silver-impregnated skin for burn wound management. *J Burn Care Rehabil* 1988;**9**(5):476-81.

29. Ersek RA, Navarro JA. Maximizing wound healing with silver-impregnated porcine xenograft. *Todays OR Nurse* 1990;**12**(12):4-9.

30. Frost M, Jackson S, Stevens P. Adsorption of bacteria onto activated charcoal cloth: an effect of potential importance in the treatment of infected wounds. *Microbios Letters* 1980;**13**:135-140.

31. Tredget EE, Shankowsky HA, Groeneveld A, Burrell R. A matched-pair, randomized study evaluating the efficacy and safety of Acticoat silver-coated dressing for the treatment of burn wounds. *J. Burn Care Rehabil.* 1998;**19**(6):531-7.

32. Gallant-Behm CL, Yin HQ, Liu S, Heggers JP, Langford RE, Olson ME, et al. Comparison of in vitro disc diffusion and time kill-kinetic assays for the evaluation of antimicrobial wound dressing efficacy. *Wound Repair Regen* 2005;**13**(4):412-21.

33. Furr JR, Russell AD, Turner TD, Andrews A. Antibacterial activity of Actisorb Plus, Actisorb and silver nitrate. *J. Hospital Infection* 1994;**27**(3):201-208.

34. Addison D, Rennison TJ. A comparison of the antimicrobial properties of silver dressings for chronic wound care.(Poster Presentation). European Wound Management Association meeting, Granada , Spain, 2002.

35. Muller G, Winkler Y, Kramer A. Antibacterial activity and endotoxin-binding capacity of Actisorb Silver 220. *J Hosp Infect* 2003;**53**(3):211-4.

36. Wright JB, Lam K, Burrell RE. Wound management in an era of increasing bacterial antibiotic resistance: a role for topical silver treatment. *Am. J. Infect .Control* 1998;**26**(6):572-7.

37. Wright JB, Lam K, Hansen D, Burrell RE. Efficacy of topical silver against fungal burn wound pathogens. *Am. J. Infect. Control* 1999;**27**(4):344-50.

38. Yin HQ, Langford R, Burrell RE. Comparative evaluation of the antimicrobial activity of ACTICOAT antimicrobial barrier dressing In Process Citation. *J. Burn Care Rehabil.* 1999;**20**(3):195-200.

39. Fraser JF, Bodman J, Sturgess R, Faoagali J, Kimble RM. An in vitro study of the anti-microbial efficacy of a 1% silver sulphadiazine and 0.2% chlorhexidine digluconate cream, 1% silver sulphadiazine cream and a silver coated dressing. *Burns* 2004;**30**(1):35-41.

40. Jones SA, Bowler PG, Walker M, Parsons D. Controlling wound bioburden with a novel silver-containing Hydrofiber dressing. *Wound Repair Regen* 2004;**12**(3):288-94.

41. Bowler PG, Jones SA, Walker M, Parsons D. Microbicidal properties of a silver-containing hydrofiber dressing against a variety of burn wound pathogens. *J Burn Care Rehabil* 2004;**25**(2):192-6.

42. Castellano JJ, Shafii SM, Ko F, Donate G, Wright TE, Mannari RJ, et al. Comparative evaluation of silver-containing antimicrobial dressings and drugs. *Int Wound J* 2007;**4**(2):114-22.

43. O'Neill MA, Vine GJ, Beezer AE, Bishop AH, Hadgraft J, Labetoulle C, et al. Antimicrobial properties of silver-containing wound dressings: a microcalorimetric study. *Int J Pharm* 2003;**263**(1-2):61-8.

44. Gaisford S, Beezer AE, Bishop AH, Walker M, Parsons D. An in vitro method for the quantitative determination of the antimicrobial efficacy of silver-containing wound dressings. *Int J Pharm* 2009;**366**(1-2):111-6.

45. Ip M, Lui SL, Poon VK, Lung I, Burd A. Antimicrobial activities of silver dressings: an in vitro comparison. *J Med Microbiol* 2006;**55**(Pt 1):59-63.

46. Holder IA, Durkee P, Supp AP, Boyce ST. Assessment of a silver-coated barrier dressing for potential use with skin grafts on excised burns. *Burns* 2003;**29**(5):445-8.

47. Edwards-Jones V. Antimicrobial and barrier effects of silver against methicillin-resistant Staphylococcus aureus. *J Wound Care* 2006;**15**(7):285-90.

48. Thomas S, McCubbin P. A comparison of the antimicrobial effects of four silver-containing dressings on three organisms. *Journal of Wound Care* 2003;**12**(3):101-107.

49. Thomas S, McCubbin P. An in vitro analysis of the antimicrobial properties of 10 silver-containing dressings. *Journal of Wound Care* 2003;**12**(8):305-8.

50. Thomas S, McCubbin P. Silver dressings: the debate continues. *Journal of Wound Care* 2003;**12**(10):420.

51. Thomas S, Ashman P. *In-vitro* testing of silver containing dressings. *Journal of Wound Care* 2004;**13**(9):392-393.

52. Walker M, Cochrane CA, Bowler PG, Parsons D, Bradshaw P. Silver deposition and tissue staining associated with wound dressings containing silver. *Ostomy Wound Manage* 2006;**52**(1):42-4, 46-50.

53. Parsons D, Bowler PG, Myles V, Jones S. Silver antimicrobial dressings in wound management: A comparison of antibacterial, physical, and chemical characteristics. *Wounds* 2005;**17**(8):222-232.

54. Brett DW. A discussion of silver as an antimicrobial agent: alleviating the confusion. *Ostomy Wound Manage* 2006;**52**(1):34-41.

55. Parsons D, Walker M, Bowler PG. Silver: clarifying the claims. *Ostomy Wound Manage* 2006;**52**(6):12,14; author reply 14, 16.

56. Percival SL, Bowler PG, Dolman J. Antimicrobial activity of silver-containing dressings on wound microorganisms using an in vitro biofilm model. *Int Wound J* 2007;**4**(2):186-91.

57. Walker M, Hobot JA, Newman GR, Bowler PG. Scanning electron microscopic examination of bacterial immobilisation in a carboxymethyl cellulose (AQUACEL((R))) and alginate dressings. *Biomaterials* 2003;**24**(5):883-90.

58. Walker M, Bowler PG, Cochrane CA. In vitro studies to show sequestration of matrix metalloproteinases by silver-containing wound care products. *Ostomy Wound Manage* 2007;**53**(9):18-25.

59. Wright JB, Lam K, Buret AG, Olson ME, Burrell RE. Early healing events in a porcine model of contaminated wounds: effects of nanocrystalline silver on matrix metalloproteinases, cell apoptosis, and healing. *Wound Repair Regen* 2002;**10**(3):141-51.

60. Nadworny PL, Wang J, Tredget EE, Burrell RE. Anti-inflammatory activity of nanocrystalline silver in a porcine contact dermatitis model. *Nanomedicine* 2008;**4**(3):241-51.

61. Chaudhry Z, Sammet S, Coffey R, Crockett A, Yuh WT, Miller S. Assessing the safety and compatibility of silver based wound dressings in a magnetic resonance environment. *Burns* 2009;**35**(8):1080-5.

62. Burrell RE, Heggers JP, Davis GJ, Wright JB. Efficacy of silver-coated dressings as bacterial barriers in a rodent burn sepsis model. *Wounds: A Compendium of Clinical Research and Practice* 1999;**11**(464-71).

63. Heggers J, Goodheart RE, Washington J, McCoy L, Carino E, Dang T, et al. Therapeutic efficacy of three silver dressings in an infected animal model. *J Burn Care Rehabil* 2005;**26**(1):53-6.

64. Ulkur E, Oncul O, Karagoz H, Celikoz B, Cavuslu S. Comparison of silver-coated dressing (Acticoat), chlorhexidine acetate 0.5% (Bactigrass), and silver sulfadiazine 1% (Silverdin) for topical antibacterial effect in Pseudomonas aeruginosa-contaminated, full-skin thickness burn wounds in rats. *J Burn Care Rehabil* 2005;**26**(5):430-3.

65. Ulkur E, Oncul O, Karagoz H, Yeniz E, Celikoz B. Comparison of silver-coated dressing (Acticoat), chlorhexidine acetate 0.5% (Bactigrass), and fusidic acid 2% (Fucidin) for topical antibacterial effect in methicillin-resistant Staphylococci-contaminated, full-skin thickness rat burn wounds. *Burns* 2005;**31**(7):874-7.

66. Bell A, Hart J. Evaluation of two absorbent silver dressings in a porcine partial-thickness excisional wound model. *J Wound Care* 2007;**16**(10):445-8, 450-3.

67. Lee JH, Chae JD, Kim DG, Hong SH, Lee WM, Ki M. [Comparison of the Efficacies of Silver-Containing Dressing Materials for Treating a Full-Thickness Rodent Wound Infected by Methicillin-resistant Staphylococcus aureus.]. *Korean J Lab Med* 2010;**30**(1):20-7.

68. Ring A, Goertz O, Muhr G, Steinau HU, Langer S. In vivo microvascular response of murine cutaneous muscle to ibuprofen-releasing polyurethane foam. *Int Wound J* 2008;**5**(3):464-9.

69. Lam PK, Chan ES, Ho WS, Liew CT. In vitro cytotoxicity testing of a nanocrystalline silver dressing (Acticoat) on cultured keratinocytes. *Br J Biomed Sci* 2004;**61**(3):125-7.

70. Poon VK, Burd A. In vitro cytotoxity of silver: implication for clinical wound care. *Burns* 2004;**30**(2):140-7.

71. Paddle-Ledinek JE, Nasa Z, Cleland HJ. Effect of different wound dressings on cell viability and proliferation. *Plast Reconstr Surg* 2006;**117**(7 Suppl):110S-118S; discussion 119S-120S.

72. Duc Q, Breetveld M, Middelkoop E, Scheper RJ, Ulrich MM, Gibbs S. A cytotoxic analysis of antiseptic medication on skin substitutes and autograft. *Br J Dermatol* 2007;**157**(1):33-40.

73. Schaller M, Laude J, Bodewaldt H, Hamm G, Korting HC. Toxicity and antimicrobial activity of a hydrocolloid dressing containing silver particles in an ex vivo model of cutaneous infection. *Skin Pharmacol Physiol* 2004;**17**(1):31-6.

74. Fredriksson C, Kratz G, Huss F. Accumulation of silver and delayed re-epithelialization in normal human skin: An ex-vivo study of different silver dressings. *Wounds* 2009;**21**(5):116-123.

75. Burd A, Kwok CH, Hung SC, Chan HS, Gu H, Lam WK, et al. A comparative study of the cytotoxicity of silver-based dressings in monolayer cell, tissue explant, and animal models. *Wound Repair Regen* 2007;**15**(1):94-104.

76. Supp AP, Neely AN, Supp DM, Warden GD, Boyce ST. Evaluation of cytotoxicity and antimicrobial activity of Acticoat Burn Dressing for management of microbial contamination in cultured skin substitutes grafted to athymic mice. *J Burn Care Rehabil* 2005;**26**(3):238-46.

77. Nadworny PL, Burrell RE. A review of assessment techniques for silver technology in wound care. Part II: Tissue culture and in vivo methods for determining antimicrobial and ant-inflammatory activity. *Journal of Wound Technology* 2008;**1**(2):14-22.

78. Agarwal A, Weis TL, Schurr MJ, Faith NG, Czuprynski CJ, McAnulty JF, et al. Surfaces modified with nanometer-thick silver-impregnated polymeric films that kill bacteria but support growth of mammalian cells. *Biomaterials* 2010;**31**(4):680-90.

79. Trop M, Novak M, Rodl S, Hellbom B, Kroell W, Goessler W. Silver-coated dressing acticoat caused raised liver enzymes and argyria-like symptoms in burn patient. *J Trauma* 2006;**60**(3):648-52.

80. Parkes A. Silver-coated dressing Acticoat. *J Trauma* 2006;**61**(1):239-40.

81. Wan AT, Conyers RA, Coombs CJ, Masterton JP. Determination of silver in blood, urine, and tissues of volunteers and burn patients. *Clin Chem* 1991;**37**(10 Pt 1):1683-7.

82. Chen J, Han CM, Yu CH. [Change in sliver metabolism after the application of nanometer silver on burn wound]. *Zhonghua Shao Shang Za Zhi* 2004;**20**(3):161-3.

83. Dunn K, Edwards-Jones V. The role of Acticoat with nanocrystalline silver in the management of burns. *Burns* 2004;**30 Suppl 1**:S1-9.

84. Vlachou E, Chipp E, Shale E, Wilson YT, Papini R, Moiemen NS. The safety of nanocrystalline silver dressings on burns: a study of systemic silver absorption. *Burns* 2007;**33**(8):979-85.

85. Hoekstra MJ. Nanoscale silver dressings in wound care: is there cause for concern? . *Journal of Wound Technology* 2008(2):60-62.

86. Varas RP, O'Keeffe T, Namias N, Pizano LR, Quintana OD, Herrero Tellachea M, et al. A prospective, randomized trial of Acticoat versus silver sulfadiazine in the treatment of partial-thickness burns: which method is less painful? *J Burn Care Rehabil* 2005;**26**(4):344-7.

87. Olson ME, Wright JB, Lam K, Burrell RE. Healing of porcine donor sites covered with silver-coated dressings [In Process Citation]. *Eur J Surg* 2000;**166**(6):486-9.

88. Innes ME, Umraw N, Fish JS, Gomez M, Cartotto RC. The use of silver coated dressings on donor site wounds: a prospective, controlled matched pair study. *Burns* 2001;**27**(6):621-7.

89. Fong J, Wood F, Fowler B. A silver coated dressing reduces the incidence of early burn wound cellulitis and associated costs of inpatient treatment: comparative patient care audits. *Burns* 2005;**31**(5):562-7.

90. Kok K, Georgeu GA, Wilson VY. The Acticoat glove-an effective dressing for the completely burnt hand: how we do it. *Burns* 2006;**32**(4):487-9.

91. Rustogi R, Mill J, Fraser JF, Kimble RM. The use of Acticoat in neonatal burns. *Burns* 2005;**31**(7):878-82.

92. Peters DA, Verchere C. Healing at home: Comparing cohorts of children with medium-sized burns treated as outpatients with in-hospital applied Acticoat to those children treated as inpatients with silver sulfadiazine. *J Burn Care Res* 2006;**27**(2):198-201.

93. Huang Y, Li X, Liao Z, Zhang G, Liu Q, Tang J, et al. A randomized comparative trial between Acticoat and SD-Ag in the treatment of residual burn wounds, including safety analysis. *Burns* 2007;**33**(2):161-6.

94. Childress BB, Berceli SA, Nelson PR, Lee WA, Ozaki CK. Impact of an absorbent silver-eluting dressing system on lower extremity revascularization wound complications. *Ann Vasc Surg* 2007;**21**(5):598-602.

95. Asz J, Asz D, Moushey R, Seigel J, Mallory SB, Foglia RP. Treatment of toxic epidermal necrolysis in a pediatric patient with a nanocrystalline silver dressing. *J Pediatr Surg* 2006;**41**(12):e9-12.

96. Bhattacharyya M, Bradley H. Management of a difficult-to-heal chronic wound infected with methycillin-resistant staphylococcus aureus in a patient with psoriasis following a complex knee surgery. *Int J Low Extrem Wounds* 2006;**5**(2):105-8.

97. Strohal R, Schelling M, Takacs M, Jurecka W, Gruber U, Offner F. Nanocrystalline silver dressings as an efficient anti-MRSA barrier: a new solution to an increasing problem. *J Hosp Infect* 2005;**60**(3):226-30.
98. Forner-Cordero I, Navarro-Monsoliu R, Munoz-Langa J, Alcober-Fuster P, Rel-Monzo P. Use of a nanocrystalline silver dressing on lymphatic ulcers in patients with chronic lymphoedema. *J Wound Care* 2007;**16**(5):235-9.
99. Sibbald RG, Contreras-Ruiz J, Coutts P, Fierheller M, Rothman A, Woo K. Bacteriology, inflammation, and healing: a study of nanocrystalline silver dressings in chronic venous leg ulcers. *Adv Skin Wound Care* 2007;**20**(10):549-58.
100. Gravante G, Caruso R, Sorge R, Nicoli F, Gentile P, Cervelli V. Nanocrystalline silver: a systematic review of randomized trials conducted on burned patients and an evidence-based assessment of potential advantages over older silver formulations. *Ann Plast Surg* 2009;**63**(2):201-5.
101. Thomas S, Fisher B, Fram PJ, Waring MJ. Odour-absorbing dressings. *Journal of Wound Care* 1998;**7**(5):246-50.
102. Mulligan CM, Bragg AJD, O'Toole OB. A controlled comparative trial of Actisorb activated charcoal cloth dressings in the community. *British Journal of Clinical Practice* 1986;**9**(1):145-8.
103. Milward PA. Comparing treatment for leg ulcers. *Nursing Times* 1991;**87**(13):70-72.
104. Leak K. PEG site infections: a novel use for Actisorb Silver 220. *Br J Community Nurs* 2002;**7**(6):321-5.
105. Stadler R. Treatment of chronic wounds with Actisorb. 2002.
106. Verdu Soriano J, Rueda Lopez J, Martinez Cuervo F, Soldevilla Agreda J. Effects of an activated charcoal silver dressing on chronic wounds with no clinical signs of infection. *J Wound Care* 2004;**13**(10):419, 421-3.
107. Kotz P, Fisher J, McCluskey P, Hartwell SD, Dharma H. Use of a new silver barrier dressing, ALLEVYN Ag in exuding chronic wounds. *Int Wound J* 2009;**6**(3):186-94.
108. Vanscheidt W, Lazareth I, Routkovsky-Norval C. Safety evaluation of a new ionic silver dressing in the management of chronic ulcers. *Wounds* 2003;**15**(11).
109. Caruso DM, Foster KN, Hermans MH, Rick C. Aquacel Ag in the management of partial-thickness burns: results of a clinical trial. *J Burn Care Rehabil* 2004;**25**(1):89-97.
110. Coutts P, Sibbald RG. The effect of a silver-containing Hydrofiber dressing on superficial wound bed and bacterial balance of chronic wounds. *Int Wound J* 2005;**2**(4):348-56.
111. Lohana P, Potokar TS. Aquacel Ag in Paediatric burns - a prospective audit. *Annals of Burns and Fire Disasters* 2006;**19**(3):144-148.
112. Caruso DM, Foster KN, Blome-Eberwein SA, Twomey JA, Herndon DN, Luterman A, et al. Randomized clinical study of Hydrofiber dressing with silver or silver sulfadiazine in the management of partial-thickness burns. *J Burn Care Res* 2006;**27**(3):298-309.
113. Paddock HN, Fabia R, Giles S, Hayes J, Lowell W, Besner GE. A silver impregnated antimicrobial dressing reduces hospital length of stay for pediatric patients with burns. *J Burn Care Res* 2007;**28**(3):409-11.
114. Paddock HN, Fabia R, Giles S, Hayes J, Lowell W, Adams D, et al. A silver-impregnated antimicrobial dressing reduces hospital costs for pediatric burn patients. *J Pediatr Surg* 2007;**42**(1):211-3.
115. Lohsiriwat V, Chuangsuwanich A. Comparison of the ionic silver-containing hydrofiber* and paraffin gauze dressing on split-thickness skin graft donor sites. *Ann Plast Surg* 2009;**62**(4):421-2.

116. Lohsiriwat V, Chuangsuwanich A. Comparison of the ionic silver-containing hydrofiber and paraffin gauze dressing on split-thickness skin graft donor sites. *Ann Plast Surg* 2009;**62**(4):421-2.

117. Jude EB, Apelqvist J, Spraul M, Martini J. Prospective randomized controlled study of Hydrofiber dressing containing ionic silver or calcium alginate dressings in non-ischaemic diabetic foot ulcers. *Diabet Med* 2007;**24**(3):280-8.

118. Stang D. The use of Aquacel Ag in the management of diabetic foot ulcers. *The Diabetic Foot* 2004;**7**(4):188-91.

119. Jurczak F, Dugre T, Johnstone A, Offori T, Vujovic Z, Hollander D. Randomised clinical trial of Hydrofiber dressing with silver versus povidone-iodine gauze in the management of open surgical and traumatic wounds. *Int Wound J* 2007;**4**(1):66-76.

120. Barnea Y, Weiss J, Gur E. A review of the applications of the hydrofiber dressing with silver (Aquacel Ag) in wound care. *Ther Clin Risk Manag* 2010;**6**:21-7.

121. Ziegler K, Gorl R, Effing J, Ellermann J, Mappes M, Otten S, et al. Reduced cellular toxicity of a new silver-containing antimicrobial dressing and clinical performance in non-healing wounds. *Skin Pharmacol Physiol* 2006;**19**(3):140-6.

122. Morgan T, Evans C, Harding K. A study to measure patient comfort and acceptance of Avance, a new polyurethane foam dressing containing silver as an antimicrobial when used to treat chronic wounds. Poster presented at the 11th European Wound Management Association Conference, Dublin,Ireland, 2001.

123. Ballard K, McGregor F. Avance: silver hydropolymer dressing for critically colonized wounds. *Br J Nurs* 2002;**11**(3):206-10.

124. Karlsmark T, Agerslev RH, Bendz SH, Larsen JR, Roed-Petersen J, Andersen KE. Clinical performance of a new silver dressing, Contreet Foam, for chronic exuding venous leg ulcers. *Journal of Wound Care* 2003;**12**(9):351-4.

125. Jorgensen B, Price P, Andersen KE, Gottrup F, Bech-Thomsen N, Scanlon E, et al. The silver-releasing foam dressing, Contreet Foam, promotes faster healing of critically colonised venous leg ulcers: a randomised, controlled trial. *Int Wound J* 2005;**2**(1):64-73.

126. Munter KC, Beele H, Russell L, Crespi A, Grochenig E, Basse P, et al. Effect of a sustained silver-releasing dressing on ulcers with delayed healing: the CONTOP study. *J Wound Care* 2006;**15**(5):199-206.

127. Dimakakos E, Katsenis K, Kalemikerakis J, Arkadopoulos N, Mylonas S, Arapoglou V, et al. Infected venous leg ulcers: management with silver-releasing foam dressing. *Wounds* 2009(1).

128. Rayman G, Rayman A, Baker NR, Jurgeviciene N, Dargis V, Sulcaite R, et al. Sustained silver-releasing dressing in the treatment of diabetic foot ulcers. *Br J Nurs* 2005;**14**(2):109-14.

129. Trial C, Darbas H, Lavigne JP, Sotto A, Simoneau G, Tillet Y, et al. Assessment of the antimicrobial effectiveness of a new silver alginate wound dressing: a RCT. *J Wound Care* 2010;**19**(1):20-6.

130. Gerry R, Kwei S, Bayer L, Breuing KH. Silver-impregnated vacuum-assisted closure in the treatment of recalcitrant venous stasis ulcers. *Ann Plast Surg* 2007;**59**(1):58-62.

131. Meuleneire F. An observational study of the use of a soft silicone silver dressing on a variety of wound types. *J Wound Care* 2008;**17**(12):535-539.

132. Barrows C. The use of antimicrobial soft silicone foam dressing in home health. *Home Healthcare Nurse* 2009;**27**(5):279-284.

133. Jorgensen B, Bech-Thomsen N, Grenov B, Gottrup F. Effect of a new silver dressing on chronic venous leg ulcers with signs of critical colonisation. *J Wound Care* 2006;**15**(3):97-100.

134. Jorgensen B, Gottrup F, Karlsmark T, Bech-Thomsen N, Sibbald RG. Combined use of an ibuprofen-releasing foam dressing and silver dressing on infected leg ulcers. *J Wound Care* 2008;**17**(5):210-4.

135. Meaume S, Vallet D, Morere MN, Teot L. Evaluation of a silver-releasing hydroalginate dressing in chronic wounds with signs of local infection. *J Wound Care* 2005;**14**(9):411-9.

136. Epstein NE. Do silver-impregnated dressings limit infections after lumbar laminectomy with instrumented fusion? *Surg Neurol* 2007;**68**(5):483-5; discussion 485.

137. Huckfeldt R, Redmond C, Mikkelson D, Finley PJ, Lowe C, Robertson J. A clinical trial to investigate the effect of silver nylon dressings on mediastinitis rates in postoperative cardiac sternotomy incisions. *Ostomy Wound Manage* 2008;**54**(10):36-41.

138. Carsin H, Wassermann D, Pannier M, Dumas R, Bohbot S. A silver sulphadiazine-impregnated lipidocolloid wound dressing to treat second-degree burns. *Journal of Wound Care* 2004;**13**(4):145-8.

139. Muangman P, Muangman S, Opasanon S, Keorochana K, Chuntrasakul C. Benefit of hydrocolloid SSD dressing in the outpatient management of partial thickness burns. *J Med Assoc Thai* 2009;**92**(10):1300-5.

140. Lazareth I, Meaume S, Sigal-Grinberg ML, Combemale P, Le Guyadec T, Zagnoli A, et al. The Role of a Silver Releasing Lipido-colloid Contact Layer in Venous Leg Ulcers Presenting Inflammatory Signs Suggesting Heavy. *Wounds* 2008;**20**(2):158-166.

141. Scanlon E, Karlsmark T, Leaper DJ, Carter K, Poulsen PB, Hart-Hansen K, et al. Cost-effective faster wound healing with a sustained silver-releasing foam dressing in delayed healing leg ulcers--a health-economic analysis. *Int Wound J* 2005;**2**(2):150-60.

142. Wang J, Smith J, Babidge W, Maddern G. Silver dressings versus other dressings for chronic wounds in a community care setting. *J Wound Care* 2007;**16**(8):352-6.

143. Cuttle L, Naidu S, Mill J, Hoskins W, Das K, Kimble RM. A retrospective cohort study of Acticoat versus Silvazine in a paediatric population. *Burns* 2007;**33**(6):701-7.

144. Jester I, Böhn I, Hannmann T, Waag K, Loff S. Comparison of two silver dressings for wound management in pediatric burns. *Wounds* 2008;**20**(11).

145. Gago M, Garcia F, Gaztelu V, Verdu J, Lopez P, Nolasco A. A comparison of three silver containing dressings in the treatment of infected chronic wounds. *Wounds* 2008;**20**(10):273-278.

146. Michaels JA, Campbell WB, King BM, Macintyre J, Palfreyman SJ, Shackley P, et al. A prospective randomised controlled trial and economic modelling of antimicrobial silver dressings versus non-adherent control dressings for venous leg ulcers: the VULCAN trial. *Health Technol Assess* 2009;**13**(56):1-114, iii.

147. McHugh GL, Moellering RC, Hopkins CC, Swartz MN. Salmonella typhimurium resistant to silver nitrate, chloramphenicol, and ampicillin. *Lancet* 1975;**1**(7901):235-40.

148. Percival SL, Bowler PG, Russell D. Bacterial resistance to silver in wound care. *J Hosp Infect* 2005;**60**(1):1-7.

149. Chopra I. The increasing use of silver-based products as antimicrobial agents: a useful development or a cause for concern? *J Antimicrob Chemother* 2007;**59**(4):587-90.

150. Percival SL, Woods E, Nutekpor M, Bowler P, Radford A, Cochrane C. Prevalence of silver resistance in bacteria isolated from diabetic foot ulcers and efficacy of silver-containing wound dressings. *Ostomy Wound Manage* 2008;**54**(3):30-40.

17. Odour Controlling Dressings

INTRODUCTION

Psychological effects of wound odour

Some wounds produce noxious odours which, even in moderate cases, can cause significant distress or embarrassment to patients and their relatives,[1] permeating the ward or domestic environment and clinging to clothing or furnishings. In extreme cases the odour can become so overpowering that it may cause an individual to withdraw from social contacts, even with family and close friends.[2-4]

According to Hack[5] wound odour has been reported to cause patients to experience feelings of shame, altered body image, embarrassment, and rejection, sometimes making them to feel less desirable as people and sexual partners. As smell greatly influences perceived taste and flavour,[4] malodour can impact upon a patient's appetite and therefore nutritional status. In extreme cases it may even induce nausea.

Assessment of wound odour

Wound odour cannot be accurately measured or quantified and is therefore highly subjective. Baker and Haig[6] devised a simple scale to characterize wound odour (Table 32), but Collier[7] has argued that the assessment of odour is very subjective and defined a malodorous wound as 'any wound assessed as being offensive in smell by either the patient, practitioner or both.'

Table 31: Assessment of wound odour

Score	Assessment
Very strong	Odour is evident upon entering the room (6 – 10 feet from the patient) with the dressing intact
Strong	Odour is evident upon entering the room (6 – 10 feet from the patient) with the dressing removed
Moderate	Odour is evident at close proximity to the patient when the dressing is intact
Slight	Odour is evident at close proximity to the patient when the dressing is removed
No odour	No odour is evident at close proximity even when the dressing is removed

The importance of odour in the assessment of patients and their wounds was recognized by Roberson *et al.*[8] who established a multi-sensorial wound care simulation experience for nursing students. They believed that exposing them to malodorous 'wounds' simulated by the addition of three 'stinky' cheeses would make the simulation more realistic for students and ultimately enhance their confidence in their ability to care for wounds.

Causes of wound odour

Wounds most commonly associated with odour production include leg ulcers and fungating (cancerous) lesions of all types.[9-10] The smell is caused by a cocktail of volatile agents that includes short chain organic acids, (n-butyric, n-valeric, n-caproic, n-heptanoic and n-caprylic) produced by anaerobic bacteria,[11] together with a mixture of amines and diamines such as cadaverine (1,5-pentanediamine) and putrescine (1,4-diaminobutane) that are produced by the metabolic processes of other proteolytic bacteria.

Organisms frequently isolated from malodorous wounds include anaerobes such as Bacteroides and Clostridium species, and numerous aerobic bacteria including Proteus, Klebsiella and Pseudomonas spp. Recent research has shown that the wound odour produced by some bacteria is specific to that species and that this may be analysed electrochemically to identify the presence of organisms such as ß-haemolytic streptococci.[12]

Management of wound odour

The most effective way of dealing with malodorous wounds is to eradicate the organisms responsible for odour production. This may be achieved in a number of ways. The administration of systemic antibiotics or antimicrobial agents may be effective in some cases, but often the nature of the wound is such that it is not possible to achieve an effective concentration of the antibiotic at the site of infection by this route, particularly in the presence of slough or necrotic tissue. Systemic antibiotics can also induce unpleasant side effects.

An alternative approach is to use some form of topical preparation, but many antiseptics are of limited value and some have been shown to adversely effect wound healing.[13-14] One agent that can provide effective odour control when applied in the form of a gel is metronidazole.[15] Research has shown that despite the fact that metronidazole is more traditionally associated with the treatment of anaerobic infections, in the concentrations used topically it also has an effect upon a range of aerobic organisms.[16]

When 68 patients with malodorous wounds were treated with 0.8% metronidazole gel for periods ranging from a few days to 15 months, odour was completely eliminated from 34 (50%) of wounds, reduced in 31 (46%) but remained unaffected in three.[17]

In a study undertaken to assess the subjective and bacteriological response to 0.75% metronidazole gel, 47 patients with foul smelling benign or malignant cutaneous lesions were assessed for smell, pain, appearance, and bacteriological profile initially and after seven and 14 days treatment. Forty-one (95%) of the 43 patients who remained in the study for 14 days reported decreased smell. Anaerobic infection, initially found in 25 (53%) of patients, was eliminated in 21 (84%).[18]

The literature relating to the use of topical metronidazole for controlling wound odour was reviewed in 1996 by Hampson[19] and in 2008 by Paul and Pieper,[20] who identified 15 publications: seven case reports/series; six descriptive longitudinal studies and two controlled clinical trials in which metronidazole was used as a 1% w/v solution or a gel containing round 0.8% w/w. The results of both reviews suggested that the antibiotic reduced or eliminated wound odour and produced an improvement in the appearance of the wound and surrounding tissue, but suggested that more formal studies were required to confirm these conclusions. Morgan[21] and Hampson[19] also raised the potential problem of the development of bacterial resistance following the widespread topical use the antibiotic.

XE "Clindamycin for controlling wound odour" A second antibiotic, Clindamycin, was used topically to prevent the odour from gauze dressings applied to postoperative maxillary bony defects in eight patients with maxillary cancer. In each case the treatment eliminated organisms such as Bacteroides and Peptostreptococcus, which were considered to be involved in odour production.[22]

Other methods for treating malodorous wounds include the use of honey and sugar,[23] applied as a powder form or formulated into a paste (see Chapter 15). Buttermilk and live yoghurt have similarly been used, in an attempt to encourage overgrowth of pathogenic organisms by lactic acid bacteria such as *Lactobacillus bulgaricus* and *Streptococcus thermophilus*.[24-26] The use of sterile maggots has also been shown in numerous studies to be an effective way of eliminating wound infection and odour from extensive necrotic wounds.

If for some reason it proves impossible to eliminate the odour-producing bacteria from a wound, it may be possible to deal with the problem by some other means. Historically wound odours were masked by burning incense and in more recent times, by the use of aerosols or air fresheners. It has even been suggested that a tray of cat litter under the bed may be of some benefit! Obviously although none of these initiatives address the underlying problem, they may make life a little more bearable for the patient and their family.

An alternative approach involves the use of a dressing that acts like a filter and absorbs the odoriferous chemicals liberated from the wound before they pass into the air. The most effective material available for this purpose is activated charcoal which is used in the manufacture of air filters, gas masks and other specialised items of military clothing. This was originally used in the form of granules, but for many applications these been replaced by a charcoal fabric such as that developed by the Chemical Defence Establishment, Porton Down; it is this material that forms the basis of most of the dressings in current use.

ACTIVATED CHARCOAL DRESSINGS

Production of activated charcoal

Activated charcoal cloth is manufactured from a suitable cellulose fabric, which is heated to about 350°C in an inert atmosphere. Under these conditions, the cellulose decomposes, leaving a residue of pure carbon. This is then activated by further heating to 800-900°C in the presence of carbon dioxide or steam, when the surface of the carbon breaks down to form large numbers of pores, some 2 nm in width.

By the end of this process the cloth is very fragile but it has been found that pre-treatment of the cellulose with a solution of certain metallic chlorides (prior to carbonisation) will reduce the loss of carbon by lowering the temperature at which activation takes place. The pre-treatment also has the effect of generating smaller pores in the fibre, which causes less damage to the fabric and prevents it falling apart.

The presence of pores increases the effective surface area of the carbon fibres, and hence their adsorptive capacity. The total area may be determined by measuring the amount of nitrogen that is required to cover the surface with a layer one molecule thick.[27] For the activated charcoal cloth that is used in the manufacture of most of the dressings, this technique gives a result of about 1300 m^2/g - the specific surface area of the fabric.

It is believed that many types of molecules, including those responsible for odour production, are attracted to the surface of the carbon and are held there (adsorbed) by electrical forces. In the main these molecules are small and detected by the nose in low concentrations in the air. A single dressing which, by virtue of the large surface area of the carbon, is capable of taking up very large numbers of molecules should therefore prove capable of removing odour over prolonged periods.

Activated charcoal dressings

The use of charcoal cloth as a dressing was first reported by Butcher *et al*. in 1976.[28] The material was incorporated into pads containing surgical gauze and a layer of a water repellent fabric which, when used in the treatment of fungating breast cancer wounds, gangrene and immediate post operative colostomies, the associated odours were said to be totally suppressed. Since Butcher's original report, numerous odour-absorbing dressings containing activated charcoal have been developed.

Actisorb Silver 220 consists of a porous spun-bonded nylon sleeve enclosing a piece of activated charcoal cloth containing 0.15% silver which is chemically bound onto the carbon. It is produced by carbonizing and activating a piece of silver-impregnated knitted fabric made from continuous filament viscose yarn. The continuous yarn is said to produce less dust than the staple yarns used in the manufacture of some other products, and the knitted structure of the cloth is claimed to make the dressing particularly conformable. The first activated charcoal dressing to be produced commercially was first marketed in the UK in 1985 as Actisorb. This original presentation did not include silver which was added in 1987 when the product was renamed Actisorb Plus. In 2000 the name of the dressing was changed once again to Actisorb Silver 220.

Askina Carbosorb comprises a thin absorbent layer bonded to a polyester-nylon nonwoven wound contact layer on one surface and a piece of charcoal cloth on the other. A second piece of nonwoven fabric bonded to the outer surface of the activated charcoal layer completes the dressing.

Carboflex is a multi-component dressing that consists of a wound contact layer composed of alginate and carboxymethylcellulose fibres, bonded to a plastic film that that has perforations designed to facilitate the passage of liquid in one direction only. Immediately behind this film are a piece of charcoal cloth and an absorbing layer of mixed fibres. A second perforated plastic layer, sealed around the perimeter to the first, completes the structure of the dressing. Carboflex is placed directly on the surface of the wound and held in place with tape or a bandage as appropriate.

Carbonet is a multi-component dressing which has both fluid and odour-absorbing properties. Unlike Actisorb Plus, the dressing can be used on its own, without a secondary dressing. The structure of Carbonet is relatively complex, consisting of six layers bonded together, as follows: a wound contact layer consisting of warp-knitted viscose, a layer of cotton/viscose absorbent wadding, a fine polyethylene net, a layer of woven activated charcoal cloth, a second layer of polyethylene net, and a layer of polyester fleece. The activated charcoal layer of Carbonet is similar in appearance and specific surface area to that of Actisorb Plus, but it is not in direct contact with the wound, and is therefore less likely to adsorb bacteria and wound toxins. Carbonet is also somewhat less conformable than Actisorb Plus, as a result of its multi-component structure.

Carbopad (now discontinued) had a polyamide wound control surface bonded to an absorbent layer backed with a piece of activated charcoal fabric and a semipermeable film.

Clinisorb consists of a piece of charcoal cloth sandwiched between two layers of absorbent viscose. Unlike some of the other charcoal dressings Clinisorb can be cut or shaped if required.

Kaltocarb (now discontinued) was a combination product, consisting of a wound contact layer of calcium alginate fibre bonded onto a woven activated charcoal cloth. The dressing was backed with a layer of a non-woven fabric composed of polyester and viscose. The dressing was claimed to combine the wound-healing properties of calcium alginate fibre with the odour-adsorbing properties of activated charcoal.

Lyofoam C consists of a piece of Lyofoam polyurethane dressing that is heat sealed to a sheet of plain polyurethane foam around the perimeter. The activated charcoal is enclosed between these two layers in the form of granules, which are bonded onto a piece of non-woven fabric. The specific surface area of the activated charcoal in Lyofoam C is significantly less than that of the charcoal cloth used in the manufacture of the other odour-absorbing dressings. However, in normal use, the charcoal layer present in Lyofoam should not become wet with wound exudate, and thus all the active sites remain available to adsorb the odour-producing chemicals in the gaseous phase.

Sorbsan Plus Carbon consists of a sheet of alginate fibre bonded to a layer of entangled absorbent viscose fibres backed with sheet of activated charcoal and a nonwoven viscose/polyester backing layer.

Vliwaktive consists of an absorbent pad with a non woven wound contact layer which also incorporates a sheet of activated charcoal fabric. Vliwaktive Ag is similar but the activated charcoal fabric is impregnated with silver. Vliwaktive Ag is also available in the form of a rope for dressing cavity wounds.

Method of use

All of the dressings described above are regarded as primary wound dressings, i.e. intended to be applied directly to the wound surface, but differences in their design and construction are important because they determine whether the activated charcoal layer is brought into intimate contact with the wound surface or held away from it by some other structural component. A further product, Denidor, once made by Jeffreys, Miller and Co. but now thought to be discontinued, consisted of a layer of charcoal fabric in an outer sleeve which was not intended to be placed in contact with the wound. The dressing was applied over the selected primary dressing immediately beneath the retaining bandage. The variation in the structure of the various products may be important for reasons that are discussed later.

Antimicrobial activity

Laboratory studies carried out by Frost et al.[29] on the original version of Actisorb revealed that when the charcoal cloth was shaken with a suspension of bacteria the number of organisms present in suspension was reduced by a factor of up to 10^5 (i.e. five log reductions) as the cells became adsorbed onto the cloth. When a similar test was carried out using a control fabric, less than one log reduction was obtained. In these tests, Gram-negative bacilli were found to be bound more firmly to the charcoal than either Gram-positive cocci or bacterial spores, both of which were subsequently released by washing. As a result of this work, it was proposed that the dressing could play an important role in reducing the bioburden of wounds such as leg ulcers, thus improving the healing environment.

These laboratory studies indicated that although many bacteria were firmly bound onto the charcoal fibres, the organisms still remained viable; a method of imparting antibacterial properties to the fabric was therefore sought. Eventually, Actisorb Plus was developed, identical to Actisorb except for the presence of silver residues which kill microorganisms that become bound to its structure.

When Actisorb Plus was shaken with bacterial suspensions as before, 5-7 log reductions in viable numbers were obtained, showing that the product performed significantly better than the original material. In a personal communication in 1988, it was revealed that these laboratory results were supported by those of an animal study in which experimental wounds on guinea pigs were inoculated with test organisms and sampled by swabbing. After 24 hours control wounds, dressed with a semipermeable film, produced counts of the order of 2×10^8 colony forming units (cfu)/swab, but wounds dressed with Actisorb gave counts around 5×10^4 cfu/swab. An even greater reduction was noted in wounds dressed with Actisorb Plus which yielded counts of 5×10^3 cfu /swab.

The antimicrobial properties of Actisorb and Actisorb Plus were compared in a series of tests undertaken in 1994 by Furr et al.[30] They showed that Actisorb Plus but not Actisorb, was able to inhibit the growth of a range of different bacteria growing on the surface of Diagnostic Sensitivity Test agar (DST). Inhibition of this activity by the sulphydryl compound, sodium thioglycollate confirmed that this antimicrobial action was due to the release of low concentrations of silver ions from the dressing into the agar.

Actisorb Silver 220 was one of ten dressings included in a laboratory comparison of silver-containing dressings published in 2003.[31] This study, which is described in more detail in Chapter 14, suggested that compared with the other silver-containing products examined, Actisorb Silver Plus exhibited very limited antimicrobial activity. This was assumed to be due principally to the low levels of silver present, around 2.5 mg/100cm^2 of dressing.

Odour absorbing properties

As described in Chapter 7 numerous methods have been described for comparing the ability of dressings containing activated charcoal to remove odours or adsorb specific molecules responsible for odour production.

In an early study Schmidt et al.[32] described a semi-quantitative assay procedure, which they used to compare the sorptive capacities of the charcoal components of some of these dressings available at that time based upon their ability to take up diethylamine from aqueous solution. Although a spurious result was obtained with Actisorb Plus, owing to the presence of silver ions, the test was able to demonstrate differences in the performance of some of the other dressings: Actisorb, for example, appeared to be considerably more active than Lyofoam C. However, as the structure and method of use of the various dressings is also very different, the results of these tests must be interpreted with care.

Subsequent workers used both chemical,[32-34] and biological materials[35-36] to test the efficacy of odour adsorbing dressings. The former technique is often favoured as the efficiency of the dressing can be determined using standard analytical techniques such as gas liquid chromatography. Determination of dressing performance using biological materials is currently restricted to more subjective methods of assessment such as the use of a human test panel. Lawrence et al,[36] adopted this second approach when they compared the odour absorbing properties of five dressings containing activated charcoal with that of a cotton gauze swab, acting as a control. A panel of volunteers were asked to assess the odour liberated from the test samples after the addition of bacterial cultures isolated from malodorous wounds. A similar approach was adopted by Griffiths et al.,[34] who also used microbiologically derived odours to test the performance of a range of products.

Some of these tests compared the dressings in the dry state, not soaked with wound fluid as in the clinical situation. For this reason the test system described in Chapter 7 was developed by SMTL in an attempt to address this important deficiency. Essentially this measures the time taken for the concentration of diethylamine, chosen to represent as a test substrate, to increase by 10 ppm above baseline values in a closed chamber over a dressing to which is applied serum spiked with the amine delivered by means of a syringe pump. Four charcoal containing dressings were tested in this way together with a standard absorbent control. Full details of this study have been reported elsewhere,[37] but a summary of the results is provided in Table 32. In this table the figures quoted represent the volume of solution that must be delivered to produce 10 ppm of diethylamine in test chamber.

Table 32: Odour absorbing properties of test samples

Dressing	Volume (ml) mean (sd)
Actisorb Plus	9.5 (1.36)
Carboflex	17.1 (1.95)
Carbonet	13.5 (2.95)
Lyofoam C	12.7 (3.48)
Release	3.9 (0.53)

In these tests all of the dressings containing activated charcoal performed better than the control although marked differences were seen between Actisorb Plus and the other dressings examined. This suggests that the odour absorbing properties of the dressing are determined by at least two factors, the physical absorbency - a function of the presence of some form of absorbent layer, and the activity of the charcoal cloth itself. Products which combine a physical absorbent with a charcoal component show enhanced performance as might be anticipated. What is not clear from the results, however, is whether the odour absorbing component of a dressing is likely to be most effective when applied directly to the surface of a wound or when it is incorporated into the structure or used as a secondary dressing.

This issue was partly addressed in a second an independent study which compared the odour absorbing properties of six different carbon dressings with a control using the identical apparatus as in the previous investigation.[38] Once again the time taken for the concentration of diethylamine to reach a predetermined value in the test chamber was determined.

The authors also measured the absorbency and air permeability of the dressing samples and from these published data, two graphs have been constructed which relate these parameters to the odour retention times for each product. The result clearly show that there is no direct relationship between these data sets confirming that the ability of the dressings to retain odour is determined by the presence and activity of the carbon fabric and is not greatly influenced by the absorbency or permeability of the dressings. Actisorb Silver 220, for example, has limited absorbency and is very permeable to air, nevertheless, it still outperformed most of the other dressings examined.

Figure 69: Relationship between absorbency and odour retention

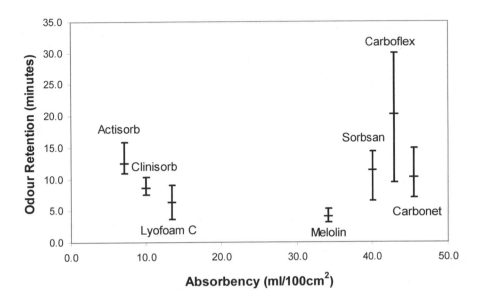

Figure 70: Relationship between permeability and odour retention

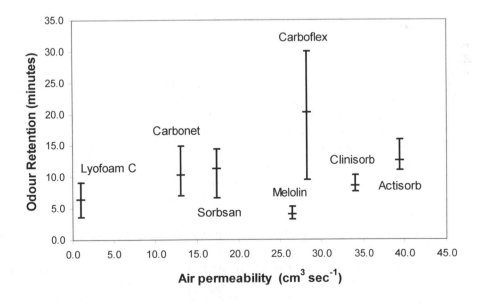

In a further series of tests the authors examined the effect of combining Actisorb Silver 220 with Melolin. This was done in two configurations with the carbon dressing placed either above or below the simple absorbent layer.

The results were somewhat surprising. When the Actisorb Silver 220 was placed beneath the Melolin the ability of the dressing to delay odour penetration was somewhat reduced from 11 - 16 to 8.5 - 9 minutes. In contrast, when the Actisorb was used as the secondary dressing the performance was enhanced, delivering a strike-through time of around 18 minutes.

These results suggest that when Actisorb Silver 220 (and presumably other types of charcoal dressings) are used simply to combat odour, it might be advantageous to use them as secondary dressings in this way. The reason for this enhanced performance is not clear but it might be due to competition for active sites with the molecular material contained in the test solution.

CLINICAL EXPERIENCE WITH CHARCOAL DRESSINGS

Despite the widespread use of activated charcoal dressings in the treatment of malodorous wounds, and the fact that since the early 1990s, many publications have made reference to their use for this application,[39-41] few clinical studies have been undertaken to examine this aspect of their performance; most publications describe their use in the treatment of leg ulcers and tend to focus upon wound healing rather than odour control per se. Also almost all published studies describe the use of the Actisorb family - very little has been published on the other charcoal containing dressings.

In one multicentre trial involving 101 patients, 97 of whom completed the study, 65 subjects with leg ulcers were allocated to treatment with Actisorb and 32 to conventional treatment (not controlled). During the course of the trial, wounds in the Actisorb group showed a mean reduction in size of 1.2 cm^2 per week, compared with only 0.2 cm^2 for the control group but this difference failed to achieve statistical significance. During the six-week treatment period, wounds dressed with Actisorb decreased in area by 28.7% compared with 11.7% for those treated conventionally. This difference was statistically significant. It was also recorded that the patients treated with Actisorb showed a significant reduction in odour, exudate, and oedema despite the fact that the largest and most longstanding ulcers were allocated to the Actisorb-treated group. In this study randomization schedules were not strictly adhered to, which accounts for the imbalance in numbers and the variation in wound size within the treatment groups.[42]

Similar benefits were reported by Wunderlich and Orfanos,[43] following a randomized controlled study involving 40 patients with venous leg ulcer. Subjects were randomized to receive either the activated charcoal dressing or a conventional treatment (zinc paste bandages). Nineteen patients in each group completed the study. Six ulcers treated with Actisorb Plus healed compared with two patients receiving conventional therapy. Statistical analysis of the results, significant differences were found in favour of the charcoal dressing group in terms of reduction of wound size and increased epithelialization (p < 0.05).

In 2002, Cassino *et al.*, reviewed treatment outcomes for 75 chronic skin lesions showing local signs of infection that were treated with Actisorb Plus, and compared them with 75 wounds dressed with moist gauze or alginate on patients who received systemic antibiotic therapy. They found that although the Actisorb Plus treatments tended to be longer (14 days compared with 10 for systemic antibiotics), there was no statistical difference in effectiveness between the two treatments. A particularly interesting finding was that 30-day recurrence rates were much higher in the antibiotic treated group (12% *cf* 1.3%). Major cost savings were also reported for the Actisorb Plus treated wounds.

The most comprehensive account of the use of Actisorb yet undertaken involved five observational studies carried out in Germany between 1996 and 2000 as part of the regulatory processes, the combined results of which were reported by Stadler in 2002.[44]

The studies involved patients with a combined total of 12444 chronic wounds of all types, many of which initially contained signs of infection. During the course of the study wounds were monitored for exudate production, odour, and the presence of necrotic tissue, fibrinous deposits and the formation of new granulation or epithelial tissue. Other parameters recorded included changes in infection rates, healing characteristics and dressing tolerability.

After initiating treatment with Actisorb, it was reported that 96% of wounds improved and 41% healed completely. Infection rates fell from 65% to 6%, and 80% of patients did not require additional medication. Dressing tolerability was also rated as excellent. Like Cassino *et al.*, Stadler concluded that Actisorb plus was very effective on infected or colonised chronic wounds with the potential to limit the use of other local antiseptics or antibiotics. A further novel application for Actisorb Silver 220 was reported by Leak[45] who described its use in the treatment of percutaneous enterostomal gastrostomy (PEG) sites when it was said to increase patient comfort, prevent over-granulation and eradicate methicillin-resistant *S. aureus* colonization and infection.

The reasons for the observed beneficial effects associated with the use of Actisorb Silver 220 are not clear. Soriano *et al.*[46] compared the effect of the dressing with that of a control treatment on the bioburden of leg ulcers. Patients were randomly assigned to treatment and monitored for two weeks. Bacterial counts were taken on admission and then after 15 days of treatment. Sixty-seven wounds were allocated to treatment with activated charcoal and 58 to treatment with the control. After two weeks 85.1% of wounds treated with the charcoal dressing showed a reduction in the number of bacteria present, compared with 62.1% of those in the control group (p = 0.003).

The possibility that Actisorb Silver 220 might reduce the bioburden of a wound could be significant, for it has long been recognised that significant numbers of microorganisms can delay or prevent closure. This was demonstrated in an early clinical leg ulcer study undertaken by Lookingbill *et al.*[47] who showed that, whilst the majority of ulcers with less than 10^5 organisms/cm^2 eventually healed, those with more than 10^5 did not. Although there is much debate concerning the definitions of infection and colonization and the significance of the presence or absence of particular microbial species, there is now a general acceptance that a bioburden of 10^5 cfu/cm^2 (or gram) is indicative of an infection or a level of colonization that is likely to adversely affect healing; in complex extremity wounds a lower value of 10 cfu/cm^2 has been suggested.[48]

Some support for the theory that Actisorb Silver 220 may have an antimicrobial effect within a wound may be drawn from the results of Frost[29] and Furr,[30] but the laboratory study conducted by Thomas *et al.*,[31] which compared the release of silver from ten different dressings failed to provide convincing evidence that the amount of silver released from Actisorb is likely to be exert a significant effect on wound microorganisms which do not come into intimate contact with the dressing. Furthermore within this study other products, not made from activated charcoal, contained (and liberated) much higher levels of silver, suggesting that these should in theory be even more effective than Actisorb in combating wound infection and promoting healing; in practice there is no clear evidence that this is the case. It is possible, therefore, that charcoal dressings, particularly those in which the activated charcoal layer is brought into intimate contact with the wound have other beneficial properties which have not yet been fully recognised or understood.

It has been the experience of the author (unpublished data) that if a charcoal dressing is tested in a cell culture system used for toxicity testing of medical devices, it appears to produce a toxic response. It is probable, however, that this apparent toxicity is due not to toxic chemicals leaching out of the dressing, but rather the uptake of essential nutrients and ions from the culture medium by the dressing which renders it unable to support the viability of the monolayer. It is entirely possible that something similar happens within the wound; is possible that the activated charcoal adsorbs proteases and bacterial toxins which are responsible for inducing or prolonging the inflammatory stage of healing and thereby exerts a positive effect upon healing rates. Some support for this theory was provided by Muller *et al.*[49] who, in a laboratory study, compared the endotoxin-binding capacity of three activated charcoal dressings, Vliwaktive, Vliwaktive Ag and Actisorb Silver 220 with that of a gauze control and found a 50% reduction in free endotoxin levels after 24 hours.

It may well be that the benefits of placing activated charcoal dressings in intimate contact with the wound surface have yet to be fully recognised and that a relatively easy and cost effective method of promoting healing has so far been largely overlooked.

REFERENCES

1. Bird C. Managing malignant fungating wounds. Prof Nurse 2000;15(4):253-6.
2. Harding KG, Cherry G, Dealey C, Turner TD, editors. Psychological consequences arising from the malodours produced by skin ulcers. Proceedings of 2nd European Conference on Advances in Wound Management; 1992; Harrogate. Macmillan magazines Ltd.
3. Cooke P. Caring for a patient with malodorous leg ulcers. Nurs Times 2006;102(44):50, 52.
4. Van Toller S. Invisible wounds: the effects of skin ulcer malodours. Journal of Wound Care 1994;3(2):103-105.
5. Hack A. Malodorous wounds--taking the patient's perspective into account. Journal of Wound Care 2003;12(8):319-21.

6. Baker PG, Haig G. Metronidazole in the treatment of chronic pressure sores and ulcers. A comparison with standard treatments in general practice. The Practitioner 1981;225:569-573.
7. Collier M. The assessment of patients with malignant fungating wounds--a holistic approach: Part 1. Nurs Times 1997;93(44):suppl 1-4.
8. Roberson DW, Neil JA, Bryant ET. Improving wound care simulation with the addition of odor: a descriptive, quasi-experimental study. Ostomy Wound Manage 2008;54(8):36-43.
9. Dowsett C. Malignant fungating wounds: assessment and management. Br J Community Nurs 2002;7(8):394-400.
10. Draper C. The management of malodour and exudate in fungating wounds. Br J Nurs 2005;14(11):S4-12.
11. Moss CW, Dees SB, Guerrant GO. Gas Chromatography of bacterial fatty acids with a fused silica capillary column. J.Clin Microbiol 1974;28:80-85.
12. Parry AD, Chadwick PR, Simon D, Oppenheim B, McCollum CN. Leg ulcer odour detection identifies beta-haemolytic streptococcal infection. Journal of Wound Care 1995;4(9):404-6.
13. Brennan SS, Foster ME, Leaper DJ. Antiseptic toxicity in wounds healing by secondary intention,. J. Hosp. Infect 1986;8:263-267.
14. Brennan SS, Leaper DJ. The effect of antiseptics on the healing wound: a study using the rabbit ear chamber. Br. J. Surg 1985;72:780-782.
15. Management of smelly tumours. Lancet 1990;335(8682):141-2.
16. Thomas S, Hay NP. The antimicrobial properties of two metronidazole medicated dressings used to treat malodorous wounds. Pharmaceutical Journal 1991;March 2:264-266.
17. Newman V. The use of metronidazole gel to control the smell of malorous lesions. Palliative Medicine 1989;3:303-305.
18. Finlay IG, Bowszyc J, Ramalau C, Gwiezdinski Z. The effect of topical 0.75% metronidazole gel on malodorous cutaneous ulcers. Journal of Pain and Symptom Management;11(3):158-162.
19. Hampson JP. The use of metronidazole in the treatment of malodorous wounds. Journal of Wound Care 1996;5(9):421-426.
20. Paul JC, Pieper BA. Topical metronidazole for the treatment of wound odor: a review of the literature. Ostomy Wound Manage 2008;54(3):18-27; quiz 28-9.
21. Morgan DA, Oppenheim B. Metronidazole use. Pharmaceutical Journal 1991;March:353.
22. Ogura T, Urade M, Matsuya T. Prevention of malodor from intraoral gauze tamponade with the topical use of clindamycin. Oral Surg Oral Med Oral Pathol 1992;74(1):58-62.
23. Chiwenga S, Dowlen H, Mannion S. Audit of the use of sugar dressings for the control of wound odour at Lilongwe Central Hospital, Malawi. Trop Doct 2009;39(1):20-2.
24. Welch LB. Buttermilk & yogurt: odor control of open lesions. Crit Care Update 1982;9(11):39-44.
25. Welch LB. Simple new remedy for the odor of open lesions. RN 1981;44(2):42-3.
26. Schulte MJ. Yogurt helps to control wound odor. Oncol Nurs Forum 1993;20(8):1262.
27. Freeman JJ, A.I. M. Nitrogen BET surface area measurement as a fingerprint method for the estimation of pore volume in active carbons. Fuel 1983;62:1090-1091.
28. Butcher G, Butcher JA, Maggs FAP. The treatment of malodorous wounds. Nurs. Mirror 1976;142:76.
29. Frost M, Jackson S, Stevens P. Adsorption of bacteria onto activated charcoal cloth: an effect of potential importance in the treatment of infected wounds. Microbios Letters 1980;13:135-140.
30. Furr JR, Russell AD, Turner TD, Andrews A. Antibacterial activity of Actisorb Plus, Actisorb and silver nitrate. J. Hospital Infection 1994;27(3):201-208.

31. Thomas S, McCubbin P. An in vitro analysis of the antimicrobial properties of 10 silver-containing dressings. Journal of Wound Care 2003;12(8):305-8.
32. Schmidt RJ, Shrestha T, Turner TD. An assay procedure to compare sorptive capacities of activated carbon dressings: the detection of impregnation with silver. J. Pharm. Pharmacol 1988;40:662-664.
33. A test method for quantifying absorbtive capacities of intact charcoal-containing wound management products. Proceedings of the 7th European Conference on Advances in Wound Management
1997; Harrogate UK.
34. Determination of malodour reduction performance in various charcoal containing dressings. Proceedings of the 7th European Conference on Advances in Wound Management, Harrogate, U.K.; 1997; Harrogate, U.K.
35. An investigation into the selective adsorption of malodour molecules onto charcoal containing dressings. Proceedings of the 7th European Conference on Advances in Wound Management, Harrogate, U.K.; 1997; Harrogate, U.K.
36. Harding KG, Cherry G, Dealey C, Turner TD, editors. Malodour and dressings containing active charcoal,. Proceedings of the 2nd European Conference on Advances in Wound Management; 1992; Harrogate, U.K. Macmillan magazines Ltd.
37. Thomas S, Fisher B, Fram PJ, Waring MJ. Odour-absorbing dressings. Journal of Wound Care 1998;7(5):246-50.
38. Lee G, Anand SC, Rajendran S, Walker I. Efficacy of commercial dressings in managing malodorous wounds. Br J Nurs 2007;16(6):S14, S16, S18-20.
39. Woodhouse P. Managing a breast wound. Nursing Timres 1992;88(12):74-75.
40. Boardman M, Mellor K. Treating a patient with a heavily exuding malodorous fungating ulcer. Journal of Wound Care 1993;2(2):74-76.
41. Young T. The challenge of managing fungating wounds. Nurseprescriber/Community Nurse 1997(October 1997):41-43.
42. Mulligan CM, Bragg AJD, O'Toole OB. A controlled comparative trial of Actisorb activated charcoal cloth dressings in the community. British Journal of Clinical Practice 1986;9(1):145-8.
43. Wunderlich U, Orfanos CE. Treatment of venous ulcera cruris with dry wound dressings. Phase overlapping use of silver impregnated activated charcoal xerodressing. Hautarzt 1991;42(7):446-50.
44. Stadler R. Treatment of chronic wounds with Actisorb. 2002.
45. Leak K. PEG site infections: a novel use for Actisorb Silver 220. Br J Community Nurs 2002;7(6):321-5.
46. Verdu Soriano J, Rueda Lopez J, Martinez Cuervo F, Soldevilla Agreda J. Effects of an activated charcoal silver dressing on chronic wounds with no clinical signs of infection. J Wound Care 2004;13(10):419, 421-3.
47. Lookingbill DP, Miller SH, Knowles RC. Bacteriology of chronic leg ulcers. Arch Dermatol 1978;114:1765-1768.
48. White R. A charcoal dressing with silver in wound infection: clinical evidence. Britsh Journal of Nursing (supplement 2) 2002;10:4-12.
49. Müller G, Abel M, Gorka M, Kramer A. Endotoxin-binding capacity of an antimicrobial silver containing,activated charcoal wound dressing – Vliwaktiv Ag. Annual Congress of European Wound Management Association(EWMA), . Prague / CZ, , 2006.

18. Silicone dressings for scar treatment

INTRODUCTION

As described in an early chapter, some wounds that fail to heal normally can form a raised hypertrophic or keloid scar, often treated by the long-term application of pressure administered by means of specially made garments.[1]

Keloids, first described in Egypt over 300 years ago, form by overgrowth of dense fibrous tissue which usually occurs following a minor skin injury. The tissue growth, which extends beyond the borders of the original injury, tends to recur after excision.

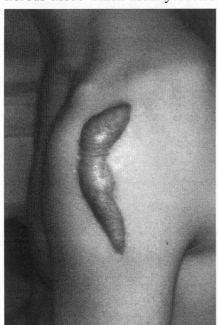

In contrast, hypertrophic scars which are common after burns and other injuries that involve the deep dermis, are characterized by erythematous, pruritic, raised fibrous lesions that are typically confined within the boundaries of the original injury. Unlike keloids, hypertrophic scars may undergo partial spontaneous resolution.

The practical problems of managing these skin defects have been reported by Carney,[2-4] Munro,[5] Eisenbeiss,[6] and Beldon,[7] and the psychological effects of scar formation described graphically by Partridge.[8]

Although the use of compression garments is still widely practiced, in 1981 it was found that the benefits of pressure therapy could be enhanced, or in some instances replaced, by the application of a sheet of silicone gel made from polydimethylsiloxane which, it was claimed, could relax or soften scar tissue thereby allowing the pressure garments and inserts to hasten their levelling effect on the hypertrophied area.[9] The use of silicone in wound treatment is not new, for silicone oil has been used as a bath for severely burned hands to facilitate exercise and physiotherapy since the late 1960s.[10]

Figure 71: A keloid scar on an old vaccination site

Silicone gel sheets are not the only products that are used for scar treatment. Davey *et al.* in a series of publications,[11-14] described the application of a dressing retention sheet such as Hypafix or Mefix, (effectively a wide piece of surgical tape) to newly grafted or healed wounds to treat or prevent hypertrophic scar formation.

Sawada and Sone[15] compared an occlusive cream, which did not contain silicone oil, with the application of Vaseline in the treatment of 31 patients with hypertrophic scars or keloid scars. They reported that in all cases the cream-treated areas demonstrated a remarkable improvement compared with those treated with Vaseline. They suggested that hydration and occlusion form the basis for the therapeutic action of this type of treatment.

Other techniques employed for treating hypertrophic and keloid scars include: a self-drying liquid silicone gel,[16-17] irradiation with lasers,[18-19] triamcinolone acetonide injections and silicone gel sheet coated earrings for keloid scars following ear piercing.[20] Magnetic disks have also been used to provide compression for this indication.[21]

A polytreatment approach has also been described which included the use of cryotherapy administered monthly for 12 months, with concomitant monthly injections of triamcinolone acetonide for three months, and the topical application of silicone gel continued for 12 months.[22]

Mederma, an aqueous hydrogel containing an extract of onion, *Allium cepa* has similarly been recommended for scar treatment. The active product in onion is quercetin, a bioflavonoid attributed with antiproliferative effects on both normal and malignant cells, and an antihistamine effect. These properties could theoretically prove beneficial in reversing the inflammatory and proliferative responses noted in hypertrophic scars. These properties were evaluated tested in an animal model by Saulis *et al.*[23] who found no significant reduction in scar hypertrophy or scar height although an improvement in dermal collagen organization was noted when Mederma-treated scars were compared with untreated controls. No significant difference in dermal vascularity or inflammation was recorded and computer analysis of scar photographs demonstrated no significant reduction in scar erythema following Mederma treatment.

Hosnuter *et al.*[24] evaluated the clinical effectiveness of this preparation, focusing on parameters such as scar height, redness, hardness, itching and pain. Sixty patients were assigned to one of three treatment groups. Group one was treated with onion extract alone, group two with silicone gel sheet alone and group three with a combination of onion extract and silicone gel sheet. The onion extract was more effective in relation to scar colour, while the silicone gel sheet was superior in decreasing the height of scar but the most effective results were obtained when the treatments were used in combination.

COMMERCIAL SILICONE DRESSINGS

Commercial silicone dressings include:

- Advasil Conform (self adherent gel sheet)
- Cica-Care (self adherent gel sheet)
- Dermatix Clear (gel sheet)
- Dermatix Fabric (fabric-backed gel sheet)
- Dermatix Gel (amorphous gel)
- Dermatix Spray
- DuraSil (gel sheet)
- Epi-Derm (self adherent gel sheet)
- Kelo-cote Gel (amorphous gel)
- Kelo-cote Spray
- Mepiform (gel sheet)
- ReJuveness (gel sheet)
- Silgel (gel sheet)
- Silgel STC-SE (topical gel)
- Sil-K(gel sheet)
- Topigel (self adherent gel sheet)

CLINICAL EXPERIENCE WITH SILICONE DRESSINGS

Results of published studies

Clinical assessments

Early experience with silicone gel was described by Quinn *et al.*[25] who treated 40 patients all of whom showed an improvement in their scars after two months. Similar benefits associated with the use of silicone gel sheets were reported by Katz[26] and Fulton,[27] who examined the effectiveness of silicone gel sheeting in the prevention and/or reduction of evolving hypertrophic scars in 20 patients who wore the dressing for at least 12 hours a day. Treated sites improved in 85% of cases and no traces of silicone were detected upon histological examination of biopsies taken from the treated areas. Chuangsuwanich *et al.*[28] evaluated a self-adhesive silicone gel sheet in the treatment of hypertrophic scars and keloids in 18 subjects. Patients were instructed to apply the dressing to their scars for at least 12 hours per day for a minimum of eight weeks. Treatment outcomes were evaluated subjectively by the patients, twelve of whom reported good results. After eight weeks the height of the scars had reduced in 12/18 patients. Two patients developed an erythematous rash around the lesions which subsided after withdrawal of the treatment.

Clinical trials

In an early formal study Ahn et al.[29] evaluated the dressings in an eight week prospective controlled trial involving 14 hypertrophic scars in 10 adults. Treated scars and untreated mirror-image or adjacent control scars were photographed, measured elastometrically before and after treatment, and biopsy specimens were also taken. Scars treated for at least 12 hours each day showed evidence of improvement after four weeks and this trend was continued during a further four weeks of treatment. Elastometric measurements revealed significant improvements in treated scars at four, eight and 12 weeks, ($p < 0.05$) and this clinical improvement persisted for at least four weeks after treatment was discontinued. The dressing was well tolerated, except for occasional transient rashes or superficial maceration, both of which resolved promptly when treatment was withdrawn. There was no histological evidence of inflammation or a foreign body reaction which suggested that silicone had entered the treated tissues. The authors concluded that the mechanism of action of silicone gel, which was apparently not related to compression, remained to be determined.

Subsequently the same authors tested the dressing in fresh surgical incisions.[30] Scar volume changes in 21 wounds were measured initially and then after one and two months when it was found that gel-treated incisions gained less volume than the control incisions at both intervals.

Camey et al.[31] studied 85 areas of scarring in 42 patients. Silastic Gel was applied to 43 areas, and 42 areas were left as controls. Objective measurements of scar elasticity were made using an extensiometer after two month of therapy. Extensibility increased in the treated group but decreased in the control group. Marked improvements were noted in gel treated wounds on the axilla, shoulder and dorsum of the foot provided that the gel was worn for at least 12 hours per day.

De Oliveira et al.[32] compared silicone with non silicone gel dressings in a controlled prospective trial in the treatment of keloids and hypertrophic scars. Patients were randomized to treatment and scar size, induration and other symptoms were evaluated before and after the treatment. Compared to the untreated controls, all of the measured parameters were significantly reduced in both silicone and non silicone-treated groups, from which the authors concluded that both treatments are equally effective in the treatment of keloids and hypertrophic scars.

Gold et al.[33] conducted a study to determine whether topical silicone gel sheeting prevents hypertrophic scars and keloids from forming following dermatologic skin surgery. Patients were stratified into two groups: those with no history of abnormal scarring (the low-risk group) and those with a history scar formation (the high-risk group). Patients within each group were then randomized to receive either routine postoperative care or treatment with topical silicone gel sheeting which was initiated 48 hours after surgery and continued for six months. In the low-risk group, no statistical difference was detected between treatment groups but in the high-risk group a statistical difference was recorded between silicone-treated and conventionally-treated patients who developed abnormal scars.

The effect of two silicone gel dressings on hypertrophic scar formation in sternotomy wounds[34] was investigated in 50 patients. For the purpose of this study each wound was divided into two parts thereby acting as its own control. By the third postoperative month, wounds treated with the silicone gels were statistically better than the controls in all parameters studied.

Silicone gel sheets were compared with massage in a study involving 45 patients with post-traumatic hypertrophic scars.[35] Wounds were randomized to treatment with silicone gel, applied for 24 hours each day for 6 months, or a period of daily massage. Regular scar assessments showed a significant difference in favour of the gel treated group in scar thickness and a nonsignificant advantage in pigmentation.

Mepiform, a self-adherent soft silicone dressing was assessed in a randomized controlled trial in which the control groups received no specific form of therapy.[36] Treatment was initiated between two and eight weeks after surgery; ten patients completed the 12-month investigation. Using the VSS as a reference, both groups were judged to have improved in appearance although patients treated with the soft silicone dressing showed greater and more rapid improvements compared with the non-treated patients.

Chernoff, et al.[37] compared the efficacy of different topical silicone preparations in the treatment of 30 patients with hypertrophic scars, keloid scars and post-laser exfoliation erythema. During the 90 day prospective study wounds were dressed either with Dermatix, a fast drying amorphous silicone gel, a silicone gel sheet, or a combination of the two treatments. Each patient had a bilateral scar that served as an untreated control. At the end of the study Dermatix treatment (or the combined use of Dermatix and silicone gel sheeting) produced superior results in terms of scar resolution and improvement compared with silicone gel sheeting alone. Wound erythema was reduced, and collagen architectural reorientation was demonstrated histologically. Both Dermatix and silicone gel sheeting reduced symptoms of itching, irritation, and skin maceration.

A liquid silicone gel was compared with zinc oxide cream in a controlled trial involving 110 patients who had undergone outpatient surgery.[38] Sixty five subjects were given the silicone gel and instructed to apply it to the wound twice daily for 60 days following the removal of their stitches. The remaining 45 subjects were provided with a zinc oxide cream and similarly instructed. Subjects were examined monthly for 3 months after surgery, then every 2 months for a total follow-up of 8 months from the date of surgery. In the gel-treated group no keloid scars were recorded and six patients (9%) developed a hypertrophic scar. In the control group five patients developed keloid scars and ten (22%) developed hypertrophic scars.

In a randomized, double-blind, placebo-controlled trial involving 38 people with hypertrophic burn scars,[39] each scar was divided into two segments. Silicone gel was applied randomly to one segment and a placebo treatment to the other. Wounds were assessed after one and four months using the VSS. After one month all scar scale measures were lower in the treated areas but only the difference in vascularity achieved significance. After 4 months, with the exception of the pain score, all scale measures were significantly lower in the silicone gel group than in the control group.

Sixty patients with hypertrophic scars were recruited into a 12-week trial.[40] Each scar was divided into two areas where were dressed with a polyurethane dressing or a silicone sheet according to the randomization schedule. The primary outcome measure was the percentage change in the overall scar index (SI) between baseline and week 12. Secondary outcome measures included objective measurements in skin colour. Patients' views on the aesthetic outcome of treatment were also recorded. Although overall both therapies achieved favourable results for all outcome measures, the improvement in the overall SI was significantly more pronounced for the polyurethane product after week four, 5.6% *vs* 15.8% (p < 0.0001) and week eight 20.2% *vs* 27.1% (p = 0.012).

Clinical reviews

A number of formal reviews of the use of silicone gel sheet and other agents in the management of hypertrophic and keloid scars have been published. Three of these concluded that there appeared to be some benefits associated with the use of silicone gel although the evidence was weak,[41-43] one suggested that surgical excision followed by postoperative intralesional steroid injection seemed to provide a reasonable treatment outcome,[44] one recommended a polytherapeutic strategy for scar management,[45] and one concluded that insufficient information was available to provide clinicians with sufficient evidence to make informed decisions.[46]

Practical problems related to the use of silicone dressings

The problems of using a silicone gel dressing in a hot climate were described by Nikkonen *et al.*[47] Persistent pruritus was encountered in 80% of patients as was skin breakdown (8%), skin rash (28%), skin maceration (16%), foul smell from the gel (4%), poor durability of the sheet (8%), failure of the sheet to improve hydration of dry scars (52%), poor patient compliance (12%) and poor response of the scar to treatment (24%) although most of these problems were eliminated by temporary interruption of treatment, more frequent washings of the gel sheet and improved skin hygiene.

Clinical experience suggests that for silicone gel sheets to function optimally they must be worn for extended periods but because of the practical/cosmetic issue related to the use of these dressings there is a natural reluctance on the part of some patients to adhere to normal protocols and timescales of usage. So *et al.*[48] conducted a study to determine whether enhanced patient education increased compliance and thereby improvement treatment outcomes. They found that patients randomized to receive conventional information only, used the dressings for 10.1 ± 7.5 h/day. Patients who received enhanced education and training, consisting of a detailed handout and videotape, used it for 21.8 ± 3.0 h/day (p < 0.001). As a result by the end of six months, scars of patients in the second group were rated significantly better than those in the first group in terms of pigmentation, height, and pliability. Patients who had used the dressings for an extended period also reported a higher degree of satisfaction with the treatment in terms of scar itch, colour, hardness and elevation.

Not all published studies involving the use of silicone dressings have reported favourable results for this type of treatment, however. Niessen *et al.*[49] compared the prophylactic effect of an occlusive silicone sheet, Sil-K, and a silicone occlusive gel Epiderm, in a bilateral breast-reduction scar model in which a control group of wounds were supported by non-occlusive surgical adhesive tape. The inframammary scars of

129 female patients were studied up to one year following surgery and in each case the width and height were measured, and the scars examined with ultrasound, laser-Doppler flowmetry. Colour measurements were also taken to act as objective indicators to distinguish between normal and exuberant scars. Three months following the operation, 64.3% of patients had a hypertrophic scar, which reduced to 56.6% after six months and 35.3% after one year. No patients developed keloid scars. Patients with an easily tanning skin, non-smokers, and individuals with an allergy were more likely to exhibit scar formation. Neither Sil-K, used in 68 patients, nor Epiderm, used in 61 totally prevented the formation of hypertrophic scars. In fact, according to the authors, if both gel treated groups were taken together scars treated with the silicone materials developed significantly more hypertrophy than those treated with the surgical paper tape. The successful use of a simple adhesive sheet in this way is consistent with the findings of Davey reported previously.

Mode of action of silicone gel

The mode of action of silicone gel has never been fully explained although several possible mechanisms have been proposed.

Effect on scar histology

Kelemen et al.[50] using light and electron microscopy examined the effect of silicone gel and intralesional steroid injections on the morphology of linear and hypertrophic scars in two groups of 12 patients over a four month period.

The first group of patients had their scars injected with diluted triamcinolone acetonide until an inactive state was achieved; the second group was treated with silicone-gel sheeting. Scars were examined every two weeks and after reaching the expected therapeutic response, inactive scars were surgically removed. The excised scars were evaluated histologically using light microscopic and electron microscopy and these investigations revealed marked differences between the samples. The treated scars showed reduced fibroblast activity and a decrease in the number of collagen fibres forming bundles. The orientation of the collagen fibres was also more variable in the silicone treated scars and more capillaries and fewer pre-capillary arteries were detected in the treated scars. Both treatments resulted in the same decrease in the Vancouver Scar Score (VSS), but the steroid treatment was more rapid in onset. The authors suggested that although clinical outcomes are comparable, the two treatments function by different mechanisms.

Hydration of stratum corneum

During the course of their clinical studies with silicone gel sheets, Quinn et al.[25,51] discounted the possible effects of temperature, pH and oxygen permeability, but proposed that the limited permeability of silicone sheet to water vapour might be a factor as the application of a dressing or membrane of lower permeability than the skin would be expected to result in the accumulation of moisture within the tissue.

Using an evaporimeter, they measured the loss of water vapour from intact skin and from skin covered with silicone gel and showed that fluid loss from the silicone-covered area was about half that recorded from normal skin. When the dressing was removed the rate of evaporation immediately increased about 10 fold before gradually returning to normal after about 20 minutes. As there was no evidence of an accumulation of fluid below the gel on the skin surface, the fluid reservoir must lie within the skin, most likely in the *stratum corneum*. The authors also noted that if silicone gel sheet was left in contact with filter paper for six hours, an oily residue was detectable on the absorbent paper leading them to speculate whether this material was capable of penetrating the skin.

Suetak *et al.*[52] also investigated the effects of silicone gel sheets on the water content of the skin, measuring evaporation from the flexor aspects of healthy volunteers for 30 min after removal of silicone gel dressings or a plastic film that had been left in place for either one or seven days. Both products increased hydration of the skin surface and when the coverings were removed there followed an initial quick and later slower process of dehydration. The increase in hydration produced by the silicone dressing was always smaller than that produced by the plastic film, but interestingly the degree of hydration became less with repetition of the silicone gel treatment. The water-holding capacity of the skin normalised after seven days of treatment with silicone gel leading the authors to conclude that the silicone sheet probably produces a favourable condition for the skin by protecting it from various environmental stimuli, while keeping it in an adequately but not over-hydrated condition. It is possible that this effect might be explained by the absorption by the *stratum corneum* of the small quantities of oil residues previously noted by Quinn.[51] which could have the effect of rendering it slightly hydrophobic thus reducing its capacity to retain moisture.

In a second paper in which she described the use of silicone gel sheet in 125 patients with 129 scars, Quinn[51] concluded, by a process of elimination, that the mode of action of the silicone dressing 'must involve a chemical factor' but acknowledged the possibility that the relatively impermeable dressing might be restoring homeostasis to the scar, thereby reducing capillary hyperaemia and secondary fibrosis resulting in hypertrophic scar formation.

Klopp *et al.*[53] compared the effects of four treatments on microcirculatory parameters including venular flow rate, total microvessel length and the number of blood cell-perfused nodal points in a defined tissue volume. They also recorded skin temperature and tissue quality in normal skin and scar tissue. The treatments they evaluated were compression used alone and compression combined with the use of a silicone sheet. These results they compared with those achieved with a self-adhesive polyurethane dressing, Cutinova Thin, with and without compression.

They found that whilst compression alone and the use of the silicone gel brought about some improvement in the appearance of the scars, for each parameter examined the combination of compression and the polyurethane dressing worn continuously for a period of eight weeks proved to be the most effective form of treatment, producing marked improvements in mature scars up to five years old.

In a subsequent publication Schmidt et al.[54] showed that acceptable results could be obtained with the same polyurethane dressing in the absence of compression even when it was only worn for twelve hours each day.

The possibility that the effects of silicone gel treatment are related solely to its limited permeability is not supported by the results of Klopp et al.[53] for although the permeability of the silicone gel sheet used in this investigation is not known, if it is assumed to broadly comparable with that tested by Quinn previously, it will be around $100 \text{ g/m}^2/24$ hours, far less than the Cutinova product.

The use of silicone gels sheets is sometimes reported to be associated with a reduction in scar pain and itching. Eishi et al.[55] used silicone gel sheets in the treatment of six patients for 24 weeks and recorded pain, itching, redness, and scar elevation every week. They also investigated the number of mast cells and Fas antigen expression in the skin of one patient before and after treatment. The pain and itching clearly decreased after 4 weeks of the silicone gel sheeting and disappeared after 12 weeks. After 24 weeks, a decrease in the number of mast cells and the enhanced expression of Fas antigen by fibroblasts in the vicinity of the scar were observed.

Effect upon blood flow

Musgrave et al.[56] postulated that silicone sheets might function by exerting an effect upon blood flow. To investigate this possibility, using a laser Doppler, they made continuous measurements of blood flow in eighteen scars and adjacent control sites in sixteen adult burn patients. Measurements were made for 5 minutes before gel application, for 30 minutes with the gel in place and for 5 minutes following removal. They also monitored and the surface temperature of the scar.

Although hypertrophic scars demonstrated higher perfusion measurements at baseline compared to control areas, the application of silicone sheeting gel did not significantly alter perfusion in either site, suggesting that the mechanism of action of silicone gel sheeting probably does not involve an effect upon blood flow. However, application of silicone gel sheeting did significantly increase the mean baseline surface temperature of the hypertrophic scar from $29 \pm 0.8°\text{ C}$ to $30.7 \pm 0.6°\text{ C}$ ($p < 0.001$) but it is considered unlikely that this effect is significant in this context as other dressings, not normally associated with hypertrophic scar treatment, such as foams, would also be likely to increase skin temperature by virtue of their thermal insulating properties.

Biochemical and cellular effects

The possible biochemical basis for the observed benefits associated with the use of silicone dressings in the treatment of hypertrophic scars has been investigated by a number of researchers.

Ricketts et al.[57] examined their effects upon the expression of key wound healing mediators and compared them with those of a hydrogel sheet dressing, Clearsite. The dressings were applied side by side on 15 hypertrophic scars and their effects compared both the clinical and molecular levels through the use of reverse transcriptase/polymerase chain reaction to evaluate effects on the expression of interleukin 8 (IL-8), basic fibroblast growth factor (bFGF), granulocyte-macrophage colony-stimulating factor (GMCSF), epidermal growth factor (EGF), transforming growth factor beta (TGF- beta), and fibronectin.

Comparable clinical improvement of the hypertrophic scars was obtained with both dressings. Treatment of hypertrophic scars resulted in increased mean levels of IL-8, bFGF, and GMCSF mRNA but mean TGF beta and fibronectin mRNAs decreased after treatment with both dressings. Comparisons between the two dressings revealed significant changes in IL-8 and fibronectin mRNA levels after treatment with Clearsite, while only fibronectin changes were significant after treatment with SGS with respect to normal skin. Only Clearsite induced significant changes in IL-8 and bFGF levels when untreated scars were compared with post-treatment lesions suggesting that the hydrogel augments collagenolysis via promotion of inflammation. The authors therefore concluded that that silicone is not a necessary component of occlusive dressings in the treatment of hypertrophic scars.

Hanasono et al.[58] examined the effect of silicone gel on the secretion of basic fibroblast growth factor (bFGF) in the laboratory using fibroblast cell cultures established from normal, keloid, and foetal skin in a serum-free medium. Serial cell counts were performed and bFGF concentrations present in the supernatant determined by enzyme-linked immunosorbent assay at 4, 24, 72, and 120 hours. No statistically significant differences in population doubling times were observed between treated and untreated specimens but statistically significant differences were detected between bFGF levels in supernatant collected from treated and untreated normal fibroblasts at all time periods. Differences in bFGF levels between treated and untreated foetal fibroblasts approached statistical significance at 72 and 120 hours. The authors concluded that silicone gel is responsible for increased bFGF levels in normal and foetal dermal fibroblasts and postulated that silicone gel treats and prevents hypertrophic scar tissue, which contains histologically normal fibroblasts, by modulating expression of growth factors such as bFGF.

Kuhn et al.[59] also used an in vitro model to study the effect of four brands of silicone sheeting on contraction of hypertrophic scar fibroblasts in a fibroblast populated collagen lattice (FPCL). Silicone sheets and pieces of Saran wrap, acting as a control, were placed over the collagen matrix. The amount of gel contraction was measured every 24 hours for five days at which time the amount of TGFbeta2 present in the culture medium was determined using an immunoassay system. A statistically significant decrease in FPCL contraction was recorded for three of the four brands of silicone sheets compared to both the untreated controls and Saran wrap treated FPCL. The immunoassay for TGFbeta2 also showed a statistically significant decrease with all four types of silicone sheeting leading the authors to conclude that silicone sheeting may act by down regulating fibroblasts and decreasing fibrogenic cytokines.

Animal studies

A small number of studies have described the use of different scar treatments in an animal model in which full-thickness wounds (down to cartilage) are produced in a rabbit ear and allowed to heal for about four weeks. By the end of this time a hypertrophic scar is formed which forms a suitable model for comparing treatments.

Saulis *et al.*[60] applied a silicone adhesive gel to scars produced in this way and measured its effect upon the Scar Elevation Index (SEI), a ratio of the scar height over normal skin, in which readings greater than 1.0 represent a raised scar. They reported that compared with untreated control, SEIs of treated ears were significantly reduced after four week treatment with silicone gel. No reduction in SEIs was recorded using non-silicone control dressings. Histological examination revealed no differences in scar cellularity, inflammation, or matrix organization between treatment groups but ultrastructural observation revealed numerous vacuoles in basal cells of control and non-silicone-treated scars that were not found in unwounded skin or silicone gel-treated scars. Because the dressings applied were similar in terms of their water vapour transmission rates, the authors discounted scar hydration as the sole mechanism of action of the silicone dressings.

Tandara *et al.*[61] also used the rabbit ear model to test the hypothesis that silicone sheeting reduces keratinocyte stimulation, decreasing dermal thickness and hence scar hypertrophy. Silicone adhesive gel sheets were applied to scars in the rabbit ear model of hypertrophic scarring 14 days post wounding for a total of 16 days. As before the SEI was recorded together with the epidermal thickness index (ETI), a ratio of the averaged epidermal height of the scar to the epidermal thickness of normal epidermis. Specific staining for anti-PCNA (proliferating cell nuclear antigen) and Masson trichrome was performed to reveal differences in scar morphology. SEIs were significantly reduced after silicone gel sheet application compared with untreated scars, corresponding to a 70% reduction in scar hypertrophy. Total occlusion reduced scar hypertrophy by 80% compared to semi-occlusion. ETIs of untreated scars were increased by more than 100% compared to uninjured skin. Silicone gel treatment significantly reduced epidermal thickness by more than 30%. The results suggested that silicone gel application at a very early onset of scarring reduced dermal and epidermal thickness apparently by reducing keratinocyte stimulation possibly stimulated by hydration of the keratinocytes.

A similar conclusion was reached by Kloeters *et al.*[62] who showed in the rabbit ear model that compared with areas dressed with a single layer of a of a semipermeable polyurethane film dressing (Tegaderm) scar formation could be reduced by 80% by the application of silicone film or five layers of Tegaderm, once again suggesting that the degree and duration of occlusion are most important for reducing scar tissue formation.

O'Shaughnessy *et al.*[63] also speculated that the mechanism of hypertrophic scar reduction using silicone gel is due to occlusion and homeostasis of the barrier layer. They adopted an established model of hypertrophic scarring using rabbits. The animals were divided into four groups and their wounds were tape-stripped or occluded with Kelo-cote (a silicone preparation that once applied dries to form a water impermeable membrane), Cavilon (a protective barrier film), or Indermil, a cyanoacrylate tissue adhesive. All wounds were harvested on day 28 and examined histologically to measure the scar elevation index (SEI), epithelial thickness, and cellularity. Inflammation in the dermis was measured by an immunohistochemical technique. Ultrastructural analysis was performed by electron microscopy.

Compared with control values, Kelocote, Cavilon, and Indermil all reduced transepidermal water loss (TEWL) while tape stripping increased TEWL. The three topical preparations also significantly decreased SEI compared with control values but tape stripping significantly increased the SEI, epithelial thickness, and cellularity. Immunostaining for macrophages showed increased density of inflammatory cells in the tape-stripped scars. Extensive inflammation and keratinocyte damage was detected in tape-stripped wounds under electron microscopy which led to an increase in scarring but unwounded skin and occlusion-treated scars did not display these characteristics. The authors concluded that hypertrophic scarring was reduced regardless of occlusive treatment applied and suggested that occlusive products function by establishing homeostasis of the epidermal barrier layer.

Together these studies provide further support for the earlier observations of Bieley and Berman,[64] who showed that a silicone free occlusive dressing, Topiclude, worn continuously for eight weeks was effective in the management of the majority of keloids, producing a reduction in height in 19 of 21 wounds examined as well a reduction in pain and pruritus in a significant proportion of patients treated.

Summary of the role of silicone dressings in scar treatment

Overall, the results of published experimental and clinical studies appear to suggest silicone in the form of gel sheets and topical preparations are able to help prevent or reduce the severity of hypertrophic scarring. Furthermore there appears to be reasonable evidence to suggest that there may be at least two mechanisms involved, increased hydration of the *stratum corneum* and a biochemical effect caused by a component or constituent of the gel itself.

It follows, however, that if a biochemical mechanisms is involved this must involve the migration of the active agent into or through the outer layers of the skin. This possibility was elegantly investigated and confirmed by Sanchez,[65] who used advanced analytical technique including MALDI-TOF/MS (Matrix Assisted Laser Desorption Ionisation-Time of Flight Mass Spectrometry) in conjunction with gel permeation chromatography to identify low molecular weight silicone species present in the polydimethylsiloxane gel which he subsequently showed in *in vitro* studies could down-regulate the proliferation of fibroblast cells and protein production.

Using highly sensitive Attenuated Total Reflectance Fourier Transform Infrared spectroscopy (ATR-FT/IR) he was also able to demonstrate that these molecules could pass through the stratum corneum of tissue explants, reaching detectable levels after 11 days. He also showed in studies of hypertrophic scars treated with medical Grade silicone gel that in some areas the low molecular weight material tended to pool, resulting in highly disorganised collagen nodules.

This excellent work by Sanchez appears to finally confirm that there is no doubt that one or more components of silicone gel act directly at a biochemical or cellular level to interfere with the growth, metabolism and morphology of fibroblast cells. It does not, however, eliminate the possibility that hydration of the stratum corneum has some benefits in this regard as suggested by studies not involving silicone dressings.

If low molecular weight silicone from other pharmaceutical or cosmetic preparations is able to pass through the skin barrier, it raises additional questions related to its eventual fate within the body and its method of elimination (if this occurs) which have yet to be addressed.

REFERENCES

1. Rayner K. The use of pressure therapy to treat hypertrophic scarring. *Journal of Wound Care* 2000;**9**(3):151-153.
2. Carney SA, Cason CG. Treating hypertrophic scars with silicone gel. *Journal of Wound Care* 1993;**2**(4):197-198.
3. Carney SA. Hypertrophic scar formation after skin injury. *Journal of Wound Care* 1993;**2**(5):299-302.
4. Carney SA, Cason CG, Gowar JP, Stevenson JH, McNee J, Groves AR, et al. Cica-Care gel sheeting in the management of hypertrophic scarring. *Burns* 1994;**20**(2):163-7.
5. Munro KJ. Treatment of hypertrophic and keloid scars. *Journal of Wound Care* 1995;**4**(5):243-5.
6. Eisenbeiss W, Peter FW, Bakhtiari C, Frenz C. Hypertrophic scars and keloids. *Journal of Wound Care* 1998;**7**(5):255-7.
7. Beldon P. Management of scarring. *Journal of Wound Care* 1999;**8**(10):509-12.
8. Partridge J. The pyschological effects of facial disfigurement. *Journal of Wound Care* 1993;**2**(3):168-171.
9. Perkins K, Davey RB, Wallis KA. Silicone gel: a new treatment for burn scars and contractures. *Burns* 1983;**9**(3):201-4.
10. Gifford D. Silicone oil for hand treatment. *Physiotherapy* 1974;**60**(11):350.
11. Davey RB, Wallis KA, Bowering K. Adhesive contact media--an update on graft fixation and burn scar management. *Burns* 1991;**17**(4):313-9.
12. Davey RB. The use of contact media for burn scar hypertrophy. *Journal of Wound Care* 1997;**6**(2):80-2.
13. Davey RB. The use of an 'adhesive contact medium' (Hypafix) for split skin graft fixation: a 12-year review. *Burns* 1997;**23**(7-8):615-9.
14. Davey RB. Burn scar contracture release: a simplified technique utilizing contact media. *Burns* 1996;**22**(5):406-8.
15. Sawada Y, Sone K. Hydration and occlusion treatment for hypertrophic scars and keloids. *Br J Plast Surg* 1992;**45**(8):599-603.
16. Lacarrubba F, Patania L, Perrotta R, Stracuzzi G, Nasca MR, Micali G. An open-label pilot study to evaluate the efficacy and tolerability of a silicone gel in the treatment of hypertrophic scars using clinical and ultrasound assessments. *J Dermatolog Treat* 2008;**19**(1):50-3.
17. Mustoe TA. Evolution of silicone therapy and mechanism of action in scar management. *Aesthetic Plast Surg* 2008;**32**(1):82-92.
18. Paquet P, Hermanns JF, Pierard GE. Effect of the 585 nm flashlamp-pumped pulsed dye laser for the treatment of keloids. *Dermatol Surg* 2001;**27**(2):171-4.
19. Kumar K, Kapoor BS, Rai P, Shukla HS. In-situ irradiation of keloid scars with Nd:YAG laser. *Journal of Wound Care* 2000;**9**(5):213-5.
20. Akoz T, Gideroglu K, Akan M. Combination of different techniques for the treatment of earlobe keloids. *Aesthetic Plast Surg* 2002;**26**(3):184-8.
21. Chang CH, Song JY, Park JH, Seo SW. The efficacy of magnetic disks for the treatment of earlobe hypertrophic scar. *Ann Plast Surg* 2005;**54**(5):566-9.

22. Boutli-Kasapidou F, Tsakiri A, Anagnostou E, Mourellou O. Hypertrophic and keloidal scars: an approach to polytherapy. *Int J Dermatol* 2005;**44**(4):324-7.

23. Saulis AS, Mogford JH, Mustoe TA. Effect of Mederma on hypertrophic scarring in the rabbit ear model. *Plast Reconstr Surg* 2002;**110**(1):177-83; discussion 184-6.

24. Hosnuter M, Payasli C, Isikdemir A, Tekerekoglu B. The effects of onion extract on hypertrophic and keloid scars. *J Wound Care* 2007;**16**(6):251-4.

25. Quinn KJ, Evans JH, Courtney JM, Gaylor JD, Reid WH. Non-pressure treatment of hypertrophic scars. *Burns Incl Therm Inj* 1985;**12**(2):102-8.

26. Katz BE. Silastic gel sheeting is found to be effective in scar therapy. *Cosmetic Dermatology* 1992(June 1992).

27. Fulton JE, Jr. Silicone gel sheeting for the prevention and management of evolving hypertrophic and keloid scars. *Dermatol Surg* 1995;**21**(11):947-51.

28. Chuangsuwanich A, Osathalert V, Muangsombut S. Self-adhesive silicone gel sheet: a treatment for hypertrophic scars and keloids. *J Med Assoc Thai* 2000;**83**(4):439-44.

29. Ahn ST, Monafo WW, Mustoe TA. Topical silicone gel: a new treatment for hypertrophic scars. *Surgery* 1989;**106**(4):781-6; discussion 786-7.

30. Ahn ST, Monafo WW, Mustoe TA. Topical silicone gel for the prevention and treatment of hypertrophic scar. *Arch Surg* 1991;**126**(4):499-504.

31. Camey SA, Cason CG, Gowar JP. Treating hypertrophic scars with silicone gel. *Journal of Wound Care* 1993;**2**(4):197-198.

32. de Oliveira GV, Nunes TA, Magna LA, Cintra ML, Kitten GT, Zarpellon S, et al. Silicone versus nonsilicone gel dressings: a controlled trial. *Dermatol Surg* 2001;**27**(8):721-6.

33. Gold MH, Foster TD, Adair MA, Burlison K, Lewis T. Prevention of hypertrophic scars and keloids by the prophylactic use of topical silicone gel sheets following a surgical procedure in an office setting. *Dermatol Surg* 2001;**27**(7):641-4.

34. Chan KY, Lau CL, Adeeb SM, Somasundaram S, Nasir-Zahari M. A randomized, placebo-controlled, double-blind, prospective clinical trial of silicone gel in prevention of hypertrophic scar development in median sternotomy wound. *Plast Reconstr Surg* 2005;**116**(4):1013-20; discussion 1021-2.

35. Li-Tsang CW, Lau JC, Choi J, Chan CC, Jianan L. A prospective randomized clinical trial to investigate the effect of silicone gel sheeting (Cica-Care) on post-traumatic hypertrophic scar among the Chinese population. *Burns* 2006;**32**(6):678-83.

36. Majan JI. Evaluation of a self-adherent soft silicone dressing for the treatment of hypertrophic postoperative scars. *J Wound Care* 2006;**15**(5):193-6.

37. Chernoff WG, Cramer H, Su-Huang S. The efficacy of topical silicone gel elastomers in the treatment of hypertrophic scars, keloid scars, and post-laser exfoliation erythema. *Aesthetic Plast Surg* 2007;**31**(5):495-500.

38. de Giorgi V, Sestini S, Mannone F, Papi F, Alfaioli B, Gori A, et al. The use of silicone gel in the treatment of fresh surgical scars: a randomized study. *Clin Exp Dermatol* 2009;**34**(6):688-93.

39. Momeni M, Hafezi F, Rahbar H, Karimi H. Effects of silicone gel on burn scars. *Burns* 2009;**35**(1):70-4.

40. Wigger-Albert W, Kuhlmann M, Wilhelm D, Mrowietz U, Eichhorn K, Ortega J, et al. Efficacy of a polyurethane dressing versus a soft silicone sheet on hypertrophic scars. *J Wound Care* 2009;**18**(5):208, 210-4.

41. Poston J. The use of silicone gel sheeting in the management of hypertrophic and keloid scars. *Journal of Wound Care* 2000;**9**(1):10-6.

42. Mustoe TA, Cooter RD, Gold MH, Hobbs FD, Ramelet AA, Shakespeare PG, et al. International clinical recommendations on scar management. *Plast Reconstr Surg* 2002;**110**(2):560-71.
43. O'Brien L, Pandit A. Silicon gel sheeting for preventing and treating hypertrophic and keloid scars. *Cochrane Database Syst Rev* 2006(1):CD003826.
44. Mofikoya BO, Adeyemo WL, Abdus-salam AA. Keloid and hypertrophic scars: a review of recent developments in pathogenesis and management. *Nig Q J Hosp Med* 2007;**17**(4):134-9.
45. Reish RG, Eriksson E. Scars: a review of emerging and currently available therapies. *Plast Reconstr Surg* 2008;**122**(4):1068-78.
46. Durani P, Bayat A. Levels of evidence for the treatment of keloid disease. *J Plast Reconstr Aesthet Surg* 2008;**61**(1):4-17.
47. Nikkonen MM, Pitkanen JM, Al-Qattan MM. Problems associated with the use of silicone gel sheeting for hypertrophic scars in the hot climate of Saudi Arabia. *Burns* 2001;**27**(5):498-501.
48. So K, Umraw N, Scott J, Campbell K, Musgrave M, Cartotto R. Effects of enhanced patient education on compliance with silicone gel sheeting and burn scar outcome: a randomized prospective study. *J Burn Care Rehabil* 2003;**24**(6):411-7; discussion 410.
49. Niessen FB, Spauwen PH, Robinson PH, Fidler V, Kon M. The use of silicone occlusive sheeting (Sil-K) and silicone occlusive gel (Epiderm) in the prevention of hypertrophic scar formation. *Plast Reconstr Surg* 1998;**102**(6):1962-72.
50. Kelemen JJ, 3rd, Cioffi WG, McManus WF, Mason AD, Jr., Pruitt BA, Jr. Burn center care for patients with toxic epidermal necrolysis see comments. *J Am Coll Surg* 1995;**180**(3):273-8.
51. Quinn KJ. Silicone gel in scar treatment. *Burns* 1987;**13 Suppl**:S33-40.
52. Suetak T, Sasai S, Zhen YX, Tagami H. Effects of silicone gel sheet on the stratum corneum hydration. *Br J Plast Surg* 2000;**53**(6):503-7.
53. Klopp R, Niemer W, Fraenkel M, von der Weth A. Effect of four treatment variants on the functional and cosmetic state of mature scars. *J Wound Care* 2000;**9**(7):319-24.
54. Schmidt A, Gassmueller J, Hughes-Formella B, Bielfeldt S. Treating hypertrophic scars for 12 or 24 hours with a self-adhesive hydroactive polyurethane dressing. *J Wound Care* 2001;**10**(5):149-53.
55. Eishi K, Bae SJ, Ogawa F, Hamasaki Y, Shimizu K, Katayama I. Silicone gel sheets relieve pain and pruritus with clinical improvement of keloid: possible target of mast cells. *J Dermatolog Treat* 2003;**14**(4):248-52.
56. Musgrave MA, Umraw N, Fish JS, Gomez M, Cartotto RC. The effect of silicone gel sheets on perfusion of hypertrophic burn scars. *J Burn Care Rehabil* 2002;**23**(3):208-14.
57. Ricketts CH, Martin L, Faria DT, Saed GM, Fivenson DP. Cytokine mRNA changes during the treatment of hypertrophic scars with silicone and nonsilicone gel dressings. *Dermatol Surg* 1996;**22**(11):955-9.
58. Hanasono MM, Lum J, Carroll LA, Mikulec AA, Koch RJ. The effect of silicone gel on basic fibroblast growth factor levels in fibroblast cell culture. *Arch Facial Plast Surg* 2004;**6**(2):88-93.
59. Kuhn MA, Moffit MR, Smith PD, Lyle WG, Ko F, Meltzer DD, et al. Silicone sheeting decreases fibroblast activity and downregulates TGFbeta2 in hypertrophic scar model. *Int J Surg Investig* 2001;**2**(6):467-74.
60. Saulis AS, Chao JD, Telser A, Mogford JE, Mustoe TA. Silicone occlusive treatment of hypertrophic scar in the rabbit model. *Aesthet Surg J* 2002;**22**(2):147-53.

61. Tandara AA, Kloeters O, Mogford JE, Mustoe TA. Hydrated keratinocytes reduce collagen synthesis by fibroblasts via paracrine mechanisms. *Wound Repair Regen* 2007;**15**(4):497-504.
62. Kloeters O, Tandara A, Mustoe TA. Hypertrophic scar model in the rabbit ear: a reproducible model for studying scar tissue behavior with new observations on silicone gel sheeting for scar reduction. *Wound Repair Regen* 2007;**15 Suppl 1**:S40-5.
63. O'Shaughnessy KD, De La Garza M, Roy NK, Mustoe TA. Homeostasis of the epidermal barrier layer: a theory of how occlusion reduces hypertrophic scarring. *Wound Repair Regen* 2009;**17**(5):700-8.
64. Bieley HC, Berman B. Effects of a water-impermeable, non-silicone-based occlusive dressing on keloids. *Journal of the American Academy of Dermatology* 1996;**35**(1):113-114.
65. Sanchez WH. PhD Thesis: Elucidating the role of silicone in the treatment of burn scars: an essential step in the development of improved treatment products. Queensland University of Technology 2006.

19. Maggot therapy

BACKGROUND TO MAGGOT THERAPY

Maggot therapy (MT), also sometimes known as larval therapy (LT), maggot debridement therapy (MDT), or biosurgery is a method of treating wounds which takes advantage of the natural propensity of maggots, the larval form of certain species of flies, to colonize wounds of humans and animals and breakdown and ingest infected or necrotic tissue thereby cleansing the wounds and eliminating infection.

Definition of myiasis

The natural infestation of wounds by maggots is called 'myiasis', a term first proposed by Hope[1] in 1840 to describe diseases in humans associated with the presence of dipterous larvae. It was subsequently redefined by Zumpt[2] as follows;

> 'The infestation of live human and vertebrate animals with dipterous larvae, which, at least for a certain period, feed on the host's dead or living tissue, liquid body-substances, or ingested food.'

Flies causing myiasis can be categorized into two groups based on the relationship with their hosts. Obligate parasites only on live hosts, but facultative parasites can develop on either live hosts or carrion.[3-5] Accidental infestations with fly larvae can sometimes occur if eggs or larvae are inhaled or swallowed inadvertently with food; these should be considered 'pseudomyiasis' rather than true parasitic myiasis.

Flies species capable of causing myiasis

Flies, unlike most other insects, have only a single pair of functional wings. They are therefore classified as Diptera, (di + pteron) 'two-winged' a description coined by Aristotle in the fourth Century BC. Blowflies (Calliphoridae) and Flesh flies (Sarcophagidae), whose larvae are commonly responsible for producing maggot infestations, probably once shared a common origin, but the habits of these two families have evolved and now include species that are specialized as breeders in dung, or as parasitoids of insects, earthworms, slugs, snails and amphibians. The adult females of both the parasitic and carrion breeding species locate a suitable site for ovipositing by locating the source of the odours of infection and tissue decay.

According to a comprehensive review by Hall and Smith,[6] flies capable of causing myiasis in man belong to one of three major families: Oestridae, Sarcophagidae, or Calliphoridae, although representatives of other families, such as Muscidae and Phoridae, also are also sometime implicated.

All 150 species of Oestridae may cause myiasis but of the approximately 1000 species of Calliphoridae and 2000 species of Sarcophagidae, only about 80 species have been reported to do so. The Oestridae have no value in maggot therapy as all are obligate parasites, generally with a high degree of host specificity. Likewise, the obligate myiasis-causing Calliphoridae, such as the Old World and New World screwworms (*Cochliomyia hominivorax* and *Chrysomya bezziana*, respectively) are definitely *not* suitable for MT because they are truly parasitic, feeding on living tissue.

The Sarcophagidae include two obligate parasites of vertebrates that can infest humans: *Wohlfahrtia magnifica* and *Wohlfahrtia vigil*. *W. magnifica* is well recognized as an agent of human myiasis, particularly in Eastern Europe, Israel, and North Africa. *W. vigil* (also known as *W. opaca*) has been reported to cause a furuncular myiasis of infants in North America, but not in Europe.

Figure 72: *Cochliomyia hominivorax*

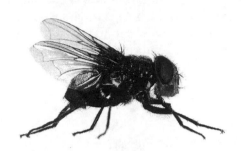

In Australia a variety of fly species have been reported to cause facultative myiasis, but the species most commonly implicated are *Calliphora* and *Sarcophaga*; in new Guinea *Chrysomya* is a primary cause.[4,7]

Photograph courtesy of Martin Hall, and copyright Natural History Museum, London

Accounts of human myiasis

Infestation of animal and human wounds of all types by maggots must have taken place for many millennia. An early written account may be found in the Bible, where it is recorded that Job complained; *'My body is clothed with worms and scabs; my skin is broken and festering.'* (Job 7:5).

Simeon the Stylite, an early Christian ascetic who lived on top of a pillar from about 420 to 495AD, was also said to have developed wounds which became infested with maggots. When these fell out he replaced them exhorting them to *'eat what God had provided'*.[8]

On the battlefield, as will be seen later, infestation of wounds with maggots was common and often beneficial. Even sailors were not immune, for at the battle of Trafalgar it is recorded how one unfortunate individual with a serious leg wound observed, *'hundreds of large red-headed maggots nearly an inch long sticking into the calf of my precious limb only their tails to be seen'*.

These maggots were thought to have come from Spanish flies that blacked the hospital which was overcrowded with wounded. The maggots were killed with a potion and the leg eventually healed.[9]

In more modern times, naturally occurring cases of myiasis in humans by facultative parasites are not unusual, but most commonly seen in young children, the elderly, the physically or mentally infirm,[10-12] or in cases of personal neglect or in settings of high fly density.

Common sites of infestation include the ear,[13] nose,[14-15] or paranasal sinuses,[16] but infestations have also been reported in the vagina,[17] tracheostomy wounds,[18] malignant wounds,[19] pin sites,[20-21] and wounds of patients with leprosy.[22-23]

Henry[24] reported an unusual case in which a 65-year-old male psychiatric patient presented with mid face swelling and purulent exudate dripping from his mouth. On intra-oral examination a large maggot-infected sinus related to the upper central incisors was discovered eating away at surrounding necrotic alveolar tissues.

Sherman[25] published the results of a multicentre, prospective observational study of urban and suburban patients who were infested with maggots. Forty-two cases of US-acquired myiasis were collected from twenty centres. Most infestations occurred within pre-existing wounds and no cases of tissue invasion were recorded. Homelessness, alcoholism, and peripheral vascular disease were frequent cofactors but two patients (5%) were hospitalized at the time of their infestation. The fly species most commonly responsible was *Phaenicia (Lucilia) sericata* but other blowflies, flesh flies, and humpbacked flies (Phoridae) were also were isolated. In six cases, two co-infesting species were identified. The results of this prospective study suggest that most cases of human myiasis are caused by non-invasive blowflies laying eggs in pre-existing wounds.

Sherman suggested that the most prudent response to such infestations is removal of the larvae to prevent tissue damage and bacterial infection, even when the maggots are known to belong to a therapeutically useful species. Although natural infestations with these maggots can have beneficial effects which may be lost when the larvae are removed, these natural infestations are uncontrolled and can, therefore, complicate ongoing medical treatment.

According to a review by Morgan,[26] over the years numerous techniques have been adopted to remove unwanted maggots from wounds including the use of fairly toxic or unpleasant agents such as chloroform and turpentine, chloroform and carbolic acid, ether, cocaine, or a mixture of camphor and chloroform followed by potassium permanganate solution. Attempts were also made to suffocate them by occluding oxygen from the wounds by the use of oil, liquid paraffin, sticking plaster pork fat or petroleum jelly.

Medico-legal importance of maggot infestations

Because maggots develop at a relatively consistent rate, it is often possible to determine the time of death of a cadaver with some accuracy based upon the nature and development of various insect species present.

Grassberger and Reiter[27] studied the development of *L. sericata* under 10 different temperature regimens, plotting the time from hatching to peak feeding against temperature. Using these data the authors suggested that it should be possible to obtain a rapid and precise estimate of the post-mortem interval when these maggots are present on a corpse. Synanthropic flies, particularly calliphorids, are initiators of carrion decomposition and as such are the primary and most accurate forensic indicators of time of death.[28]

An earlier account of maggots being used in this way was provided by McClellan in 1931,[29] although according to a fascinating review by Greenberg,[28] forensic entomology might actually have begun in China in the 13th Century!

Fly species used for medical applications

Considerable caution must be exercised when selecting maggots for clinical use as only a relatively small number of species have been used medicinally. The most widely used is a blowfly, the greenbottle *L. sericata* (Figure 73), although treatment with other facultative calliphorids, have also been described in the literature.

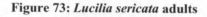

Figure 73: *Lucilia sericata* adults

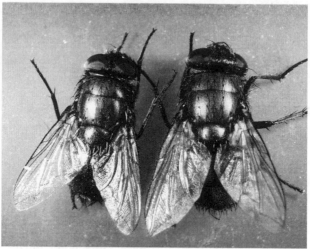

(Male on left)

A sarcophagid, *Wohlfahrtia nuba*, was successfully employed by Grantham-Hill[30] in the Sudan, but this organism was observed to feed on healthy tissue at the margin of the wound if all necrotic tissue was exhausted. In contrast Weil *et al.*[31] reported that that larvae of *L. sericata* starved on clean granulation tissue and suggested that they were, therefore, ideally suited for MT. Other authors, however, have suggested (incorrectly) that this species may occasionally feed on healthy human tissue.[32]

Sarcophaga bullata was used successfully in the US, but details about its relative risks and benefits are not known. Similarly, *Sarcophaga crassipalpis*, found infesting bed sores in an elderly patient in Italy, and *Boettcherisca peregrina*, found infesting a parotid gland papillary adenocarcinoma, could possibly be candidates for MT.

A major problem with the Sarcophagidae as a group, however, is that females deposit live larvae, and these are much more difficult to sterilise than eggs.

Some calliphorids cannot be used therapeutically due to their propensity to cause malign myiasis: these include *Cochliomyia macellaria*, *Chrysomya megacephala* and *Lucilia cuprina*. With careful management, however, even these three species might someday have a role in MT as an apparently non-pathogenic strain of *L. cuprina* has already been used with some success.[33] Interestingly, *L. sericata*, the species used most commonly in MT today, is a serious pest to the sheep industry of the UK, Europe and New Zealand. Called 'sheep strike,' myiasis in sheep due to *Lucilia* can be fatal in cases of heavy infestation due to ammonia toxicity and alkalosis.

HISTORY OF MAGGOT THERAPY

Throughout the millennia, the popularity of maggot therapy has ebbed and flowed a process which was elegantly summarized by Sir William Osler, M.D. in 1902 who concluded that;

> 'The philosophies of one age become the absurdities of the next, and the foolishness of yesterday has become the wisdom of tomorrow'.

Maggot therapy in antiquity

According to Kumar,[34] one of the earliest accounts of MT was provided in India by Sushruta around 600 BC. In his surgical treatise *Sushruta Samhita*, he described how flies could be induced to deposit worms (maggots) onto tumours and thereafter eat away the affected tissue thus:

> 'Nispava, pinyaka (molasses), and paste of kulattha (herbal medicine) added with more meat and water of curd (whey) made a nice paste and was applied on the tumor so that flies shall swarm to it and krimi (worms/maggots) develop there and eat away the tumor. When only a small remnant (of the tumor) remains after the worms have eaten, the area should be scraped and burnt by fire; or if the base (of the tumor) is small it can be kept encircled (for some days) with thin sheets of tin, copper, lead, and iron.'

Primitive societies have also long recognized that the larvae of certain flies can have beneficial effects upon the healing of infected wounds. In the early part of the 20th Century, the Ngemba tribe of New South Wales, Australia, commonly used maggots to cleanse suppurating or gangrenous wounds and it is said that the aborigines traced this practice back to their remote ancestors.[35-36]

The Hill Peoples of Northern Burma were observed during World War II placing maggots on a wound then covering them with mud and wet grass and the Mayans of Central America ceremoniously exposed dressings of beef blood to the sun before applying them to certain superficial tumours when, after a few days, the dressings were expected to pulsate with maggots.[31,36]

Maggots in military conflicts

The opportunistic infestation of wounds, particularly those sustained in battle, has similarly been observed throughout the centuries. Goldstein, in two fascinating reviews of the early history of maggots in wound care,[37-38] quoted the words of Ambroise Paré (1509-1590), Chief Surgeon to Charles IX and Henri III, who recorded that in the battle of St. Quentin (1557) maggots frequently infested suppurating wounds and promoted wound cleansing. Paré described one treatment thus;

> 'After some months space a great number of worms came forth by the rotten bone, which moved to hasten the separation and falling away of the putrid bones ..... the patient recovered beyond all men's expectation.'.

According to Goldstein, Napoleon's Surgeon in Chief, Baron Dominic Larrey, also reported that when maggots developed in battle injuries, they prevented the development of infection and accelerated healing, describing his observations thus;

> 'These insects, so far from being injurious to their wounds, promoted rather their cicatrization by cutting short the process of nature and causing the separation of cellular eschars which they devoured. These larvae are indeed greedy only after putrefying substances and never touched the parts endowed with life.'

There is no evidence, however, that Larrey deliberately introduced maggots into his patients' wounds.

Maggots in the American Civil War

During the American Civil War, a Confederate medical officer Joseph Jones, quoted by Chernin,[39] described the beneficial effects of wound myiasis as follows;

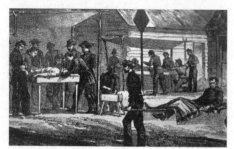

> 'I have frequently seen neglected wounds filled with maggots, as far as my experience extends, these worms only destroy dead tissues, and do not injure specifically the well parts. I have heard surgeons affirm that a gangrenous wound which has been thoroughly cleansed by maggots heals more rapidly than if it had been left to itself.'

According to Baer[40] and McLellan,[41] the Confederate surgeon J. Zacharias, may have been the first western physician to intentionally introduce maggots into wounds for the purpose of cleaning or debriding them. In his paper Baer quotes Zacharias as stating:

> 'During my service in the hospital in Danville, Virginia, I first used maggots to remove the decayed tissue in hospital gangrene and with eminent satisfaction. In a single day would clean a wound much better than any agents we had at our command.... I am sure I saved many lives by their use, escaped septicaemia, and had rapid recoveries.'

Maggots in the First World War

The ability of maggots to cleanse battlefield injuries was also reported during the First World War. Kampmeier,[42] in his autobiography, recalled how one surgeon, Walter Pugh, who had seen service on the western front used 'sterile maggots' in a Salt Lake City Hospital in the early 1920s - apparently obtaining them from a commercial source. He introduced the maggots directly into the wound, protecting the surrounding skin with Vaseline. Remarkably he never described his experiences in the medical literature.

This honour was to fall to William Baer (1872-1931), Clinical Professor of Orthopaedic Surgery at the Johns Hopkins School of Medicine in Maryland.[40] Baer described how, during the First World War, he had treated two wounded soldiers who had remained overlooked on the battlefield for seven days having sustained compound fractures of the femur and large flesh wounds of the abdomen and scrotum. On arrival at the hospital they showed no sign of fever or septicaemia despite the very serious nature of their injuries and their prolonged exposure to the elements without food or water. On removal of their clothing Baer found *'thousands and thousands of maggots that filled the entire wounded area.'* When these were removed, to Baer's surprise the wounds looked very healthy with obvious signs of healing; this at a time when the mortality rate for compound fractures of the femur was about 75-80%. He stated,

> *'There was practically no bare bone to be seen and the internal structure of the wounded bone as well as the surrounding parts was entirely covered with most beautiful pink granulation tissue that one could imagine.'*

Support for Baer's observations was provided by Crile & Martin,[43] who also reported that soldiers whose wounds were infested with maggots did far better than their wounded comrades who wounds were not similarly afflicted.

Early use of maggots in civilian practice

Following his wartime experiences, in 1928 Baer treated four children with intractable bone infections (osteomyelitis) at the Children's Hospital in Baltimore.[40] Initially his use of unsterilized maggots was very successful and all wounds healed within six weeks. Encouraged by these results, Baer began to use the technique more widely, but unfortunately several of his patients developed tetanus and he concluded that it would be necessary to use sterile maggots for future work and devoted considerable efforts to developing a suitable sterilization process.

Initially he attempted to sterilize the maggots themselves by first exposing them to full strength hydrogen peroxide for two hours, and then immersing them in mercuric chloride solution 1 in 1000. Although he was able to demonstrate that this process effectively sterilized the outer surface of the larvae, viable bacteria persisted within the insects' gut. He then decided to sterilize the outer surface of the eggs, believing correctly that the contents were sterile. He tried many different solutions including mercuric chloride, phenol, alcohol, mercurochrome, gentian violet, hexylresorcinol and silver nitrate. These efforts were more successful at achieving sterility, but most also proved lethal to the eggs. Eventually a technique was developed which involved the use a solution containing mercuric chloride 1 in 1000, 25% alcohol and 0.5% hydrochloric acid.

Initially maggots were used principally for the treatment of osteomyelitis,[31-32,41,44-52] and in some instances it was reported that their use led to rapid regeneration of bone 'that approximates more closely to normal bone structure than any of the hitherto accepted methods of treatment'.[53]

Most of these early publications described the use of maggots in the treatment of infections of the long bones, but Oschsenhirt and Komara[54] described a complicated technique involving the production of a cage or denture into which maggots could be introduced to treat osteomyelitis of the mandible. Four patients were treated in this way, apparently with complete success.

Maggots were not used exclusively for osteomyelitis, however, as their wound cleansing abilities were also utilised in soft tissue injuries. Ferguson and McLaughlin[55] described how they were used to treat including carbuncles leg ulcers gangrene and other minor wounds concluding that;

> 'Except for excision, maggot therapy is probably the most rapid method of removing sloughing soft tissue, and maggot action alone gives a more complete result than can be obtained by excision and without injury to recovering tissue'.

In the absence of any other equally effective treatment maggots became so popular in the USA that *L. sericata* larvae were produced by Lederle Corporation[56] and sold for $5 per 1000 (now equivalent to about $100).

The general acceptability of MT was confirmed in the mid-1930s by Robinson who surveyed 947 North American surgeons known to have employed the treatment.[57] Of the 605 responding surgeons who had treated 5750 patients, 91.2% expressed a favourable opinion; only 4.4% expressed an unfavourable view. The most common complaints raised by surveyed practitioners were the cost of the maggots, the time and effort required to construct the maggot dressings, and the degree of discomfort suffered by patients. Robinson's paper also included a list of 54 other articles on MT that had been published by that time. Other than Baer's cases of tetanus and one case of erysipelas, thought to be associated with the use of non-sterile larvae,[31] no other serious adverse reactions were reported.

A somewhat critical view of Baer's observations and publications was expressed by Martin and Heeks[58] who doubted that maggots could act as 'disinfecting agents' suggesting that they offered little benefit in the treatment of osteomyelitis.

Maggots in the treatment of tuberculosis

An even more bizarre historical application for maggots has recently been reported by Wainwright *et al.*[59] who described how, in the early 1900s, a farmer called Arthur Bryant set up a 'maggotorium' where those suffering from pulmonary TB could sit and breathe maggot fumes in the hope of improving their condition.

Each year Bryant would grow maggots on 15-25 tons of meat the smell of which could be detected three miles away. Consumptives would sit in the maggotorium beside troughs of maggots 'to inhale the fumes and pass the time reading chatting or playing card games'. According to testimonials produced by grateful patients, the treatment appeared to be very successful and these claims were given some support by independent tests undertaken by the Bradford city analyst of the time who, although initially sceptical, analysed the gases liberated by the maggots and showed that they contained a mixture of volatiles including traces of indol and skatol (methyl indol) together with much larger quantities of ammonia and triethanolamine which he subsequently showed were able to destroy microorganisms within a few hours. These observations led him to believe that the treatment could have some scientific basis.

In their recent paper Wainwright and his colleagues describe how they tested fumes produced by the maggots of a variety of fly species against *Mycobacterium phlei*, a non-pathogenic model used as a substitute of the more dangerous *Mycobacterium tuberculosis* and found them to be markedly inhibitory leading them to conclude that might be some scientific rationale behind the claims made by Bryant and his patients. Interestingly, however, the fumes appeared not to inhibit the growth of *S. aureus*. As far as is known, maggot inhalation therapy is not currently employed anywhere in the world at this time!

The decline of maggot therapy

The first half of the 20th Century marked the beginning of the antibiotic era. By 1940, sulphonamides already were available, and Chain *et al.*[60] had discovered the methods for mass-producing Fleming's penicillin. As a result, by the mid-1940s, maggot therapy had virtually ceased, except as a treatment of last resort,[61-62] due largely to the ready availability of the new wonder drug and general improvements in surgical and wound management techniques and materials.

In what must be regarded as one of the major misjudgements in the history of wound management, Wainwright,[63] in 1988, summarised the status of MT thus;

> ' ....fortunately maggot therapy is now relegated to a historical backwater, of interest more for its bizarre nature than its effect on the course of medical science....a therapy the demise of which no one is likely to mourn...'

In fact Wainwright's pronouncement about the demise of the technique was premature, for in the last decade of the 20th Century maggot therapy began a significant renaissance and still continues to grow in popularity.

Development of modern maggot therapy

In the late 1980s, Sherman, an infectious diseases fellow at the University of California with a background in entomology, became interested in MT and began to employ the technique in the treatment of pressure ulcers and other chronic wounds. The results of his preliminary investigations indicated that MT offered several advantages over other wound treatments currently then employed.[64]

In Europe, in late 1995, an NHS hospital department in South Wales established a maggot breeding facility called the Biosurgical Research Unit (BRU) and soon afterwards published an account of the use of sterile maggots in a variety of wound types.[65] In 2001 the BRU achieved a 'Queens Award for Innovation' for its work in this area[66] and in 2005 it was spun out of the NHS to form a commercial company called Zoobiotic. By late 2006 the facility had supplied over 70,000 vials containing some 20 million maggots for the treatment of an estimated 30,000 patients.

Prior to 2004 the production of maggots for clinical use was unregulated anywhere in the world but in September 2001 the BRU made a successful submission to the European Medicines Evaluation Agency (EMEA) to have maggots classified as a 'Medicinal Product' at which time they were given Part B status in accordance with

Annex II to Council Regulation (EEC) No. 2309/93. In the USA in January 2004, the Food and Drug Administration decided to classify maggots as Medical Devices. These regulatory changes meant that the production of maggots for clinical use, together with the literature and claims that were made for them, were, for the first time, subject to the same requirements as other products intended for the treatment of wounds in humans and animals.

A maggot production facility was also established at an early date in the Hadassah Hospital in Jerusalem,[67] and by 1999 it was reported to have treated over 70 patients in this and other affiliated units.

Thereafter maggot production facilities were established in several other centres throughout the world including Holland and Germany and the technique has gained widespread use with advocates in France, Sweden, Belgium, Denmark, Poland and the Ukraine. In April 2010, Zoobiotic acquired Biomonde, thereby becoming the largest manufacturer/distributor of medical maggots worldwide.

Some sources have suggested that British special forces are taught the value of maggots when working in the field, and an American author has published a booklet that makes reference to the value of maggots in modern military and survival medicine.[68]

In 1996, an 'International Biotherapy Society' was founded 'to investigate and develop the use of living organisms, or their products, in tissue repair,' and the first in a series of highly successful international conferences on MT and other similar topics also took place in that year.[69]

BASIC BIOLOGY OF *LUCILIA SERICATA*

Life history

In the wild an adult fly lays large numbers of eggs in clusters or 'rafts' on organic matter such as that present in suppurating wounds or carrion but for medical use a more appropriate protein source is selected which may be sterilized, typically liver or egg. The eggs hatch within a few hours, and the recently-emerged maggots are small enough to pass through the eye of a large needle (Figure 74).

The newly hatched maggots produce a powerful mixture of proteolytic enzymes which break down dead tissue to a semi-liquid form which is then reabsorbed and digested. In order to maximize the potential of this extra-corporeal digestive process, the larvae tend to congregate into groups and feed in the head-down position, concentrating initially on small defects or holes in the tissue.

The larvae increase in size very rapidly; they moult twice, and these moults differentiate them into three recognised growth stages or 'instars'. When fully grown - usually after about 5 days, depending upon the temperature - they cease feeding, leave the food source, and seek a dry place to pupate.

The puparium is formed from the hardened larval skin on which structures such as the posterior spiracles (holes through which the larvae breathe) are still visible. The adult fly develops within this puparium and emerges by rupturing the skin with the ptilinum, a bladder-like organ that is temporarily extruded from the head. The rate of development of the adult fly within the puparium is temperature dependent. Under adverse conditions, development may be arrested for weeks or even months.

The newly emerged adult bears little resemblance to the familiar greenbottle, but within a short while the wings expand and the body takes on its familiar green hue: the life cycle is thus complete.

Figure 74: Life cycle of *L.sericata*

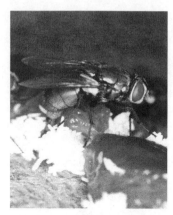

Adult fly laying eggs on liver

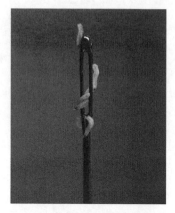

Newly hatched larvae are approximately 1-2 mm long

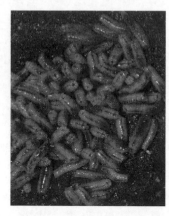

Maggots feed in groups in the 'head-down' position

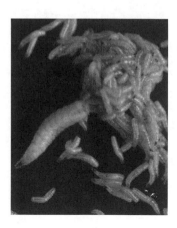

Maggots rapidly increase in size over a period of 4-5 days

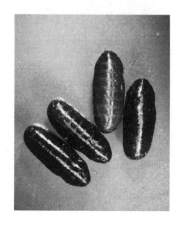

When fully grown maggots cease feeding and pupate

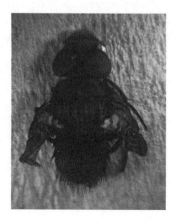

A newly hatched fly with the ptilinum clearly visible

Important anatomical features

General morphology

This description of maggot morphology is drawn from a comprehensive description previously published by Hall *et al.*[70]

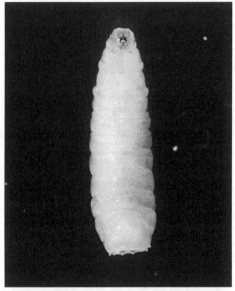

Figure 75: General morphology

A larva (maggot) of L. sericata has a typical calliphorid form with a body pointed at the anterior end and truncated posteriorly. It comprises 12 segments: a small head, incompletely divided from a prothoracic segment, followed by a mesothoracic, a metathoracic and eight abdominal segments.

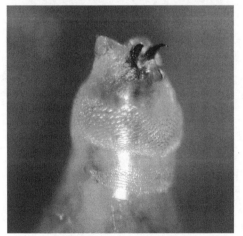

Figure 76: Structure of head

The thorax and abdomen are not clearly differentiated. The anterior (head) end is divided ventrally into two cephalic lobes with a mouth opening at the base of the furrow. The mouthparts consist of hooks and associated sclerites to which the muscles are attached. The head also has two pairs of peg-like sensory organs.

The respiratory system

The maggot has a simple yet effective respiratory system, and is capable of breathing through both ends of its body.

Figure 77: Structure of the respiratory system

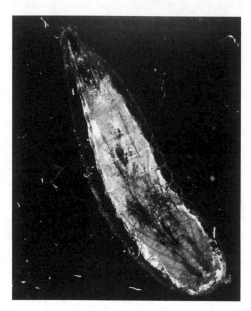

Respiration takes place through spiracles, which are simple external openings to the internal tracheal network.

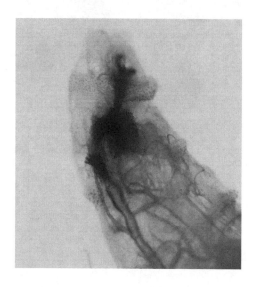

A pair of anterior spiracles is present on the prothoracic segment, which have finger-like projections, imparting a vague resemblance to a glove or flippers.

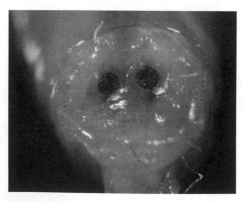

The 12th or terminal segment has a pair of caudal or posterior spiracles, the structure of which can be used for taxonomic purposes. The position of these spiracles is important for they enable the insect to feed with its head immersed in liquid without drowning.

The anatomy of the digestive tract

The digestive tract is tubular, highly convoluted and, according to Robinson,[71] 90 - 95 mm in length, some 6 - 7 times the length of a full grown maggot. It consists of three principal sections each of which fulfils a particular digestive function. This may be illustrated by reference to a drawing of the structure of the gut of the blowfly *Phormia regina* published by Fletcher and Haub in 1933.[72]

Figure 78: Structure of a maggot's gut

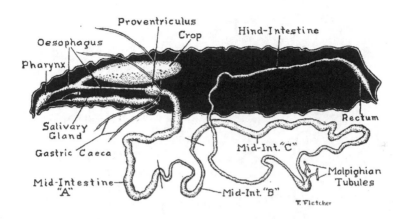

Image reproduced courtesy of the Ohio Academy of Science

The foregut extends from the mouth at the anterior end, and includes a short, very narrow, oesophagus which is attached to the pharynx into which also opens the salivary gland. Part way along the oesophagus is the entrance to the crop, effectively a large sac or reservoir for retaining undigested food. This lies along the back and, when full of ingested material, is clearly visible through the dorsal surface. The oesophagus enters the stomach through an enlarged muscular crop or proventriculus.

The midgut or 'stomach', also known as the mesenteron, (or mid-intestine in the diagram above) is long, about 60-65 mm comprising about two thirds of the length of the entire tract. It is here that most of the digestive processes take place. It too is histologically and functionally divided into three sections: the fore-, mid-, and hind-stomach. At the distal end of the midgut are the Malpighian tubes responsible for the production and excretion of uric acid and it is at this point that the midgut joins the hindgut, the region where faecal material is formed and water reabsorbed from the faecal mass.

The gut is very convoluted; the hind-gut is coiled outside the midgut, extending forward as far as the proventriculus before returning to the anus.[73]

The significance of the structure of the gut is considered in a more detail in the section on mechanism of action.

PRODUCTION AND USE OF MEDICAL MAGGOTS

Maggot production techniques

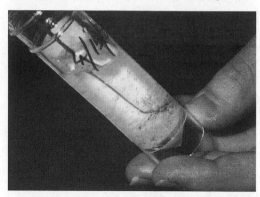

Figure 79: Separating eggs prior to sterilisation

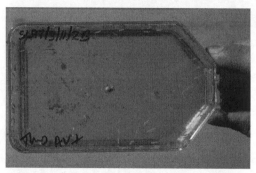

Figure 80: Maggots growing on sterile agar

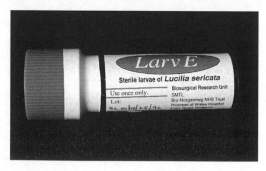

Figure 81: A vial of maggots

The techniques used to produce medical maggots vary from centre to centre and in some instances involve proprietary technology, but in essence the procedures used are broadly similar to those described by the early workers in the field.[31,33,41,44-49,74-77]

Flies are kept in suitable cages fed with sugar and water and presented with suitable materials upon which to lay their eggs - typically liver, egg, or some other suitable protein source. The external surface of an egg is normally very heavily contaminated with bacteria, which must be removed or killed if the emerging larvae are to remain sterile.

After collection the eggs are mechanically separated, cleansed, and chemically treated (sterilized) under aseptic conditions. Historically, a commonly used method consisted of pretreating the eggs with Dakin's solution (dilute sodium hypochlorite, or bleach) followed by immersion in mercuric chloride or formaldehyde. Simmons[76] reported satisfactory sterilisation using 5% formalin and 1% sodium hydroxide but even this did not kill all spore forming bacteria such as *Cl. perfringens* or *Cl. tetanii*.

The treated eggs are then transferred aseptically into sterile vessels containing an appropriate substrate such as agar to which has been added a protein source which will sustain the maggots without allowing them to grow too rapidly.

Before being approved for clinical use, the newly hatched maggots should be subjected to appropriate microbiological investigations to ensure either complete sterility or freedom from specific pathogenic organisms.

Modern maggot production techniques have been described by several authors,[78-83] but probably the most graphic and comprehensive account of the process appeared in a special supplement to the Journal of Wound Care published in 1996.[65]

Because of the very large bioburden present on the eggs prior to processing, a surface sterilising technique does not provided the required level of assurance for a sterile pharmaceutical preparation.

An alternative production technique, which could provide the required level of confidence in the sterility of the final product, involves the production of a colony of flies free from microorganisms which are kept under sterile conditions in a pharmaceutical clean room facility. Once the sterility of such a colony is confirmed, the eggs laid by the flies on a suitable sterile food source would also be bacteria free and thus not require the time-consuming and potentially ineffective chemical sterilisation process.

The concept of producing insects in this way is not novel. Greenberg[78] described three classes of insects with a modified microbiological population as follows: aposymbiotic - free of cellular symbiotes but not of intestinal microbes; aseptic - free of intestinal microbes but not symbiotes; and axenic - free of demonstrable cellular and intestinal microbes.

It is the axenic group that would be required for medical maggot production. This process is not without its problems as everything that comes into contact with the fly colony must be sterile including the food, water, egg laying medium and even the air that the insects breathe. A specially designed disposable cage designed for this purpose is described in a patent number GB2436199 (A); entitled 'Apparatus and an improved method for the production of and growth of sterile fly larvae.

Examples of artificial food sources which supply all the necessary nutrients for the insects have also been described in the literature,[84-87] but a formulation is required that can be shown to be free of viruses and other infective agents, which can also be sterilized by gamma irradiation prior to use.

METHOD OF APPLICATION

Free-range maggots

Over the years, numerous techniques and dressing systems have been described for ensuring that maggots, once applied, are contained within the area of the wound. Some of these systems were difficult to construct and almost certainly very uncomfortable to wear. Child et al.[45] used a piece of 80 mesh brass net set in a foam frame secured to the skin. Others, including Weil,[31] and Mckeever,[49] adopted a similar approach using copper mesh or milk strainer wire held in place with adhesive tape.

Self retaining metal[31] or glass devices[49] were also described which were used to hold wounds open during therapy, allowing free drainage of exudate whilst providing the maggots easy access to all areas.

Ochsenhirt and Komara[54] described a complex technique for intraoral treatment, involving dentures incorporating tubes which extended out of the mouth through which the larvae were introduced - a technique which, unsurprisingly, did not appear to gain widespread popularity!

A less drastic approach for normal skin wounds involved the use of layers of crinoline or gauze,[33] sometimes secured in place around the wound margins with Unna's Paste - a mixture of zinc oxide, gelatin, glycerin, and water.[51]

As part of the application process, Livingston[46] recommended exposing the maggots, once applied, to a bright light in order to drive them deep into the wound, but this was considered unnecessary by Robinson[88] who also emphasized the need to control the number of larvae applied, proposing that as few as 6 might be sufficient for a finger tip injury although 500-600 may be required for more extensive wounds

Large quantities of larval enzymes can cause significant excoriation if they are allowed to run onto unprotected skin around the margin of a wound. In severe cases this resembles a superficial burn, but like such an injury, this will rapidly resolve over a few days.[65] Robinson[88] who had also encountered this problem, suggested that the surrounding skin should be covered to protect it from larval secretions and to eliminate the tickling sensation caused by the maggots' movements. He considered that the collodion proposed by Weil et al.[31] and adhesive plaster advocated by Child,[45] were not suitable as they tended to separate from the skin once wet. He suggested that a liquid adhesive system described by Buchman and Blair,[47] or the Unna's paste described by Jewett,[51] would both be far more satisfactory for this purpose.

In more recent years several different types of maggot dressings have been described, constructed from readily available dressing materials.[89-93] In 1998 Thomas et al.[94] published an illustrated application guide using a model wound which showed each individual step involved in the production of a maggot dressing.

For small wounds the guide suggested that a tracing of the wound may be prepared on a sterile plastic sheet to form a template which is then used to cut out a matching wound-sized hole from a hydrocolloid dressing, a self-adhesive wafer with a semipermeable film on the outer surface although the use of a tracing may be omitted if required.

This hydrocolloid sheet protects the intact skin from irritation by the maggots' proteolytic enzymes and protects the patient from sensing the movement of the larvae. It also forms a base to which adhesives tapes can be fixed with causing damage to the skin.

Using a small volume of sterile saline, the sterile maggots are then irrigated out of the container in which they are supplied onto a piece of sterile fine mesh nylon net placed upon an absorbent layer such as a nonwoven swab. This absorbent layer draws away excess fluid leaving the maggots in small heap on the surface of the nylon mesh. This is then inverted over the wound and the edges stuck to the hydrocolloid using a waterproof adhesive tape. This dressing system effectively forms a little 'cage' that retains the maggots in the wound, allowing them to breathe whilst facilitating drainage of the liquefied necrotic tissue and serous exudate. The entire process is extremely simple, taking only a few moments to perform. The dressing is finally covered with a simple absorbent pad held in place with adhesive tape or a bandage. A layer of moist gauze is sometimes placed over the net under the absorbent pad to prevent the young maggots from drying out in the early stages of their development. For areas that are more difficult to dress, such as the toes or feet, the nylon mesh is supplied heat sealed into a bag or sleeve that is taped to strips of hydrocolloid dressing placed above and/or below the wound. For patients whose skin is too fragile to permit the use of adhesive dressings, or patients who are allergic to hydrocolloid dressings, a zinc oxide paste can be used to protect the skin and form a seal with the nylon net, a technique formally similar to that formally used by Jewett.[51]

The quantity of maggots applied is determined by the size of the wound and the amount of necrotic tissue present. Originally a maximum of about 10 maggots per cm^2 was suggest as recommended by Robinson,[88] but provided the surrounding skin is well protected, the maximum number of maggots applied is probably not critical. It is more cost effective to use a large number of maggots for a short period of time than a small number for an extended period. A simple calculator which provided some broad guidance on the number of maggots to be applied to different sized wounds was published in 2001.[95]

The dressing is removed from the wound one to three days later by which time the maggots are usually fully developed and typically about 8 mm long. The removal process is relatively simple, the outer dressing is simply peeled away and any maggots remaining in the wound are collected with forceps or a gloved hand as they attempt to escape. The dressing together with the maggots should be sealed in a plastic bag and disposed of in the manner customary for other potentially infectious dressings and waste. Depending upon the condition of the wound, a fresh batch of larvae or a conventional dressing may then be applied.

Figure 82: Formation of a simple maggot dressing

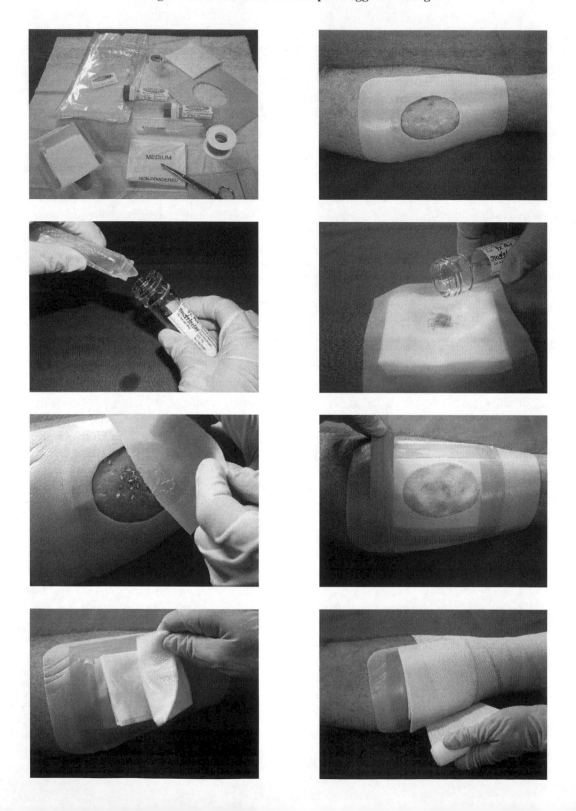

Figure 83: Formation of a maggot 'sleeve' dressing'

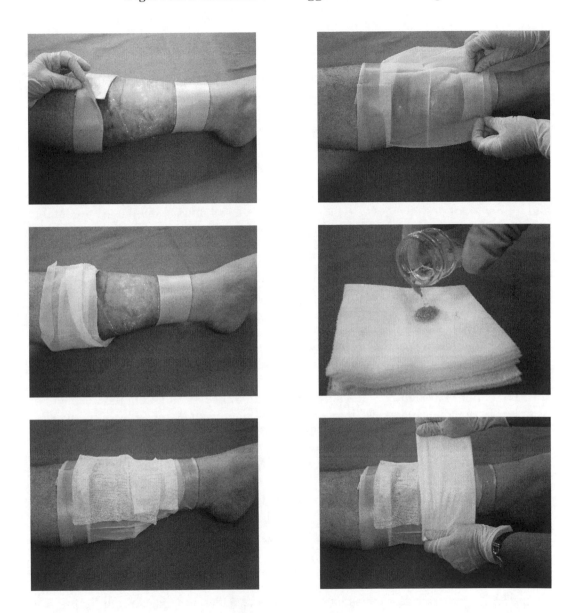

When dressing toes or digits, a modification to this technique may be used in which a suitably sized closed bag is applied to the relevant area, taking care to protect the skin surrounding the area to be treated by the application of a suitable barrier cream.

Maggots in bags

There is no doubt that many people find the idea of having maggots applied to their wounds distasteful, particularly given their association with decay, death and disease. This feeling of revulsion may be reinforced by the sight of the creatures crawling disappearing in small sinuses or apparently burrowing into dead tissue.

In an attempt to overcome this problem, an alternative application technique was devised in which the maggots are supplied in bags constructed from a fine nylon mesh or layers of polyvinyl alcohol foam sheet 0.5-mm thick. The bags which also contain a small cube of spacer material to prevent them collapsing are applied directly to the wound and held in place with a suitable secondary dressing. In this way, application and removal of the maggots is facilitated and, depending upon the nature of the material from which the bag is constructed, the enclosed maggots are either partially or totally obscured from view.

The theory behind the use of these bags is that the enzymes which are produced in prodigious quantities by the maggots are released into the wound to exert their biological effect but the creatures themselves are not able to wander freely over the wound surface. These bags were first produced commercially by Biomonde and marketed as 'Biobags'.[96]

Whilst maggots contained in this way might be expected to function reasonably well on an open wound, the advantages of convenience and increased patient or doctor acceptability associated with this presentation are likely to be offset by a reduction in speed of action. Furthermore the value of the bags will be of limited in the treatment of narrow cavity wounds, sinuses, or wounds with a significant degree of undermining.

Laboratory studies, supported by clinical experience,[97] suggested that the growth rate, and therefore the efficacy of maggots contained in simple foam or net bags is impaired compared with the free-range variety and this observation was supported by the results of a 64 patient study reported by Steenvoorde et al.[98] who showed that patients treated with free-range maggots had significantly better outcomes than those dressed with the simple bags, 79.6% vs 46.7% (p = 0.028), and required fewer treatments, 2.4 vs 4.3 (p = 0.028). Specifically in the contained group 6/15 patients eventually needed major amputation compared with on 6/54 in the free-range group. Lerch et al.[99] placed both free-range and bagged maggots on agar plates inoculated with a strain of E. coli that produces a green fluorescent protein and recorded the time taken for the fluorescent organisms to become detectable in the insects gut. In the case of the free-range maggots the bacteria were detectable after 3 minutes and reached maximum intensity after 5 minutes (± 0.1 min). Maggots contained in vinyl bags showed no evidence of fluorescence after 5 minutes and did not reach maximum fluorescence for 25 minutes. Examination of frozen sections of the maggots gut under the microscope showed a gradual decrease in fluorescence from the crop, which fluoresced strongly to the posterior gut where no evidence of fluorescence was detected. In contrast to the above, Blake et al.[100] found no difference between the nutritional activity of maggots that were allowed to crawl freely over their food source with those confined within a Biobag and concluded that the debridement efficiency of the two presentations was comparable.

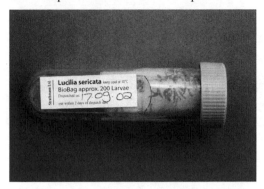

Figure 84: A net 'Biobag' in transit container

A significant improvement to these early bags resulted from research work undertaken by Zoobiotic which involved the production of a maggot bag which also contained substantial quantities of small chips made from hydrophilic polyurethane foam. Called a 'Biofoam' dressing it is claimed to combine the proven advantages of free-range maggots with the clinical benefits of absorbent foam used in many conventional products.

Laboratory studies revealed, somewhat unexpectedly, that the presence of the foam chips markedly increased both the survival and growth rate of the maggots contained within the bags when they were placed on a food source such as liver. An even more unexpected observation was that there appeared to be a direct correlation between maggot development and the total mass of foam present. The reason for this is not clear, but one explanation may be that the foam removes excess wound fluid which otherwise has the effect of diluting the maggots externalised secretions. It is also possible that the physical environment produced by the closely packed moist foam chips also in some way facilitates maggot development. The dressing can either be left undisturbed for the duration of the treatment which may last 2 - 5 days, or be removed to allow regular inspection of the wound then replaced if required – something that is not possible with free-range maggots.

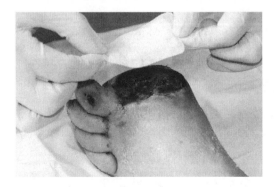

Figure 85: Application of a Biofoam Dressing

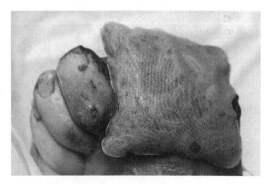

Figure 86: Biofoam dressing prior to removal four days later

MECHANISM OF ACTION

The maggot 'active principle'

According to an historical account in paper by Maseritz,[101] the biological activity of maggot secretions was first investigated by Fabre in 1894, who observed that they brought about rapid liquefaction of coagulated albumin - an activity he attributed to the secretion of pepsin. Maseritz described how Guyénot in 1906 made extracts of maggots and their salivary glands but failed to demonstrate activity against proteins, carbohydrates or fats. He did, however, isolate a microorganism which he showed was capable of liquefying protein and therefore attributed the digestive activity associated with maggots to this organism, a conclusion subsequently apparently supported by the work of Bogdanow. In 1911 Wollman produced evidence which suggested that the autoclaving process previously used by both Guyénot and Bogdanow to produce the test substrates in a sterile form, had rendered them resistant to the maggots' enzymes thus leading them to make an incorrect assumption. In 1931 the issue was resolved when Hobson[102] finally demonstrated the presence of a proteolytic enzyme in the excreta and gut of *L. sericata* capable of digesting gelatin, elastin and white fibrous tissue collagen.

Maseritz himself investigated the effects of the secretions of *Phormia regina* on preparations of bone from human ribs and showed that they contained an enzyme capable of digesting collagen, the organic component of bone. He also screened an emulsion prepared from intact maggots for antimicrobial activity but found that far from inhibiting bacterial growth the emulsion actually facilitated it. It is perhaps surprising that he did not also test the maggot secretions he had collected for the first part of his study for antimicrobial activity as these may well have produced a different result.

During the 1930s, various attempts were made to isolate and identify the biologically active chemical agents or agents assumed to be present in maggot secretions. Livingston in 1932[103-104] described the treatment of 567 patients using MT alone, or in combination with 'maggot active principle' which he produced by grinding live maggots of *L. sericata* in sterile saline. He also used a polyvalent vaccine of pyogenic organisms suspended in the maggot principle as a vehicle administered intra-muscularly. This technique was said to produce a success rate of 88%, 38% higher than control cases treated by other methods. Perhaps not surprisingly, this was associated with significant systemic reactions, and eventually abandoned.

Elia,[105] commenting upon the work of Livingston, suggested that the active principle was in fact an enzyme, possibly pepsin, which liquefies their food source which the maggots then ingest by suction. Responding to this letter Livingston stated that that maggots do not feed entirely by suction as they also have a pair of mandibles or hooks which they use to disrupt tissue, releasing small particles which can be identified within their crop.[106] He also stated that the active principle could not be pepsin as suggested by Elia as the secretions are alkaline, and pepsin does not work under these conditions.

Robinson in 1933[107] neatly summarized the benefits of maggots therapy, stating that the treatment removed necrotic tissue, facilitated drainage, promoted the production of granulation tissue and combated infection. Each of these roles is considered in more detail below.

Wound debridement activity

Necrophagous larvae feed on dead tissue, cellular debris, and serous drainage (exudate) of corpses or necrotic wounds. Crile[43] in 1917 commented:

> *'The maggots live on devitalized tissue and if they destroy that tissue,*
> *they do in time what the surgical operation does'*

As previously identified, contrary to popular belief, maggots do not have teeth and therefore cannot actively 'chew away' dead tissue. They feed mainly by a process of extracorporeal digestion, producing secretions containing powerful collagenases and trypsin-like and chymotrypsin-like enzymes which rapidly breakdown dead tissue into a semi-liquid form that the creatures can ingest.[72-73,102,108-113] Because of this mode of action they have previously be likened to 'living chemical factories',[114] or 'carpet shampooers'.[115]

Casu et al.[116-117] purified two chymotrypsin-like serine proteases from the secretory and excretory material of first instar larvae of L. cuprina. At least one of these proteases was thought to degrade collagen, confirming the earlier observations of Ziffren.[110] Young et al.[118-119] showed that secretions produced by newly hatched larvae of L. cuprina change quite dramatically over a short period of time and although a wide range of proteases are produced at all time points examined, some appear to be developmentally regulated and also appear to be influenced by the nature of the substrate upon which the maggots are feeding. They also showed that most of this activity is lost in the presence of serine protease inhibitors, a finding consistent with that of Schmidtchen et al.[120] who demonstrated the production of 20 - 50 kDa serine proteinases by L. sericata both in the laboratory and in patients receiving MT.

When Chambers et al.[121] examined maggots' secretions using class-specific substrates and inhibitors they were able to identify three classes of proteolytic enzymes. The predominant activity was due to serine proteinases (pH optima 8-9) belonging to two different subclasses, trypsin-like and chymotrypsin like, with a weaker aspartyl proteinase (pH 5) and a metalloproteinase (pH 9) with exopeptidase characteristics also present.

They then used extracellular matrix components of skin as substrates and showed that the secretions were capable of solubilising fibrin clots and degrading fibronectin, laminin and acid-solubilised collagen types I and III. This activity was inhibited by the addition of phenylmethylsulphonyl fluoride but not 4-amidiminophenyl-methylsulphonyl fluoride, indicating that degradation was due to the 'chymotrypsin-like' serine proteinase present. The trypsin-like activity did not appear to play a major role in ECM degradation but may have other as yet unidentified activity within the wound.

Antibacterial activity

In their natural environment blowfly larvae feed upon material which is very heavily contaminated with microorganisms of all types. For the maggots to compete and survive they must be able to tolerate, if not eradicate, these potential pathogens.

In an early review published in 1926, Duncan[122] recorded how other workers in the first twenty years of the 20th Century had shown that many insect species were capable of killing organisms taken into their gut whilst feeding, and that this activity was due to the presence of one or more unidentified molecules or 'active principles'. A similar view was expressed by Hobson in a number of publications.[73,123]

Livingston and Prince[103] claimed to have demonstrated bactericidal activity in a filtered extract prepared from crushed maggots, but other workers[101,107,124] subsequently disputed this claim.

Robinson *et al.*[71,107] dissected maggots that had been feeding on necrotic tissue to examine the distribution of bacteria within their alimentary tract. In all the specimens examined, abundant bacterial growth was found in the fore-stomach but no growth at all was detected in the intestine; an intermediate area called the hind-stomach showed slight growth in one third of cases. A progressive destruction of bacteria was therefore found to take place in the alimentary canal. It is perhaps significant that the majority of this activity is found in the hind-stomach, a region which Hobson had earlier demonstrated possessed marked proteolytic activity.

The fact that bacteria are lysed as they pass through the insects' gut was elegantly confirmed by Mumcuoglu *et al.*[125] who used a laser scanning confocal microscope to investigate the fate of green fluorescent protein-producing *E. coli* as they passed through the alimentary tract of sterile maggots of *L. sericata*. A computer program was used to analyze the intensity of the fluorescence and to quantify the number of bacteria.

They found that the crop and the anterior midgut were the most heavily infected areas of the intestine. A significant decrease in the amount of bacteria was observed in the posterior midgut. The number of bacteria decreased even more significantly in the anterior hindgut and practically no bacteria were seen in the posterior end, near the anus.

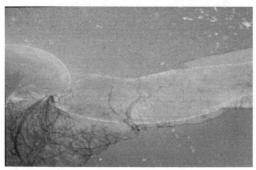
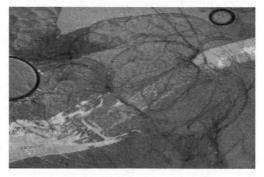

Figure 87: Anterior midgut   **Figure 88: Posterior hindgut**

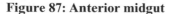

Photographs courtesy of Kosta Mumcuoglu

The viability of the bacteria in the different parts of the gut was also examined by a microbiological method and it was found that in the insects examined, 66.7% of the crops, 52.8% of the midguts, 55.6% of the anterior hindguts, and 17.8% of posterior hindguts contained viable bacteria. The results of both these experimental techniques were consistent with the earlier observations of Robinson that the majority of bacteria (*E. coli* in this instance) were destroyed in the midgut. Most of the remaining bacteria were killed in the hindgut, indicating that the faeces were either sterile or contained only small numbers of viable organisms.

Some early authors also suggested that wound exudate, abundant in response to the activity of the maggots, facilitated the irrigation of bacteria out of wounds[126] and that the alkalinity of maggot-treated wounds contributed to wound disinfection. Baer[40] was the first to demonstrate that wound fluid was alkaline during MT, and Messer and McClellan[127] believed that ammonia secreted by the maggots was the cause. Subsequently, ammonia and ammonium derivatives such as ammonium bicarbonate were suggested as the factors responsible for disinfection and wound-healing.[128-129] Stewart's studies led him to conclude that calcium and calcium carbonate produced by the maggots killed bacteria directly, stimulated phagocytosis, and possibly promoted the growth of granulation tissue.[32]

Simmons, in 1935,[130-131] showed the presence of antimicrobial activity in excretions collected from both sterile and non-sterile maggots of *L. sericata* and Pavillard and Wright[132] in 1957 isolated and partially purified a substance from the secretions of non-sterile *Phormia terraenovae* larvae which killed *S. pyogenes* and *S. pneumoniae* (pneumococcus). *S. aureus* was much less sensitive to this substance and *E. coli* and *P. vulgaris* were both highly resistant. Injection of this isolate into mice protected the mice from the lethal effects of intraperitoneal injections of pneumococcus. Unfortunately, Pavillard and Wright never identified the chemical structure of this agent.

Thomas *et al.*,[133] similarly showed that secretions collected from sterile maggots also possessed marked antimicrobial activity against *Streptococcus* A and B and *S. aureus*. Some activity was also detected against *Pseudomonas sp.* and a clinical isolate of a resistant strain of *S. aureus* (MRSA). No evidence of inhibition was recorded against *Enterococcus* or the Gram-negative bacteria *E. coli* and *Proteus*. No attempts were made in this preliminary study to isolate or identify the agent or agents responsible for the observed antimicrobial activity and the possibility of a significant pH effect could not be ruled out. Elevated pH alone, however, could not be entirely responsible for the inhibitory effects of larval secretions as *S. aureus* was able to grow in broth buffered to pH 9.

The effect of maggot therapy on the bioburden of the wounds of 16 patients successfully treated with an average of seven courses of maggot therapy for an average of 27 days was reported by Steenvoorde and Jukema.[134] Most patients were treated for osteomyelitis, with trauma being the principal causative factor. Overall MT was found to be more effective in wounds infected with Gram-positive organisms than Gram-negative bacteria which were cultured more often after maggot treatment than before it (p = 0.001), although the authors noted that increasing the number of maggots applied appeared to reverse this trend.

Jaklic *et al.*[135] examined the effect of maggot secretions on a different bacterial species in both *in vitro* and *in vivo* studies and once again found that they were most effective against Gram-positive organisms such as *S. aureus* but less effective against Gram-negative organisms especially Proteus spp. and Pseudomonas spp. Bacteria from the genus Vagococcus were found to be totally resistant to the secretions.

Kerridge *et al.*[136] and Bexfield[137-138] also showed that secretions from *L. sericata* were active against a range of potentially pathogenic and antibiotic resistant organisms.

It is likely the results of all these laboratory-based investigations actually represent a significant *underestimate* of the ability of maggots to overcome infection *in vivo*. In such situations secretions are produced continuously by the feeding larvae, resulting in much higher concentrations of the active agents. The laboratory test methods also take no account of the ability of actively feeding larvae to ingest bacteria and destroy them in their gut as described by Robinson and Norwood[107] and Mumcuoglu.[125]

This second, and possibly more important mechanism, may explain the reported ability of maggots to eliminate clinical infection from wounds caused by MRSA[139-140] and pseudomonas, - organisms that are less susceptible to their externalised secretions under laboratory conditions. In such situations, however, it is important to ensure that a sufficient number of maggots are present in the wound to exert an antimicrobial effect.

In 1968, Greenberg[141] suggested that the ability of maggots to kill bacteria was due to metabolic products of *P. mirabilis*, a commensal of the larval gut. These chemicals, which he called 'mirabilicides', were highly lethal to Gram-positive and Gram-negative bacteria under acidic conditions. Some support for this theory was provided by Erdmann and Khalil,[142-143] who subsequently identified two antibacterial substances, phenylacetic acid and phenylacetaldehyde, which were produced by *P. mirabilis* isolated from the gut of screwworm larvae (*C. hominivorax*).

However, the results of laboratory studies involving secretions collected from sterile maggots,[139-140,144] clearly show that Greenberg's hypothesis that the antimicrobial activity of maggot secretions was due to metabolic activity of a gut commensal was incorrect, although it is entirely possible that sterile maggots when applied to a wound may become colonised with this organism which may further enhance their ability to kill other microbial species *in vivo*.

The limited antimicrobial action of maggot secretions against Pseudomonas was investigated in laboratory study which paid particular attention to the quorum-sensing (QS)-regulated virulence.[145] The maggots were challenged with *P. aeruginosa* wild-type (WT) PAO1 tagged with green fluorescent protein (GFP) and a GFP-tagged *P. aeruginosa* QS-deficient mutant in different concentrations. Maggots were killed in the presence of WT PAO1 whereas the challenge with the QS mutant showed a survival reduction of approximately 25 % compared to negative controls. Furthermore, ingestion of bacteria by the maggots was lower in the presence of WT PAO1 compared to the PAO1 mutant. When the maggot excretions/secretions (ES) were assayed for the presence of QS inhibitors only high doses of ES showed inhibition of QS in *P. aeruginosa*. The authors therefore concluded that *P. aeruginosa* was toxic to *L. sericata* maggots confirming the clinical observations reported previously.

It has long been recognised that insects have well established defence mechanisms against bacterial infections. The injection of bacterial cultures induces the presence of antibacterial peptides, termed 'insect defensins' in the insects' blood.[146-147] These antibacterial peptides usually exceed 3 kDa and some of them have been produced commercially. A comprehensive review of the antimicrobial peptides isolated from a host of invertebrates including flesh flies, was published by Salzet in 2005.[148]

In one study published by Bexfield et al.,[137] examination of secretions collected from sterile L. sericata revealed that the active molecule(s) are heat stable and protease resistant. They are also slightly alkaline, with the majority of samples examined in the range pH 8.2 - 8.3. A negative correlation between pH and bacterial activity was noted suggesting that those samples with the highest pH had the greatest antibacterial activity. Adjusting the pH of the individual samples did not negate these initial differences. Fractionation of the secretions revealed two discrete antibacterial activities associated with the 500 Da - 10 kDa and < 500 Da fractions but only the < 500 Da fraction exhibited significant activity against MRSA. This low molecular weight molecule is too small to be one of the many the previously described low-M_r insect peptides but it is similar in size to β-alanyl-tyrosine (252 Da) an antimicrobial dipeptide isolated from the larvae of the fleshfly Neobellieria bullata and N-β-alanyl-5-S-glutathionyl-3,4-dihydroxy-phenylalanine, 5-S-GAD, (573 Da) from the adult fleshfly Sarcophaga peregine.

The mechanism of action of the low molecular fraction from L. sericata was examined in a further study by the same group,[138] which once again confirmed that that the molecule has broad spectrum activity. It was also found to induce marked morphological changes in individual cells of Bacillus cereus, resulting in extensive bacterial filamentation compared with controls. In the case of E. coli, cells exposed to the extracts became rounded taking on a lemon or racket shape; tests also showed that the secretions exert either static or cidal effects depending on the bacterial species in question.

Kerridge et al.[136] also investigated the antibacterial properties of L. sericata secretions. They similarly reported the presence of a small (< 1 kDa) antibacterial factor(s) which possessed the spectrum of activity previously reported. They found the secretions to be highly stable as a freeze dried preparation and suggested that it might offer benefits in the treatment of MRSA infections.

Cerovsky et al.[149] isolated and characterised a novel homologue of insect defensin which they designated lucifensin (Lucilia defensins) from the extracts of various tissues (gut, salivary glands, fat body, haemolymph) of L. sericata larvae and from their excretions/secretions. This they found to be very similar to sapecin and other dipteran defensins and assumed that it is the key antimicrobial component that protects the maggots from infection in their normal feeding environment. They proposed that 'lucifensin' is that long-sought larger molecular weight antimicrobial factor of the L. sericata excretions/secretions which are believed to be responsible for the insects' ability to kill pathogenic organisms in clinical practice.

Effect upon biofilm formation

As previously described, a major contribution to the development of infection by some species of bacteria is the formation of a biofilm, an aggregate of microorganisms in which individual cells become bound to a surface and to each other within a complex matrix of extracellular polymeric substances. Van der Plas et al.[150] examined the effects of maggot secretions on biofilm production by *S. aureus* and *P. aeruginosa* using microtitre plate assays, and upon bacterial viability using *in vitro* killing and radial diffusion assays, and on quorum sensing systems using specific reporter bacteria. They found that as little as 0.2 µg of secretions prevented *S. aureus* biofilm formation and 2 µg rapidly degraded existing biofilms. In contrast, the secretions initially promoted biofilm formation by *P. aeruginosa*, but after 10 h the biofilms collapsed. Boiling of the secretions abrogated their effects on *S. aureus* biofilms but not those produced by *P. aeruginosa*, indicating that different molecules within the secretions are responsible for the observed effects. The activity did not involve bacterial killing or quorum sensing systems.

In a follow up study[151] the same researches demonstrated assessed the effect of combinations of maggot secretions and antibiotics on *S. aureus* biofilms and on the survival of the bacteria released from the biofilms. They found that Vancomycin and daptomycin dose-dependently enhanced biofilm formation, but clindamycin reduced *S. aureus* biofilm size. The addition of maggot secretions to the test system caused a complete biofilm breakdown rendering the bacteria released susceptible to the antibiotics.

The ability of maggots' secretions to breakdown biofilms on polyethylene, titanium, and stainless steel was investigated by Cazander et al.[152] using secretions of first and third instar maggots of *L. sericata*. They showed that they not only prevented biofilm formation, but even helped to break it down once formed, and suggested that these findings may have implications for the treatment of infections associated with orthopaedic implants.

Stimulation of wound healing

The rapid development of healthy granulation tissue in maggot-treated wounds has for centuries led some practitioners to speculate that maggots actually stimulate wounds to heal more quickly. It was initially suggested that the secretions that were responsible for the antimicrobial effect could also account for the growth-promoting activity of maggots and it was even claimed that the abundant growth of granulation tissue was, at least in part, a response to the physical stimulation of the maggots crawling over the wound,[47] although this is now considered unlikely.

Allantoin, (2,5-Dioxo-4-imidazolidinyl) urea, first isolated from comfrey root, was isolated from maggot secretions,[153] where it occurs as a product of purine metabolism. It was suggested that this molecule, which is still used today in some cosmetics and pharmaceuticals, was at least partly responsible for the beneficial effects of maggots' secretions on wound healing.[154-155] Ammonium bicarbonate[129] and urea were also found to be present and as a result various mixture of these,[129,155] and other agents including picric acid,[156] were proposed as alternatives to live maggots. In 1977 Lewy[157] criticized Horn's use of maggots for wound debridement,[61] citing his own earlier experimental work with urea in 1937, suggesting that this might have been equally as effective, a suggestion which Gates et al. subsequently repudiated.[158]

Potential mechanisms by which maggot secretions may influence wound healing have been investigated by a number of research groups. Early evidence emerged from the work of Prete,[159] who assessed the growth promoting effects of maggot secretions on mammalian tissue by exposing them to human fibroblasts in culture in the presence and absence of epidermal growth factor (EGF) and recombinant interleukin-6 (IL-6). Alimentary secretions were found to stimulate fibroblast growth as determined by ^{3}H-thymidine incorporation but only to about 10% of the maximum increase produced by EGF. She also showed that the addition of maggot secretions to EGF and IL-6-stimulated fibroblasts further increased their growth rate, suggesting that these secretions stimulate cell development by a different mechanism from that of EGF.

Horobin et al.[160-162] investigated the effects of larval secretions upon human dermal fibroblasts and extracellular matrix proteins and showed that they reduced fibroblast cell adhesion and promoted cell migration over extracellular matrix (ECM) component surfaces such as fibronectin and collagen, an effect which was associated with their proteolytic activity; degradation of the ECM by larval secretion was thought to lead to the formation of bioactive peptides which could modulate fibroblast behaviour. The same research group subsequently incorporated maggot secretions into a hydrogel which they applied to fibroblasts and keratinocytes in a laboratory wound model and showed that this presentation, like the native secretion, was capable of promoting cell migration, (and therefore it is assumed wound closure), without exerting a significant mitogenic effect.[163]

Wang et al.[164] in a randomized control study examined the influence of maggot secretions on expression of bFGF and connective tissue growth factor (CTGF) in a wound model in rats with induced diabetes mellitus. Compared with the control wounds, those treated with the maggot secretions were clean and healed rapidly. In the control group 60% of wounds became infected with S. aureus but none of the wounds in the treated group showed signs of infection. Wounds treated with maggot secretions also produced elevated expressions of bFGF and CTFG in ulcers ($p < 0.05$).

Van der Plas et al.[150] assessed the effects of maggot secretions on functional activities of human neutrophils and found that they inhibited elastase release and H_2O_2 production by activated neutrophils in a dose-depend fashion. The secretions did not affect phagocytosis and intracellular killing of C. albicans by neutrophils. Based upon these and other observations, the authors suggested that the beneficial effects of maggots on chronic wounds may be explained in part by inhibition of multiple pro-inflammatory responses of activated neutrophils. These conclusions were subsequently supported by Pecivova et al.[165] who also examined the effect of salivary glands extracts (SGE) of maggots on opsonized zymosan stimulated whole blood chemiluminescence (CL), superoxide generation and myeloperoxidase (MPO) release from human neutrophils. Crude SGE extracts had no significant effect either on superoxide generation and MPO release from isolated unstimulated human neutrophils or on activity of isolated enzymes but significantly decreased opsonized zymosan stimulated blood CL, superoxide generation and MPO release. Like Van der Plas *et al.* they proposed that the beneficial effects of maggot therapy might involve a reduction in the generation and release of neutrophil-derived pro-inflammatory factors, while neither phagocytosis nor subsequent apoptosis is disturbed. Brandner *et al.*[166] confirmed that maggot secretions had a stimulatory effect upon wound healing rates using an '*ex vivo*' porcine wound healing model which involved biopsies taken from pig ears removed from animals slaughtered for human consumption.

The ability of maggot secretions to promote the cellular processes involved in wound healing, and which have been observed in many clinical studies as the enhanced production of granulation tissue, were investigated in eight patients using contact-free remittance spectroscopy, a technique which objectively measures changes in chronic wounds associated with enhanced blood supply and the formation of granulation tissue. The remittance spectra of maggot treated wounds showed an improvement of tissue oxygenation as revealed by the characteristic oxygen doublet peak which the authors suggested, argue for a positive effect of larval secretions on tissue oxygenation, oedema and the formation of red granulation tissue.[167]

A more specialist potential application for maggot secretions was described by Zhang *et al.*[168] who found that the homogenate product from disinfected maggot larvae can promote wound nerve regeneration and suggested that this could be used with advantage as an external layer outside a chitosan tube applied as a biocompatible and biodegradable bilateral guide for nerve repair

In 1936, Livingston[104] suggested that no simple group of chemicals could replace the complex nature of maggot secretions and despite the progress that has been made to date on the isolation and identification of some of the active agents produced by these creatures, it still seems unlikely that these can be as effective as the creatures themselves in cleansing, disinfecting and promoting the growth of new tissue.

EARLY ACCOUNTS OF THE USE OF MAGGOT THERAPY

The early maggot therapy literature contains many references to the successful treatment of chronic or acutely infected soft tissue injuries, including those infected with *C. welchii* (*C. perfringens*) the 'gas bacillus'. Wounds treated with maggots included abscesses,[31] carbuncles,[33] leg ulcers,[55] pressure ulcers, mastoiditis[61] and compound fractures.[33] However, in the early days maggots were primarily used in the treatment of osteomyelitis,[31,33,40-41,45-47,50,52,55,103,106] and although unable to digest or liquefy dead bone (sequestra) they were said to facilitate its separation at the interface with normal bone, leaving behind clean healthy granulation tissue.[31] Very many dramatic accounts of the use of MT appear in the literature summarized by Pomeranz,[53] who stated that following maggot therapy;

> *'The end product approximates more closely to normal bone structure than any of the hitherto accepted methods of treatment'.*

It was also claimed repeatedly that in addition to removing devitalized tissue, the application of maggots had a positive effect upon the speed of wound healing. This was first noted by Larrey in 1829 who reported that when maggots developed in wounds sustained in battle, they prevented the development of infection and accelerated healing.[169] This view was also shared by Baer[40] and Fine[33] who stated that;

> *'Maggots produce rapid and thorough debridement and stimulate granulation tissue production' and 'When debridement is complete, fewer maggots are used and their function at this time is to complete to keep the wound clean and promote healing.'*

Weil *et al.*[31] the first to coin the term 'larval therapy' also asserted that;

> *'Coincident with the removal of necrotic and devitalized soft structures, is the development of highly vascular granulation tissue which excretes abundant serum and which may be looked upon as a very beneficial factor in wound defence in this form of therapy. ... The apposition of wound margins following larval therapy brings about a rapid development of granulation tissue, which can often be noted within a few hours'.*

Maggots appear to have another interesting and potentially very valuable ability; they are able to destroy unhealthy or abnormal tissue leaving healthy tissue in its place. Weil *et al.*[31] observed,

> *'When the larvae come into contact with exuberant and edematous granulations, they attack it vigorously, and remove it as any other abnormal structure, after which the change to healthy granulation tissue soon occurs. We have observed that the larvae will attack almost any type of abnormal viable structure, including malignant tissue as well as devitalized soft or bony tissues.'*

This they illustrated by reference to two cases of inoperable breast cancer and two sarcomas of the thigh.

> *'On admission, each breast ulcer measured the approximate size of half a dollar with the malignant tissue presenting itself upon a level with the surrounding skin. There was extensive invasion of almost the entire breast substance. Following four implantation of larvae, in one case there was observed an excavation of the underlying malignant tissues for a depth of 3.5-4 cm but with only slight variation in the size of the original skin opening. As the larvae cleared away the malignant tissue, clean healthy granulation tissue appeared, the odour disappeared and the wound attempted to close.'*

The remaining cases showed a similar response and the authors concluded that malignant tissue has a very weak defence against the activity of larvae.

Subsequently, Bunkis *et al.*[170] and Reames *et al.*[171] described the benefits of debridement and odour control resulting from accidental myiasis of head and neck tumours, and Seaquist and colleagues[172] also reported benefits from naturally occurring *Phormia regina* myiasis in a malignant lesion although this infestation was accompanied by pain.

MODERN MAGGOT THERAPY

Rationale for use

According to one estimate,[173] the management of chronic wounds costs the National Health Service about £1bn per annum, a figure that takes no account of the sociological or economic consequences suffered by patients with wounds such as leg or diabetic ulcers.

Many new treatments have been developed to facilitate the management of these and other soft tissue injuries, including: growth factors, proteinase inhibitors, gene therapy and skin substitutes of various types. Conventional dressings and wound management materials are also becoming more sophisticated and technologically advanced, replacing more basic products that have a simple absorptive function. Given all of these new developments, the question might reasonably be asked, why, in the 21st Century, are maggots still being used to treat wounds of all descriptions?

The answer is simple - if these expensive new treatments are to function optimally they must be applied to wounds free from infection or necrotic tissue, for according to Falanga,[174] the application of expensive new dressings or skin substitutes to an inadequately prepared wound is doomed to failure, a massive waste of time and resources. Leading clinicians and some manufacturers of wound dressings have therefore come to recognize that wound bed preparation is a key factor in determining treatment outcomes and a variety of dressings and pharmaceutical agents are promoted for this purpose. Experience suggests that the application of maggots remains the most rapid and cost-effective treatment available for debriding all types of infected or necrotic wounds.

Early experience

The background to the use of MT, and its introduction into the United States was described in early publications by Pechter and Sherman[175] and Sherman et al.,[64,81-82,176-177] whilst early accounts of the use of the technique in Europe were published by Thomas et al.[65,90,115,178]

As the treatment gained popularity, numerous other papers appeared in the literature and whilst some of these are reviews or digests of previously published articles,[90,179-191] others describe the successful use of maggots in specific therapeutic areas,[192] or describe the treatment of one or more patients with wounds of differing aetiology.[115,193-200] Several letters have also appeared in medical journals extolling the virtues of maggot therapy.[201-204]

Mumcuoglu et al.[205] described how they treated 25 patients with 35 wounds of various types including pressure ulcers and leg ulcers that had been present for between one and 90 months. Maggots were applied two to five times weekly and replaced every one to two days. Complete debridement was achieved in 38 wounds (88.4%). One wound remained unchanged the remaining four showed some improvement. In five patients who were scheduled for amputation, the operation was prevented by the use of the maggots.

Wolff and Hansson[206] similarly investigated the value of MT in 74 patients with wounds of different aetiologies and reported that 86% of wounds were successfully cleansed. Treatment reduced wound pain in one quarter of subjects but 34% experienced increased pain during treatment. Odour was reduced in 58% of 31 foul smelling wounds.

The somewhat unusual nature of maggot therapy meant that initially it tended to be reserved for used in the hospital environment, but in as the potential benefits of the treatment became more widely recognized it also began to be used in the community both in the USA[207] and in the UK[208-209] when MT became reimbursable on prescriptions written by registered general medical practitioners. At this time detailed advice was provided on the ordering, storage and disposal of maggots once they had been removed from the wound.[210]

Orthopaedic wounds

Given that much of the early literature on maggot therapy described their application in the treatment of orthopaedic wounds, it is perhaps not surprising that a number of more recent publications have similarly reported how they have been used to treat non-healing post-surgical orthopaedic wounds and in some instances prevent an amputation.

The ability of maggots to cleanse necrotic wounds following knee arthroplasty and thereby facilitate healing whilst eliminating the need for further surgery has twice been reported.[211-212] and Jukema et al.[213] described their use in eleven patients with a variety of orthopaedic wounds which they treated with both free-range and bagged maggots, concluding that the use of the maggots aided tissue remodelling and cure. Experience with use of maggots in the treatment of an infected amputation stump confirmed the importance of continuing therapy until the wound is completely free of necrotic material, for premature termination may cause the wound to deteriorate, necessitating more prolonged treatment than might otherwise have been the case.[214]

Diabetic ulcers

In the UK an estimated 84,000 patients have ulcers associated with diabetes, 76% (64,000) of which are primarily neuropathic or neuroischaemic in origin. Diabetic ulcers often contain a significant quantity of necrotic material and readily become infected. It is estimated that 15% of all diabetic patients who develop ulcers will eventually require an amputation of the toe, foot or leg. The total annual cost of managing diabetic peripheral neuropathy (DPN) and its sequelae is estimated to be around £300m.

When treating such wounds it is imperative that the wound is cleansed of dead tissue and bacteria as rapidly as possible, tasks for which maggots are ideally suited if surgical debridement is not an option. It is for this reason that the treatment of the diabetic foot is regarded as potentially the most important indication for this form of treatment.

An early account of the highly successful use of maggots in this way was provided by Stoddard et al. in 1995,[215] who described the use of maggots in a patient with bilateral non-healing ulcers under the first metatarsal heads caused by ischaemic or occlusive disease; an insidious collagen vascular disease such as early scleroderma was also suspected though not confirmed. Both ulcers had been present for a minimum of five years; one ulcer was treated with maggots, the other with conventional treatment and the wounds photographed weekly. After 14 weeks treatment, the ulcer dressed with maggots had virtually closed but the other ulcer showed no improvement despite continual conventional inpatient dressing changes. The authors concluded that, at a time when medical cost containment is a critical issue, MT offers a viable alternative for treating non-healing wounds.

Evans in 1997[216] described how maggots brought about a dramatic improvement in the quality of life of a terminally patient with very extensive weeping necrosis of the foot for whom radical surgery was not an option. The maggots removed all the necrotic toes leaving healthy granulation tissue in their place. Steenvoorde et al.[217] reported similar benefits associated with the use of maggots in a palliative setting and both cases illustrate the remarkable activity of the larval enzymes to remove large quantities of necrotic tissue, combat wound odour and even reduce wound-related pain.

This ability was utilized by Rayman et al.[218] and Johnson[219] who used maggots to assist in the removal on gangrenous toes whilst preserving adjacent viable tissue when surgical intervention was not an option. Prior to the treatment the patient had been in considerable pain and unable to mobilize and his wound was also highly offensive which caused him to become withdrawn. Following larval therapy the pain and odour were eliminated with a consequent improvement in his quality of life. In a second paper Johnson described how maggots were used to help differentiate between dead and salvageable tissue to minimize the requirement for repeat surgery.[220] Other case studies followed,[221-223] and several authors described how maggots could be employed as one of numerous modalities in the treatment of diabetic foot wounds,[224] particularly in the presence of malodour.[225]

Mumcuoglu et al.[67] also described the long term use of maggots in the treatment of gangrene of the foot as result of which a patient, who had previously been encouraged to have an amputation, was able to walk again.

A further instance of maggots preventing amputation was described by Murray et al.,[226] who reported how maggots were used to debride a necrotic dorso-plantar ulcer that extended deeply into the inter-digital space in a diabetic patient with Wegener's granulomatosis, a vasculitic condition that affects small and medium arteries. The wound was initially so severe that amputation was advised by the medical staff but this possibility was rejected by the patient. The maggot treatment was very effective, cleaning the wound very rapidly which then went on to heal completely within 13 weeks.

Some publications have recorded the use of maggots in larger groups of patients or in more formal studies. Mumcuoglu et al.[227] summarised the results of the treatment of 22 patients with a total of 27 ulcers of mean duration 10.3 months (range 1 - 48 months) for whom all forms of treatment had proved unsuccessful. Complete debridement was achieved in 18 wounds (66.7%), significant debridement in six wounds (22.2%), and partial debridement in two wounds. Only one wound remained unchanged. Twelve wounds were fully cleansed in one week and the average treatment period was two weeks. Of 14 wounds that that did not receive presurgical maggot treatment, eight became infected postoperatively but none of five wounds that received maggot treatment preoperatively subsequently became infected.

Sherman[228] assessed the efficacy of MT for treating foot and leg ulcers in diabetic patients who had failed to respond to conventional therapy by comparing changes in necrotic and total surface area of chronic wounds treated with either MT or standard (control) surgical or nonsurgical therapy.

In a cohort of 18 patients with 20 non healing ulcers, six wounds were treated with conventional therapy, six with MT, and eight were first provided with conventional therapy, followed by MT. During the first 14 days of conventional therapy there was no significant debridement of necrotic tissue; but during the same period with MT, necrotic tissue decreased by an average of 4.1 cm^2 (p = 0.02). After 4 weeks maggot-treated wounds were completely debrided, but conventionally treated wounds were still covered with necrotic tissue over 33% of their surface after 5 weeks of treatment (p = 0.001). The use of maggots also associated accelerated the growth of granulation tissue and improved healing rates.

Tantawi et al.[229] similarly evaluated MT in the management of ten diabetic patients with a total of 13 foot ulcers unresponsive to conventional treatment and surgical intervention. Consecutive diabetic patients with foot wounds presenting at the vascular surgery unit and the diabetic foot unit of Alexandria Main University Hospital were enrolled into an open uncontrolled study. Maggots of L. sericata were applied to the ulcers for three days per week and changes in the percentage of necrotic tissue and ulcer surface area were recorded weekly during the 12 week follow-up period. A semi-quantitative technique was used to assess the bacterial bioburden before and after treatment. The mean baseline ulcer surface area was 23.5 cm^2 (range 1.3 - 63.1), and the mean percentage of necrotic tissue was 74.9% (range 29.9 - 100). Complete debridement was achieved in all ulcers in a mean of 1.9 weeks (range 1 - 4). Five ulcers (38.5%) were completely debrided with one three-day treatment cycle. The mean reduction in ulcer size was significant at 90.2%, and this occurred in a mean of 8.1 weeks (range 2 - 12). Full wound healing occurred in 11 ulcers (84.6%) within a mean of 7.3 weeks (range 2 - 10). The bacterial load of all ulcers reduced sharply after the first MDT cycle to below 10^5.

Armstrong et al.[230] used a case-control model to compare the efficacy of maggot debridement therapy in 30 non-ambulatory patients with 30 age and sex matched historical controls (72.2 ± 6.8 years, mean ± s.d). All patients had peripheral vascular disease and neuroischaemic diabetic foot wounds (University of Texas Grade C or D). Twenty-seven patients (45%) healed during 6 months of review. Healings rates in the two treatment groups were 57% vs 33% for maggot treated and conventionally treated wounds respectively but this difference did not achieve significance. Of patients who healed, time to healing was significantly shorter in the MT than in the control group (18.5 ± 4.8 versus 22.4 ± 4.4 weeks). Approximately one in five patients (22%) required a high-level, above-the-foot, amputation. Patients in the control group were three times as likely to undergo amputation (33% vs 10%). Although there was no significant difference in infection prevalence in patients undergoing MT versus controls (80% vs 60%), there were significantly more antibiotic-free days during follow-up in patients who received MT (126.8 ± 30.3 vs 81.9 ± 42.1 days). The authors concluded that maggot debridement therapy reduces short-term morbidity in non-ambulatory patients with diabetic foot wounds

Most of the studies so far described make reference to the use of free-range maggots, but in 2006 Lodge et al.[231] described a dramatic case study in which maggots in net bags packed with foam chips (Biofoam Dressings) were used to treat an infected amputation site. The patient was an elderly gentleman with complex medical and surgical problems who was threatened with a further amputation following removal of the halux. The maggots were initially applied simply to achieve debridement, but because of the dramatic improvement and accelerated healing which occurred, treatment was continued until the wound was virtually closed. This is believed to be the first time that maggots have been used in this way.

Pressure ulcers.

Pressure ulcers also represent a significant clinical and financial burden to the healthcare system and these wounds, like diabetic ulcers frequently contain necrotic tissue. In an early publication Sherman[177] described a small prospective study in which MT was evaluated in patients with spinal cord injuries. Twenty patients were treated, eight of whom were followed for three weeks before applying maggots. Of the ulcers with > 20% coverage of necrotic tissue, none were more that half cleansed by the time MT was initiated but following the use of maggots all were cleansed within 1.4 weeks. More importantly, the average change in wound are prior to maggot treatment was an increase of 21.8%; during maggot treatment the change was a decrease in size of 22% (p = 0.001).

This publication was followed by a second in 2002[232] which described treatment outcomes for a cohort of 103 patients with 145 pressure ulcers. In this study, 61 ulcers in 50 patients received MT at some point in their monitored course; 84 ulcers in 70 patients did not. Debridement and wound healing could be quantified for 43 maggot treated wounds and 49 treated conventionally. Of the wounds treated with maggots 80% were completely debrided compared with 48% treated conventionally (p = 0.021). In the 31 wounds previously monitored prior to MT the amount of necrotic material decreased by 0.2 cm^2 per week and while total wound area increased by 1.2 cm^2 per week. During maggot treatment necrotic tissue decreased by 0.8 cm^2 per week (p = 0.003) and wound area decreased by 1.2 cm^2 per week (p = 0.001). These two publications, which support the conclusions of numerous other case studies,[178,233-234] provide powerful evidence of the value of maggots for this indication

Burns

Patients with burns frequently present with wounds covered with a layer of necrotic tissue which has to be removed before healing can progress normally. If surgery is not an option, MT may be indicated for this purpose.

Namias et al.[235] described how maggots were used for limb salvage in the treatment of 9% TBSA burns on the lower legs of a subject whose boots had caught fire when sleeping by a campfire. Two attempts at full thickness excision and autografting failed because of the presence of unrecognized residual nonviable tissue which could not be successfully removed because it was intermingled with viable tissue and tendons on the dorsa of the feet. For courses of maggots therapy were applied after which the wounds became free of necrotic material and granulation tissue began to migrate over the exposed bone. The wounds could then be closed surgically.

Similar success with maggot treatment was reported when it was used to debride an extensive burn to the dorsum of a foot caused by the excessive use of a microwaved 'wheat-filled' heat bag.[236] A short review of the role of maggots in wound care, which also contained some brief illustrated case histories, was published by Edwards.[237]

Leg ulcers

Like other types of wounds leg ulcers, irrespective of aetiology, commonly contain large quantities of necrotic tissue which must be removed before healing can commence. Maggot therapy is just one of the treatments which may be used for this purpose,[238] and numerous publications have described their use for this indication.[239-242]

In 2002 Kotb et al.[198] described how they used maggots to treat 20 patients with 30 ulcers. Complete debridement was achieved in 19 patients (95%) in the remaining patient debridement was described as significant (90% of wound free of slough). After maggot therapy granulation tissue was seen in wounds of all patients. Sixteen patients (80%) had a single application of maggots but 3 patients (15%) required two cycles.

The authors followed up 10 patients with 17 ulcers and found that the average area of the wounds had reduced from 57.7 cm^2 to 17.19 cm^2 in an average of 18 days following the start of treatment, leading the authors to conclude that maggot therapy is a rapid, efficient, safe, simple, and cost effective method for the treatment of venous ulcers.

The first prospective randomized controlled trial involving maggots and leg ulcers was undertaken by Wayman et al.[243-244] in 2000 in which they compared debridement rates achieved with MT with those obtained with the use of a hydrogel dressing. Twelve patients were recruited and randomized to treatment either with maggots or Intrasite Gel, commonly regarded as a standard technique for promoting autolytic wound debridement. All wounds dressed with maggots were cleansed with a single application of maggots lasting about 3 days, but after one month only 2 of the wounds dressed with gel were fully cleansed. Despite the small numbers of patients involved, the difference in the speed of debridement recorded with the two treatments made this result statistically significantly. Patients dressed with also maggots required fewer visits to achieve debridement that those dressed with gel; median values 19 vs 3 days ($p < 0.05$). The debridement rates quoted for wounds dressed with gel in this study (2/6, 33%) are consistent with those of other published clinical trials involving hydrogels.[114]

In 2004 a trial to examine the effect of maggot therapy on leg ulcers was initiated by the Centre for Evidence Based Nursing, University of York. This study which was originally planned to include 600 patients with venous leg ulcers,[245] was closed down hen only 267 patients had been treated.[246-247] Despite the fact that the design of the study was badly flawed and choice of endpoint (wound healing) was inappropriate for a product intended to achieve debridement,[248] the results once again confirmed the superiority of larval therapy over a hydrogel when used as a debriding agent. The median time to debridement with loose maggots was 14 days, (95% confidence interval 10 to 17) compared with 28 days for the Biomonde bagged maggots, (c.i. 13 to 25) and 72 days (72 (c.i. 56 to 131) for the hydrogel. The duration of treatment was on average 30 days longer in the hydrogel arm than the larval therapy arms (43 vs 12 days). The Biobag was not included in this trial.

Miscellaneous wounds

The use of maggots has also been described in a variety of other wound types. In 1997 Chaffrey[249] applied them to an extensive necrotic area on the posterior aspect of a calf extending from the knee to the Achilles tendon which resulted from an infected insect bite. After weeks of unsuccessful treatment with conventional therapies, the wound was successfully cleansed by five applications of maggots after which it progressed uneventfully towards healing.

A 43-year-old man was treated with maggots for a traumatic degloving injury to his foot followed by a transmetatarsal amputation because of the extensive soft tissue loss. Frequent regular sharp debridements produced little improvement in the wound bed so two cycles of MT were provided which painlessly debrided the tissues exposing a healthy granulating wound base. The wound subsequently head uneventfully requiring no further surgical intervention.[250]

Gacheru[251] described the use of maggots as an adjunct to surgery, in the treatment of a diabetic patient with extensive bilateral necrotising fasciitis. After a period of management with conventional materials, treatment with maggots was initiated, initially on one leg whilst the other was treated with silver sulphadiazine cream. The improvement in the maggot treated wound was such, however, that at the end of three days maggots were applied to both legs. Following this treatment it was recorded that both wounds were cleansed so effectively that it was possible to close them surgically.

Maggots were similarly used following surgery in a case of necrotizing fasciitis in the neck region.[252] After 48 hours a marked improvement was noted and the wound subsequently closed by secondary intention within six weeks.

Steenvoorde et al.[253] described the use of maggots in 15 patients with necrotizing fasciitis and showed that this treatment reduced the requirement for repeated surgical intervention. An average of 45 Biobags was applied per patient (range 9 - 100) and the average maggot treatment period was 17 days (range 3 - 38 days). Overall patients required an average of 2.9 surgical debridements (range 1 - 6) but the number of surgical debridements was statistically less in patients where maggots were applied within 9 days after diagnosis, 1.8 vs 4.1 (p = 0.001).

Maggots were also used with some success in the treatment of skin lesions caused by calciphylaxis, a rare condition generally associated with end-stage renal failure,[254-255] and was one of a series of measures employed to treat a large ulcer caused by pyoderma gangrenosum.[256] Renner et al.,[257] however, reported that in two patients with this condition who were receiving immunosuppressive therapy, the maggots failed to survive which led to a failure of the treatment.

A couple of papers have similarly described how maggots were successful used to debride malignant wounds and thereby help to reduce the odour commonly associated with this condition.[258-259]

In 2007, Sherman et al.[260] published the results of a survey to assess the use of maggots in 'off label' indications in the USA, described as indications other than simple debridement of wounds listed on the product label. Twelve respondents treated a total of 544 wounds, 131 (24%) of which were rare or off-label applications. These included: stimulation of epithelialization in clean but nonhealing wounds, disinfection odour and drainage control, determination of tissue viability, debridement of acute burns, necrotic tumours, ischemic ulcers and debridement of a variety of unusual sites including the glans penis, joints, pleural space, and peritoneal cavity.

In 2007, Steenvoorde et al.[261] published the results of a prospective study designed to determine which patient and wound characteristics were most likely to influence the outcomes of maggot treatment. A total of 101 patients with 117 infected wounds with signs of gangrenous or necrotic tissue thought suitable for MT were enrolled over a three year period, most of whom were treated with maggots as a last resort. Seventy two patients (71%) were classified according to the American Society of Anaesthesiologists (ASA) classification system as III or IV. Of the 116 wounds treated 60 healed completely, 12 healed almost completely and 6 were clean at least at last follow-up, resulting in a successful outcome in 67% of treatments. All 24 traumatic wounds healed completely but 13 wounds associated with septic arthritis failed to heal and 50% of these resulted in a major amputation. According to a multivariate analysis, chronic limb ischaemia, the depth of the wound, and age (≥ 60 years) negatively influenced outcomes. Treatment outcomes appeared not to be influenced by gender, obesity, diabetes mellitus, smoking, ASA-classification, location of the wound, wound size or wound duration.

Maggots and MRSA.

Wound infections caused by antibiotic resistant microorganisms represent a serious clinical problem. Possibly the first account of the use of maggots in the treatment of wounds infected by MRSA was given by Jones and Thomas in 1997.[178] An 82 year old gentleman presented with a small pressure ulcer on his elbow which on careful examination revealed the presence of significant tracking and undermining. The wound, which was very sloughy and MRSA positive, was dressed with a single application of maggots and when these were removed several days later the wound was completely free of slough with clear evidence of fresh granulation tissue present. A second swab taken at this time revealed that the MRSA had also been eliminated.

A similar account of the use of maggots in a non-healing wound infected with MRSA was provided by Wolff and Hansson in 1999.[262] Shortly afterwards Thomas et al.,[139] described how MT was used in the treatment of five patients whose wounds were infected or colonized with this organism. Despite the fact that the wounds had in some instances been treated unsuccessfully for up to 18 months with conventional therapies, the maggots were able to eliminate the bacterium from all the wounds in an average of 4 days. It was suggested that the use of maggots therefore represents a highly cost-effective method for managing the MRSA problem without further adding to the problems of antibiotic resistance. An abridged version of this study was published in the nursing press.[140]

In 2006 Bowling et al.[263] described how, when 13 patients with diabetic ulcers containing MRSA were treated with maggots, the organism was eliminated from all but one of the wounds after a mean of three applications with a mean duration of 19 days. The authors suggested that this compared very favourably with the 28 weeks required to achieve the same effect with conventional treatments. These results are consistent with and support the results of laboratory studies which indicate that maggot secretions are able to destroy MRSA in vitro.

Maggots in third world countries

The relatively low cost of maggot production at a basic level, makes it an attractive proposition for use in third world countries with very limited healthcare resources.[264] It has also been suggested that the therapy may prove to be of some value in treating a variety of tropical skin ulcers including cutaneous Leishmaniasis if the results of animal studies are replicated in humans.[265] Some of the practical problems of implementing MT in the third world have been discussed previously.[266-267]

Maggot surveys

Courtenay et al.,[268] carried out a prospective study using a structured questionnaire to collate information upon 70 patients who were treated with maggots in nine different hospital around the United Kingdom. Most of the wounds were leg ulcers; 16 were arterial, 11 venous, 11 diabetic, and 9 of mixed pathology. The average wound area was 80 cm^2, including 52 cm^2 of slough and necrotic tissue and 8 cm^2 of granulation tissue. Wound exudate was moderate or copious in 52, and 53 were malodorous. 39 patients were in moderate or severe pain primarily caused by ischaemia, and 49 wounds were infected.

The maggots were left on the wounds for a mean of 3 days, being changed an average of three times before treatment was complete. In only 2 out of the 70 cases the maggots failed to survive in the wound. Twenty three patients reported pain during MT, severe in 6, moderate in 11, mild in 6. Twelve of these patients had arterial ulcers and 8 had venous ulcers. The pain usually developed with 48 - 72 hours from the start of treatment. Bleeding was evident in 24 patients;[r] in none was it serious. Pyrexia during MT was observed in 5 patients.

After MT, 30 of the wounds were fully debrided, 20 were partially debrided and 8 were unchanged. In one case the wound had deteriorated.[a] The average wound size was reduced by nearly 5% and the area of slough and necrotic tissue by 68%. The area of granulation tissue increased by 21 cm^2 or 26%. The number of wounds with copious or moderate exudate declined from 52 to 32 a reduction of 33%. Wound odour was reduced in 43 wounds (81%) and 27 (69%) patients had less pain. Bacterial growth was recorded in 49 wounds (70%) at the start of the study. After MT only 16 wounds were investigated microbiologically and in 5 of these no bacterial growth was detected. There were no cases reported in which antibiotics had to be used after application of the larvae. In the opinion of nurse practitioners, MT reduced hospital stay in 24 (34%) of the patients, prevented surgery in 19 (27%), avoided hospital admission in 11 (16%) and reduced the need for antibiotics in 18 (26%). They thought that MT had played a major role in management of 63 (90%) of the wounds treated with MT.

At one stage, in 1997, simple questionnaires were sent out with all containers of maggots purchased from the Biosurgical Research Unit in South Wales to obtain information on the types of wounds being treated and the success rates achieved. An analysis of the first 100 forms returned indicated that treatment with maggots was at least partially successful in 90% of cases. Of 35 of patients, whose wounds were fully cleansed by the application of maggots, this was achieved in 25 instances with only one or two applications of maggots; this is equivalent to about 4 - 6 days treatment. About one third of patients experienced increased pain following application of maggots and 86% of treated patients had granulation tissue present in their wounds after treatment.

The results of the largest survey undertaken on the use of maggots were published in 2002.[269] This described an analysis of data returned to the Biosurgical Research Unit

---

[r] It is quote common for exudate from wounds dressed with maggots to be discoloured and it is possible that this is what was being reported here. Frank bleeding from maggot treated wounds is actually relatively uncommon.

[a] The numbers in this paper do not appear to add up correctly

on 'yellow cards' supplied with each container of maggots. These requested information on treatment times and outcomes, pain and number of applications of maggots applied to each wound. A total of 343 cards were returned for analysis equivalent to around 2% of those sent out. Fifty-one percent of patients were female and 43% male, the sex of the remaining 4% was not recorded. The majority of treated wounds (37%) were leg ulcers, but significant numbers of diabetic ulcers (25%) and pressure sores (20%) were also dressed with maggots. The remaining wounds were of varying aetiology or not identified.

Most wounds, about 90%, were described as 'sloughy' although a significant number also contained necrotic tissue. Not surprisingly, many wounds were also described as infected or malodorous.

Fifty-six percent of wounds only had a single application of maggots; a further 28% had two applications. Seven percent of wounds had three applications and the remainder four or more. Four percent of cards were incomplete.

The majority of wounds, about 68%, had a maximum of two applications of maggots. Twenty five percent of wounds were fully cleansed with a single application of maggots and a further 58% were improved by the treatment. Only four percent of wounds were said to have deteriorated during maggot therapy.

Twenty five percent of patients experienced increased discomfort with maggots although 17% reported a reduction in pain. An increase in wound pain was most likely to occur in patients with leg ulcers, confirming the results of previous observations that patients with ischaemic leg ulcers often required additional analgesia when treated with maggots. A reduction in pain was most commonly noted with pressure sores.

A total of 60 'adverse events' were recorded. Of these, 27 related to increased wound pain, and 7 to bleeding from the wound. In one case it was reported that a patient was pyrexial during maggot therapy. The remainder of the adverse events included poor survival of the maggots, problems with escapees and irritation of surrounding skin by wound exudate.

When clinicians were asked to rate the success of the maggot treatment, 248 (72%) rated the treatment as good or very good. Only 33 individuals (11%) rated it as poor or very poor. In most instances this was largely due to maggots failing to survive (16), escaping (3), or causing pain (3).

Financial implications

A number of publications have considered the financial implications of maggot treatment. In their small-scale study, Wayman et al.[243-244] determined that the total cost of materials, excluding nursing time, of successfully treating six patients with maggots was £471.21 compared with £639.12 for achieving debridement in two patients in the gel-treated group. The total material costs to successfully debride one wound dressed with maggots was therefore £69.53, (£417.21÷6) and that the average cost of successfully debriding one wound dressed with gel was £319.56. (£639.12÷2). If nursing costs were also included, these figures increased to £81.98 and £503.29 respectively.

Trudgian[270] in 2002 calculated that maggots therapy resulted in an estimated saving in surgical and prosthetic limb costs of over £3000 in an individual who was scheduled to undergo a secondary amputation for an infected stump wound which was prevented by the application of maggots.

Following a comparison of published debridement rates achieved with maggot therapy compared with those achieved with hydrogel dressings, Thomas[271] calculated that if maggots were to be used as the debridement treatment of choice for the estimated 334,000 pressure ulcers, diabetic ulcers and leg ulcers that are treated each year in the United Kingdom, it could reduce total treatment time by an astonishing 6.9 million days and result in a theoretical financial saving of nearly £162m.

CONTRAINDICATIONS AND SIDE EFFECTS

A review of the literature reveals no significant risks or adverse events related directly to the clinical use of medical maggots, although the following potential side effects have been reported.

Bleeding

Potentially the most serious potential side effect of maggot therapy is excessive bleeding caused by damage to a blood vessel as a result of the maggots foraging activity. Although it is not uncommon to find exudate from wounds dressed with maggots containing traces of blood, in most cases this is very limited. Steenvoorde *et al.*[272] treated 41 patients with maggots, eight with Biobags the remainder with free-range maggots. In total four patients treated with free-range maggots, three of whom were receiving anticoagulant or antiplatelet therapy experienced mild bleeding one of whom required to be admitted to hospital. No patients treated with confined maggots experienced bleeding problems. These findings appear to support the advice provided in the instruction leaflets supplied by the BRU which recommended that caution should be observed when using free-range maggots on patients receiving anticoagulant therapy.

It might be assumed that individuals suffering from haemophilia are at particular risk of suffering a significant bleed during maggot therapy but Rojo *et al.*[273] determined that MT was indicated for wound debridement in a patient with this condition who was not a candidate for surgery. Treatment was uneventful and total closure of the wound was eventually achieved. In such situations the risk posed by MT may well be les than that associated with surgery or surgical debridement, but to reduce the chances of a major bleed to a minimum, the treatment should probably be administered whilst the patient is hospitalized or under constant medical supervision.

For most patients, the risk of a serious bleed is very small although instances have occurred in the past. In 2008 it was recorded how a patient required admission to hospital and fluid replacement therapy when on maggot therapy.[274]

It should also be noted, however, that leg ulcers can bleed spontaneously and profusely, even in the absence of maggots. The author is personally aware of one occasion when a patient who was scheduled to receive maggot therapy exsanguinated from a spontaneous bleed in a leg ulcer prior to the scheduled application of maggots. Had this occurred a couple of days later, after the maggots had been applied, they would undoubtedly have been blamed.

Pyrexia

A transient pyrexia of 2 - 4°F is sometimes associated with maggot usage. This was reported by Fine[33] Weil,[31] McLellan[41] and Buchman[47] who suggested that this was due to 'the opening of chronically infected lymphatics' but it has also been recorded in more recent times. Its aetiology has never been satisfactorily explained but it is possible, that it might be due to the absorption of pyrogenic material that is released from the cell walls of Gram-negative bacteria that are lysed during their passage through the maggots' gut.

Pain and discomfort

The most common patient complaint is physical discomfort. This can vary from mild 'picking' sensation to pain that is so severe that it leads to premature termination of the treatment. Experience with the technique in the UK suggests that such pain is most commonly associated with the use of free-range maggots in the treatment of ischaemic limbs. It has also been noted that the pain increases with time as the maggots increase in size.[183]

It is postulated that the pain may be due, at least in part, to an increase in wound pH known to result from the metabolic activity of the maggots for it is generally eliminated immediately the maggots are washed out of the wound. If wound related pain becomes a serious problem the use of potent analgesics should be considered.

Several authors have investigated the effect of maggot therapy on wound pain. Wolff et al.[206] in a study involving 74 patients found 34% of maggot-treated patients felt increased pain during treatment, 25% less pain and 41% no difference in pain.

Steenvoorde et al.[272] in a retrospective study used a visual analogue scale (VAS) to record pain experienced by 41 patients treated with MDT (22 men and 19 women). Patients were provided with paracetamol (1 g three times daily), and Duragesic (fentanyl) patches (25 µg/hr every three days, and 50 µg/hr patches the day before the dressing change). Maggots were applied using the contained or the free-range techniques. The results of the study indicated that diabetic patients experienced the same degree of pain before and during MDT. Eight out of 20 non-diabetic patients experienced more pain during MDT than before; the remaining non-diabetic patients had the same amount of pain before and during the therapy. The difference between diabetic and non-diabetic patients was statistically significant ($p < 0.05$) for all applications combined. The authors concluded that in 78% of patients (29/37) pain can be adequately treated with analgesic therapy. However, if pain is unmanageable in the outpatient department, hospital admission should be considered using the contained method of application or, in the worst case scenario, cessation of treatment.

Generally, however, and perhaps surprisingly, despite the pain issue, patient acceptance of the technique has been very high.

Skin reactions

Larval enzymes produced within a wound can cause a brisk erythema or even erosion of the outer layers of the epidermis if they are allowed to spread onto surrounding skin which is not adequately protected.[65]

Once the enzymes come into contact with living tissue in the epidermis they appear to be inactivated, presumably by proteolytic enzyme inhibitors found in serum and healthy tissue and no further tissue damage takes place.

Figure 89: Erythema caused by maggot secretions

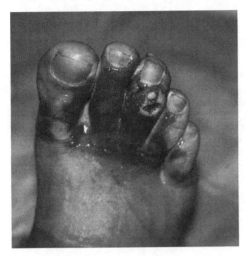

Damaged caused by the application of an excessive number of maggots

In the case shown opposite, the skin reaction resolved very quickly and the two wounds on the toe healed uneventfully.

A rather more unusual skin reaction was reported in a 53 year old fisherman who developed hyperkeratotic desquamative dermatitis of his hands mainly involving the pulps of the thumb and index finger of both hands which was shown to be due to coelomic fluid from maggots used as bait.[275] This reaction has never been reported from maggots used clinical, perhaps because the maggots remain intact and exposure times are relatively limited.

Infection

Because flies contain large numbers of microorganisms both on their body and within their gut, there exists a very real possibility that at least some of these bacterial species will be transferred to their progeny unless adequate procedures are put in place to prevent this occurring as previously described. This topic was addressed in a series of publications by Greenberg.[276-279] Contamination of wounds with maggot-transmitted bacteria is therefore a real possibility if these procedures are not strictly adhered followed. In 2002, in Switzerland, Nuesch *et al.*[280] reported that five of 24 patients (21%) developed bloodstream infections which could be traced back to the use of contaminated maggots. Four were caused by *Providencia stuartii* and one *C. albicans*. Once the disinfecting procedure of the maggots was optimized and the fly species was changed from *Protophormia terraenovae* to *L. sericata* no further cases of sepsis occurred in a cohort of 45 patients. No other episodes of infection have been reported since 'sterile' or medical grade maggots have been generally adopted.

Experiments with poliomyelitis virus and Coxsackie viruses conducted in 1952 showed that if flies were fed on infected material the viruses could be detected in their gut for a number of days. However, poliomyelitis virus could not be isolated from flies which developed from maggots that were fed infected material.[281]

The possibility that fly larvae and pupae could act as vectors of scrapie was investigated by Post et al.[282] They showed that infected samples of either form fed to hamsters would transmit the disease, indicating a conservation of infectivity in larvae and pupae suggesting that prion diseases, possibly including bovine spongiform encephalopathy, might be transmitted by flies in different developmental stages even after death. However, they considered the possibility that the insect could replicate infectivity to be unlikely because the relevant encoding gene has not been identified in any insect.

Together these findings suggest that there is a negligible risk of transmission of human viruses or prions from maggots obtained from an established colony of flies that have passed through a large number of generations provided that they are effectively isolated from any external source of contamination.

Ammonia toxicity

In sheep experimentally infested with 16,000 larvae, systemic illness has been associated with ammonia toxicity[283] resulting from the absorption of maggot-secreted ammonia into the blood stream. Sheep struck by parasitic *Lucilia cuprina* display a rapid increase in temperature and respiratory rate, accompanied by loss of weight and appetite.[284] Ammonia toxicity is theoretically possible in humans, although MT generally utilizes far fewer larvae.

EXAMPLES ILLUSTRATING THE USE OF MAGGOTS IN CLINICAL PRACTICE

Free-range maggots

The first case study illustrates both the effectiveness and specificity of maggot secretions when used for the debridement of wounds. A seriously ill gentleman with extensive ulcerated areas to both legs and feet was given two applications of maggots, lasting a total of six days after which his wounds were s fully cleansed of slough leaving the blood vessels on the surface of the exposed tissue undamaged.

Figure 90: Case study illustrating the use of free range maggots

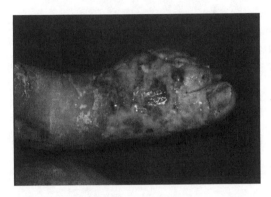
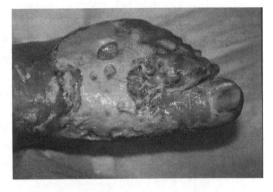

Foot prior to application of maggots showing extensive poorly demarcated areas of necrosis

Foot after one application of maggots showing clear evidence of significant debridement

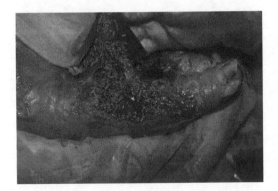
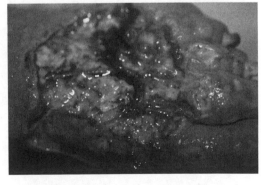

Removal of second application of maggots

Close up of wound showing intact blood vessels on almost fully cleansed wound surface

Maggots in bags, the Biofoam dressing

The second case study illustrates how the maggots and foam chips appear to act synergistically, facilitating rapid debridement of a vasculitic ulcer. These photographs are particularly interesting as they facilitate a direct comparison of the effects of the Biobag and Aquacel Ag, a CMC fibre dressing containing silver ions.

Because the wound was a little to large to be covered with a single Biobag a piece of the silver dressing was placed over the remaining area. When both dressings were removed three days later a marked improvement in the portion of the wound covered with the Biobag was clearly visible. In contrast there was no evidence of improvement in that portion of the wound dressed with Aquacel Ag. After two further applications of the Biobag the wound was fully cleansed, making considerable progress towards healing with clear evidence of the formation of new granulation tissue.

The speed of action of the Biofoam bags in this and numerous other sloughy and necrotic wounds was remarkable, and in the view of the author, based upon experience with large numbers of patients, is at least equivalent to that of free range maggots. It is also much faster than with the standard Biomonde Biobag which, according to the results of the York study (page 602), took twice as long as free-range maggots to bring about complete debridement.

Figure 91: Case study illustrating the use of the Biofoam dressing

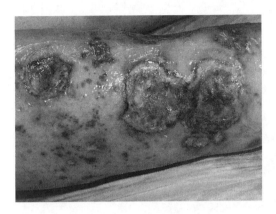

Vasculitic ulcer before maggot treatment

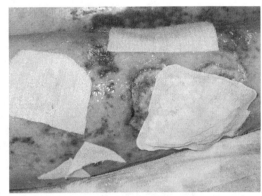

Application of Biofoam and Aquacel dressings

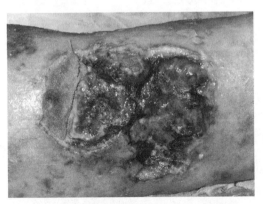

Wound on Day 3, after removal of Biofoam dressing

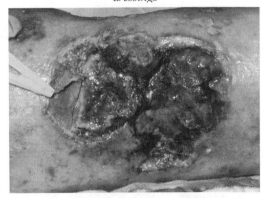

Wound on Day 3, showing removal of Aquacel

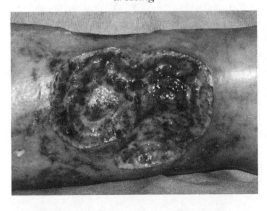

Wound on Day 6 after second Biofoam treatment

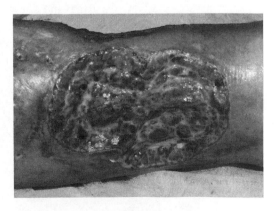

Wound on Day 13 after two further Biofoam treatments now showing clear signs of healing

PRACTICAL PROBLEMS ASSOCIATED WITH MAGGOT THERAPY

Clinical acceptability

The prospect of having live creatures introduced into a wound that feed upon dead tissue is not something that everyone is prepared to accept. Nevertheless, despite the common association of maggots with dirt and decay, experience suggests that most patients are prepared to accept the treatment once it has been fully explained to them. Kitching[285] examined patients perceptions and experiences of larval therapy in a phenomenological study in which six recently treated patients were interviewed using an open, unstructured approach. The author concluded that the therapy is acceptable to most patients if adequate attention is given to aspects that might repulse them. Factors that influenced patients to accept the treatment included: the nurse-patient relationship and the importance of informed choice and autonomy, disillusionment with previous treatments and the problems of living with a chronic wound which led to feelings of hopelessness particularly related to expectations of recurrence and a reduced quality of life. All six patients stated that their negative feelings about the therapy disappeared once it had started, adding that they would not hesitate to have the treatment again.

Failure of maggots to survive within a wound

> 'A maggot must be born i' the rotten cheese to like it.'

(George Eliot in Adam Bede).

Sometimes maggots fail to survive or develop properly within a wound. McKeever[49] suggested that this could be due to the creatures maggots drowning due to poor drainage but an alternative explanation is that the pH of the wound is not suitable for the young larvae. Hobson[73] showed that secretions of Lucilia larvae contain proteolytic enzymes which function optimally at pH 8.5. As conditions become progressively more acidic the enzyme activity is reduced. It is possible, therefore, that in a wound with a relatively low pH, the enzymes will be unable to breakdown the necrotic tissue and the maggots will therefore starve to death. Some support for this theory was provided by Wilson et al.[50] who showed that maggots do not survive well in an acid environment.

Experiences in the Biosurgical Research Unit identified that transport and storage conditions could adversely affect the survival or subsequent activity of young maggots, a consideration that was addressed by Rosales et al.[286] who developed a simple technique to determine what they termed the 'maggot motility index' which they believed could be used to predict the viability or effectiveness of maggots prior to their application into the wound. This involved selecting ten maggots at random and placing them on a translucent grid; thereafter their total excursion in 30 seconds was measured in mm/min. These data were used to assist in determining optimal storage conditions and shelf life.

Effects of concomitant treatments

Antibiotics

As maggots are often used in the treatment of infected wounds, it is inevitable that they will sometimes be applied to patients who are receiving concomitant antibiotic therapy. Sherman et al.[287] therefore examined the effects upon maggot development of seven commonly used antibiotics: ampicillin, cefazolin, ceftizoxime, clindamycin, gentamicin, mezlocillin and vancomycin in concentrations of 1,10,100 and 1000 times the average minimum bactericidal or bacteriostatic concentration. They observed that in media with cefazolin and gentamicin, inhibition only occurred at concentration in excess of 100 and 1000 times the normal therapeutic levels respectively. They therefore concluded that larval growth and development should be unimpeded by therapeutic doses of the products examined and therefore there was no reason why maggots should not be applied to patients on antibiotic therapy.

Hydrogels

Many wounds will have been dressed with a number of different products before maggots are first introduced. In many instances, these will include one of the amorphous hydrogels that are widely used for promoting autolytic wound debridement. Clinical experience has indicated, however, that if larvae are applied to wounds containing hydrogel residues, these materials can have an adverse effect upon larval survival or development.

A study was therefore undertaken to examine the effects of different hydrogels upon the viability and growth rate of maggots feeding upon mixtures containing varying proportions of gel and macerated liver.[288] The results revealed that some hydrogels have a marked effect upon the larvae. With Granugel, Intrasite, Nugel and Sterigel, increasing concentrations of hydrogel reduced larval growth and produced a marked increase in mortality. Less inhibition was noted with Aquaform although development of the larvae was still reduced at all concentrations of gel examined. In marked contrast, the growth of larvae applied to mixtures of liver containing 20% and 40% of Purilon gel was substantially increased compared with control values. The gel itself does not act as a food source for larvae, for in a further study, maggots placed upon Purilon gel in the absence of liver all failed to develop and died. The reason for the difference in growth of larvae applied to Purilon as compared with other hydrogels appears to be due, at least in part, to the absence of propylene glycol. This material is added to the gels to act as a humectant and preservative, to stop the gel from drying out in use and to prevent the growth of microorganisms.

The addition of water both to the liver/gel mixture and liver alone also reduced survival and growth rate of the larvae. Maggots feed by secreting enzymes; these dissolve dead tissue resulting in the production of a liquid 'soup', which they subsequently ingest. In the presence of excess liquid, it is postulated that if the maggots do not drown, their digestive enzymes become diluted and therefore rendered less effective. The increased larval development observed with increasing quantities of Purilon gel may be attributed to the ability of the gel to absorb excess fluid from the blended liver, resulting in the formation of an increasingly cohesive mass. Some additional support for this theory may be drawn from the observation that Aquaform, like Purilon, reduced the fluidity of the macerated liver more effectively than the remainder of the gels examined. The adverse effect of a very moist substrate upon larval survival may explain why MT is sometimes of limited efficacy in very heavily exuding wounds. (These findings also support the proposition that the foam chips contained within the Biofoam dressings facilitate maggot development by removing excess fluid as previously described.)

The results of this investigation suggested that that all traces of hydrogels containing propylene glycol should be removed from a wound prior to the application of maggots.

X-Rays

In a further unpublished study, maggots were exposed to X-rays using doses that were orders of magnitude greater than those used clinically. No effects on larval development were observed, indicating that maggots do not have to be removed from wounds prior to x-ray investigations.

MAGGOTS IN VETERINARY PRACTICE

Despite the widespread acceptance of maggots in human medicine, the use of maggots in veterinary practice remains limited. This may be due in part to a natural reluctance on the part of vets to deliberately introduce maggots into the wounds of their patients when a significant part of their activity may be related to the treatment of some animal species, notably sheep and pet rabbits, for natural infestations which can cause major tissue damage. Nevertheless, concern over antibiotic resistance and the increase in demand for organic husbandry and residue-free meat and milk, suggest that it is an option which merits serious consideration.[289]

A few papers have been published which describe the use of maggots in the treatment of a number of animal species but particularly in cattle and equids. One of the earliest references describes how maggots were used to treat actinomycosis in a six year old Guernsey bull,[290] and in 2001 Bell and Thomas[291] successfully used maggots to treat panniculitis in an aged donkey.

Sherman et al.[292] in 2007, published the results of a survey of veterinary practitioners in the USA who had used MT. Between 1997 and 2003, 13 horses were treated by eight veterinarians who used MDT to control infection or debride wounds, which could not easily be reached surgically or were not responding to conventional therapy. Seven animals were lame, and six were expected to require euthanasia. Following maggot therapy, all infections were eradicated or controlled, and only one horse had to be euthanized. No adverse events were attributed to maggot therapy for any of these cases, other than presumed discomfort during therapy.

Morrison[293] similarly described how maggots were used to treat 108 podiatry cases of varying aetiology in an equine hospital, with very good results.

Maggots have also been used to treat a variety of small animals. Sherman *et al.*[294] reported that the eight vets previously surveyed had also treated at least two dogs, four cats and one rabbit, most commonly to effect debridement and control infection, especially if the wound failed to respond to conventional medical and/or surgical therapy. The practitioners concerned considered the treatment to be safe and often beneficial, often preventing the need for amputation and euthanasia. The present author is also personally aware of the successful use of maggots in the treatment of two horses, a goat and several dogs.

MYTHS AND LEGENDS RELATED TO MAGGOT THERAPY

Over the years a number of misconceptions related to the use of maggots have appeared in the literature or have been put forward in lectures and elsewhere. Also a number of questions related to the use of maggots are sometimes raised by potential patients or users the answers to which are as follows;

- Maggots of *L. sericata* will not attack or burrow into healthy tissue although the proteolytic enzymes that they produce can occasionally cause irritation to unprotected skin.
- Maggots will not turn into flies within a wound as it takes about 10-14 days for a newly hatched maggot to complete its life cycle and turn into a fly. As dressings are normally changed every 3-4 days any fully grown maggots should be removed well before they are ready to pupate. Furthermore maggots like somewhere dry and warm to pupate so they will attempt to leave the moist environment of the wound in order to do so.
- Maggots cannot lay eggs in a wound as only adult flies can reproduce or lay eggs.
- Most people are unaware of the presence of even free-range maggots in the wounds although a small number of patients claim that they can feel them. If full grown maggots are allowed to get onto intact skin surrounding a wound they may tickle but this can be easily prevented by the application of an appropriate dressing system.
- In most instances, the application of a compression bandage should not interfere with the action of maggots provided they receive sufficient air to breathe.
- Most practitioners stop maggot therapy when the wound is clean and free of necrotic tissue, but there is some evidence to suggest that, for chronic wounds, it may be beneficial to continue treatment, possibly with smaller numbers of maggots, until granulation is well established.
- Individual maggots do not have to be counted into or out of a wound. This is totally unnecessary and virtually impossible to do. Furthermore, it is not uncommon for a proportion of the maggots that applied to a wound to fail to survive. This means that, even if it were possible count large numbers of maggots into a wound, (an almost impossible task), this number would not correlate with the number of full grown maggots that were recovered after

several days treatment.

- Some practitioners recommend that a maggot dressing should be moistened on a daily basis to prevent the maggots from drying out. Although very young maggots are quite delicate and susceptible to desiccation, after about the first 24 hours they become much more resistant to dehydration and generally do not require the application of any additional liquid.

- It is normally recommended that free-range maggots should be left on the wound for three days but maggots contained bags may be left in place for longer if required.

- Patients undergoing treatment with maggots should not immerse their wound in water or sit with the affected area too close to a source of heat, particularly in the first 24 hours after application as there is a possibility that the creatures might dry out and die. Care should also be taken when maggots are applied to weight bearing areas such as the feet or buttocks. Ambulant patients receiving MT on a leg ulcer, for example, may continue to live normally and go about their daily business as usual.

- There have been no reports of adverse interactions between maggot treatment and any form of medication, although it is recommended that patients receiving anticoagulant therapy should be carefully monitored during treatment.

- In the unlikely event that some maggots will remain undetected within the depths of a wound, these will certainly be found the next time the dressing is removed.

- Maggots and the associated dressing residues once removed from a wound should be double-bagged in the appropriate clinical waste bags and sent for disposal in the usual manner in accordance with local practice. If the bags are not incinerated, and the maggots complete their life cycle and turn into flies, these will soon die within the plastic bags. Given the fact that wild green bottles normally lay eggs on carrion, it is not considered that flies that develop from maggots removed from wounds will represent an additional health hazard.

REFERENCES

1. Hope FW. On insects and their larvae occasionally found in the human body. . *Trans. R. Entomol. Soc.* 1840. ; 2 : :256-271.
2. Zumpt F. *Myiasis in Man and Animals in the Old World: A Textbook for Physicians, Veterinarians and Zoologists.* London: Butterworth, 1965.
3. Norris KR. Myiasis in humans. *Medical Journal of Australia* 1989;150:235-237.
4. Hall M, Wall R. Myiasis of Humans and Domestic Animals. *Advances in Parasitology* 1995;35:257-334.
5. Burgess IF. Myiasis: maggot infestation. *Nurs Times* 2003;99(13):51-3.
6. Hall MJW, Smith KGV. Diptera causing myiasis in man. In: Lane RP, Crosskey RW, editors. *Medical Insects and Arachnids.* London: Chapman & Hall, 1995:429-469.
7. Lee DJ. Human myiasis in Australia. *Medical Journal of Australia* 1968;1:170-172.
8. Rowbotham TJ. Surgical maggots letter; comment. *Journal of Hospital Infection* 1995;29(4):311-2.
9. Clayton T, Craig P. *Trafalgar:The Men, the Battle,the Storm,* 2005.
10. King AB, Flynn KJ. Maggot therapy revisited: a case study. *Dermatology Nursing* 1991;3(2):100-102.
11. Chigusa Y, Kirinoki M, Yokoi H, Matsuda H, Okada K, Yanadora A, et al. Two cases of wound myiasis due to lucilia sericata and L. illustris (Diptera Calliphoridae). *Medical Entomology and Zoology* 1996;47:73-76.
12. Chigusa Y, Matsumoto J, Kirinoki M, Kawai S, Matsuda H, Oikawa A, et al. A case of wound myiasis due to Lucilia sericata (Diptera Calliphoridae) in a patient suffering from alcoholism and mental deterioration. *Medical Entomology and Zoology* 1996;49:125-127.
13. Brauneck HWF. A case of human myiasis. *British Medical Journal* 1949;16:1335.
14. Hira PR, Assad RM, Okasha G, Al-Ali FM, Iqbal J, Mutawali KE, et al. Myiasis in Kuwait: nosocomial infections caused by lucilia sericata and Megaselia scalaris. *Am J Trop Med Hyg* 2004;70(4):386-9.
15. Sood VP, Kakar PK, Wattal BL. Myiasis in otorhinolaryngology with entomological aspects. *Journal of Laryngology and Otology* 1976;90:393-399.
16. Daniel M, Sramova H, Zalabska E. Lucilia sericata (Diptera: Calliphoridae) causing hospital-acquired myiasis of a traumatic wound see comments. *Journal of Hospital Infection* 1994;28(2):149-52.
17. Shaunik A. Pelvic organ myiasis. *Obstet Gynecol* 2006;107(2 Pt 2):501-3.
18. Bhatia ML, Dutta K. Myiasis of the tracheostomy wound. *Journal of Laryngology and Otology* 1965;79:907-911.
19. Joo CY, Kim JB. Nosocomial submandibular infections with dipterous fly larvae. *Korean J Parasitol* 2001;39(3):255-60.
20. Verettas DA, Chatzipapas CN, Drosos GI, Xarchas KC, Staikos C, Chloropoulou P, et al. Maggot infestation (myiasis) of external fixation pin sites in diabetic patients. *Trans R Soc Trop Med Hyg* 2008;102(9):950-2.
21. Paris LA, Viscarret M, Uban C, Vargas J, Rodriguez-Morales AJ. Pin-site myiasis: a rare complication of a treated open fracture of tibia. *Surg Infect (Larchmt)* 2008;9(3):403-6.
22. Shwe T. Myiasis in necrotic tissue of a leprosy patient. *Leprosy Review* 1987;58:306.
23. Sreevasts, Malaviya GN, Husain S, Girdhar A, Bhat HR, Girdhar BK. Preliminary observations on myiasis in leprosy patients. *Leprosy Review* 1990;61:375-378.

24. Henry J. Oral Myiasis: A Case Study. *Dental Update* 1996;Nov:372-373.

25. Sherman RA. Wound myiasis in urban and suburban united states. *Arch Intern Med* 2000;160(13):2004-14.

26. Morgan D. Myiasis: the rise and fall of maggot therapy. *Journal of Tissue Viability* 1995;5(2):43-51.

27. Grassberger M, Reiter C. Effect of temperature on Lucilia sericata (Diptera: Calliphoridae) development with special reference to the isomegalen- and isomorphen- diagram. *Forensic Sci Int* 2001;120(1-2):32-6.

28. Greenberg B. Flies as Forensic Indicators. *Journal of Medical Entomology* 1991;28(5):565-577.

29. McClellan RH. Medicolegal use of maggots, (Letter to the Editor). *Journal of the American Medical Association* 1931;96(26):2226.

30. Grantham-Hill C. Preliminary note on the treatment of infected wounds with the larva of Wohlfartia nuba. *Trans. Roy. Soc. Trop. Med. Hyg (London)* 1933;27:93-98.

31. Weil GC, Simon RJ, Sweadner WR. A biological, bacteriological and clinical study of larval or maggot therapy in the treatment of acute and chronic pyogenic infections. *American Journal of Surgery* 1933;19:36-48.

32. Stewart MA. The role of Lucilia sericata Meig. larvae in osteomyelitis wounds. *Annals of Tropical Medicine and Parasitology* 1934;28:445-460.

33. Fine A, Alexander H. Maggot therapy - technique and clinical application. *Journal of Bone and Joint Surgery* 1934;16:572-582.

34. Kumar P. Limited Access Dressing and Maggots. *Wounds* 2009;21(June 6th).

35. Dunbar GK. Notes on the Ngemba tribe of the Central Darling River of Western New South Wales. *Mankind* 1944;3:177.

36. Root-Bernstein R, Root-Bernstein M. *Honey, mud, maggots, and other medical marvels*. 1999 ed. London: Macmillan, 1999.

37. Goldstein HI. Maggots in the treatment of wound and bone infections. *Journal of Bone and Joint Surgery* 1931;13:476-478.

38. Goldstein HI. Live maggots in the treatment of chronic osteomyelitis, tuberculous abscesses, discharging wounds, leg ulcers and discharging inoperable carcinoma. *Internat. Clinics* 1932;4:269-282.

39. Chernin E. Surgical Maggots. *Southern Medical Journal* 1986;79(9):1143-1145.

40. Baer WS. The treatment of chronic osteomyelitis with the maggot (larva of the blow fly). *Journal of Bone and Joint Surgery* 1931;13(July):438-475.

41. McLellan NW. The Maggot treatment of osteomyelitis. *Canadian Medical Association Journal* 1932;27:256-260.

42. Kampmeier RH. Surgical maggots (letter). *Southern Medical Journal* 1987;80(5):666.

43. Crile G, Martin E. Clinical Congress of Surgeons of North America, "War Session". *Journal of the American Medical Association* 1917;69:1538-41.

44. Murdoch FF, Smart TL. A method of producing sterile blowfly larvae for surgical use. *United States Naval Medical Bulletin* 1931;29:406-417.

45. Child FS, Roberts EF. The treatment of chronic osteomyelitis with live maggots. *New York State Journal of Medicine* 1931;31:937-943.

46. Livingston SK. Maggots in the treatment of chronic osteomyelitis, infected wounds, and compound fractures. An analysis based on the treatment of one hundred cases with a preliminary report on the isolation and use of the active principle. *Surgery, Gynecology and Obstetrics* 1932;54:702-706.

47. Buchman J, Blair JE. Maggots and their use in the treatment of chronic osteomyelitis. *Surgery, Gynecology and Obstetrics* 1932;55:177-190.

48. Miller DF, Doan CA, Wilson EH. The treatment of osteomyelitis (infection of bone) with fly larvae. *Ohio Journal of Science* 1932;32:1.

49. McKeever DC. Maggots in treatment of osteomyelitis. A simple inexpensive method. *Journal of Bone and Joint Surgery* 1933;15:85-93.

50. Wilson EH, Doan CA, Miller DF. The Baer maggot treatment of osteomyelitis - Preliminary report of 26 cases. *Journal of the American Medical Association* 1932;98:1149-1152.

51. Jewett EL. The use of Unna's paste in the maggot treatment of osteomyelitis. *Journal of Bone and Joint Surgery* 1933;15:513-515.

52. Buchman J. The rationale of the treatment of chronic osteomyelitis with special reference to maggot therapy. *Annals of Surgery* 1934;99:251-259.

53. Pomeranz MM. Peculiar regeneration of bone, following maggot treatment of osteomyelitis. *Radiology* 1932;19:212-214.

54. Ochsenhirt NC, Komara MA. Treatment of osteomyelitis of mandible by intraoral maggot-therapy. *Journal of Dental Research* 1933;13:245-246.

55. Ferguson LK, McLaughlin CW. Maggot Therapy - A rapid method of removing necrotic tissues. *American Journal of Surgery* 1935;29:72-84.

56. Puckner WA. New and nonofficial remedies, surgical maggots-Lederle. *Journal of the American Medical Association* 1932;98(5):401.

57. Robinson W. Progress of maggot therapy in the United States and Canada in the treatment of suppurative diseases. *American Journal of Surgery* 1935;29:67-71.

58. Martin W. Maggots and osteomyelitis. *Annals of Surgery* 1932;96:930-950.

59. Wainwright M, Laswd A, Alharbi S. When maggot fumes cured tuberculosis. *Microbiologist* 2007;8(1):33-35.

60. Chain E, Florey HW, Gardner AD, Heatley HG, Jenning MA, Orr-Ewing J, et al. Penecillin as a chemotherapeutic agent. *Lancet* 1940;2:226-228.

61. Horn KL, Cobb AH, Gates GA. Maggot therapy for subacute mastoiditis. *Archives of Otolaryngology* 1976;102:377-379.

62. Teich S, Myers RAM. Maggot therapy for severe skin infections. *Southern Medical Journal* 1986;79:1153-1155.

63. Wainwright M. Maggot therapy - a backwater in the fight against bacterial infection. *Pharm. Hist.* 1988;30:19-26.

64. Sherman RA, Wyle F, Vulpe M, Levsen L, Castillo L. The utility of maggot therapy for treating pressure sores. *Journal of the American Paraplegia Society* 1993;16(4):269-270.

65. Thomas S, Jones M, Shutler S, Jones S. Using larvae in modern wound management. *Journal of Wound Care* 1996;5(2):60-9.

66. Anon. Maggots and Viagra win Queen's Awards. *Pharmaceutical Journal* 2001;266:571.

67. Mumcuoglu KY, Lipo M, Ioffe-Uspensky I, Miller J, Galun R. Maggot therapy for gangrene and osteomyelitis. *Harefuah* 1997;132(5):323-5.

68. Craig GK. Primative treatments. *U.S. Army Special Forces Handbook*. Colarado: Paladin Press, 1988.

69. Fear-Price M. 1st World Conference on Biosurgery. *Nursing Care* 1996;Nov:18-19.

70. British Standard 7505: Elastic properties of extensible bandages.

71. Robinson W, Norwood VH. Destruction of pyogenic bacteria in the alimentary tract of surgical maggots implanted in infected wounds. *Journal of Laboratory and Clinical Medicine* 1934;19:581-586.

72. Fletcher F, Haub J, G. Digestion in blowfly larvae, Phormia regina Meigen, used in the treatment of osteomyelitis. *Ohio Journal of Science* 1933;33(2):101.

73. Hobson RP. Studies on the nutrition of blowfly larvae. I. Structure and function of the alimentary tract. *Journal of Experimental Biology* 1931;8(2):109-123.

74. Simmons SW. Surgical maggots in the treatment of infected wounds: a convenient blowfly cage. *J. Econ. Entomol.* 1932;25:1191-1193.

75. Robinson W, Simmons SW. Effects of low temperature retardation in the culture of sterile maggots for surgical use. *Journal of Laboratory and Clinical Medicine* 1934;19:683-689.

76. Simmons SW. Sterilization of blowfly eggs in the culture of surgical maggots for use in the treatment of pyogenic infections. *American Journal of Surgery* 1934;25:140-147.

77. Robinson W. Improved methods in the culture of sterile maggots for surgical use. *Journal of Laboratory and Clinical Medicine* 1934;20:77-85.

78. Greenberg B. Gnotobiotic insects in biomedical research. In: Miyakawa M, Luckey TD, editors. *Advances in Germfree Research and Gnotobiology*, 1968:410-416.

79. Greenberg B. Sterilising procedures and Agents, Antibiotics and Inhibitors in Mass Rearing of Insects. *Bulletin of the Entomological Society of America* 1970;16:31-36.

80. Daniels S, Simkiss K, Smith RH. A simple larval diet for population studies on the blowfly Lucilia sericata (Diptera: Calliphoridae). *Med Vet Entomol* 1991;5(3):283-92.

81. Sherman RA, My-Tien -Tran J. A simple, sterile food source for rearing the larvae of Lucilia sericata (Diptera: Calliphoridae). *Medical and Veterinary Entomology* 1995;89:000-000.

82. Sherman RA, Wyle FA. Low-cost, low-maintenance rearing of maggots in hospitals, clinics and schools. *Am J Trop Med Hyg* 1995;00:000-000.

83. Wolff H, Hansson C. Rearing larvae of Lucilia sericata for chronic ulcer treatment--an improved method. *Acta Derm Venereol* 2005;85(2):126-31.

84. Michelbacher AE, Hoskins WM, Herms WB. The nutrition of flesh fly larvae, Lucilia sericata (Meigen). *Journal of Experimental Zoology* 1932;64:109-131.

85. Tenquist JD. Rearing of Lucilia sericata (Diptera: Calliphoridae) in a modified musca domestica medium. *New Zealand Entomologist* 1971; 5(1):30-31.

86. Chaudhury MF, Alvarez LA, Lopez Velazquez L. A new meatless diet for adult screwworm (Diptera: Calliphoridae). *J Econ Entomol* 2000;93(4):1398-401.

87. Tachibana S-I, Numata H. An artificial diet for blow fly larvae, Lucilia sericata (Meigen) (Diptera: Calliphoridae). *Applied Entomology and Zoology* 2001;36:521-523.

88. Robinson W. Suggestions to facilitate the use of surgical maggots in suppurative infections. *American Journal of Surgery* 1934;25:525.

89. Sherman RA. A new dressing design for use with maggot therapy. *Plastic and Reconstructive Surgery* 1997;100(2):451-6.

90. Thomas S, Jones M, Andrews A. The use of fly larvae in the treatment of wounds. *Nursing Standard* 1997;12(12):54-59.

91. Shutler SD, Jones M, Thomas S. Management of a fungating breast wound. *Journal of Wound Care* 1997;6(5):213-4.

92. Thomas S, Jones M. *The use of sterile maggots in wound management.* Ipswich: Wound Care Society, 1999.

93. Armstrong DG, Mossel J, Short B, Nixon BP, Knowles EA, Boulton AJM. Maggot debridement therapy A primer. *Journal of the American Podiatric Medical Association* 2002;92(7):398-401.

94. Thomas S, Jones M, Andrews AM. The use of larval therapy in wound management. *Journal of Wound Care* 1998;7(10):521-524.

95. Thomas S, Jones M, Wynn K, Fowler T. The current status of maggot therapy in wound healing. *British Journal of Nursing (supplement)* 2001;10(22):s5-s12.

96. Grassberger M, Fleischmann W. The biobag - a new device for the application of medicinal maggots. *Dermatology* 2002;204(4):306.

97. Thomas S, Wynn K, Fowler T, Jones M. The effect of containment on the properties of sterile maggots. *British Journal of Nursing (supplement)* 2002;11(12):S21-S28.

98. Steenvoorde P, Jacobi CE, Oskam J. Maggot debridement therapy: free-range or contained? An in-vivo study. *Adv Skin Wound Care* 2005;18(8):430-5.

99. Lerch K, Linde HJ, Lehn N, Grifka J. Bacteria ingestion by blowfly larvae: an in vitro study. *Dermatology* 2003;207(4):362-6.

100. Blake FA, Abromeit N, Bubenheim M, Li L, Schmelzle R. The biosurgical wound debridement: experimental investigation of efficiency and practicability. *Wound Repair Regen* 2007;15(5):756-61.

101. Maseritz IH. Digestion of bone by larvae of Phormia regina. Its relationship to bacteria. *Archives of Surgery* 1934;28:589-607.

102. Hobson RP. On an enzyme from blowfly larvae. (Lucilia Sericata) which digests collagen in alkaline solution. *Biochemical Journal* 1931;25:1458, 1931.

103. Livingston SK, Prince LH. The treatment of chronic osteomyelitis with special reference to the use of the maggot active principle. *Journal of the American Medical Association* 1932;98:1143-1149.

104. Livingston SK. The therapeutic active principle of maggots with a description of its clinical application in 567 cases. *Journal of Bone and Joint Surgery* 1936;18:751-756.

105. Elia S. Maggot treatment of osteomyelitis (Letter). *Journal of the American Medical Association* 1932;98(18):1585.

106. Livingston SK. Maggot treatment of osteomyelitis (letter). *Journal of the American Medical Association* 1932;98(18):1585-1586.

107. Robinson W, Norwood VH. The role of surgical maggots in the disinfection of osteomyelitis and other infected wounds. *Journal of Bone and Joint Surgery* 1933;15:409-412.

108. Baer WS. Sacro-iliac joint; Arthritis Deformans: viable antiseptic in chronic osteomyelitis. *Proceedings of the International Assembly Inter-State Postgraduate Medical Association North America (1929)* 1929;5:365.

109. Baer WS. The use of viable antiseptic in the treatment of osteomyelitis. *Southern Medical Journal* 1929;22:382-383.

110. Ziffren SE, Heist HE, Womack NAMSC. The secretion of collagenase by maggots and its implication. *Annals of Surgery* 1953;138:932-934.

111. Fraser A, Ring RA, Stewart RK. Intestinal proteinases in an insect, Calliphora vomitoria L. *Nature* 1961;4806:999-1000.

112. Pendola S, Greenberg B. Substrate-specific Analysis of Proteolytic Enzymes in the Larval Midgut of Calliphora vicina. *Annals of the Entomological Society of America* 1975;68(2):341-345.

113. Vistnes LM, Lee R, Ksander GA. Proteolytic activity of blowfly larvae secretions in experimental burns. *Surgery* 1981;90:825-841.

114. Thomas S. A wriggling remedy. *Chemistry and Industry* 1998(17):680-683.

115. Thomas S, Jones M, Shutler S, Andrews A. Wound care. All you need to know about ... maggots. *Nursing Times* 1996;92(46):63-6, 68, 70 passim.

116. Casu RE, Pearson RD, Jarmey JM, Cadogan LC, Riding GA, Tellam RL. Excretory/secretory chymotrypsin from Lucilia Cuprina: purification, enzymatic specificity and amino avid sequence deduced from mRNA. *Insect Molecular Biology* 1994;3(4):201-211.

117. Casu RE, Eisemann CH, Vuocolo T, Tellam RL. The major excretory/secretory protease from Lucilia cuprina larvae is also gut digestive protease. *International Journal of Parasitology* 1996;26(6):623-628.

118. Young AR, Mancuso N, Meeusen EN, Bowles VM. Characterisation of proteases involved in egg hatching of the sheep blowfly, *Lucilia cuprina*. *International Journal of Parasitology* 2000;30(8):925-932.

119. Young AR, Mesusen NT, Bowles VM. Characterisation of ES products involved in wound initiation by Lucilia cuprina larvae. *International Journal of Parasitology* 1996;26(3):245-252.

120. Schmidtchen A, Wolff H, Rydengard V, Hansson C. Detection of serine proteases secreted by Lucilia sericata in vitro and during treatment of a chronic leg ulcer. *Acta Derm Venereol* 2003;83(4):310-1.

121. Chambers L, Woodrow S, Brown AP, Harris PD, Phillips D, Hall M, et al. Degradation of extracellular matrix components by defined proteinases from the greenbottle larva Lucilia sericata used for the clinical debridement of non-healing wounds. *Br J Dermatol* 2003;148(1):14-23.

122. Duncan JT. On a bactericidal principle present in the alimentary canal of insects and arachnids. *Parasitology* 1926;18:238-252.

123. Hobson RP. Studies on the nutrition of blowfly larvae. II. Role of the intestinal flora in digestion. *Journal of Experimental Biology* 1932;9:128-138.

124. Slocum MA, McClellan RH, Messer FC. Studies on the nutrition of blowfly larvae. 1 Structure and function of the alimentary tract action of blowfly maggots in the treatment of chronic osteomyelitis. *Pennsylvannia Medical Journal* 1933;36:570-573.

125. Mumcuoglu KY, Miller J, Mumcuoglu M, Friger M, Tarshis M. Destruction of bacteria in the digestive tract of the maggot of *Lucilia sericata* (Diptera: Calliphoridae). *Journal of Medical Entomology* 2001;38(2):161-166.

126. Robinson W. The use of blowfly larvae in the treatment of infected wounds. *Annals of the Entomological Society of America* 1933;26:270-276.

127. Messer FC, McClellan RH. Surgical maggots. A study of their functions in wound healing. *Journal of Laboratory and Clinical Medicine* 1935;20:1219.

128. Robinson W, Baker FL. The enzyme urease and occurrence of ammonia in maggot infected wounds. *Journal of Parasitology* 1939;25:149-155.

129. Robinson W. Ammonium bicarbonate secreted by surgical maggots stimulates healing in purulent wounds. *American Journal of Surgery* 1940;47:111-115.

130. Simmons SW. The bactericidal properties of excretions of the maggot of Lucilia sericata. *Bull Entomol Res* 1935;26:559-563.

131. Simmons SW. A bactericidal principle in excretions of surgical maggots which destroys important etiological agents of pyogenic infections. *Journal of Bacteriology* 1935;30:253-267.

132. Pavillard ER, Wright EA. An antibiotic from maggots. *Nature* 1957;180:916-917.

133. Thomas S, Andrews AM, Hay NP, Bourgoise S. The anti-microbial activity of maggot secretions: results of a preliminary study. *Journal of Tissue Viability* 1999;9(4):127-132.

134. Steenvoorde P, Jukema GN. The antimicrobial activity of maggots: in-vivo results. *Journal of Tissue Viability* 2004;14(3):97-101.

135. Jaklic D, Lapanje A, Zupancic K, Smrke D, Gunde-Cimerman N. Selective antimicrobial activity of maggots against pathogenic bacteria. *J Med Microbiol* 2008;57(Pt 5):617-25.

136. Kerridge A, Lappin-Scott H, Stevens JR. Antibacterial properties of larval secretions of the blowfly, Lucilia sericata. *Medical and Veterinary Entomology* 2005;19(3):333-337.

137. Bexfield A, Nigam Y, Thomas S, Ratcliffe NA. Detection and partial characterisation of two antibacterial factors from the excretions/secretions of the medicinal maggot Lucilia sericata and their activity against methicillin-resistant Staphylococcus aureus (MRSA). *Microbes Infect* 2004;6(14):1297-304.

138. Bexfield A, Bond AE, Roberts EC, Dudley E, Nigam Y, Thomas S, et al. The antibacterial activity against MRSA strains and other bacteria of a <500Da fraction from maggot excretions/secretions of Lucilia sericata (Diptera: Calliphoridae). *Microbes Infect* 2008;10:325-333.

139. Thomas S, Jones M. *Maggots and the battle against MRSA*. Bridgend: SMTL, 2000.

140. Thomas S, Jones M. Maggots can benefit patients with MRSA. *Practice Nurse* 2000;20(2):101-104.

141. Greenberg B. Model for destruction of bacteria in the midgut of blow fly maggots. *Journal of Medical Entomology* 1968;5(1):31-38.

142. Erdmann GR, Bromel M, Gassner G, Freeman TP, Fischer A. Antibacterial activity demonstrated by culture filtrates of *Proteus mirabilis* isolated from screwworm (*Cochliomyia Hominivorax*) (Diptera: Calliphoridae) larvae. *Journal of Medical Entomology* 1984;21(2):159-164.

143. Erdmann GR, Khalil SKW. Isolation and identification of two antibacterial agents produced by a strain of proteus mirabilis isolated from larvae of the screwwork (Cochliomyia Hominivorax) (Diptera: Calliphoridae). *Journal of Medical Entomology* 1986;23(2):208-211.

144. Freidman E, Shaharabany M, Ravin S, Golomb E, Gollop N, Ioffe-Uspensky I, et al. Partially purified antibacterial agent from maggots displays a wide range of antibacterial activity. *Presented at the Int. Conf. on Biotherapy, 3rd, Jerusalem, Israel.* 1998.

145. Andersen AS, Joergensen B, Bjarnsholt T, Johansen H, Karlsmark T, Givskov M, et al. Quorum-sensing-regulated virulence factors in Pseudomonas aeruginosa are toxic to Lucilia sericata maggots. *Microbiology* 2010;156(Pt 2):400-7.

146. Hoffman JA, Hetru C. Insect defensins: inducible antibacterial peptides. *Immunology Today* 1992;13(10):411-415.

147. Hoffman JA, Reichart J, Hetru C. Innate immunity in higher insects. *Current Opinion in Immunology* 1996;8:8-13.

148. Salzet M. Neuropeptide-derived antimicrobial peptides from invertibrates for biomedical applications. *Current Medicinal Chemistry* 2005;12.

149. Cerovsky V, Zdarek J, Fucik V, Monincova L, Voburka Z, Bem R. Lucifensin, the long-sought antimicrobial factor of medicinal maggots of the blowfly Lucilia sericata. *Cell Mol Life Sci* 2010;67(3):455-66.

150. van der Plas MJ, van der Does AM, Baldry M, Dogterom-Ballering HC, van Gulpen C, van Dissel JT, et al. Maggot excretions/secretions inhibit multiple neutrophil pro-inflammatory responses. *Microbes Infect* 2007;9(4):507-14.

151. van der Plas MJ, Dambrot C, Dogterom-Ballering HC, Kruithof S, van Dissel JT, Nibbering PH. Combinations of maggot excretions/secretions and antibiotics are effective against Staphylococcus aureus biofilms and the bacteria derived therefrom. *J Antimicrob Chemother* 2010.

152. Cazander G, van Veen KE, Bouwman LH, Bernards AT, Jukema GN. The influence of maggot excretions on PAO1 biofilm formation on different biomaterials. *Clin Orthop Relat Res* 2009;467(2):536-45.

153. Brown AWA. The nitrogen metabolism of an insect (Lucilia sericata Mg.) Uric acid, allantoin and uricase. *Biochem J.* 1938;32(5):895–902.

154. Robinson W. Stimulation of healing in non-healing wounds by allantoin occurring in maggot secretions and of wide biological distribution. *Journal of Bone and Joint Surgery* 1935;17:267-271.

155. The healing properties of allantoin and urea discovered through the use of maggots in human wounds. Ann Rep Smithsonian institution, Washington, DC, US Government Printing Office.; 1938.

156. Stewart MA. A new treatment of osteomyelitis - preliminary report. *Surgery, Gynecology and Obstetrics* 1934;58:155-165.
157. Lewy B. Maggot therapy. *Arch Otolaryngol* 1977;103:310.
158. Gates GA, Horn KL, Cobb AH. Maggot therapy. *Arch Otolaryngol* 1977;103:310-311.
159. Prete P. Growth effects of *Phaenicia sericata* larval extracts on fibroblasts: mechanism for wound healing by maggot therapy. *Life Sciences* 1997;60(8):505-510.
160. Horobin AJ, Pritchard DI, Shakesheff KM. How do larvae of Lucilia sericata initiate human wound healing? *European Cells and Materials* 2002;4 (Suppl. 2.):69.
161. Horobin AJ, Shakesheff KM, Woodrow S, Pritchard DI. Maggots and wound healing: The effects of Lucilia sericata larval secretions upon human dermal fibroblasts. *European Cells and Materials* 2003;Vol. 6. (Suppl. 2):3.
162. Horobin AJ, Shakesheff KM, Woodrow S, Robinson C, Pritchard DI. Maggots and wound healing: an investigation of the effects of secretions from *Lucilia sericata* larvae upon interactions between human dermal fibroblasts and extracellular matrix components. *British Journal of Dermatology* 2003;148:923-933.
163. Smith AG, Powis RA, Pritchard DI, Britland ST. Greenbottle (*Lucilia sericata*) Larval Secretions Delivered from a Prototype Hydrogel Wound Dressing Accelerate the Closure of Model Wounds. *Biotechnol. Prog.* 2006.
164. Wang S, Lv D, Wang Y, Wang J. Influence of maggot secretion on expression of bFGF and connective tissue growth factor in ulcer tissue of diabetes mellitus rat and antibacterium study. *Zhongguo Xiu Fu Chong Jian Wai Ke Za Zhi* 2008;22(4):472-5.
165. Pecivova J, Macickova T, Takac P, Kovacsova M, Cupanikova D, Kozanek M. Effect of the extract from salivary glands of Lucilia sericata on human neutrophils. *Neuro Endocrinol Lett* 2008;29(5):794-7.
166. Brandner JM, Houdek P, Quitschau T, Siemann-Harms U, Ohnemus U, Willhardt I, et al. An ex-vivo model to evaluate dressings & drugs for wound healing. *EWMA Journal* 2006;6(2):11-15.
167. Wollina U, Liebold K, Schmidt WD, Hartmann M, Fassler D. Biosurgery supports granulation and debridement in chronic wounds-- clinical data and remittance spectroscopy measurement. *Int J Dermatol* 2002;41(10):635-9.
168. Zhang Z, Wang S, Tian X, Zhao Z, Zhang J, Lv D. A new effective scaffold to facilitate peripheral nerve regeneration: chitosan tube coated with maggot homogenate product. *Med Hypotheses* 2010;74(1):12-4.
169. Larrey DJ. *Observations on wounds and their complications by erysipelas, gangrene and tetanus, Clinique. chirurgucale. 51-52 (Nov.) 1829 translated from the French by E.F. Rivinus. Des vers ou larves de la mouche bleue, Chez Gabon, Paris,.* Philadelphia: Key, Mielke and Biddle,, 1832.
170. Bunkis MD, Gherini S, Walton R. Maggot therapy revisited. *Western Journal of Medicine* 1985;142:554-556.
171. Reames MK, Christensen C, Luce EA. The use of maggots in wound debridement. *Annals of Plastic Surgery* 1988;21(4):388-91.
172. Seaquist ER, Henry TR, Cheong E, Theologides A. Phormia regina myiasis in a malignant wound. *Minn Med* 1983;66:409-410.
173. Harding KG, Morris HL, Patel GK. Healing chronic wounds. *British Medical Journal* 2002;324:160-163.
174. Falanga V. Classifications for wound bed preparation and stimulation of chronic wounds. *Wound Repair Regeneration* 2000;8(5):347-352.
175. Pechter EA, Sherman RA. Maggot therapy: the surgical metamorphosis. *Plastic and Reconstructive Surgery* 1983;72(4):567-70.

176. Sherman RS, Pechter EA. Maggot therapy: a review of the therapeutic applications of fly larvae in human medicine, especially for treating osteomyelitis. *Medical and Veterinary Entomology* 1988;2:225-230.

177. Sherman RA, Wyle F, Vulpe M. Maggot therapy for treating pressure ulcers in spinal cord injury patients. *Journal of Spinal Cord Medicine* 1995;18(2):71-74.

178. Jones M, Thomas S. Wound cleansing - a therapy revisited. *Journal of Tissue Viability* 1997;7(4):119-121.

179. Mulder JB. The medical marvels of maggots. *J Am Vet Med Assoc* 1989;195(11):1497-9.

180. Editorial. Sterile maggots used in wound management. *Pharmaceutical Journal* 1995;255:803.

181. Graner JL. S.K. Livingston and the maggot therapy of wounds. *Military Medicine* 1997;162(4):296-300.

182. Sherman RA. Maggot Debridement in Modern Medicine. *Infections in Medicine* 1998;15(September):651-656.

183. Courtenay M. The use of larval therapy in wound management in the UK. *Journal of Wound Care* 1999;8(4):177-9.

184. Courtenay M, Church JC, Ryan TJ. Larva therapy in wound management. *J R Soc Med* 2000;93(2):72-4.

185. Courtenay M. Larva therapy. *Nursing Times* 2001;97(16):38.

186. Bonn D. Maggot therapy: an alternative for wound infection. *Lancet* 2000;356(Sptember 30):1174.

187. Thomas S. Sterile maggots and the preparation of the wound bed. In: Cherry G, Harding KG, Ryan TJ, editors. *Wound bed preparation*. London: Royal Society of Medicine Press Limited, 2001:59-65.

188. Galeano M, Ioli V, Colonna M, Risitano G. Maggot therapy for treatment of osteomyelitis and deep wounds: an old remedy for an actual problem. *Plast Reconstr Surg* 2001;108(7):2178-9.

189. Sherman RA, Hall MJ, Thomas S. Medicinal maggots: an ancient remedy for some contemporary afflictions. *Annual Review of Entomology* 2000;45:55-81.

190. Beasley WD, Hirst G. Making a meal of MRSA-the role of biosurgery in hospital-acquired infection. *J Hosp Infect* 2004;56(1):6-9.

191. Whitaker IS, Twine C, Whitaker MJ, Welck M, Brown CS, Shandall A. Larval therapy from antiquity to the present day: mechanisms of action, clinical applications and future potential. *Postgrad Med J* 2007;83(980):409-13.

192. Thomas S. New treatments for diabetic foot ulcers (c) larval therapy. In: Boulton AJM, Connor H, Cavanagh PR, editors. *The Foot in Diabetes, 3rd edition*: John Wiley & Sons Ltd, 2000:185-191.

193. Boon H, Freeman L, Unsworth J. Larvae help debridement. *Nursing Times* 1996;92(46):76-80.

194. Jones M, Thomas S. Larval therapy. *Nursing Standard* 2000;14(20):47-51.

195. Mumcuoglu KY. Clinical applications for maggots in wound care. *Am J Clin Dermatol* 2001;2(4):219-27.

196. Jones M. Maggots in Wound Care. *Nurse 2 Nurse* 2001:36-37.

197. Thomas S. Maggots in wound care. *Update* 2002(11 April 2002):464-467.

198. Kotb MM, Tantawi TI, Gohar YM, Beshara FMS, Fatthalla SSA. The medicinal use of maggots in the management of venous stasis ulcers and diabetic foot ulcers. *Bulletin of Alexandria Faculty of Medicine* 2002;37(2):205-214.

199. Graninger M, Grassberger M, Galehr E, Huemer F, Gruschina E, Minar E, et al. Biosurgical debridement facilitates healing of chronic skin ulcers. *Archives of Internal Medicine* 2002;162:1906-1907.

200. Tanyuksel M, Araz E, Dundar K, Uzun G, Gumus T, Alten B, et al. Maggot debridement therapy in the treatment of chronic wounds in a military hospital setup in Turkey. *Dermatology* 2005;210(2):115-8.

201. Jarvis A. Maggot therapy (letter). *Lancet* 2000;356(December 9):2016.

202. Thomas S, Andrews A, Jones M, Church J. Maggots are useful in treating infected or necrotic wounds [letter; comment]. *Bmj* 1999;318(7186):807-8.

203. Summers JB, Kaminski JM. Management of pressure ulcers. *Jama* 2003;289(17):2210; author reply 2210-1.

204. Summers JB, Kaminski J. Maggot debridement therapy for diabetic necrotic foot. *Am Fam Physician* 2003;68(12):2327, 2330; author reply 2330.

205. Mumcuoglu KY, Ingber A, Gilead L, Stessman J, Friedmann R, Schulman H, et al. Maggot therapy for the treatment of intractable wounds. *Int J Dermatol* 1999;38(8):623-7.

206. Wolff H, Hansson C. Larval therapy - an effective method of ulcer debridement. *Clin Exp Dermatol* 2003;28(2):134-7.

207. Sherman RA, Sherman J, Gilead L, Lipo M, Mumcuoglu KY. Maggot debridement therapy in outpatients. *Arch Phys Med Rehabil* 2001;82(9):1226-9. t&artType=abs&id=aapmr0821226&target=.

208. MacDougall KM, Rodgers FR. A case study using larval therapy in the community setting. *Br J Nurs* 2004;13(5):255-60.

209. Green T. Larval therapy in the community-challenge or opportunity. *Nurse2Nurse Magazine* 2004;4(4):51-52.

210. Thomas S. Advice for community pharmacists on how to order and dispose of maggots. *Pharmaceutical Journal* 2004;272:222-223.

211. Thomas S. The use of sterile maggots in wound management. *Nursing Times* 2002;98(36):45-46.

212. Townley WA, Jain A, Healy C. Maggot debridement therapy to avoid prosthesis removal in an infected total knee arthroplasty. *J Wound Care* 2006;15(2):78-9.

213. Jukema GN, Menon AG, Bernards AT, Steenvoorde P, Taheri Rastegar A, van Dissel JT. Amputation-sparing treatment by nature: "surgical" maggots revisited. *Clin Infect Dis* 2002;35(12):1566-71.

214. Thomas S. The use of maggot therapy in an infected amputation wound. *Irish Nurse* 2003;6(3):26-28.

215. Stoddard SR, Sherman RM, Mason BE, Pelsang DJ. Maggot debridement therapy - an alternative treatment for nonhealing ulcers. *Journal of the American Podiatric Medical Association* 1995;85(4):218-221.

216. Evans H. A treatment of last resort. *Nursing Times* 1997;93(23):62-64,65.

217. Steenvoorde P, van Doorn LP, Jacobi CE, Oskam J. Maggot debridement therapy in the palliative setting. *Am J Hosp Palliat Care* 2007;24(4):308-10.

218. Rayman A, Stansfield G, Woolard T, Mackie A, Rayman G. Use of larvae in the treatment of the diabetic necrotic foot. *The Diabetic Foot* 1998;1(1):7-13.

219. Johnson S. Larval therapy in the treatment of wounds: case history. *British Journal of Community Nursing* 1999;4(6):293-295.

220. Johnson S. Using larva therapy to debride an ischaemic toe. *Nursing Times* 2001;97(16):39-40.

221. Knowles A, Findlow A, Jackson N. Management of a diabetic foot ulcer using larval therapy. *Nurs Stand* 2001;16(6):73-6.

222. Yates I, Fox I, Crewdson M, Woodyer AB. Larvae - a key member of the multidisciplinary foot team. *The Diabetic Foot* 2003;6(4):166171.

223. Wollina U, Karte K, Herold C, Looks A. Biosurgery in wound healing - the renaissance of maggot therapy. *European Academy of Dermatology and Venerology* 2000;14:285-89.

224. Edmonds M. Adjunctive treatments for wound healing in the diabetic foot. *The Diabetic Foot* 2006;9(3):128-134.

225. Murray F. Malodour in diabetic foot wounds. *The Diabetic Foot* 2005;8(3):122-132.

226. Murray F, Benbow M. Diabetic foot ulcer associated with Wegener's granulomatosis. *Journal of Wound Care* 1999;8(8):377-378.

227. Mumcuoglu KY, Ingber A, Gilead L, Stessman J, Friedmann R, Schulman H, et al. Maggot therapy for the treatment of diabetic foot ulcers [letter]. *Diabetes Care* 1998;21(11):2030-1.

228. Sherman RA. Maggot therapy for treating diabetic foot ulcers unresponsive to conventional therapy. *Diabetes Care* 2003;26(2):446-51.

229. Tantawi TI, Gohar YM, Kotb MM, Beshara FM, El-Naggar MM. Clinical and microbiological efficacy of MDT in the treatment of diabetic foot ulcers. *J Wound Care* 2007;16(9):379-83.

230. Armstrong DG, Salas P, Short B, Martin BR, Kimbriel HR, Nixon BP, et al. Maggot therapy in "lower-extremity hospice" wound care: fewer amputations and more antibiotic-free days. *J Am Podiatr Med Assoc* 2005;95(3):254-7.

231. Lodge A, Jones M, Thomas S. Maggots 'n' Chips: a novel approach to the treatment of diabetic ulcers. *British Journal of Community Nursing, Wound Care Supplement,* 2006;11(12):S23 - S26.

232. Sherman RA. Maggot versus conservative debridement therapy for the treatment of pressure ulcers. *Wound Repair and Regeneration* 2002;10(4):208-214.

233. Semple L. Use of larval therapy to treat a diabetic patient's pressure ulcer. *British Journal of Nursing, Tissue Viability Supplement* 2003;12(15):S6-S13.

234. Johnstone A. Management of infection and exudation after larval debridement of a heel pressure ulcer. *Wounds UK*.

235. Namias N, Varela JE, Varas RP, Quintana O, Ward CG. Biodebridement: a case report of maggot therapy for limb salvage after fourth-degree burns. *J Burn Care Rehabil* 2000;21(3):254-7.

236. Thornton D, Berry M. Maggot therapy in an acute burn. *Scottish Nurse* 2002;7(4):14-16.

237. Edwards J. Larval therapy in full thickness burns. *Journal of Community Nursing* 2006;20(11):33-38.

238. Davies C, Turton G, Woolfrey G, Elley R, Taylor M. Exploring debridement options for chronic venous leg ulcers. *Britsh Journal of Nursing* 2005;14(7):393-397.

239. Sherman RA, My-Tien-Tran J, Sullivan R. Maggot therapy for venous stasis ulcers. *Archives of Dermatology* 1996;132:254-256.

240. Jones M, Champion A. Nature's Way. *Nursing Times* 1998;94(34):75-76.

241. Sherman RA. Maggot Therapy for Foot and Leg Wounds. *International Journal of Lower Extremity Wounds* 2002;1(2):135-142.

242. Newton H. The multiprofessional treatment of a patient with arterial leg ulceration. *Wound Essentials* 2006;1(1):64-65.

243. Wayman J, Nirojogi V, Walker A, Sowinski A, Walker MA. The cost effectiveness of larval therapy in venous ulcers. *Journal of Tissue Viability* 2000;10(3):91-94.

244. Wayman J, Nirojogi V, Walker A, Sowinski A, Walker MA. The cost effectiveness of larval therapy in venous ulcers Erratum. *Journal of Tissue Viability* 2001;11(1):51.

245. Raynor P. A new clinical trial of the effect of larval therapy. *Journal of Tissue Viability* 2004;14(3):104-105.

246. Soares MO, Iglesias CP, Bland JM, Cullum N, Dumville JC, Nelson EA, et al. Cost effectiveness analysis of larval therapy for leg ulcers. *BMJ* 2009;338:b825.

247. Dumville JC, Worthy G, Bland JM, Cullum N, Dowson C, Iglesias C, et al. Larval therapy for leg ulcers (VenUS II): randomised controlled trial. *BMJ* 2009;338:b773.

248. Sherman RA, Mumcuoglu K. 2009.

249. Chaffrey R. *Case study: Larval therapy for an infected insect bite.* 1997

250. Husain ZS, Fallat LM. Maggot therapy for wound debridement in a traumatic foot-degloving injury: a case report. *J Foot Ankle Surg* 2003;42(6):371-6.

251. Gacheru I. A case report: The use of maggots in wound treatment. *The Nairobi Hospital Proceedings* 1998;2(4):234-238.

252. Dunn C, Raghavan U, Pfleiderer AG. The use of maggots in head and neck necrotizing fasciitis. *J Laryngol Otol* 2002;116(1):70-2.

253. Steenvoorde P, Jacobi CE, Wong CY, Jukema GN. Maggot debridement therapy in necrotizing fasciitis reduces the number of surgical debridements.
Report on 15 treated patients. . *Wounds* 2007;19(3):73-7.

254. Tittlebach J, Graefe T, Wollina U. Painful ulcers in calciphylaxis - combined treatment with maggot therapy and oral pentoxyfillin. *Journal of Dermatological Treatment* 2001;12:211-214.

255. Pliquett RU, Schwock J, Paschke R, Achenbach H. Calciphylaxis in chronic, non-dialysis-dependent renal disease. *BMC Nephrol* 2003;4(1):8.

256. Kelly J. Pyoderma gangraenosum: exploring the treatment options. *Journal of Wound Care* 2001;10(4):125-128.

257. Renner R, Treudler R, Simon JC. Maggots do not survive in pyoderma gangrenosum. *Dermatology* 2008;217(3):241-3.

258. Jones M, Thomas S. A case history describing the use of sterile larvae (maggots) in a malignant wound. *World Wide Wounds* 1998.

259. Sealby N. The use of maggot therapy in the treatment of a malignant foot wound. *Br J Community Nurs* 2004;9(3):S16-9.

260. Sherman RA, Shapiro CE, Yang RM. Maggot therapy for problematic wounds: uncommon and off-label applications. *Adv Skin Wound Care* 2007;20(11):602-10.

261. Steenvoorde P, Jacobi CE, Van Doorn L, Oskam J. Maggot debridement therapy of infected ulcers: patient and wound factors influencing outcome - a study on 101 patients with 117 wounds. *Ann R Coll Surg Engl* 2007;89(6):596-602.

262. Wolff H, Hansson C. Larval therapy for a leg ulcer with methicillin-resistant Staphylococcus aureus [letter]. *Acta Derm Venereol* 1999;79(4):320-1.

263. Bowling FL, Salgami EV, Boulton AJ. Larval therapy: a novel treatment in eliminating methicillin-resistant Staphylococcus aureus from diabetic foot ulcers. *Diabetes Care* 2007;30(2):370-1.

264. Stokes K. Biosurgery: how maggots are making a comeback in mainstream medicine. *Biotech.Ghana* 2004;3(1):3-4.

265. Arrivillaga J, Rodriguez J, Oviedo M. Preliminary evaluation of maggot (Diptera: Calliphoridae) therapy as a potential treatment for leishmaniasis ulcers. *Biomedica* 2008;28(2):305-10.

266. Fadaak H. Maggot debridement therapy. *Burns* 2003;29(1):96.

267. Summers JB, Kaminski J. Maggot debridement therapy (MDT) for burn wounds. *Burns* 2003;29(5):501-2.

268. Courtenay M. Larval therapy in the management of wounds: clinical update. *British Journal of Community Nursing* 1999;4(6):290-292.

269. Thomas S, McCubbin P. Use of maggots in the care of wounds. *Hospital Pharmacist* 2002;9(9):267-271.

270. Trudgian J. Evaluating the benefits of larval therapy. *Nursing Standard* 2002;16(22):65-73.

271. Thomas S. The cost of managing chronic wounds in the UK with particular emphasis on maggot debridement therapy. *Journal of Wound Care* 2006;15(10):465-469.

272. Steenvoorde P, Budding T, Oskam J. Determining pain levels in patients treated with maggot debridement therapy. *Journal of Wound Care* 2005;14(10):485-488.

273. Rojo S, Geraghty S. Hemophilia and maggots: from hospital admission to healed wound. *Ostomy Wound Manage* 2004;50(4):30, 32, 34.

274. Steenvoorde P, van Doorn LP. Maggot debridement therapy: serious bleeding can occur: report of a case. *J Wound Ostomy Continence Nurs* 2008;35(4):412-4.

275. Virgili A, Ligrone L, Bacilieri S, Corazza M. Protein contact dermatitis in a fisherman using maggots of a flesh fly as bait. *Contact Dermatitis* 2001;44(4):262-3.

276. Greenberg B. Persistence of bacteria in the developmental stages of the housefly. 1. Survival of Enteric Pathogens in the Normal and Aseptically Reated Host. *Am. J. Trop. Med & Hyg.* 1959;8:405-411.

277. Greenberg B. Persistence of bacteria in the developmental stages of the housefly. II Quantitative study of the host-contaminant relationship in flies breeding under natural conditions. *Am. J. Trop. Med. & Hyg.* 1959;8:412-416.

278. Greenberg B. Persistence of bacteria in the developmental stages of the housefly. III. Quantitative distribution in Prepupae and Pupae. *Am J Trop Med Hyg* 1959;8:613-617.

279. Greenberg B, Migglano V. Host contaminant biology of muscoid flies IV. Microbial competition in a blowfly. *Journal of Insect Pathology* 1960;2:44-54.

280. Nuesch R, Rahm G, Rudin W, Steffen I, Frei R, Rufli T, et al. Clustering of bloodstream infections during maggot debridement therapy using contaminated larvae of Protophormia terraenovae. *Infection* 2002;30(5):306-9.

281. Melnick JL, Penner LR. The survival of poliomyelitis and Coxsackie viruses following their ingestion by flies. *J. Exper. Med.* 1952;96:255-271.

282. Post K, Riesner D, Walldorf V, Mehlhorn H. Fly larvae and pupae as vectors for scrapie. *Lancet* 1999;354(9194):1969-70.

283. Guerrini VH. Ammonia toxicity and alkalosis in sheep infested by Lucilia cuprina larvae. *International Journal for Parasitology* 1988;18(1):79-81.

284. Broadmeadow M, Gibson JE, Dimmock CK, Thomas RJ, O'Sullivan BM. The pathogenesis of flystrike in sheep. *Wool Technol. Sheep Breed.* 1984;32:28-32.

285. Kitching M. Patients' perceptions and experiences of larval therapy. *Journal of Wound Care* 2004;13(1):25-29.

286. Rosales A, Vazquez JR, Short B, Kimbriel HR, Claxton MJ, Nixon BP, et al. Use of a maggot motility index to evaluate survival of therapeutic larvae. *J Am Podiatr Med Assoc* 2004;94(4):353-5.

287. Sherman RA, Wyle FA, L.Thrupp. Effects of seven antibiotics on the growth and development of Phaenicia sericata (Diptera: Calliphoridae) larvae. *Journal of Medical Entomology* 1995;32(5):646-649.

288. Thomas S, Andrews AM. The effect of hydrogel dressings on maggot development. *Journal of Wound Care* 1999;8(2):75-77.

289. Jones G, Wall R. Maggot-therapy in veterinary medicine. *Res Vet Sci* 2008;85(2):394-8.

290. Dicke RJ. Maggot therapy of actinomycosis. *J Econ Entomol* 1953;46(4):706-707.

291. Bell NJ, Thomas S. Use of sterile maggots to treat panniculitis in an aged donkey. *Veterinary Record* 2001;149:768-770.
292. Sherman RA, Morrison S, Ng D. Maggot debridement therapy for serious horse wounds - a survey of practitioners. *Vet J* 2007;174(1):86-91.
293. Morrison SE. AAEP Convention: How to use sterile maggot debridement therapy for foot infections of the horse. In: Brown K, editor. *AAEP*. Seattle Washington, 2005:461-464.
294. Sherman RA, Stevens H, Ng D, Iversen E. Treating wounds in small animals with maggot debridement therapy: a survey of practitioners. *Vet J* 2007;173(1):138-43.

20. Negative pressure wound therapy

HISTORICAL BACKGROUND

Negative Pressure Wound Therapy (NPWT) also known as vacuum assisted closure (VAC), Vacuum therapy, vacuum sealing or simply topical negative pressure therapy is a sophisticated development of a standard surgical procedure: the application of vacuum assisted drainage to remove blood or serous fluid from a wound or operation site and thereby reduce the risk of bacterial contamination.

In a review of the use of drains in orthopaedic surgery, Gaines and Dunbar[1] recount how simple wound drains in varying forms have been used at least since the time of Hippocrates (460-377 BC). They also describe how Ambrose Pare (1510-1590), a pioneer of surgical drainage, used cannulated lead tubes, which he called 'tentes' for drainage and debridement, suggesting that he may have been the first to apply this technique to orthopaedic procedures.

Subsequently the microbiological studies of Joseph Lister and Robert Koch suggested that they may be a sound basis for excess removing fluid from wounds which could potentially become infected with bacteria, accordingly from the late 19th Century until the mid 20th Century, gravity-type open drain systems were used extensively for this purpose.

It was not until the middle of the 20th Century that drains were developed which could be used successfully with an applied vacuum, leading to the development of closed drainage systems, which were demonstrably superior to open or gravity systems for reducing wound complications as well as helping to bring about apposition of the wound margins to facilitate healing.[2]

An alternative early use of negative pressure to promote healing was described by Johnson,[3] who used it when applying skin grafts to donor site. His approach was relatively simple: a piece of fine mesh gauze impregnated with ointment was applied directly to the graft and covered with dry gauze. A suction drain, connected to a suitable vacuum source, was placed over the top and the entire assembly covered with an occlusive membrane. Johnson claimed that as the suction was applied, any air or exudate trapped between the graft and the wound surface was removed with the result that the graft was brought into intimate contact with the wound surface across its entire area, thereby increasing the likelihood of a successful graft 'take'.

A similar technique was described by Jeter et al.,[4] for managing patients with draining wounds or fistulae. They reported that it increased rate of granulation and re-epithelialization and concluded that, compared with conventional treatments, the suction technique enhanced wound closure, prevented skin damage and reduced nursing time and treatment costs. Like Johnson et al., Jeter and colleagues employed wall suction or Emerson vacuum devices to generate negative pressure in the wound.

In 1991 Argenta and Morykwas filed a patent in the US in which they described a closed vacuum wound closure technique, which utilized foam instead of the cotton gauze employed by earlier workers.

DEVELOPMENT OF NPWT

An early account of the clinical use of sub-atmospheric pressure to promote debridement and healing of granulating wounds was provided by Fleischmann et al. in 1993,[5] following his successful use of this technique in 15 patients with open fractures. They observed that the treatment resulted in 'efficient cleaning and conditioning of the wound, with marked proliferation of granulation tissue'. No bone infections occurred in any of these patients although one developed a soft tissue infection, which subsequently resolved with further treatment.

In two further papers, Fleischmann described the treatment of 25 patients with a compartment syndrome of the lower limb,[6] and 313 patients with acute and chronic infections of various types.[7]

Further early success with topical negative pressure treatment in Germany was reported by Muller,[8] following the treatment of 300 patients with infected wounds, and in 1998 Kovacs et al.[9] described how 'vacuum sealing' could be used for the treatment of chronic radiation ulcers.

The results of a prospective trial involving 45 patients with soft tissue injuries including sacral pressure ulcers, acute traumatic soft tissue defects and infected soft tissue defects following rigid stabilisation of lower extremity fractures were described by Mullner et al.[10] They reported that in 38/45 patients (84%), the use of the vacuum sealing technique following irrigation and debridement decreased the dimensions of the initial wound, thus facilitating healing time and the eradication of any pre-existing infection.

In the first published studies, negative pressure within a wound was achieved by the use of conventional means such as a wall suction apparatus or surgical vacuum bottles, but as Banwell et al.[11] described, both of these are associated with practical problems in terms of the delivery, control and maintenance of the required levels of negative pressure.

In 1995, these problems were largely resolved by Kinetic Concepts Inc. (KCI) who introduced a commercial system for promoting vacuum assisted closure into the United States. This subsequently became known throughout the world as the V.A.C. system.

The heart of the system was a microprocessor-controlled vacuum unit capable of providing controlled levels of continuous or intermittent sub-atmospheric pressure ranging from 25 to 200 mmHg.

The technique proved an outstanding clinical and commercial success. Over 3 million patients worldwide have been treated in this way, and according to some internet sources the global Negative Pressure Wound Therapy (NPWT) market, which was valued at $640m in 2009, is forecast to grow by 8.2% annually for the next seven years to reach $1.1 billion in 2016.

A simple basic search of the PubMed Medline database identified over 600 references that appear to be related to this topic. When these are grouped by the year of publication, they reveal exponential growth in the interest in this topic Figure 92.

Figure 92: Publications on NPWT by year

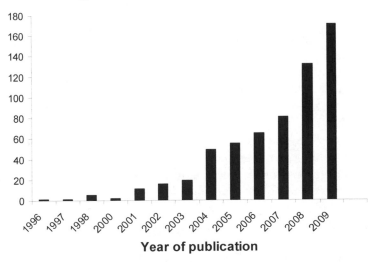

Year of publication

As might be anticipated, the value of the NPWT market attracted the attention of other medical device companies, but their attempts to introduce competitive products were strongly resisted by KCI, resulting in numerous legal battles around the world. Eventually other companies won the right to produce NPWT systems and, as a result, numerous different systems have been developed although not all are available in all markets. Those identified to date include:

- **Convatec**
  - o Eugenex System
- **KCI**
  - o ActiV.A.C. (lightweight portable system for ambulatory patients)
  - o InfoV.A.C. (system designed for the acute care environment)
  - o V.A.C. Freedom (system designed for long term care environments)
- **Ohio Medical Corp**
  - o MoblVac System
- **Mölnlycke**
  - o Avance
- **Prospera**
  - o Prospera
- **Smith and Nephew**
  - o EZCare
  - o Vista (portable system)
  - o Renasys
- **Talley Medical**
  - o Venturi

These systems differ not only in the design of the hardware, but also in the nature of the disposables that are used with each. These include gauze and various types of foam, some of which include silver compounds.

METHOD OF USE

To function correctly, the vacuum source must generate a fluidic pathway between the foam or gauze placed within the wound and the container or reservoir in which it will subsequently be contained, Furthermore as seals, including that formed by the outer adhesive membrane to the skin, must be completely airtight.

Obtaining such a seal can be particularly difficult near the anus or vagina or where the surrounding skin is moist. These problems can sometimes be overcome by the use of a hydrocolloid dressing such as Duoderm,[12] which is first applied around the wound and used as a base for the adhesive membrane, Greer et al.[13]

The basic technique for performing a simple dressing is illustrated in Figure 93 which shows how it was used following debridement by maggot therapy to dress a knee wound following an arthroplasty. The wound was initially heavily infected and the metalwork of the joint was clearly visible in the base of the wound.

Stages in formation of a NPWT dressing

- A suitably sized piece of foam is selected together with an adhesive film and drainage tube (a).
- The foam is cut to the approximate size of the wound with scissors and placed gently into position (b).
- The perforated drain tube is then located on top of the foam and a second piece of foam placed over the top (c.). (For shallower wounds, a single piece of foam may be used and the drainage tube is inserted inside it).
- The foam, together with the first few inches of the drainage tube and the surrounding area of healthy skin, is then covered with the adhesive transparent membrane ensuring that the membrane forms a good seal both with the skin and the drainage tube (d).
- The distal end of the drain is connected to the vacuum source which is programmed to produce the required level of pressure.
- Once the vacuum is switched on, the air is sucked out of the foam causing it to collapse inwards drawing the edges of the wound inwards (e) until closure is obtained (f).

Figure 93: Stages in the formation of a simple NPWT dressing system

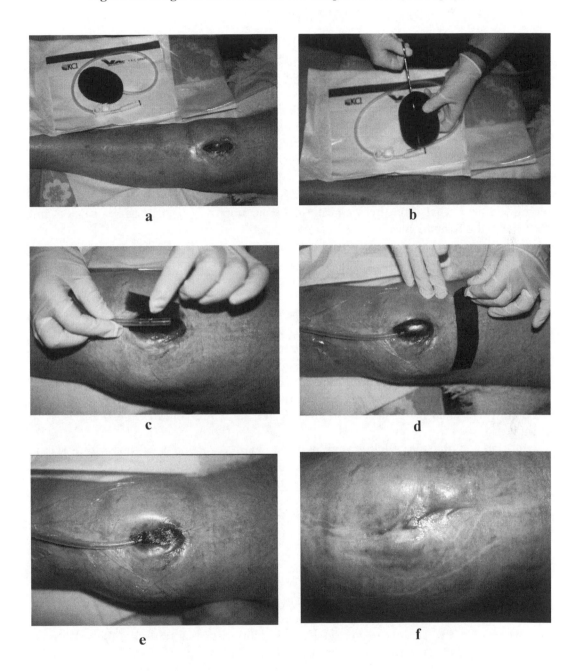

CLINICAL EXPERIENCE WITH NPWT

As previously indicated the literature on NPWT is extensive and contains many case reports, reviews, and trials of varying complexity and quality. They include accounts of the use of the therapy in a variety of wound types including extensive degloving injuries,[14-15] infected sternotomy wounds,[16-18] and various soft tissue injuries prior to surgical closure, grafting or reconstructive surgery.[19-20] Brief details of some of these publications are provided below by way of example.

Argenta and Morykwas[12] described how 296 out of 300 wounds of mixed aetiology treated with NPWT responded favourably to treatment. The wounds were treated until completely closed, or covered with a split-thickness skin graft, or a flap was rotated into the health, granulating would bed. They considered the principal advantages of the technique to be that it removes chronic oedema, improves local tissue perfusion and stimulates the formation of granulation tissue.

Smith et al,[21] in a retrospective review, described the use of VAC over a four-year period in 93 patients who required open abdomen management for a variety of conditions, concluding that, with careful subsequent management, good patient outcomes could be achieved. They therefore recommended vacuum assisted closure as the treatment method of choice for open abdomen management and temporary abdominal closure.

NPWT has also been described in the treatment of donor sites, particularly in areas that are difficult to manage using conventional techniques,[20] such as those on the radial forearm.[22] It has been reported that as many as one third of all patients undergoing radial forearm free flaps develop complications, including exposed tendons, and it has been suggested that these individuals may derive particular benefit from the use of the therapy.[23]

Similarly with split thickness skin grafts in the treatment of burns, NPWT is claimed to be particularly useful for body sites with irregular or deep contours such as the perineum, hand or axilla.[24-25] In all these situations the vacuum helps to hold the graft securely onto the wound bed thus preventing pooling of tissue fluid which would otherwise make the graft unstable. If the technique is applied to donor sites, some authors recommend the use of a low adherent wound contact layer such as Adaptic or paraffin gauze beneath the foam layer.[20,22]

Molnar et al.,[26] described how they used NPWT in conjunction with skin grafts to treat four patients with full thickness loss of the scalp following a burn injury or excision of an extensive carcinoma. Normally, if such wounds cannot be closed with a flap, the outer surface of the skull is removed to obtain punctate bleeding and a skin graft is applied a week or two later once granulation tissue has started to form. Without this delay the graft take is usually very poor, but with the use of NPWT it was possible to apply a successful skin graft immediately after the initial operation.

Numerous case histories describing the successful use of NWPT in a variety of nonhealing or chronic wounds have also been published. These include a recalcitrant below knee amputation wound and a suspected brown recluse spider bite,[27] a bite from a cantharid beetle,[28] dog bites,[29] hidradenitis suppurativa,[30] pressure sores,[13,31-33] leg ulcers,[34] and a group of 30 patients with longstanding wounds that were deemed unsuitable for reconstructive surgery, 26 of whom responded favourably to the treatment.[35]

Given the widespread adoption of this technique and the considerable expenditure it has attracted, it is not surprising that over the years a number of systematic reviews have been undertaken to assess its value in a more objective fashion. Some of these reviews are identified below.

- Evans and Land[36] in 2001 identified two small RCT which provided weak evidence to suggest that NPWT may be superior to saline-gauze dressings in terms of wound healing.

- In 2007 Wasiak and Cleland[37] concluded that there was insufficient quality data to demonstrate differences between NPWT and conventional therapy dressings in the treatment of partial thickness burns.

- Gregor et al.[38] in 2008 reviewed seven RCTs and 10 non-RCTs. Although overall the quality of the trials was poor, significant differences in favour of NPWT for time to wound closure or incidence of wound closure were shown in 2 of 5 RCTs and 2 of 4 non-RCTs. The authors concluded that although there is some indication that NPWT may improve wound healing; the body of evidence available is insufficient to clearly prove an additional clinical benefit of NPWT. They also identified that the large number of prematurely terminated and unpublished trials on this topic was a potential cause for concern.

- Peinemann et al. in 2008[39] similarly expressed reservation about potential publication bias caused by lack of access to unpublished study results relating to this therapy.

- Hinchcliffe et al.[40] in 2008, following a systematic review of the effectiveness of interventions to enhance the healing of chronic ulcers of the foot in diabetes, concluded that NPWT 'may promote healing of post-operative wounds'.

- Noble-Bell et al. in 2008[41] similarly concluded that whilst there was evidence that NPWT therapy was more effective than conventional dressing for the treatment of diabetic foot ulcers, the quality of the studies was weak.

- Ubbink et al. in 2008[42] reviewed seven trials involving 205 participants with chronic wounds in which NPWT was compared with five different comparator treatments. They found that the studies had methodological flaws and produced data that did not demonstrate a beneficial effect of NPWT on wound healing. In their review, they also made reference to earlier systematic reviews published by Mendonca[43] and Pham[44] both of which were more favourable to NPWT. They suggested, however, that this could be due to the fact that these authors included data from non-randomised studies which are highly susceptible to bias.

- In a second review, Ubbink *et al.*[45] evaluated NPWT in both acute and chronic wounds, once again concluding that the technique did not bring about earlier complete wound healing. They did report, however, a 1-10 day reduction in the time needed to prepare a wound for secondary closure surgery. Once again they concluded that there was little evidence to support the use of TNP in the treatment of wounds
- Vikatmaa *et al.*[46] 2008 identified 14 RCTs involving patients with a variety of wound types only two of which were classified as 'high-quality' studies, the remainder were classified as having poor internal validity. In all studies NPWT was found to be at least as effective and in some cases more effective than the control treatment although the authors stressed the need for further high quality RCTs.

As with systematic reviews undertaken in other wound management areas, in the main these fail to demonstrate any strong evidence to support the use of the therapy in question. This is due, at least in part, to the lack of clinical studies which met the stringent requirements for inclusion. Nevertheless it is difficult to understand how such an expensive and, in some ways, inconvenient therapy could continue to grow so rapidly in popularity unless it actually delivered sound clinical benefits when used in the treatment of problem wounds as judged by the tens of thousands of healthcare professionals who have adopted its use in their daily clinical practice.

Furthermore, the types of patients who are most likely to benefit from this form of treatment are those with complex, advanced or difficult to manage wounds for whom the prognosis is poor. These types of patients are generally excluded from randomized controlled studies for practical or ethical reasons.

COST IMPLICATIONS OF TREATMENT

The cost of VAC therapy is not insignificant, for in addition to the purchase cost or hire charges for the machine itself, it is necessary to purchase disposables including dressings, drainage tubes, canisters and adhesive films. Nevertheless, numerous authors have suggested that efficacy of the technique is such that it is actually cost effective in practice.

In a retrospective study Philbeck *et al.*,[47] compared treatment costs of NPWT with those of more conventional therapies, by comparing healing rates achieved with the vacuum technique with those recorded for similar wounds in a previously published study. Treatment records of 1032 Medicare patients with 1,170 NPWT-treated wounds of all types, that had failed to respond to previous interventions, were reviewed.

From these data, the healing rates of patients nursed on a low air loss surface (LAL) with 43 pressure ulcers (stages III and IV) located on the trochanter and trunk were abstracted and compared with previously published values for a comparable group of patients, also nursed on a LAL surface, whose wounds were dressed with saline-gauze packs. Prior to treatment, the area of NPWT-dressed lesions was 22.2cm^2 compared with 4.3cm^2 for the comparators. Wounds dressed with NPWT closed at an average of

$0.23 cm^2$ per day compared with $0.09 cm^2$ for the historical controls. Using these healing rates they calculated that the time to heal a group of patients with wounds 22.2 cm^2 in area would be 97 days with NPWT and cost $14,546, compared with 247 days with traditional therapy at a cost of $23,465. Whilst acknowledging all the limitations of their study, the authors concluded that negative pressure therapy is an "effective treatment modality for a variety of chronic wounds" producing healing in certain types of pressure ulcers 61% faster than saline soaked gauze whilst reducing costs by 38%.

Le Franc et al.[48] also used retrospective data to compare NPWT with moist wound dressings for preparing open-leg fractures prior to reconstructive surgery involving graft or flap formation. Preparation time was, on average, 20 days shorter for patient treated with NPWT (p = 0.026). Hospital costs were very significantly lower for patients being treated with NPWT (p = 0.02). In absolute terms this cost reduced on average by 6000 Euros per patient (> 60%). The incremental cost-effectiveness ratio is of the order of 164 Euros per day of wound preparation.

Other studies which predicted financial advantages in favour of NPWT include a variety of wound type including diabetic ulcers,[49-50] infected wounds,[51] and surgical wounds[52]

The time at which NPWT is initiated may be significant. Kaplan et al.[53] used retrospective data to study the clinical and cost-effective benefits of using NPWT at an early stage, Day 1 or Day 2 of treatment, compared with initiating on Day 3 or later in the management of traumatic wounds. For wound treated early, 518 patient records were included and for the wounds treated later 1000 records were reviewed. They found that early-group patients had fewer hospital inpatient days (10.6 vs 20.6 days; p < 0.0001) and fewer treatment days (5.1 vs 6.0 days; p = 0.0498). They also required a shorter stay in an intensive care unit (ICU) (5.3 vs 12.4 days; p < 0.0001), but had higher ICU admission rates (51.5 vs 44.5%; p = 0.0091) than the late group.

Compared with late-treated group patients, patients treated promptly had lower total and variable costs per patient discharge ($43,956 vs $32,175; p < 0.0001 and $22,891 vs $15,805; p < 0.0001, respectively) suggesting that that early intervention with NPWT has potential clinical and cost-effective benefits for the treatment of traumatic wounds. These conclusions were supported by the results of a second study published by Baharestani et al.[54]

COMPARISONS BETWEEN NWPT SYSTEMS

Home-made systems

Because of the very significant costs associated with the original VAC system, a number of clinical centres have attempted to devise cheaper 'home-made' versions using readily-available materials and resources.

Hu et al.[55] compared two kinds of NPWT in 44 inpatients with acute, subacute, and chronic wounds. Subjects were divided into a simplified NPWT group, Group A, and the conventional NPWT group, Group B, using a random number table.

Wounds of patients in Group A were treated with gauze and continuous suction with hospital central negative pressure (-10.64 kPa) for 24 h but wounds of patients in

Group B were treated with a commercial system involving a foam dressing and intermittent suction. (-16.63 kPa) for 24 h. Gross wound condition, treatment time, survival rates of skin graft and flap, changes of bacterial species on wound, treatment cost, and ratio of side effects between two groups were compared. No significant differences were detected between the two groups in respect of gross wound condition, and treatment outcomes. Treatment times for the two groups were 29 ± 12 vs 26 ± 13 days for Groups A and B respectively, ($p > 0.05$).

As expected, treatment costs for Group A were significantly lower than for Group B (374 ± 134 vs 9825 ± 4956 yen; $p < 0.01$) but more side effects were observed in Group A than Group B (33.3% vs 5.0%; $p < 0.05$). The authors concluded that although the simplified system is cheaper, it has the potential to cause more side effects including nosocomial infections.

The costs of using a 'home-made' NPWT system were also compared with those of a commercial system by Rozen et al.[56] who devised used a single cut foam sheet, a conventional disposable closed-system suction drain and an adhesive film to dress split skin grafts in nine consecutive patients. In all nine patients, there was a 100% take of the graft, with no partial or complete loss. Cost analysis demonstrated a minimum treatment cost of $577 over 5 days compared to an estimated $3180 for a commercial system: a net saving of $2603 per patient, leading the authors to conclude that the use of a simple suction drain is a cheap and safe alternative to commercial dressings for the treatment of lower limb split skin grafts.

Choice of primary dressing

The original V.A.C. system exclusively made use of grey hydrophobic, reticulated open-cell polyurethane foam with a pore size of 400 - 600 μm.

The hydrophobic nature of this material means that it does not 'absorb' exudate as such; it simply allows it free-passage throughout its structure under the influence of the partial vacuum produced within the closed system over the wound. A version of this foam containing silver is also available.

In some situations, however, over-exuberant production of granulation tissue can result in this cellular material becoming incorporated into the structure of the foam, resulting in damage or trauma on removal. An additional type of white foam was therefore introduced which is made from hydrophilic polyvinyl alcohol and is indicated for use in situations where adherence is judged to be a real or potential problem. This alternative foam is described as 'non-reticulated' with a higher-density cell structure and a pore size of 200 - 1000 μm.

Because of the legal issue around the KCI patent, specifically the use of foam as a wound contact material, alternative commercial forms of NPWT were introduced which made use of cotton gauze as described previously by Jeter et al.[4]

The relative merits of foam and cotton have become the subject of some debate and to a large extent the matter currently remains unresolved. From a theoretical point of view foam should be superior to gauze for a number of reasons: it is more resilient, has a large volume for packing cavities, and does not shed particles and fibres in the way that cotton does. In contrast gauze may be used more easily over larger areas of tissue and it is claimed by some that it conforms better to wounds with an uneven base.

Resent changes in the legal situation with regard to the KCI patent now means that other manufacturers are free to offer foam dressings as part of their NPWT systems so the situation is likely to change once again. Readers who wish to obtain more up-to-date information on this topic are advised to contact the companies concerned for details of the products on offer.

MODE OF ACTION

In early studies no attempts were made to investigate the physiological basis for the benefits of NPWT, or to determine the optimum levels of pressure required. Initially it was assumed that the system functioned by removing excess wound fluid which might contain inflammatory mediators or microorganisms which might otherwise inhibit healing.

In a seminal paper Morykwas et al.,[57] published the results of series of animal studies in which deep circular defects, 2.5 cm in diameter, on the backs of pigs were dressed with open-cell polyurethane-ether foam with a pore size ranging from 400-600 μm. In their first series of experiments, a laser Doppler technique was used to measure blood flow in the subcutaneous tissue and muscle which surrounded the wounds as these were exposed to increasing levels of negative pressure applied both continuously and intermittently.

Their results indicated that whilst an increase in blood flow equivalent to four times the baseline value occurred with negative pressure values of 125 mmHg, blood flow was inhibited by the application of negative pressures of 400 mmHg and above. A negative pressure value of 125 mmHg was therefore selected for use in subsequent studies.

The rate of granulation tissue production under negative pressure was determined using the same model by measuring the reduction in wound volume over time. Compared with control wounds dressed with saline soaked gauze, significantly increased rates of granulation tissue formation occurred with both continuous (63.3 ± 26.1%) and intermittent (103% ± 35.3%) application of negative pressure.

Fabian et al.,[58] using the rabbit ear model, provided further hard evidence for the stimulatory effects of sub-atmospheric pressure on the production of granulation tissue and also demonstrated a trend to enhanced epithelialisation.

In experimental partial-thickness burns in pigs, sub-atmospheric pressure was shown to prevent progressive tissue damage in the zone of stasis that surrounds the area of the initial injury. This effect was demonstrable within 12 hours following injury, with treatment times of as little as six hours being sufficient to exert a measurable effect.[59] The authors proposed that NPWT removed of oedematous fluid containing suspended cellular debris, osmotically active molecules and biochemical mediators, released following the initial injury, which may prevent or inhibit normal blood flow in the local area.

The observation that intermittent or cycled treatment appears more effective than continuous therapy is interesting although the reasons for this are not fully understood. Two possible explanations were advanced by Philbeck et al.[47] They suggested that intermittent cycling results in rhythmic perfusion of the tissue which is maintained because the process of capillary autoregulation is not activated. They also suggested that as cells which are undergoing mitosis must go through a cycle of rest, cellular component production and division, constant stimulation may cause the cells to 'ignore' the stimulus which thus become ineffective. Intermittent stimulation allows the cells time to rest and prepare for the next cycle. For this reason it is suggested that cyclical negative pressure should be used clinically, although some authors suggest that this may follow a 48-hour period of continuous vacuum, which is presumably applied to exert a rapid initial cleansing effect.[16,31]

As part of their study, Morykwas et al.[57] also undertook some basic microbiological investigations which they claimed suggested that compared with control values, tissue bacterial counts of vacuum-treated wounds may decrease after four days. In the final part of the same study NPWT was found to increase flap survival by 21% compared to control values.

As a result of all of these investigations, the authors postulated that multiple mechanisms might be responsible for these observed effects. In particular, they suggested that removal of interstitial fluid decreases localised oedema and increases blood flow, which in turn decreases tissue bacterial levels. They also suggested that the application of sub-atmospheric pressure produces mechanical deformation or stress within the tissue resulting in protein and matrix molecule synthesis.

The importance of cell deformation and its stimulatory effect on proliferation has been recognized in other areas but in this context formed the subject of a study undertaken by Saxena et al.,[60] who hypothesize that application of micromechanical forces to wounds in vivo can promote wound healing through this cell shape-dependent, mechanical control mechanism. They therefore created a computer model (finite element) of a wound and simulated the effects of NPWT, i.e. varying pressure, pore diameter, and pore volume fraction, to study the effects of vacuum-induced material deformations. When the results from the computer wound model were compared with histological sections of wounds treated with NPWT they found that most elements stretched by the application of negative pressure experienced deformations of 5 to 20 percent strain, values comparable with in vitro strain levels known to promote cellular proliferation. They also showed that the deformation predicted by the model were similar in morphology to the surface undulations observed in histological cross-sections of the wounds. The authors therefore hypothesized that the tissue deformation produced by NPWT stretches individual cells, thereby promoting proliferation in the wound microenvironment as previously suggested by Morykwas et al.[57]

The effect of NPWT with a foam wound insert on capillary formation and MMP activity was examined by Greene et al.[61] in a clinical study in which NPWT was administered to the chronic wounds of 3 debilitated patients. Tissue obtained from wound areas with and without foam contact was examined to determine microvessel density and MMP activity by immunohistochemistry and zymography. The authors showed that during the first week of treatment the microvessel density of wounds treated with NPWT was significantly higher than the areas not covered by foam, $4.5\% \pm 0.8$ *vs* $1.6\% \pm 0.1$ (p = 0.05). During the second week the corresponding values were $2.7\% \pm 0.3$ *vs* $1.3\% \pm 0.1$ respectively (p = 0.03). MMP-9/NGAL (neutrophil gelatinase-associated lipocalin), MMP-9, latent MMP-2, and active MMP-2 were all reduced by 15%-76% in wounds treated with NPWT providing strong supporting evidence for the mode of action of the technique proposed by earlier authors.

Scherer *et al.*[62] evaluated the importance of the various components of a foam based NPWT system in a full-thickness wound model in diabetic mice. Groups of wounds were treated with an occlusive dressing, subatmospheric pressure at 125 mmHg, and a piece of polyurethane foam without and with downward compression.

Seven days after injury, the wounds treated as above were examined by a two-dimensional immunohistochemical staging system based on blood vessel density (CD31) and cell proliferation (Ki67).

Wounds exposed to polyurethane foam in compressed and uncompressed dressings or to the vacuum-assisted closure device showed a two-fold increase in vascularity compared with the occlusive dressing group (p < 0.05). The vacuum-assisted closure device in addition stimulated cell proliferation, with up to 82 percent Ki67-positive nuclei, compared with the other groups. Direct measurements of wound surface deformations showed significant microstrains in the vacuum-assisted closure and foam in compressed dressing groups (60% and 16%, respectively) compared with all other groups.

The authors concluded that these data provide confirmatory evidence for proposed mechanism of action of NPWT and suggested that their wound model represented a useful and reproducible experimental platform with which to evaluate performance of wound healing devices.

In a second study, the same research group [63] used the same model to revisit the issue of the importance of the duration of treatment. They compared the effects of an occlusive dressing used alone, the NPWT used for 6 or 12 hours, or applied periodically for 4 hours every other day, or allowed to run continuously for 7 days. As before, wound closure and tissue response were evaluated by macroscopic, histological, and immunohistochemical analyses on day 7.

Compared with continuous treatment, wound closure was significantly faster after short initial vacuum-assisted closure in the 6-hour and 12-hour treated groups. Compared with the dressing-alone controls, increased granulation tissue was detected in the 12-hour group (2.4-fold increase) and in those treated periodically for 4 hours every other day (3.2-fold increase).

Significant stimulation of cell proliferation was seen after all vacuum-assisted closure patterns (3.6 - 5.3-fold increase); whereas angiogenesis was augmented only after the device was applied for 4 hour periods. Three treatments of 4 hours showed a superior angiogenic effect compared with short initial applications as in the 6-hour and 12-hour groups. The authors therefore concluded that short vacuum-assisted closure treatment induced an extended biological response in the wound. A total of 12 hours of periodically applied vacuum-assisted closure reached a similar wound tissue response as continuously applied vacuum-assisted closure for 7 days, findings which may have important implications for the design of future devices.

Fabian et al.,[58] in a well controlled animal study, investigated the possibility that subatmospheric pressure might act synergistically with hyperbaric oxygen (HBO2). They found, however, that although negative pressure increased the rate of healing compared with control values, HBO2 therapy did not offer any significant benefit.

THE FUTURE OF NPWT

Although numerous papers have been published that suggest that the technique may have an important role to play in the management of many types of chronic or infected wounds, the cost of the system is such that some clinicians may be reluctant to use it until further prospective studies have been undertaken to demonstrate its cost effectiveness in routine use.

Even in the absence of such studies, however, few would argue that the technique does not have a role to play in the management of extensive cavity wounds that cannot be surgically closed and are too large to be dressed with conventional dressings. The system may also be of value in the management of heavily exuding wounds, including those with lymphatic involvement.

The principal indications and contraindications to the use of NPWT are summarised below. In addition, for obvious reasons, special precautions should be observed when using the technique where haemostasis is difficult, in the presence of active bleeding or in the treatment of patients receiving anticoagulant therapy.

An excellent summary on the indications and contraindications for NPWT was published in the form of a consensus document in 2008. [64]

REFERENCES

1. Gaines RJ, Dunbar RP. The use of surgical drains in orthopedics. *Orthopedics* 2008;**31**(7):702-5.
2. Raffl AB. The use of negative pressure under skin flaps after radical mastectomy. *Ann Surg* 1952;**136**(6):1048.
3. Johnson FE. An improved technique for skin graft placement using a suction drain. *Surgery, Gynaecology and Obstetrics* 1984;**159**(6):585-586.
4. Jeter K, Tintle T, Chariker M. Managing draining wounds and fistulae: new and established methods . . In: Krasnr D, editor. *Chronic Wound Care*. King of Prussia, Pennsylvania: Health Management Publications, Inc., 1990:240-246.
5. Fleischmann W, Strecker W, Bombelli M, Kinzl L. Vacuum sealing as treatment of soft tissue damage in open fractures. *Unfallchirurg* 1993;**96**(9):488-92.
6. Fleischmann W, Lang E, Kinzl L. Vacuum assisted wound closure after dermatofasciotomy of the lower extremity. *Unfallchirurg* 1996;**99**(4):283-7.
7. Fleischmann W, Lang E, Russ M. Treatment of infection by vacuum sealing. *Unfallchirurg* 1997;**100**(4):301-4.
8. Muller G. Vacuum dressing in septic wound treatment. *Langenbecks Arch Chir Suppl Kongressbd* 1997;**114**:537-41.

9. Kovacs L, Kloppel M, Geishauser S, Schmiedl S, Biemer E. Vacuum sealing: a new and promising regimen in the therapy of radiation ulcers. *British Journal of Surgery* 1998;**85**:70.

10. Mullner T, Mrkonjic L, Kwasny O, Vecsei V. The use of negative pressure to promote the healing of tissue defects: a clinical trial using the vacuum sealing technique. *Br J Plast Surg* 1997;**50**(3):194-9.

11. Banwell P, Withey S, Holten I. The use of negative pressure to promote healing. *British Journal of Plastic Surgery* 1998;**51**(1):79.

12. Argenta LC, Morykwas MJ. Vacuum-assisted closure: a new method for wound control and treatment: clinical experience. *Ann Plast Surg* 1997;**38**(6):563-76; discussion 577.

13. Greer SE, Duthie E, Cartolano B, Koehler KM, Maydick-Youngberg D, Longaker MT. Techniques for applying subatmospheric pressure dressing to wounds in difficult regions of anatomy. *J Wound Ostomy Continence Nurs* 1999;**26**(5):250-3.

14. Meara JG, Guo L, Smith JD, Pribaz JJ, Breuing KH, Orgill DP. Vacuum-assisted closure in the treatment of degloving injuries. *Ann Plast Surg* 1999;**42**(6):589-94.

15. DeFranzo AJ, Marks MW, Argenta LC, Genecov DG. Vacuum-Assisted Closure for the treatment of degloving injuries. *Plastic and Reconstructive Surgery* 1999;**104**(7):2145-8.

16. Tang AT, Ohri SK, Haw MP. Novel application of vacuum assisted closure technique to the treatment of sternotomy wound infection. *Eur J Cardiothorac Surg* 2000;**17**(4):482-4.

17. Obdeijn MC, de Lange MY, Lichtendahl DH, de Boer WJ. Vacuum-assisted closure in the treatment of poststernotomy mediastinitis. *Ann Thorac Surg* 1999;**68**(6):2358-60.

18. Tang AT, Okri SK, Haw MP. Vacuum-assisted closure to treat deep sternal wound infection following cardiac surgery. *Journal of Wound Care* 2000;**9**(5):229-230.

19. Avery C, Pereira J, Moody A, Whitworth I. Clinical experience with the negative pressure wound dressing. *Br J Oral Maxillofac Surg* 2000;**38**(4):343-5.

20. Blackburn JH, Boemi L, Hall WW, Jeffords K, Hauck RM, Banducci DR, et al. Negative-pressure dressings as a bolster for skin grafts. *Ann Plast Surg* 1998;**40**(5):453-7.

21. Smith LA, Barker DE, Chase CW, Somberg LB, Brock WB, Burns RP. Vacuum pack technique of temporary abdominal closure: a four-year experience. *Am Surg* 1997;**63**(12):1102-7; discussion 1107-8.

22. Avery C, Pereira J, Moody A, Gargiulo M, Whitworth I. Negative pressure wound dressing of the radial forearm donor site. *Int J Oral Maxillofac Surg* 2000;**29**(3):198-200.

23. Greer SE, Longaker MT, Margiotta M, Mathews AJ, Kasabian A. The use of subatmospheric pressure dressing for the coverage of radial forearm free flap donor-site exposed tendon complications. *Ann Plast Surg* 1999;**43**(5):551-4.

24. Schneider AM, Morykwas MJ, Argenta LC. A new and reliable method of securing skin grafts to the difficult recipient bed. *Journal of Plastic & Reconstructive Surgery* 1998;**102**(4):1195-8.

25. Pfau M, Rennekampff HO, Schaller HE. Skin graft fixation by vacuum assisted topical foam dressing. *Journal of Burn Care and Rehabilitation* 2000;**21**(1):1.

26. Molnar JA, DeFranzo AJ, Marks MW. Single-stage approach to skin grafting the exposed skull. *Plastic and Reconstructive Surgery* 2000;**105**(1):174-7.

27. Mendez-Eastman S. Negative pressure wound therapy. *Plast Surg Nurs* 1998;**18**(1):27-9, 33-7.

28. von Gossler CM, Horch RE. Rapid aggressive soft-tissue necrosis after beetle bite can be treated by radical necrectomy and vacuum suction-assisted closure. *J Cutan Med Surg* 2000;**4**(4):219-22.

29. Brown KM, Harper FV, Aston WJ, O'Keefe PA, Cameron CR. Vacuum-assisted closure in the treatment of a 9-year-old child with severe and multiple dog bite injuries of the thorax. *Ann Thorac Surg* 2001;**72**(4):1409-10.

30. Elwood ET, Bolitho DG. Negative-pressure dressings in the treatment of hidradenitis suppurativa. *Ann Plast Surg* 2001;**46**(1):49-51.
31. Collier M. Know how: A guide to vacuum-assisted closure (VAC). *Nurs Times* 1997;**93**(5):32-3.
32. Deva AK, Siu C, Nettle WJ. Vacuum-assisted closure of a sacral pressure sore. *Journal of Wound Care* 1997;**6**(7):311-2.
33. Baynham SA, Kohlman P, Katner HP. Treating stage IV pressure ulcers with negative pressure therapy: a case report. *Ostomy Wound Manage* 1999;**45**(4):28-32, 34-5.
34. Mendez-Eastman S. Use of hyper-baric oxygen and negative pressure therapy in the multidisciplinary care of a patient with non- healing wounds. *Journal of Wound, Ostomy and Continence Nursing* 1999;**26**(2):67-76.
35. Deva AK, Buckland GH, Fisher E, Liew SC, Merten S, McGlynn M, et al. Topical negative pressure in wound management. *Med J Aust* 2000;**173**(3):128-31.
36. Evans D, Land L. Topical negative pressure for treating chronic wounds: a systematic review. *Br J Plast Surg* 2001;**54**(3):238-42.
37. Wasiak J, Cleland H. Topical negative pressure (TNP) for partial thickness burns. *Cochrane Database Syst Rev* 2007(3):CD006215.
38. Gregor S, Maegele M, Sauerland S, Krahn JF, Peinemann F, Lange S. Negative pressure wound therapy: a vacuum of evidence? *Arch Surg* 2008;**143**(2):189-96.
39. Peinemann F, McGauran N, Sauerland S, Lange S. Negative pressure wound therapy: potential publication bias caused by lack of access to unpublished study results data. *BMC Med Res Methodol* 2008;**8**:4.
40. Hinchliffe RJ, Valk GD, Apelqvist J, Armstrong DG, Bakker K, Game FL, et al. A systematic review of the effectiveness of interventions to enhance the healing of chronic ulcers of the foot in diabetes. *Diabetes Metab Res Rev* 2008;**24 Suppl 1**:S119-44.
41. Noble-Bell G, Forbes A. A systematic review of the effectiveness of negative pressure wound therapy in the management of diabetes foot ulcers. *Int Wound J* 2008;**5**(2):233-42.
42. Ubbink DT, Westerbos SJ, Evans D, Land L, Vermeulen H. Topical negative pressure for treating chronic wounds. *Cochrane Database Syst Rev* 2008(3):CD001898.
43. Mendonca DA, Papini R, Price PE. Negative-pressure wound therapy: a snapshot of the evidence. *Int Wound J* 2006;**3**(4):261-71.
44. Pham CT, Middleton PF, Maddern GJ. The safety and efficacy of topical negative pressure in non-healing wounds: a systematic review. *J Wound Care* 2006;**15**(6):240-50.
45. Ubbink DT, Westerbos SJ, Nelson EA, Vermeulen H. A systematic review of topical negative pressure therapy for acute and chronic wounds. *Br J Surg* 2008;**95**(6):685-92.
46. Vikatmaa P, Juutilainen V, Kuukasjarvi P, Malmivaara A. Negative pressure wound therapy: a systematic review on effectiveness and safety. *Eur J Vasc Endovasc Surg* 2008;**36**(4):438-48.
47. Philbeck TE, Whittington KT, Millsap MH, Briones RB, Wight DG, Schroeder WJ. The clinical and cost effectiveness of externally applied negative pressure wound therapy in the treatment of wounds in home healthcare Medicare patients. *Ostomy/Wound Management,* 1999;**45**(11):41-50.
48. Le Franc B, Sellal O, Grimandi G, Duteille F. [Cost-effectiveness analysis of vacuum-assisted closure in the surgical wound bed preparation of soft tissue injuries.]. *Ann Chir Plast Esthet* 2009.
49. Apelqvist J, Armstrong DG, Lavery LA, Boulton AJ. Resource utilization and economic costs of care based on a randomized trial of vacuum-assisted closure therapy in the treatment of diabetic foot wounds. *Am J Surg* 2008;**195**(6):782-8.

50. Flack S, Apelqvist J, Keith M, Trueman P, Williams D. An economic evaluation of VAC therapy compared with wound dressings in the treatment of diabetic foot ulcers. *J Wound Care* 2008;**17**(2):71-8.
51. Gabriel A, Shores J, Heinrich C, Baqai W, Kalina S, Sogioka N, et al. Negative pressure wound therapy with instillation: a pilot study describing a new method for treating infected wounds. *Int Wound J* 2008;**5**(3):399-413.
52. Moues CM, van den Bemd GJ, Meerding WJ, Hovius SE. An economic evaluation of the use of TNP on full-thickness wounds. *J Wound Care* 2005;**14**(5):224-7.
53. Kaplan M, Daly D, Stemkowski S. Early intervention of negative pressure wound therapy using Vacuum-Assisted Closure in trauma patients: impact on hospital length of stay and cost. *Adv Skin Wound Care* 2009;**22**(3):128-32.
54. Baharestani MM, Houliston-Otto DB, Barnes S. Early versus late initiation of negative pressure wound therapy: examining the impact on home care length of stay. *Ostomy Wound Manage* 2008;**54**(11):48-53.
55. Hu KX, Zhang HW, Zhou F, Yao G, Shi JP, Wang LF, et al. [A comparative study of the clinical effects between two kinds of negative-pressure wound therapy]. *Zhonghua Shao Shang Za Zhi* 2009;**25**(4):253-7.
56. Rozen WM, Shahbaz S, Morsi A. An improved alternative to vacuum-assisted closure (VAC) as a negative pressure dressing in lower limb split skin grafting: a clinical trial. *J Plast Reconstr Aesthet Surg* 2008;**61**(3):334-7.
57. Morykwas MJ, Argenta LC, Shelton-Brown EI, McGuirt W. Vacuum-assisted closure: a new method for wound control and treatment: animal studies and basic foundation. *Ann Plast Surg* 1997;**38**(6):553-62.
58. Fabian TS, Kaufman HJ, Lett ED, Thomas JB, Rawl DK, Lewis PL, et al. The evaluation of subatmospheric pressure and hyperbaric oxygen in ischemic full-thickness wound healing. *Am Surg* 2000;**66**(12):1136-43.
59. Morykwas MJ, David LR, Schneider AM, Whang C, Jennings DA, Canty C, et al. Use of sub-atmospheric pressure to prevent progression of partial-thickness burns in a swine model. *Journal of Burn Care and Rehabilitation* 1999;**20**(1):15-21.
60. Saxena V, Hwang CW, Huang S, Eichbaum Q, Ingber D, Orgill DP. Vacuum-assisted closure: microdeformations of wounds and cell proliferation. *Plast Reconstr Surg* 2004;**114**(5):1086-96; discussion 1097-8.
61. Greene AK, Puder M, Roy R, Arsenault D, Kwei S, Moses MA, et al. Microdeformational wound therapy: effects on angiogenesis and matrix metalloproteinases in chronic wounds of 3 debilitated patients. *Ann Plast Surg* 2006;**56**(4):418-22.
62. Scherer SS, Pietramaggiori G, Mathews JC, Prsa MJ, Huang S, Orgill DP. The mechanism of action of the vacuum-assisted closure device. *Plast Reconstr Surg* 2008;**122**(3):786-97.
63. Scherer SS, Pietramaggiori G, Mathews JC, Orgill DP. Short periodic applications of the vacuum-assisted closure device cause an extended tissue response in the diabetic mouse model. *Plast Reconstr Surg* 2009;**124**(5):1458-65.
64. Calne S, editor. *Vacuum assisted closure:recommendations for use. A consensus document.* London: Medical Education Partnership (MEP) London, 2008.

21. Dressing Selection

FACTORS THAT IMPACT UPON DRESSING SELECTION

The choice of an appropriate dressing or dressing system for a specific wound is determined by a number of factors. These include:

Condition of the wound
    Necrotic/Sloughy
    Dry/exuding
    Epithelializing
    Infected
    Overgranulating
    Malodorous
    Malignant
    Painful

Aim of treatment
    Facilitate healing
    Promote debridement
    Combat infection
    Absorb exudate or donate moisture
    Relieve pain
    Prevent or treat scarring
    Combat odour
    Provide concealment

Condition of surrounding skin
    Fragile
    Macerated

Influence of aetiology
    Is external compression indicated
      or contraindicated
    Does the wound have a realistic
      prospect of healing or is
      palliative treatment required
    Are specific topical therapies
      indicated e.g. use of steroids
      antibiotics etc

Practical considerations
    Cost
    Availability (reimbursement
      issues)

Anatomical location
    Difficult to dress
    Dressings affect use of normal
      clothing or shoes etc

The importance of some of these factors is discussed below. It is important to recognize, however, that this chapter is *not* intended to provide detailed advice on the management of specific types of wounds such as leg ulcers or pressure ulcers for example, as many excellent texts have been published on these and related topics.

Rather it seeks to illustrate how the key properties of particular dressings, may be made best utilized to provide the optimum conditions for the treatment of some types of problem wounds at a particular point in their healing cycle. It also attempts to show how an inappropriate dressing choice can adversely affect wound healing. To this end, wounds have been categorized according to their condition, using the simple black-yellow-red-pink colour classification system as a guide.

It is also important to emphasise that before any form of topical treatment is administered, every patient should be subjected to a thorough examination by a suitably qualified practitioner to identify and address any underlying medical/surgical conditions in so far as this may be possible.

BLACK NECROTIC WOUNDS

Wounds linked to a disease state

Black necrotic tissue is formed when previously healthy tissue dies and becomes dehydrated or desiccated. This can be due to a number of factors, but is most commonly caused by local ischaemia induced either by occlusion of a major blood vessel or capillary network, perhaps associated with diabetes or some other metabolic or clinical disorder.

Alternatively ischaemia can be caused by occlusion of blood vessels by unrelieved locally-applied external pressure when soft tissue is compressed between bone and an unyielding surface such as a hard chair or mattress, leading to the formation of a pressure ulcer (pressure sore).

For any necrotic wound it is therefore clearly important to identify the underlying cause, as this will to a large extent determine the nature of the treatment applied. In some instances, however, like that shown in Figure 94, no treatment is either indicated or required.

Figure 94: A necrotic toe before and after auto-amputation

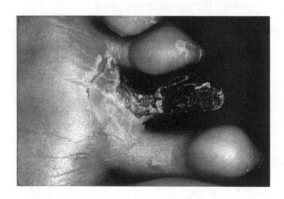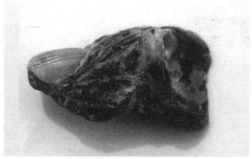

In the example shown above an entire toe has become devitalized, due, it is assumed, to an interruption to the local blood supply. In this instance the toe can safely be left to auto-amputate, although there remains a real possibility that further problems caused by ischaemia may later develop in adjacent tissue. During this process the affected digit should be kept dry to prevent maceration and reduce the possibility of infection. The separation process can be relatively pain free, causing the patient little or no discomfort.

The prognosis when larger areas of tissue are affected in this way is much less favourable, typical resulting in major surgery or amputation, particularly if infection is present.

Figure 95 shows the extensive necrotic areas that developed on both feet of a patient with advanced vascular disease. The gentleman concerned was in considerable continuous pain, which was greatly exacerbated when the affected areas were dressed.

In this instance the wounds were kept as dry as possible, and an effective low-adherent silicone dressing applied until a surgical referral could be arranged.

Figure 95: Extensive areas of dry necrosis caused by ischaemia

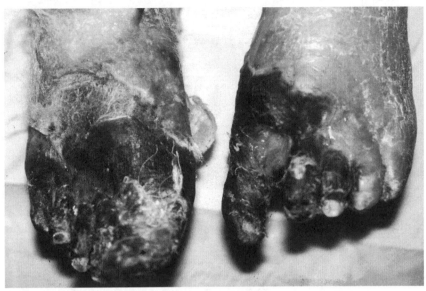

Sometimes the necrotic tissue does not dry out and in these circumstances proteolytic bacteria begin to liquefy the dead tissue, a process which can generate a noxious odour and potentially lead to a serious infection (Figure 96).

Figure 96: Area of wet necrosis associated with diabetes

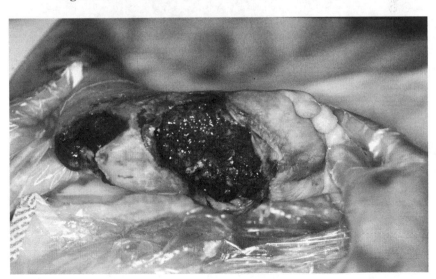

Other medical conditions, such as system lupus erythematosus, can also cause local ischaemia, which may result in widespread necrosis of limbs and digits.

Figure 97 records extensive damage, caused by this condition, which resulted in the loss of one digit and major damage to the remaining ones. The entire area was weeping and extremely painful, so an alginate dressing was applied to absorb the exudate. This also offered the advantage that it could be easily removed by irrigation with saline solution, thereby minimising the need for direct physical contact with the affected area.

With this treatment, despite the extensive tissue damage, remarkably some evidence of the formation of new granulation tissue was visible in the wound at the interface between the junction of the damaged and healthy tissue.

Figure 97: Necrosis associated with systemic lupus erythematosus

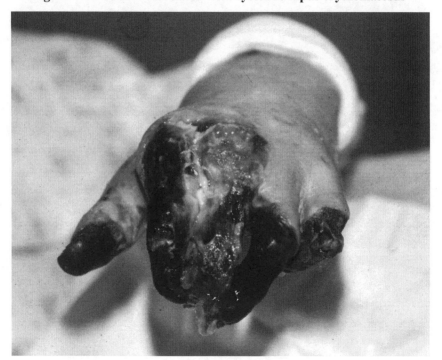

In the types of wounds so far identified, it is thought by some to be inappropriate to attempt debridement using dressings that promote autolysis, although some experts believe that some necrotic wounds, including those associated with diabetes, can be successfully cleansed using medical maggots, a view which is supported by numerous publications.

A further type of necrotic wound, which is fortunately becoming much less common, is that associated with meningitis caused by Neisseria meningitidis. This can lead to vaso-occlusion, secondary to disseminated intravascular coagulation, DIC, (the formation of multiple fibrin leukocyte-platelet clots), and a suppurative inflammatory response caused by endotoxins that attach to endothelial cells of the vascular tissue resulting in extravasation and the development of the characteristic purple patches. In severe cases these vascular changes can lead to death, and in those patients who survive, formation of necrotic lesions requiring deforming autoamputation of digits or limbs.

Figure 98: Lesions characteristic of an infection caused by
Neisseria meningitides

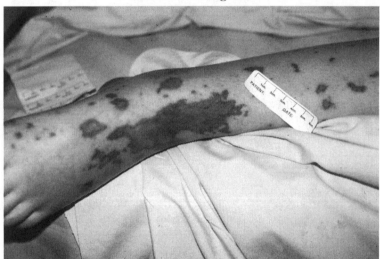

Experience has shown that the use of dressings that prevent desiccation of these purple areas can help to limit tissue damage, reduce scarring and in some instance, perhaps even eliminate the need to amputate digits. One patient with this condition, who developed multiple lesions all over her body, was very successfully treated by the use of hydrocolloid dressings and plastic gloves filled with hydrogel to facilitate healing and minimize scarring of the hands.

Wounds caused by pressure

Skin changes caused by unrelieved pressure can take variety of forms as previously described in Chapter 2. These range from small superficial areas of damage that heal in

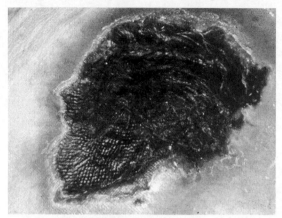

a couple of days to very large lesions that require surgical intervention to achieve closure. Such wounds also vary in appearance. If the intact epidermis has become completely dehydrated it takes on a black leathery or mummified appearance (Figure 99), but if the process is incomplete, the dead tissue may be light brown to olive green in colour.

If this necrotic layer is removed it frequently reveals a cavity filled with soft yellow/brown material commonly referred to as 'slough' (see later).

Figure 99: Pressure area covered with necrotic epidermis

In contrast to the black necrotic wounds previously described, most practitioners agree that some form of debridement of pressure ulcers is required to initiate the healing process. In some instances surgical debridement in theatre may be indicated, but many patients who develop extensive areas of pressure damage are too unwell to undergo this procedure. In such instances, sharp debridement involving the use of surgical scissors or a blade (Figure 100), may offer an acceptable alternative approach. .

Where surgical intervention is not indicated, debridement may be achieved by the application of dressings that maintain a moist environment to rehydrate the necrotic tissue in order to soften it and thus initiate autolysis

This process can be promoted either by the use of amorphous hydrogels, which are thought to donate moisture directly to the dead tissue, or by the application of a relatively impermeable product which functions by preventing the loss of moisture from the skin by evaporation. Some

Figure 100: Sharp debridement of a pressure ulcer with a blade

hydrocolloid dressings are ideally suited for this purpose, for as described in Chapter 12, they are impermeable to moisture vapour in their intact state.

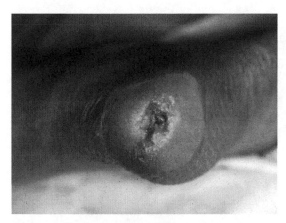

Figure 101: Rehydration of dry skin around a pressure ulcer by a hydrocolloid dressing

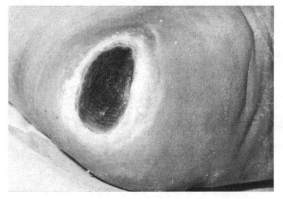

Figure 102: Partially rehydrated necrotic tissue with evidence of maceration

Film dressings, and those made from polyurethane foam, are less suitable for this indication as they are frequently highly permeable to water vapour and therefore do not facilitate tissue rehydration. The effect of hydrocolloid dressing on the hydration, and therefore the appearance, of otherwise dry skin is graphically illustrated in Figure 101

A patient with a pressure ulcer on their heel has had the wound dressed with a piece of Granuflex to promote debridement and facilitate the production of granulation tissue. In the figure that area of skin which has been covered by the dressing is clearly visible and shows clear evidence of rehydration, although there is no evidence of maceration due to the ability of the hydrocolloid adhesive base to absorb any excess moisture present. Contrast this with Figure 102, where the application of saline soaks to a pressure ulcer has led to maceration of the periwound skin.

Once the necrotic cap has been removed from a wound, it may be possible to get some idea of the extent of the underlying damage, although this may not be possible if the wound contains significant residues of necrotic soft tissue.

YELLOW SLOUGHY WOUNDS

As previously indicated, wounds such as pressure ulcers often contain necrotic muscle and fat which is exposed when the necrotic epidermal layer is removed. In many instances, provided that sufficient moisture is present, this soft material, commonly referred to as 'slough' separates also from the underlying healthy tissue by autolysis, often revealing small bubbles of newly formed granulation tissue (Figure 103).

This process is presumably also facilitated by the action of proteolytic bacteria present within the wound, and it is interesting to speculate if the action of these organisms is inhibited by the application of topical antimicrobial agents, thereby delaying the debridement process.

Despite the considerable size of some pressure ulcers and the often poor state of health of the patient, it is remarkable how rapidly such wounds can improve once the

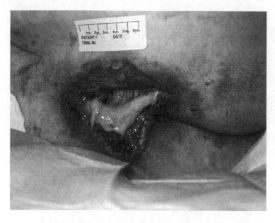

Figure 103: Spontaneous separation of slough in a large pressure ulcer

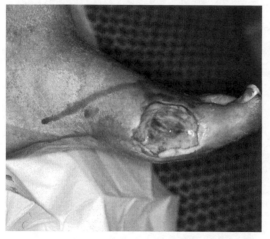

Figure 104: Slough covered diabetic ulcer

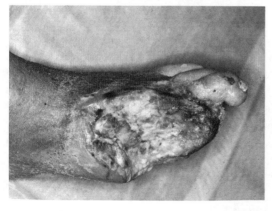

Figure 105: Infected, slough-covered surgical wound

underlying problem has been addressed. Often the largest, most unpleasant looking pressure ulcers show the presence of healthy granulation tissue beneath the foul smelling necrotic material covering the wound surface which is revealed as the partially liquefied material comes away.

Unfortunately, however, the removal of slough is not always so straight-forward.

Diabetic ulcers (Figure 104), and leg or foot ulcers associated with ischaemia, can be much harder to debride due to the fact that, unlike pressure ulcers, the wounds are caused by an underlying medical condition which is not always easily rectified.

Sometime a thick viscous yellow covering develops on a previously clean wound (Figure 105). This consists principally of a mixture of fibrin and pus which in turn contains bacterial cell, leucocytes and significant quantities of deoxyribonucleo-protein. If exposed to the air, this viscous covering can dry out, taking on a hard 'crusty' appearance.

The presence of this layer is frequently associated with, or indicative of, the presence of infection and is typified by the wound shown in Figure 105.

This particular surgical site developed an anaerobic infection, producing an odour that was detectable throughout a large ward. The smell was eventually controlled by the use of a hydrogel containing 0.8% metronidazole.

In these hard-to-cleanse wounds, dressings that promote autolytic debridement are often of limited effectiveness, and alternative treatments may therefore be required. Although numerous proprietary preparations are available for this purpose, including various enzymatic agents and chemical preparations that are claimed to degrade sloughy tissue, the results achieved with these preparations can be also be disappointing and in some studies they have

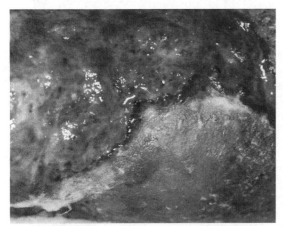

failed to demonstrate any significant advantage over hydrogels or hydrocolloids. It is in such situations that the use of maggots may prove beneficial.

In some instances a number of treatments may be used consecutively. For example, a hydrocolloid or hydrogel may initially be applied to an extensive pressure area for a couple of days to soften the dead tissue, followed by sharp debridement to remove the necrotic epidermis. Finally a couple of cycles of medical maggots may be applied to complete the cleansing process The slough and necrotic material so far described material

Figure 106: Fibrinous membrane being displaced by advancing epithelial edge

should not be confused with the thin, highly adherent and almost translucent fibrinous covering that is sometimes encountered in granulating wounds. This fibrinous layer is not indicative of infection and is frequently a predictor of good wound healing. Epithelial cells from the advancing wound margin readily grow beneath this fibrinous layer which is thus progressively displaced (Figure 106).

RED GRANULATING WOUNDS

Cavity wounds

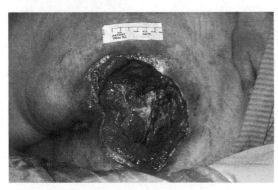

Once a wound has been freed of slough and necrotic tissue, a cavity is revealed, the depth of which can vary from a few millimeters to ten centimetres or more (Figure 107). Before this defect can become covered with new epithelium, it must first be filled with granulation tissue to bring it up to the approximate level of the surrounding skin. For much of the 20th century cavity wounds and

Figure 107: An extensive Grade 4 pressure ulcer largely free of necrotic tissue

sinuses were firmly packed with gauze, sometimes impregnated with white soft paraffin or soaked in saline or antiseptic agents including sodium hypochlorite solution, or proflavine lotion or cream. This procedure was believed to be essential to facilitate healing and prevent premature wound closure that would result in the formation of a sinus or enclosed cavity.

So widely held was this belief, that it was not uncommon to see even narrow wounds totally filled with tightly packed ribbon gauze, which undoubtedly caused the patient considerable pain upon insertion and even more upon removal.

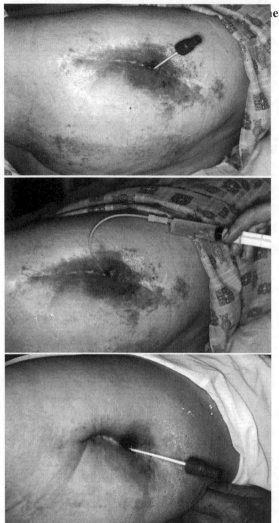

Despite the almost universal nature of this practice, a review of the literature has revealed no solid evidence to support this procedure. Whilst it is probably appropriate to ensure that potentially contaminated exudate is not allowed to accumulate and stagnate within a cavity wound, this may be achieved without the introduction of excessive amounts of packing.

One an alternative approach to the management of sinus wounds is shown in Figure 108. A sinus that developed following orthopaedic surgery was initially dressed with ribbon gauze soaked in proflavine cream in the traditional manner. Apart from the pain associated with this procedure, the periwound skin had become inflamed due to a reaction to lanolin, a component of the proflavine cream. The opening of the wound also looked unhealthy with little sign of healing. An alternative management strategy was therefore adopted in which the wound was dressed with an amorphous hydrogel dressing, which was introduced into the wound using a syringe and quill. In this way it was possible to ensure that the wound was completely filled with gel right down to the base. Removal of the gel was easily accomplished by flushing the wound with sterile saline using the same technique.

As a result of this change in treatment the periwound skin rapidly improved as did the appearance of the wound itself and the patient's pain was also virtually eliminated using this method.

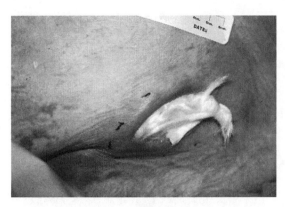

Figure 109: A Grade 4 pressure ulcer dressed with alginate fibre

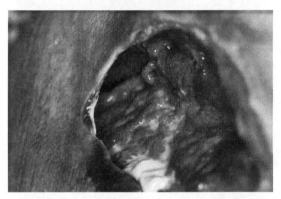

Figure 110: Granulation tissue forming in a pressure ulcer with significant undermining

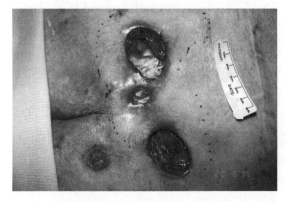

Figure 111: Three interconnected pressure ulcers showing extent of undermining

For slightly larger cavity wounds there are numerous treatment options available. These include the use of dressings specifically designed for the purpose made from hydrophilic polymers such as alginate and CMC which can be rolled up, or otherwise inserted into cavity wounds, to facilitate exudate removal (Figure 109).

For most cavity wounds the precise choice of dressing is determined by the nature and depth of the wound.

A large open cavity might be dressed with alginate or CMC sheets applied to the wound surface and covered with an appropriate absorbent secondary dressing such as cotton gauze or an absorbent dressing pad. In this way the alginate forms an effective low-adherent wound contact layer which can be easily removed without causing pain or trauma.

If infection is present or suspected a product containing an antimicrobial agent such as silver might be indicated, but the wisdom of using these materials routinely without good reason must be questioned.

For smaller cavities an Allevyn Cavity Wound Dressing might be appropriate as these are easy to introduce and remove, but for shallower wounds or sinuses, an amorphous hydrogel may be considered, particularly if the wound is relatively dry.

With pressure ulcers in particular, the size of the opening may not indicate the full extent of tissue damage, and in some instances considerable under-mining may be present (Figure 110).

The extent of undermining may be determined by the use of a sterile probe which is pushed gently under the skin to determine the extent of the damage.

When such a procedure was carried on a patient with multiple, apparently discrete, pressure ulcers it was found that at least three of the wounds were interconnected.

Using an indelible marker it is possible to record the extent of the undermining to facilitate dressing changes (Figure 111) and thereby monitor progress towards healing.

The most recent and arguably the most effective treatment for cavity wounds involves the use of NPTW as described in a previous chapter.

The technique has grown in popularity and is now considered by many to be the optimum method of dealing with such lesions. Despite its undoubted efficacy, the principal drawback with this method is the requirement to use, and in some instances, carry about, a vacuum pump controlled by a piece of sophisticated electronic equipment. For this reason negative pressure wound therapy (NPWT) is probably currently best suited to hospitalized or relatively immobile patients with large cavity wounds or wounds that have failed to respond to more conventional dressings.

Superficial granulating wounds

Some granulating wounds are of limited depth and therefore not normally described as cavity wounds. Most burns, donor sites and leg ulcers fall into this category, although the latter can vary in area from a few square millimetres to extensive lesions that involve most of the lower leg. Many pressure ulcers are also of limited depth and even the most extensive examples eventually become superficial wounds as they progress towards healing thereby necessitating a change of dressing.

In the early stages of healing many wounds produce copious amounts of exudate, particularly if an infection develops or the wound becomes critically colonised with pathogenic bacteria. At this stage a dressing or dressing system is required which is capable of absorbing or otherwise dealing with the problem of fluid production as effectively as possible. Later, as exudate production diminishes, a dressing capable of maintaining a moist wound environment may be indicated.

This approach is illustrated in Figure 112. A large dehisced abdominal wound that initially contained a significant quantity of slough was first dressed with alginate sheets backed with absorbent dressings to absorb wound fluid and promote debridement and the formation of granulation tissue. As the wound decreased in depth, and exudate production diminished, the alginate treatment became less appropriate so a hydrocolloid dressing was applied until complete closure was achieved.

This type of wound might well also be considered suitable for negative pressure wound therapy.

Figure 112: A large dehisced abdominal wound, sequentially dressed with alginate and hydrocolloid to optimize healing

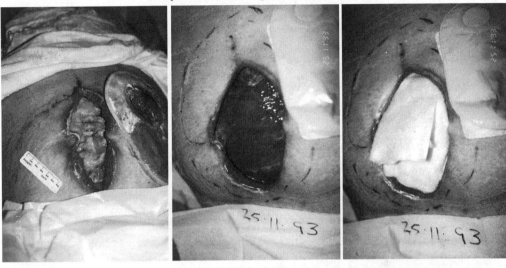

| **Wound prior to alginate treatment (4-11-93)** | **Wound after 3 weeks treatment (25-11-93)** | **Showing alginate in position (25-11-93)** |

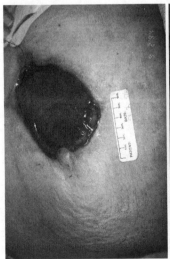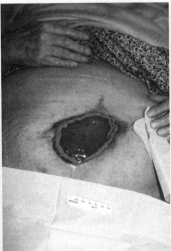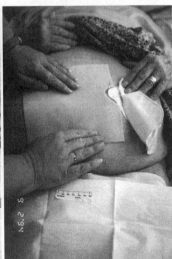

| **Wound now dressed with hydrocolloid (9-2-94)** | **Hydrocolloid paste seal in position (9-2-94)** | **Application of hydrocolloid (9-2-94)** |

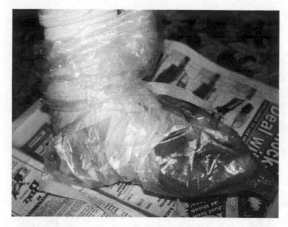

Figure 113: A community patient's attempt to cope with the problems of exudate production

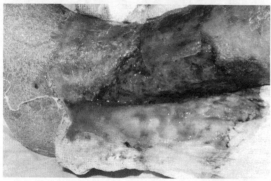

Figure 114: Inappropriate use of hydrogel sheet dressing in the treatment of a heavily exuding leg ulcer

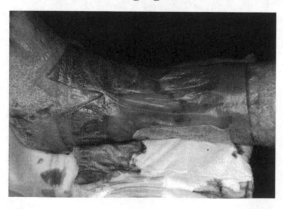

Figure 115: Inappropriate use of hydrocolloid dressing in treatment of a heavily exuding leg ulcer

It should be noted that a similar outcome could have been achieved by continuing the use of the alginate as a primary dressing but modifying the secondary dressing to conserve moisture within the dressing system.

A similar approach should be adopted in the treatment of all other types of superficial wounds, ensuring that the fluid handling properties of the chosen system are appropriate for the wound at that stage in the healing cycle.

Failure to address this issue can result in significant practical problems for the patient (Figure 113) and produce potentially serious consequences for a successful treatment outcome (Figure 114 and Figure 115).

Although alginate and CMC dressings can and have been used successfully in the treatment of exuding leg ulcers for example, for this indication they are often now replaced by hydrophilic polyurethane foam dressings which combine absorbency and moisture vapour permeability to maximize their fluid handling capability.

As with cavity wounds an accurate diagnosis is essential when determining the treatment of leg ulcers. For venous ulcers the application of sustained graduated pressure is a key element of their management but for wounds that are ischaemic in origin, the application of high levels of pressure could have very serious consequences.

The possibility that an ulcer can be a manifestation of some other underlying medical disorder must also not be ignored.

Figure 116: Bilateral ulcers caused by pyoderma gangrenosum

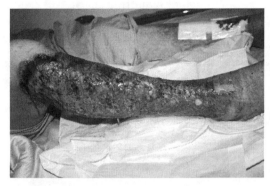

Legs on presentation, March 20th

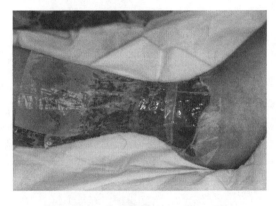

Tegapore applied to leg, May 28th

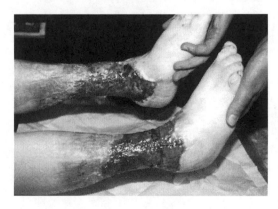

Clear progress towards healing, July 9th

One such condition is pyoderma gangrenosum, a rare condition that affects about 1 in 100,000 of the population. The aetiology of the disease is not well understood, but the condition is often found in individuals with ulcerative colitis, Crohn's disease and other disorders of the immune system.

One form results in the formation of skin lesions that vary in size and location, but which typically possess a purple coloured border. First line treatment involves the use of corticosteroids and cyclosporine.

A patient with this condition, who had not been correctly diagnosed until referred for expert dermatological review, presented with extensive lesions involving both lower legs (Figure 116).

The ulcerated areas were extremely painful, particularly during dressing changes making the individual concerned extremely apprehensive about this procedure. For this reason the decision was taken to dress his legs with Tegapore, (now Tegaderm Contact), a fine mesh woven nylon net as a low-adherent, free draining wound contact material. This material, which has no intrinsic absorbency, allows free passage of exudate into a secondary absorbent layer, provided that the dressing is carefully applied and maintained in intimate contact with the wound surface.

The rationale behind this choice was that the net could be left *in situ* for an extended period whilst the outer layer of absorbent pads could be changed on a regular basis without disturbing the wound or causing the patient unnecessary pain. Both legs were dressed in this way and over a period of months they progressed uneventfully to healing, causing minimal discomfort to the patient.

Figure 117: Treatment of an ulcerated haemangioma

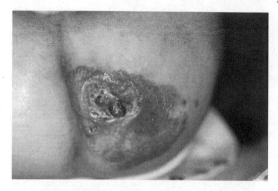

Haemangioma on the buttock of a young baby

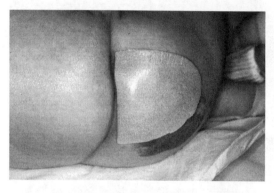

Application of a tailored hydrocolloid sheet

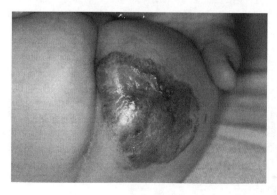

After about a week the wound has closed with the hydrocolloid treatment

A further type of distressing ulcerative condition is a haemangioma, a benign self-involuting tumour encountered in infancy. This condition is not usually serious or life threatening, but if the tumour ulcerates it can become a problem, particularly if it occurs in the diaper area as shown in Figure 117.

In the case shown, the proximity of the wound to the baby's anus meant that it was continually became contaminated with faecal material, which was a source of distress both to the parents and the infant when the wound had to be cleansed.

In this instance the treatment priority was to protect the wound from contamination. A hydrocolloid sheet was therefore selected as the dressing of choice as this could be easily tailored to fit the area and, once it place, it would prevent contamination and facilitate cleansing or bathing.

Somewhat unexpectedly, following the use of the hydrocolloid, closure of the wound also occurred within a few days.

The ability of hydrocolloid dressings to form an effective seal on periwound skin which is capable of resisting short term immersion in water makes them ideally suited for this type of application provided that the wound itself is not exuding too heavily.

If significant quantities of exudate are produced, some, but by no means all, self-adhesive foam island dressings may be used in this way, although these are unlikely to be as water resistant (wash proof) as the hydrocolloids.

PINK EPITHELIALIZING WOUNDS

Once the process of granulation is well advanced the final visible stage of healing involves the migration of epithelial cells from the wound margin over the newly formed wound bed, a process which is facilitate by the provision of a moist environment. This process is particularly easy to see on dark skin as melanin, produced by melanocytes present in the stratum basale, is not present in the migrating epithelial cells.

Figure 118: Wound healing in heavily pigmented skin showing the advancing epithelial edge

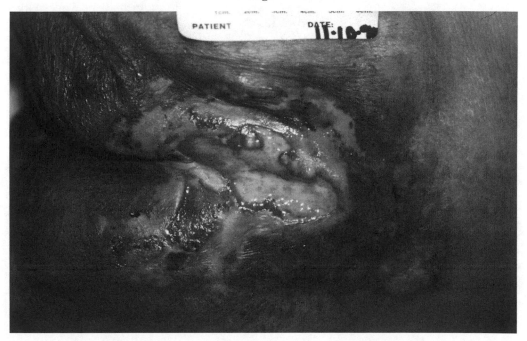

The newly formed epithelial layer is fragile and easily damaged so a dressing system is required that does not adhere and cause trauma upon removal.

In some individuals even normal skin is particularly fragile, as in the case of the elderly, or those receiving steroids or radiotherapy. The skin of patients who suffer from the genetic disorder, epidermolysis bullosa (EB) is particularly at risk as they can develop blisters, often as a result of minor trauma, which is caused by separation of the component layers of the skin. Several types of EB have been described: intra-epidermal, junctional (between the epidermis and dermis) and intradermal. Depending upon the type, the symptoms vary from mild seasonal blistering to a life-threatening condition, often with large areas of skin loss that can involve the oral, gastrointestinal, or respiratory tract. Sometimes the fingernails are lost and webbing can form between the digits. Because the skin of individuals with EB is so fragile, the use of adhesive

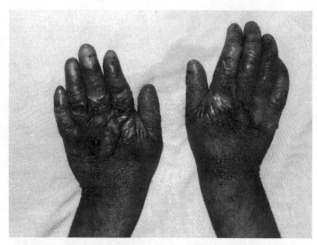

Figure 119: Epidermolysis bullosa showing papery skin and loss of fingernails

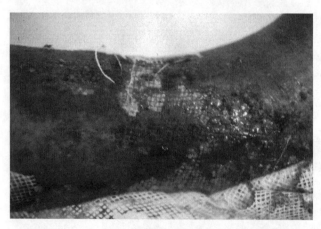

Figure 120: Evidence of adherence and fibre los from paraffin gauze dressing

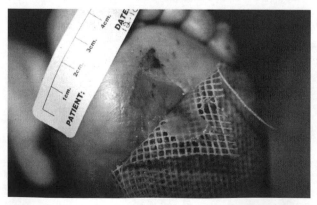

Figure 121: Large area of epithelium removed by adherence to paraffin gauze dressing

dressings should be avoided, as removal may cause further traumatic injuries. In some forms of EB it may even be necessary to dress non-blistered areas to prevent blister formation. Once a blister has formed, it is recommended that it be lanced and all fluid gently expelled to prevent it from extending. At this stage a dressing which does not damage the skin should be applied and held in place with a bandage – not adhesive tape.

The problems caused by adherence of dressings to the surface of all types of healing wounds has been recognized for centuries, and many attempts made to overcome the problems by coating fabrics with a variety of greasy agents; the most familiar of which are the paraffin impregnated fabric dressings, historically used extensively by plastic surgeons for dressing donor sites.

Despite their widespread use, the performance of this material is far from optimal, and numerous attempts have been made to develop improved forms of low-adherent dressing including the simple Knitted Viscose Primary Dressing, perforated plastic films, nylon net materials (Tegaderm Contact) and, arguably the most successful of all, products impregnated with a silicone gel such as NA Ultra and Mepitel.

Simple semipermeable poly-urethane film dressings can also be employed to dress lightly-exuding superficial wounds as the adhesive on the film will not adhere to the moist wound base. Similarly hydrocolloid dressings can also be used but there exists a slight tendency for these materials to promote the development of excess granulation tissue due, it is assumed, to their relatively low permeability to oxygen.

MALIGNANT WOUNDS

Malignant or fungating wounds, although relatively uncommon, present major problems both to patients and those responsible for their care. They are most often associated with carcinoma of the female breast (Figure 122), but can also arise from other internal malignancies and may develop at the site of the original lesion or elsewhere as a result of infiltration of skin epithelium by cancerous cells.

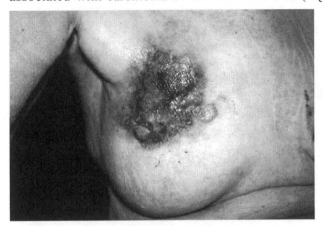

Figure 122: Fungating breast wound

From these, a tumour develops and increases in size until it loses its vascularity when capillary rupture occurs followed by necrosis. Radiotherapy may reduce the size of the resultant area, but such wounds are frequently not expected to heal, may bleed profusely when dressings are changed and often become infected with anaerobic organisms that produce volatile fatty acids with a pungent odour that can be a source of great embarrassment and distress to the patient and their relatives.

The literature contains limited information or advice on the management of fungating wounds as most authors concentrate primarily on methods of controlling the odour by means of agents as varied as icing sugar, honey, or live yoghurt which has been applied in an attempt to encourage overgrowth of

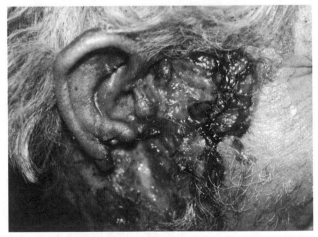

Figure 123: Facial carcinoma

pathogenic organisms by lactic acid bacteria such as *Lactobacillus bulgaricus* and *Streptococcus thermophilus*. Metronidazole is also useful for this indication. It can be given systemically but is more commonly applied topically in the form of gel. When used in this way is active against both aerobic and anaerobic organisms present in these wounds.

The other major problem with fungating wounds is the amount of exudate they produce. Whilst it may be possible to address this problem by the use of absorbent dressing or pads, if the wound is located on the trunk or breast, management of facial lesions (Figure 123) is much more difficult.

INFECTED WOUNDS

Infected or not infected?

The diagnosis and treatment of infected wounds represents a significant challenge for the wound-care practitioner.

In soft tissue, a diagnosis of infection is normally suggested by the presence of the cardinal signs of inflammation identified by Celsus (*circa* 25 BC - 50 AD) as; calor (warmth), dolor (pain), tumor (swelling) and rubor (redness and hyperaemia).

Whilst these indicators might apply to regions of cellulitis around the margin of a wound, they cannot be used to assist with a diagnosis of infection within a wound itself for obvious reasons.

Similarly, visual examination of a wound at a single point in time may not be sufficient to confirm (or exclude) the presence of an infection as appearances can be deceptive.

For example, a wound is sometimes described as 'infected' if it contains a significant amount of slough, or is a source of an unpleasant odour, but both of these signs can be misinterpreted.

Sloughy tissue is often present in pressure ulcers but may only be revealed once the outer layer of necrotic epidermis is removed. Such wounds can also produce a very unpleasant odour due to the presence of proteolytic bacteria.

Nevertheless, despite their unpleasant appearance, providing the underlying cause has been addressed, pressure ulcers usually progress rapidly towards healing as the dead tissue separates by autolysis as previous described. In these wounds the presence of slough is therefore not indicative of infection or delayed healing and therefore the use of antimicrobial agents is not necessarily indicated.

In contrast, the development of a malodorous yellow covering on a previously clean surgical site or granulating wound bed may well reveal an infection that requires urgent attention (see Figure 105).

Conversely some acute wounds, not associated with any particular aetiology which might be expected to impair healing, can appear relatively normal but stubbornly refuse to progress towards closure due to the presence of a significant bioburden.

Qualitative microbiological studies may be of some assistance when assessing such wounds, but even these can be misleading as bacteria can be isolated from almost all wounds in varying numbers which frequently appear to have little effect upon the healing process.

The bacterial population of a wound can also change over time, complicating the position still further: Gram-negative organisms tend to predominate in wet wounds, but Gram-positive organisms may do better in drier wounds.

Quantitative microbiological investigations are sometimes useful in confirming the presence of infection but such procedures are expensive and are often of limited value.

Causes of wound infection

The ability of bacteria to delay healing is determined by numerous factors including the nature and virulence of the organism, the number present and the ability of the patient's immune system to withstand the challenge that these organisms represent.

Recognizing that the relationship between a wound and its bacterial bioburden is complex one, four definitions have been derived which define the bacterial status of a wound as follows:

- **Contamination** - the presence of bacteria which do not increase in number or cause clinical problems
- **Colonization** - multiplication of the bacterial population with any apparent adverse clinical effects
- **Critical colonization** - multiplication of the bacterial population causing a delay in wound healing, sometimes associated with increased pain but no overt host reaction
- **Infection** - delayed healing and disruption of tissue or caused by the presence of microorganisms

In practice, however, these definitions are of limited practical value to a clinical practitioner. Whilst, from a clinical examination alone, it is possible to determine with some certainty that a particular wound is rapidly deteriorating and therefore may truly be classed as 'infected', it is much less easy to differentiate between colonization and critical colonization.

For all practical purposes a much simpler classification system may be preferred in which wounds are divided into those that are healing normally (allowing for aetiological effects), and those which have suffered a microbiological insult causing healing to be halted or delayed.

Regularly monitoring of a wound's dimensions should enable such a problem to be identified relatively quickly. Alternatively, in many wounds careful examination of the wound margin alone might be sufficient.

Closure is normally achieved by the formation of a thin translucent border of newly formed epithelium which migrates across the wound bed. This new tissue is particularly susceptible to infection so if it is clearly visible and healthy the bioburden of the wound is unlikely to be causing a significant problem.

If such an edge is normally clearly visible, but becomes disrupted or disappears at some point, it may indicate or predict the presence of a clinical problem (infection). This type of advancing epithelial edge can often even be seen in wounds that contain significant amounts of sloughy tissue (Figure 124), confirming that the presence of this material does not necessarily impact negatively on wound healing.

Other potential indicators of localized infection include changes in pain or odour levels, formation of granulation tissue that is very friable and bleeds easily, changes to the appearance of the wound bed (including the formation of pockets or bridging) and increased or altered exudate production.

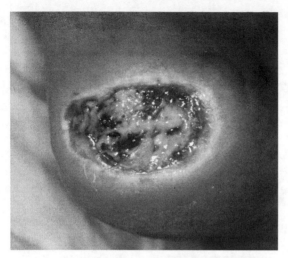

Figure 124: Wound showing clear evidence of epithelial migration even in presence of sloughy tissue

Location of infection

An important, but perhaps poorly understood aspect of the impact that bacteria may have upon wound healing relates to the precise location of the organisms within the wound.

Firstly organisms may find their way deep into the cellular structure of the wound bed causing tissue damage that results in deterioration of the wound and, possibly, the development of cellulitis. Such organisms are unlikely to be affected by topical antimicrobials, but will potentially be killed by systemic antibiotics delivered directly to the site *via* the vascular system.

A second possibility is that bacteria can attach themselves to the wound surface and form a protective covering or biofilm around themselves which is impervious to many antiseptic agents. These protected cells may produce toxins which when liberated into the wound, can produce cell death and prevent healing.

Finally, significant numbers of pathogenic organisms may develop within sloughy or dead tissue. As this material does not have a blood supply, systemic antibiotics may not be delivered in sufficient concentration to exert any significant effect.

In the second and third scenarios some form of local treatment may be indicated to remove the sloughy tissue and destroy the biofilm. Other than surgical intervention, maggot therapy is probably the most effective way of achieving this.

Treatment of infection

If there is evidence to suggest that wound healing is being delayed by the presence of bacteria, the clinician has to determine the most appropriate course of treatment. If cellulitis is present, or there are any other signs of systemic infection (including pyrexia, lymphangitis, changed cell counts or general malaise) then systemic antibiotics are normally indicated, the choice of which should be determined by appropriate microbiological investigation and local policies for the control of infection.

If all the above signs are absent, local treatment alone may be attempted. This generally involves the removal of slough and necrosis, or if the wound bed is already relatively free of slough, the application of a topical antiseptic agent in the form of a dressing or soak. Antibiotics including framycetin and fusidic acid were also widely used in the past, but these have now been largely set aside because of the twin problems of the development of skin reactions and bacterial resistance. Mupirocin is sometimes employed for antibiotic resistant strains of bacteria, including MRSA.

The antibacterial agents now most commonly used contain povidone iodine, chlorhexidine and polyhexanide (poly-hexamethylene biguanide) but the most widely used medicated dressings are currently those based upon silver technology.

Influence of wound condition on choice of dressing

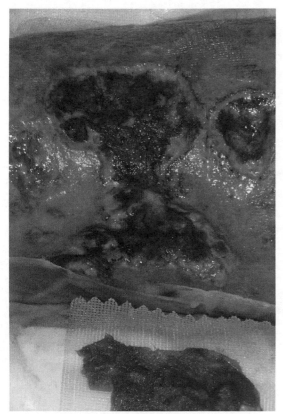

Figure 125: Surface of slough stained black following using of a silver releasing dressing

The ability of a dressing to combat or prevent infection will be greatly influenced by the condition of the wound. In the case of slough-covered wounds, it is postulated that silver dressings are likely to be of very little value, for given the highly reactive nature of the silver ions, it is unlikely that these will penetrate far into the bulk of the slough before they become chemically bound and therefore inactivated. Some evidence for this proposition is provided in Figure 125 which clearly shows how the outer surface of a sloughy wound has been stained black by interaction with silver ions.

As there is also no evidence that silver dressings have any wound debriding activity whatsoever, they should not be used as debriding agents.

The manufacturers of many silver-containing and iodine-based products are very cautious about making claims for the ability of their products to combat existing wound infections, suggesting that in some cases (but by no means all) they can be applied to infected wounds but only as part of a package of care, which probably involves the administration of system antibiotics.

In general, the literature contains little evidence to support the use of medicated dressings as primary treatments for existing wound infections. Indeed most published studies have compared antimicrobial dressings with an unmedicated product in selected non-infected wound types, such as burns, by recording the number of infections that subsequently developed in both treatment groups. In this sense the dressings are being used to prevent rather than treat wound infections.

The clinical benefits that result from the use of silver-containing dressings are also open to debate. Some studies suggest that they do assist healing whilst other fairly large studies could find no such effect, particularly in the treatment of leg ulcers.

Overall, therefore, it appears therefore that silver dressings are probably greatly overused, often applied in situations where they are neither indicated nor likely to be of significant clinical or financial benefit: practitioners should therefore be more discriminating in the use of these and other antimicrobial dressings,

22. Buyer's guide

This chapter contains a list of wound management materials, most but not all of which have been discussed within the text. The information is presented in two sections. In the first the products are listed alphabetically and each is given a two or three digit manufacturer's or distributor's code. In the second section the codes are listed alphabetically, with contact details of the companies concerned.

LIST OF PRODUCTS IN ALPHABETICAL ORDER

Acticoat	SN	Algisite M	SN
Acticoat 7	SN	Algisite M Rope	SN
Acticoat Absorbent	SN	Algivon	ADV
Acticoat Moisture Control	SN	Algosteril	SN
ActiFast	ACT	Algosteril Rope	SN
Actiform Cool	ACT	Alione	COL
Actilite	ACT	Alldress	MOL
Actisorb Silver 220	SYS	Allevyn Adhesive	SN
Activheal Alginate	AMS	Allevyn Ag Adhesive	SN
Activheal Alginate Rope	AMS	Allevyn Ag Non-adhesive	SN
Activheal Aquafiber	AMS	Allevyn Cavity	SN
Activheal Aquafiber Rope	AMS	Allevyn Compression	SN
Activheal Flexipore	AMS	Allevyn Gentle	SN
Activheal Foam Island	AMS	Allevyn Gentle Border	SN
Activheal Foam Non-Adhesive	AMS	Allevyn Heel	SN
Activheal Hydrocolloid	AMS	Allevyn Lite	SN
Activheal Hydrocolloid Foam Backed	AMS	Allevyn Non-adhesive	SN
		Allevyn Plus	SN
Activheal Hydrogel	AMS	Allevyn Plus Adhesive	SN
Activon Tube	AMS	Allevyn Plus Cavity	SN
Activon Tulle	AMS	Allevyn Thin	SN
ActiWrap	ACT	Allevyn Tracheostomy	SN
Actrys	AGU	AMD Foam	COV
Adaptic Digit	SYS	Anabact	CHS
Adva-co	ADV	Apligraft	ORG
Advadraw	ADV	Aquacel	CON
Advadraw Spiral	ADV	Aquacel Ag	CON
Advasil	ADV	Aquacel Ag ribbon	CON
Advasil conform	ADV	Aquacel ribbon	CON
Advasozorb Border	ADV	Aquaclear	HAR
Advasozorb Plus	ADV	Aquaflo	COV
Algisite Ag	SN		

Aquaform	ASP	Carrgauze	CRN
Aquagel	LOD	Catrix	LES
Aquasorb	DRL	Cavi-Care	SN
Aquasorb Border	DRL	Cavilon	3M
Arglaes	ASP	Cellona Undercast Padding	ACT
Aserbine	GOL	Central Gard	ASP
Askina Biofilm Transparent	BRA	Cerdak Aerocloth	CER
Askina Calgitrol Ag	BRA	Cerdak Aerofilm	CER
Askina Carbosorb	BRA	Cerdak basic	CER
Askina Derm	BRA	Cerdak Cavity	CER
Askina Foam	BRA	Cestra Primary	ROB
Askina Foam Cavity	BRA	Cica-care	SN
Askina Gel	BRA	Cica-plaie	SN
Askina Heel	BRA	Citrugel	ADV
Askina Pad	BRA	Clearsite	ZZZ
Askina Sorb	BRA	Clinishield	CLI
Askina Transparent	BRA	Clinsorb	CLI
Atrauman	HAR	Coban	3M
Atrauman Ag	HAR	Collatek Foam	HUM
Avance	MOL	Collatek Foam	HUM
Avance A	MOL	Collatek Hydrocolloid Particles	HUM
Bactigras	SN	Collatek Hydrocolloid sheet	HUM
Bactroban	GSK	Collatek Hydrogel	HUM
Bard Absorbtion Dressing	ZZZ	Combiderm	CON
Betadine Dry Powder Spray	MOL	Combiderm N	CON
Biatain	COL	Comfeel Paste	COL
Biatain Adhesive	COL	Comfeel Plus	COL
Biatain Adhesive Ag	COL	Comfeel Plus Contour	COL
Biatain Ag	COL	Comfeel Plus PRD	COL
Biatain Contour	COL	Comfeel Plus Transparent	COL
Biatain Heel	COL	Comfeel Skin Care	COL
Biatain Sacral	COL	Conotrane	AST
Biatain Soft-Hold	COL	Contreet	COL
Biatain-IBU	COL	Contreet Foam Filler	COL
Biobrane	SN	Coolie	ZER
Bioclusive	SYS	Copa Foam	COV
Blisterfilm	COV	Copa Island	COV
Branolind	HAR	Copa Plus	COV
BreakAway Wound Dressing	BOR	Coraderm	ZZZ
Cadesorb	SN	Cosmopor E	HAR
Carboflex	CON	Coverflex	HAR
Carbonet	SN	Curafil	COV
Carbopad VC	SYN	Curafil Gel	COV
Carrasyn gel	CRN	Curafoam Island	COV

Curafoam Plus	COV	Elta Hydrovase	SAP
Curagel	COV	Elta Impregnated gauze	SAP
Curagel Island	COV	Elta Wound gel	SAP
Curasalt	COV	Ensure it	ZZZ
Curasorb	COV	Epi-Derm	BDM
Curasorb Plus	COV	Epi-fix	ASP
Curasorb Rope	COV	Epigard	ZZZ
Curasorb ZN	COV	Epiglu	SCH
Curiosin	RIC	Epilock	ZZZ
Curity	COV	Epi-lock	ZZZ
Cuticell Classic	BSN	Episil	ADV
Cutifilm	SN	Episil Absorbent	ADV
Cutimed Sorbact	BSN	Exu Dry	SN
Cutinova Hydro Border	SN	EZ DERM	BRN
Cutisorb LA	BSN	Flamazine	SN
C-View	ASP	Flaminal Forte	ARK
Debrisan	ZZZ	Flaminal Hydro	ARK
Dermabond	ETH	Flexderm	BER
Dermafilm	VYG	Flexigran Gel	A1P
Dermafilm	VYG	Flexzan	DOW
Dermal pads	SPE	Geliperm	GEI
Dermanet	DRL	Gentell Hydrogel	GLL
Dermarite	VYG	Granuflex	CON
Dermatell	GLL	Granuflex Bordered	CON
Dermatell Secure	GLL	Granuflex Paste	CON
Dermatix Clear	MDP	Granugel	CON
Dermatix Fabric	MDP	Grassolind	HAR
Dermatix Gel	MDP	Hioxyl Cream	FER
Dermatix Silicone Gel	DER	Hyaff	FID
Dermatix Silicone Sheet Clear	DER	Hydrocoll	HAR
Drisorb	SYN	Hydrocoll Border	HAR
Duoderm Extra Thin	CON	Hydrocoll Thin	HAR
Duoderm Signal	CON	Hydrofilm Plus	HAR
Durasil	DON	Hydrosorb	HAR
E Z Derm	EUR	Hydrosorb Comfort	HAR
EasI-V	ASP	Hydrotul	HAR
Eclypse	ADV	Hypafix Tape	BSN
Eclypse Adherent	ADV	Hypergel	MOL
Elasto-Gel	SWT	Inadine	SYS
Elset	MOL	Indermil	COV
Elset S	MOL	Interpose	FMG
Elta Film	FIN	Intrasite Conformable	SN
Elta Foam	FIN	Intrasite Gel	SN
Elta Gel	FIN	Ioban 2	3M

Iodoflex	SN	Melgisorb	MOL
Iodosorb Ointment	SN	Melgisorb Cavity	MOL
Iodosorb Powder	SN	Melladem Plus	SAN
Iodozyme	ARC	Melladerm Gel	SAN
IV 3000	SN	Melladerm Plus	SAN
Jelonet	SN	Melolin	SN
K Lite	URG	Melolite	SN
Kaltoclude	ZZZ	Mepiform	MOL
Kaltogel	ZZZ	Mepilex	MOL
Kaltostat	CON	Mepilex Ag	MOL
Kaltostat Cavity	CON	Mepilex Border	MOL
Kelo-cote Spray	ABT	Mepilex Border Lite	MOL
Kerraboot	ARK	Mepilex Heel	MOL
LarvE	ZOO	Mepilex Lite	MOL
LarvE Biofoam Dressing	ZOO	Mepilex Sacrum	MOL
LBF No sting	CLI	Mepilex Transfer	MOL
Leukomed	BSN	Mepitac	MOL
Leukomed T	BSN	Mepitel	MOL
Leukomed T plus	BSN	Mepore Film	MOL
Liquiband	AMS	Mepore Film and Pad	MOL
Lomatuell	LOH	Mepore Ultra	MOL
Lyofoam	MOL	Mesalt	MOL
Lyofoam C	MOL	Mesitran	ASP
Lyofoam Extra	MOL	Mesitran Border	ASP
Lyofoam Extra Adhesive	MOL	Mesitran Mesh	ASP
Lyofoam Extra T	MOL	Mesitran Ointment	ASP
Lyofoam T	MOL	Mesitran Ointment S	ASP
M&M Tulle	MAL	Mesoft	MOL
Matriderm	EUR	Mesorb	MOL
Maxgel	MAX	Metalline	LOH
Maxsorb Extra	MED	Mother Mates	COV
Medgel	EUR	Myskin	ALT
Medifil Gel	HUM	N-A Dressing	SYS
Medifil Particles	HUM	N-A Ultra	SYS
Medihoney Antibacteral Medical Honey	MHO	Neosport	NEO
		Neotulle	NEO
Medihoney Antibacterial Alginate	MHO	Niko Fix	ASP
		Normlgel	MOL
Medihoney Antibacterial honey tulle	MHO	Normlgel Impregnated gauze	MOL
		Novagel	EUR
Medihoney Barrier Cream	MHO	Novogel	FOR
Medihoney Gel Sheet	MHO	N-Terface	WIN
Medipore+ Pads	3M	Nu-derm	SYS
Medisafe	NEO	Nu-gel	SYS
Mefix	MOL		

Suprasorb A	LOH	Ultec pro	COV
Suprasorb c	LOH	Unitulle	ZZZ
Suprasorb F	LOH	Urgosorb	URG
Suprasorb G	LOH	Urgosorb Pad	URG
Suprasorb H	LOH	Urgosorb Rope	URG
Suprasorb M	LOH	Urgosorb Silver Rope	URG
Suprasorb M PHMB	LOH	Urgotul	URG
Suprasorb P	LOH	Urgotul Duo	URG
Suprasorb X	LOH	Urgotul Silver	URG
Surgicel	J&J	Urgotul SSD	URG
Surgipad	SYS	Urogosorb Silver	URG
Surgisis	COO	Vacunet	PRO
Synthaderm	ZZZ	Vacuskin	PRO
Tegaderm + Pad	3M	Vacutex	PRO
Tegaderm Absorbent Clear Acrylic Dressing	3M	Varidase	ZZZ
		Vaseline Petrolatum Gauze	COV
Tegaderm Alginate	3M	Veloderm	MDI
Tegaderm Contact	3M	Versiva	CON
Tegaderm Film Dresing	3M	Versiva XC	CON
Tegaderm Foam	3M	Vigilon	BAR
Tegaderm Foam adhesive	3M	Visiband	CON
Tegaderm heel	3M	Wound dres	COL
Tegaderm Hydrocolloid	3M	Xeroflow	COV
Tegaderm Matrix	3M	Xeroform	COV
Tegaderm Thin	3M	Zetuvit	HAR
Tegagel	3M		
Telfa	COV		
Telfa Island	COV		
Telfa Max	COV		
Telfa Plus	COV		
Tenderwet	HAR		
Tielle	SYS		
Tielle Lite	SYS		
Tielle Packing	SYS		
Tielle Plus	SYS		
Tielle Plus Heel	SYS		
Topigel	INA		
Topper	SYS		
Traumacel	BSR		
Transorbent	ASP		
Tricotex	SN		
Trufoam NA	ASP		
Trufoam SA	ASP		
Ultec Pro	COV		

MANUFACTURERS' CONTACT DETAILS

3M   3M Health Care Ltd, 3M House, Morley St , Loughborough , Leics, LE11 1EF, (0)1509 611611

A1P   Al Pharmaceuticals Plc , Units 20+21 Easter Park, Site 8A Beam Reach , Ferry Lane , South Rainham, Essex, RM13 9BP, (0)1708 528 900

ABT   ABT Healthcare UK Ltd, Springwood Booths Hall, Booths Park, Chelford Rd, Knutsford, Ches, WA16 8QZ, (0)1565 757783

ACT   Activa Healthcare, 1 Lancaster Park, Newborough Rd, Needwood, Burton-upon-Trent, Staffs, DE13 9PD, 0845 0606707

ADV   Advancis Medical Ltd, Lowmoor Business Park, Kirkby-in-Ashfield, Notts, NG17 7JZ, (0)1623 751500

AGU   Aguettant, The Barn, 41a Main Road, Cleeve, Somerset, BS49 4NZ, (0)1934 835 694

AHS   Associated Hospital Supplies, 4a Sherwood Road, Bromsgrove, Worcs, B60 3DR, (0)1527 876776

ALT   Altrika Ltd, The Innovation Centre, 217 Portobello, Sheffield, Yorks, S1 4DP, (0)114 2220985

AMS   Advanced Medical Soutions, Premier Park, 33 Road One, Winsford Industrial Estate, Winsford, Cheshire, CW7 3RT, 08444 125 755

ARC   Archimed, Colworth Science Park, Sharnbrook, Bedford, Beds, MK44 1LQ, (0)1234 782 870

ARK   Ark Therapeutics Group Plc, 79 New Cavendish St, London, W1W 6XB, (0)20 7388 7722

ASP   Aspen Medical Europe Ltd, Thornhill Rd, Redditch, Worcs, B98 7NL, (0)1527 587 700

AST   Astellas Pharma Europe Ltd, Lovett House, Lovett Road, Staines, Middx, TW18 3AZ, (0)1784 419400

BAR   Bard Medical Division, 8195 Industrial Boulevard, Covington, Georgia, 30014, 770-784-6100

BDM   Biodermis, 6000 S. Eastern, Suite 9-D, Las Vegas, Vevada, 89119, 800-322-3729

BER   Bertek Pharmaceuticals, 12720 Barry Ashford Drive, Sugar Land, Texas, 77478, 281-240-1000

BOR   Boracchia + associates, 3920 Cypress Drive, Petaluma, California, 94954, 707-765-3100

BRA   B Braun (Medical) Ltd, Brookdale Rd, Thorncliffe Park Estate, Chapeltown, Sheffield, Yorks, S35 2PW, (0)114 225 9000

BRN Brennen Medical LLC, 1290 Hammond Road, ST. Paul, Minnesota, 55110, 651-429-7413

BSI Biomed Sciences Inc, 7584 Morris Court, Suite 218, Allentown, Pensylvania, PA18106, 610-530-3193

BSN BSN Medical Ltd, PO Box 258, Willerby, Hull, Yorks, HU10 6WT, 0845 1223 600

BSR Bioster a.s., TEJN 621, 664 71 Veverská, Bítýška, Czech Republic,

CDM CD Medical Ltd, Aston Grange, Oker, Matlock, Derbys, DE4 2JJ, (0)1629 733 860

CER Cerdak, Distributed in UK by Clinimed,

CHS Cambridge Healthcare Supplies, Unit 14D Wendover Rd, Rackheath Industrial Estate, Norwich, Norfolk, NR13 6LH, (0)1603735200

CLI CliniMed Ltd, Cavell House, Knaves Beech Way, Loudwater, High Wycombe, Bucks, HP10 9QY, (0)1628 850 100

CLS Clinisupplies Ltd, 9 Crystal Way, Elmgrove Rd, Harrow, Middx, HA12HP, (0)20 8863 4168

COL Coloplast Ltd, Peterborough Business Park, Peterborough, Cambs, PE2 6FX, (0)1733 342000

CON ConvaTec Ltd, Harrington House, Milton Rd, Ickenham, Uxbridge, Middx, UB10 8PU, (0)1895 628 400

COO Cook Medical Inc, P.O. Box 4195, Bloomington, IN 47402-4195, 812-239-2235

COV Covidien (UK) Ltd, Ashwood, Chineham Business Park, Crockford Lane, Basingstoke, Hants, RG24 8EH, (0)1329 224000

CRN Carrington Laboratoies Inc, 2001 Walnut Hill Lane, Irving, Texas, 75038, 972-518-1300

DEG Degania Silicone Ltd, Degania Bet, 15130, Israel, 972-4-6755100

DER Dermatix, see Meda Pharmaceuticals,

DON Donell Super-Skin, PO Box 471, Bardstown, Kentucky, 40004, 502-331-0241

DRL Deroyal, 200 DeBusk Lane, Powell, TN37849, 865-362-1357

EAS Easigrip Ltd, Unit 13, Scar Bank, Millers Rd, Warks, CV34 5DB, (0)1926 497 108

FID Fidia farmaceutici S.p.A., Via Ponte della Fabbrica 3/A, 35031 Abano, Terme (PD), Italy, (+39) 049 8232111

FMC   Ferris Mfg Corp, Distributed by Aspen medical,

FOR   Ford Medical Associates Ltd, 8 Wyndham Way, Orchard Heights, Ashford, Kent, TN25 4PZ, (0)1233 633 224

FRO   Frontier Multigate, Newbridge Rd Industrial Estate, Blackwood, Gwent, NP12 2YL, (0)1495 233050

GEI   Geistlich Pharma, Newton Bank, Long Lane, Chester, Ches, CH2 2PF, (0)1244 347 534

GLL   Gentell, Inc., 3600 Boundbrook Ave., Trevose, PA, 19053, 215-364-3600

HAR   Paul Hartmann Ltd, Unit P2 Parklands, Heywood Distribution Park, Pilsworth Rd, Heywood, Lancs, OL10 2TT, (0)1706 363 200

HMR   Hoechst Marion Roussel,

HOL   Hollister Ltd, Rectory Road, 42 Broad Street, Wokingham, Berks, RG40 1AB, (0)118 989 5000

HUM   Human BioSciences, Inc., 940 Clopper Road, Gaithersburg, Maryland, 20878,

J&J   Johnson & Johnson Medical, Coronation Rd, Ascot, Berks, 5L5 9EY, (0)1344 871000

JAN   Janssen-Cilag Ltd, PO Box 79, Saunderton, High Wycombe, Hants, HPI4 4HJ, (0)1494 567 444

KCI   KCI Medical Ltd, KCI House, Langford Business Park, Langford Locks, Kidlington, Oxon, OX5 1GF, (0)1865 840 600

LOH   Lohmann & Rauscher, See Activa Healthcare,

MAL   Malam Laboratories, 37 Oakwood Drive, Bolton, Lanc, BL1 5EE, (0)1204841285

MAX   Maxford Medical Technology Co. Ltd.,

MDI   Medestea Internazionale S.p.A., Via Cernaia 31, 10121 Torino, (TO), Italy, Tel. +39.011.5156611

MED   Medline Industries, Inc., One Medline Place, Mundelein, Illinois, 60060,

MHO   Medihoney (Europe) Ltd, 200 Brook Drive, Green Park, Reading, Berks, RG2 6UB, 0800 071 3912

MOL   Molnlycke Health Care Ltd, The Arenson Centre, Arenson Way, Dunstable, Herts, LU5 5UL, (0)161 777 2628

MON   Monarch Pharmaceuticals, King Pharmaceuticals Inc., 501 Fifth Street, Bristol, Tennessee, 37620,

NAG	Nagor Ltd, PO Box 21, Global House, Isle of Man Business Park, Douglas, Isle of Man, IM99 1AX, (0)1624 625556
NEO	Neomedic Ltd, 112-114 Hallowell Road, Northwood, Middx, HA6 3ED, (0)1923 836379
NOV	Novartis Consumer Health UK Ltd, Wimblehurst Road, Horsham, West Sussex, RH12 5AB, (0)1403 210211
OMI	Omikron Scientific Limited, Rehovot, Israel,
ORG	Organogenesis Inc, 150 Dan Road, Canton, Mass 02021, 781-575-0775
PRO	Protex Healthcare (UK) Ltd, Unit 5, Molly Millars Lane, Wokingham, Berks, RG41 2Q2, 08700 114 112_
REJ	Rejuveness, 28 Clinton Street STE 6, Saratoga Springs, New York, 12866, 518-584-5017
RHC	Richardson Healthcare, Richardson House, Crondal Rd, Coventry, Warks, CV7 9NH, 08700 111126
ROB	Robinson Healthcare Ltd, Lawn Rd, Carlton-in-Lindrick Industrial Estate, Worksop, Notts, S819LB, (0)1909 7350(0)1
SAN	Sanomed Manufacturing B.V, Smoutweg 4-008, 4524 EK Sluis, Netherlands, 0032 50393627
SAP	Swiss American Products, 2055 Luna Rd, Carrollton, Texas, 75006, 972-385-2900
SHE	Shermond, Castle House, Sea View Way, Woodingdean, Brighton, Sx, BN2 6NT, 0870 242 7701
SN	Smith and Nephew Healthcare Ltd, Healthcare House, Goulton St, Hull, Yorks, HU3 4DJ, (0)1482 222 200
SOR	Sorbion, c/o H&R Healthcare Ltd, Melton Court, Gibson Lane, Melton, Hull, Yorks, HU14 3HH, (0)1482 638491
SPE	Spenco Healthcare International Ltd, Brian Royd Mills, Saddleworth Road, Halifax, Yorks, HX4 8NF, (0)1422 378569
SYN	Synergy Healthcare (UK) Ltd, Lion Mil, lFitton St, Royton, Oldham, Lancs, OL2 5JX, (0)161 624 5641
SYS	Systagenix Wound Management, 1st Floor, 2 City Place, Beehive Ring Road, Gatwick Airport, Sx, RH6 0PA, (0)1293 842000
URG	Urgo Ltd, Sullington Rd, Shepshed, Loughborough, Leics, LE12 9JJ, (0)1509 502051
VAL	Valeant Pharmaceuticals Ltd, Cedarwood, Chineham Business Park, Crockford Lane, Basingstoke, Hants, RG24 8WD, (0)1256 707 744
VC	Vernon-Carus Ltd, 1 Western Avenue, Matrix Park, Chorley, Lancs, PR77NB, (0)1772 299 900

VYG	Vygon UK, Bridge Road, Cirencester, Gloucs, GL7 1PT, (0)1285 6500293
VYG	VYGON S A, 5-11 Rue Adeline, Ecouen, Île-de-France, 95440,
WCA	Wallace Cameron Ltd, 26 Netherhall Rd, Netherton Industrial Estate, Wishaw, Lanarkshire, ML2 OJG, (0)1698 354 600
WIN	Winfield Laboratories, Inc., P.O. Box 832297, ., Richardson, Texas, 75083,
ZER	Zeroderma Ltd, The Manor House, Victors Barns, Northampton Rd, Brixworth, Northants, NN6 9DQ, (0)1604 889 855
ZOO	ZooBiotic Ltd, Units 2-4 Dunraven Business Park, Coychurch Road, Bridgend, Mid Glam, CF31 3AP, 0845 2301810
MDP	Meda Pharmaceuticals Ltd, Skyway House, Pasonage Road, Takeley, Bishop's Stortford, Herts, CM22 6PU, 0800 783 4995
RIC	Richter Gedeon PLC, Budapest 10, 27th POB, u-1475, Hungary, 36 1-431-4000
LES	Lescarden Inc, 420 Lexington Ave, Suite 212, New York, New York, 10170, 212-687-1051

23. Index

A